Lecture Notes in Electrical Engineering

Volume 784

The book series *Lecture Notes in Electrical Engineering* (LNEE) publishes the latest developments in Electrical Engineering - quickly, informally and in high quality. While original research reported in proceedings and monographs has traditionally formed the core of LNEE, we also encourage authors to submit books devoted to supporting student education and professional training in the various fields and applications areas of electrical engineering. The series cover classical and emerging topics concerning:

- Communication Engineering, Information Theory and Networks
- Electronics Engineering and Microelectronics
- Signal, Image and Speech Processing
- Wireless and Mobile Communication
- Circuits and Systems
- Energy Systems, Power Electronics and Electrical Machines
- Electro-optical Engineering
- Instrumentation Engineering
- Avionics Engineering
- Control Systems
- Internet-of-Things and Cybersecurity
- Biomedical Devices, MEMS and NEMS

For general information about this book series, comments or suggestions, please contact leontina.dicecco@springer.com.

To submit a proposal or request further information, please contact the Publishing Editor in your country:

China

Jasmine Dou, Editor (jasmine.dou@springer.com)

India, Japan, Rest of Asia

Swati Meherishi, Editorial Director (Swati.Meherishi@springer.com)

Southeast Asia, Australia, New Zealand

Ramesh Nath Premnath, Editor (ramesh.premnath@springernature.com)

USA, Canada:

Michael Luby, Senior Editor (michael.luby@springer.com)

All other Countries:

Leontina Di Cecco, Senior Editor (leontina.dicecco@springer.com)

**** This series is indexed by EI Compendex and Scopus databases. ****

More information about this series at http://www.springer.com/series/7818

Ruidan Su · Yu-Dong Zhang ·
Han Liu
Editors

Proceedings of 2021 International Conference on Medical Imaging and Computer-Aided Diagnosis (MICAD 2021)

Medical Imaging and Computer-Aided Diagnosis

Springer

Editors
Ruidan Su
Shanghai Advanced Research Institute
Chinese Academy of Sciences
Shanghai, China

Yu-Dong Zhang
Department of Informatics
University of Leicester
Leicester, UK

Han Liu
College of Computer Science
and Software Engineering
Shenzhen University
Shenzhen, Guangdong, China

ISSN 1876-1100 ISSN 1876-1119 (electronic)
Lecture Notes in Electrical Engineering
ISBN 978-981-16-3879-4 ISBN 978-981-16-3880-0 (eBook)
https://doi.org/10.1007/978-981-16-3880-0

This Springer imprint is published by the registered company Springer Nature Singapore Pte Ltd.
The registered company address is: 152 Beach Road, #21-01/04 Gateway East, Singapore 189721, Singapore

Preface

Welcome to the Proceedings of the 2021 International Conference on Medical Imaging and Computer-Aided Diagnosis (MICAD 2021) which was held virtually on March 25–26, 2021. MICAD is an annual conference which aims to provide a communication platform for top scholars, engineers, scientists, as well as graduate students to share ideas and discuss the latest technology in medical imaging and computer-aided diagnosis or related fields such as artificial intelligence and machine learning, to encourage growth, raising the profile of this multidisciplinary field with an ever-increasing real-world applicability.

The diverse range of topics reflects the growth in development and application of medical imaging and computer-aided diagnosis. The main topics covered in the proceedings are (i) computer-aided detection/diagnosis, (ii) automated medical image analysis, (iii) medical image segmentation, registration and reconstruction, and (iv) machine learning and deep learning.

MICAD 2021 received submissions from 16 countries, in total, 80 full papers, and each paper was reviewed by at least three reviewers in a standard peer-review process. Based on the recommendation by three independent referees, finally 45 papers were accepted for MICAD 2021 (acceptance rate of 56%).

Many people have collaborated and worked hard to produce successful MICAD 2021. First, we would like to thank all the authors for submitting their papers to the conference, for their presentations and discussions during the conference. Our thanks go to program committee members and reviewers, who carried out the most difficult work by carefully evaluating the submitted papers. Our special thanks to James Duncan (Yale University, USA), Leo Joskowicz (The Hebrew University of Jerusalem, Israel), Alejandro F Frangi (University of Leeds, UK), Joseph M. Reinhardt (The University of Iowa, IA, USA), Le Lu (PAII Inc., Bethesda Research Lab, Maryland, USA), Erik Meijering (University of New South Wales, Australia), Tanveer Syeda-Mahmood (Medical Sieve Radiology Grand Challenge Almaden Research Center, IBM), Raphael Sznitman (University of Bern, Switzerland), Robin Strand (Uppsala University, Sweden), Kensaku Mori (Nagoya University, Japan), Ayelet Akselrod-Ballin (Zebra Medical Vision Ltd.), and David Golan (Viz. ai) for the exciting keynote talks. We express our sincere thanks to the organizing committee chairs for helping us to formulate a rich technical program. We hope you enjoy the proceedings of MICAD 2021.

With warmest regards,

Ruidan Su

Organization

General Chair

Ruidan Su	Shanghai Advanced Research Institute, Chinese Academy of Sciences, Shanghai, China

General Co-chair

Yu-dong Zhang	University of Leicester, UK

Program Chairs

Alejandro F. Frangi	University of Leeds, UK
Joseph M. Reinhardt	The University of Iowa, IA, USA
Han Liu	Shenzhen University, China
Ryuji Hamamoto	Representative Director, Japanese Association for Medical Artificial Intelligence (JMAI), Japan

Publication Chair

Ruidan Su	Shanghai Advanced Research Institute, Chinese Academy of Sciences, Shanghai, China

Supporting Academic Organizations

Japanese Association for Medical Artificial Intelligence (JMAI)

Technical Program Committee

Zakaria Belhachmi	Université Haute Alsace, France
Qiang (Shawn) Cheng	University of Kentucky, USA

Sourav Dhar	Sikkim Manipal University, India
Jan Ehrhardt	Institute for Medical Informatics, University of Lübeck, Germany
Smain Femmam	IEEE Senior Member, University of Haute-Alsace, France
Linlin Gao	Ningbo University, China
Maroun Geryes	Lebanese University, Lebanon
Yuzhu Guo	Beihang University, China
Zhiwei Huang	National University of Singapore, Singapore
Yuankai Huo	Vanderbilt University, USA
Sujatha Krishnamoorthy	Wenzhou-Kean University, China
Yuan Liang	University of California, Los Angeles, USA
Cheng Lu	Case Western Reserve University, USA
Na Ma	Shanghai Advanced Research Institute, Chinese Academy of Sciences, Shanghai, China
Mahsa Mohaghegh	Auckland University of Technology, New Zealand
Xiang Pan	Jiangnan University, China
Luca Parisi	Coventry University, UK
Sivarama Krishnan Rajaraman	Lister Hill National Center for Biomedical Communications (LHNCBC), National Library of Medicine (NLM), National Institutes of Health (NIH), India
Su Ruan	LITIS Laboratory, University of Rouen, France
Francesco Rundo	STMicroelectronics S.R.L., Catania, Italy
Rachel Sparks	King's College London, UK
Vinesh Sukumar	University of Idaho, USA
Gunasekar Thangarasu	Linton University College, Malaysia
Gennaro Vessio	University of Bari, Italy
Jichuan Xiong	Nanjing University of Science and Technology, China
Lequan Yu	Stanford University, USA
Yitian Zhao	iMED China Group at Cixi Institute of Biomedical Engineering, Ningbo Institute of Industrial Technology, Chinese Academy of Sciences, China
Yuyao Zhang	ShanghaiTech University, China
Jun Zhuang	Indiana University–Purdue University at Indianapolis (IUPUI), USA

Contents

Computer-Aided Detection/Diagnosis

Medical Imaging

A Dual Supervision Guided Attentional Network for Multimodal MR Brain Tumor Segmentation

Tongxue Zhou[1,2,3], Stéphane Canu[1,3], Pierre Vera[4], and Su Ruan[2,3](✉)

[1] INSA Rouen, LITIS - Apprentissage, 76800 Rouen, France
[2] Université de Rouen Normandie, LITIS - QuantIF, 76183 Rouen, France
su.ruan@univ-rouen.fr
[3] Normandie Univ., INSA Rouen, UNIROUEN, UNIHAVRE, LITIS, Rouen, France
[4] Department of Nuclear Medicine, Henri Becquerel Cancer Center, 76038 Rouen, France

Abstract. Early diagnosis and treatment of brain tumor is critical for the recovery of the patients. However, it is challenged by the various brain anatomy structure, low image contrast and fuzzy contour. In this paper, we present a dual supervision guided attentional network for multimodal brain tumor segmentation. The backbone is a multi-encoder based U-Net. The multiple independent encoders are used to obtain individual feature representation from each modality. A dual attention fusion block is proposed to extract the most informative feature representation from different modalities. It consists of a spatial attention module and a modality attention module. Since the same brain tumor regions can be observed in the different modalities, therefore, the spatial feature representations from different modalities can provide the complementary feature representations for segmentation. To this end, a spatial attention based supervision is introduced to enable hierarchical learning of the multi-scale feature representations, and also to provide addition constraint for the segmentation decoder. In addition, an image reconstruction based another supervision is integrated to the network to regularize the encoders. The ablation experiments and the visualization results evaluated on BraTS 2019 dataset prove that the proposed method can achieve promising results.

Keywords: Brain tumor segmentation · Fusion · Deep supervision · Deep learning · MRI

1 Introduction

A brain tumor is one of the most aggressive cancers in the world. There are 700,000 people living with a primary brain tumor in the United States, it's predicted that 18,020 people will die because of the malignant brain tumor in 2020. Therefore, early diagnosis and treatment is critical for recovery of the brain tumor patient. Magnetic resonance imaging (MRI) [1] is a common imaging technique to measure the tumor because it uses magnetic fields to produce detailed images without radiation. And different MR modalities such as Fluid Attenuation Inversion Recovery (FLAIR), contrast enhanced T1-weighted (T1c), T1-weighted (T1), and T2-weighted (T2) images can provide complimentary information for accurate segmentation. However, MR brain tumor segmentation still faces with

R. Su et al. (Eds.): MICAD 2021, LNEE 784, pp. 3–11, 2022.
https://doi.org/10.1007/978-981-16-3880-0_1

various challenges due to the various brain anatomy structure between patients, and the fuzzy tumor contour due to low contrast. Figure 1 shows a case in BraTS 2019 dataset.

In recent years, automatic brain tumor segmentation based on deep learning has gained much attention, and there are many related works [2–4]. However, multi-modal brain tumor segmentation is still confronted with some challenges. The first challenge is how to exploit the individual feature representation of each modality due to the different image characteristics between modalities. The segmentation network architectures can be generally grouped into single-encoder-based network and multi-encoder-based network. And the multi-encoder-based method can provide more accurate segmentation results than the single-encoder-based one [5, 6]. To this end, we used the multi-encoder based U-Net [7] to extract individual feature representation of each modality. The second challenge is how to fuse the complementary features to enhance the segmentation result. Inspired by the spatial and channel SE (scSE) blocks [8, 9], we proposed a dual attention fusion block to exploit the most useful feature representation. It consists of a modality attention module and a spatial attention module. Considering a fact that the location of brain tumor region is the same in different modalities, the multi-scale spatial feature representations are used as a deep supervision path to guide the network to extract tumor related features. In addition, the reconstruction decoders are used as another supervision path to provide additional guidance to the shared encoders.

There are four contributions in our work: 1) A dual supervision guided attentional network is proposed to segment multimodal brain tumor in MRI. 2) A dual attention fusion block is applied to extract the most discriminative feature representation for segmentation. 3) A dual deep supervision strategy is proposed to guide the model to emphasize on the interested regions to improve the segmentation performance. 4) The experiments evaluated on BraTS 2019 dataset prove that the proposed method can outperform the state-of-the-art methods.

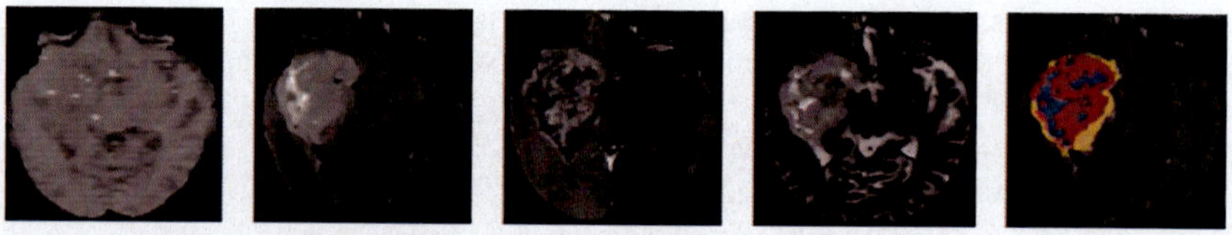

Fig. 1. A case from BraTS 2019 dataset. The left four columns are the input modalities: T1, FLAIR, T1c, T2, the fifth column is the real annotations. Blue: non-enhancing tumor and necrotic regions, yellow: edema region, red: enhancing tumor region.

2 Method

The proposed network framework is depicted in Fig. 2. It consists of four parts: encoders, fusion block, segmentation decoder and two auxiliary deep supervision paths. Let x_i represents the input images, where $x_i = \{x_F, x_{T1}, x_{T1c}, x_{T2}\}$. The four individual encoders can be denoted as f_{en}^i. At the endpoint of the encoders, we can obtain four individual feature representations F_i, $F_i = f_{en}^i(x_i, \theta_i)$, where θ is the parameters of the encoders.

To obtain the most important feature representations from different modalities, a dual attention fusion block f_{att} is introduced. It includes a modality attention module f_m and a spatial attention module f_s, $f_{att} = f_m \oplus f_s$, where $\oplus$ is element-wise summation. It first concatenates the four individual feature representations F_i and then re-weight the feature represents along modality path and spatial path according to their contribution for the segmentation to achieve the fused representations f_f. Then the fused feature representation is guided by two novel deep supervision paths (f_{re} and f_{sa}) to obtain the segmentation.

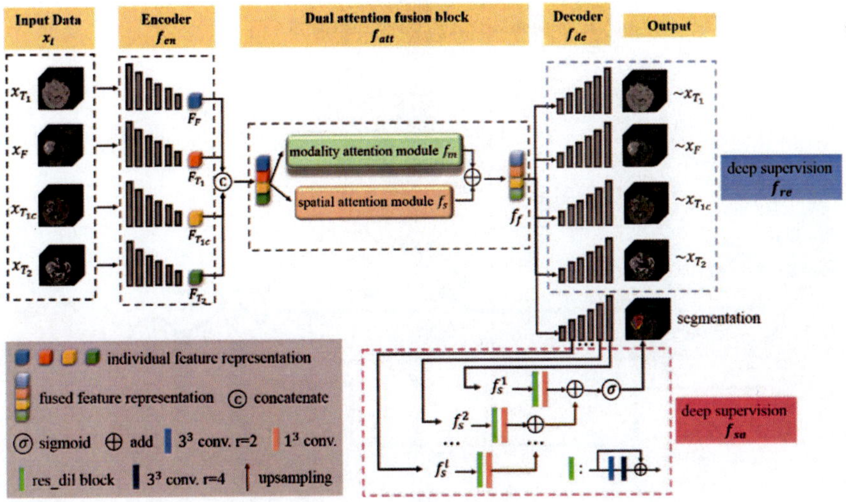

Fig. 2. The overview of our proposed network architecture.

2.1 Encoder and Decoder

The four individual encoders are used to extract the individual feature representations from the modalities. They have the same architecture, which consists of a convolutional block and a res_dil block. The res_dil block can increase the receptive field, which is a combination of residual block and dilated convolutions. The decoder starts with an up-sampling layer and a convolution. And the skip connection is used to integrate the upsampled semantic features with the shallow features from the encoder. Following that, the res_dil block is used. All the convolutions used are $3 \times 3 \times 3$.

2.2 Dual Attention Fusion Block

The key challenge of multimodal segmentation is to fuse the different modality information and utilize the complimentary feature information. Therefore, we proposed a dual attention fusion block, which consists of a modality attention module and a spatial attention module. The former one is to distinguish the contribution of each modality, and the latter one is to extract the useful spatial information to boost the segmentation result. The architecture is shown in Fig. 3. First, the concatenation is used to combine the four independent feature representations F_i to obtain the input feature representation, then they are passed to the dual attention fusion block. In the modality attention module f_m, the global average pooling is used to transform the input feature representation to four hidden nodes, then two fully connected layers are used to produce the modality weight based on the contribution of each modality for the final segmentation. In the spatial attention module f_s, a $1 \times 1 \times 1$ convolution is introduced to get the spatial weights. Finally, the two attentional feature representations are obtained by multiplied with the input feature representation, and the fused feature representation f_f is achieved by integrating the two attentional feature representations.

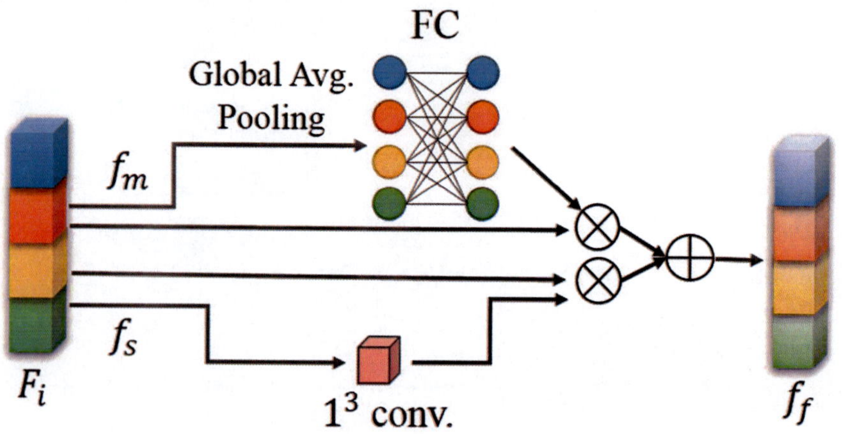

Fig. 3. The architecture of dual attention fusion block.

2.3 Dual Supervision Strategy

Since the different MR modalities from the same patient have the same brain tumor regions, it is intuitive that utilizing the spatial feature information of different modalities to guide the network to achieve better performance. Based on the spatial attention module, we proposed a spatial attention based deep supervision f_{sa}. We first extract spatial feature representations at different levels of the network, and then we can predict the multi-scale segmentation results using these spatial feature representations. Finally, we integrate all the multi-scale segmentation results by element-wise summation to obtain the segmentation, $Segmentation = f_{de}(f_f) \oplus \sum_{l=1}^{N} f_s^l$, f_s^l is the spatial attention feature representation of layer l, $N = 5$. In addition, a reconstruction based supervision f_{re} is introduced to the network, $x_i = f_{re}(f_f)$. These additional decoders can help regularize the shared encoders. In addition, it can cope with the limitation of input images. The architecture of the dual supervision strategy is described in Fig. 2 (highlighted in blue and pink).

2.4 The Choice of Loss Function

A hybrid loss is introduced to train our network, defined in Eq. 1. L_d is the dice loss for segmentation, and L_r is the Mean Absolute Error (MAE) for reconstruction, β is the weighting parameter, $\beta = 0.3$.

$$L = L_d + \beta L_r \tag{1}$$

$$L_d = 1 - 2\frac{\sum_{c=1}^{C}\sum_{n=1}^{N} P_i^c T_i^c}{\sum_{c=1}^{C}\sum_{n=1}^{N}(P_i^c + T_i^c)} \tag{2}$$

$$L_r = \sum_{i=1}^{M} MAE\|r_i(f) - x_{i1}\| \tag{3}$$

where N denotes the number of the examples, C denotes the number of the classes, P_i^c and T_i^c are the probabilities of voxel i belonging to class c. M is the number of modality, r is the reconstruction path, f is the fused representation, x is the input modality.

3 Experiments

3.1 Dataset and Implementation Details

The BraTS 2019 dataset is applied to validate our method. The training set includes 335 cases, the validation set has 125 cases with hidden ground truth. Each case includes four modalities: FLAIR, T1, T2 and T1c, and the three target segmentation regions are Whole Tumor (WT), Tumor Core (TC) and Enhancing Tumor (ET). The N4ITK method [10] and normalization are applied as the pre-processing. The original image size is $155 \times 240 \times 240$, we cropped and resized them to $128 \times 128 \times 128$. The network is implemented by Keras with an Nvidia GPU Quadro P5000 (16G), and Adam optimizer is used. The initial learning rate is 5e−4, and it will be half reduced when the validation loss is not improved during 10 epochs. Early stopping is used to avoid over-fitting if the validation loss is not improved in consecutive 50 epochs.

3.2 Evaluation Metrics

All the prediction results are uploaded to the public evaluation system[1] based on Dice Score and Hausdorff Distance. Dice Score (DSC) is to calculate the overlap rate of prediction results and ground truth. Hausdorff distance (HD) is to evaluate the boundaries of the prediction results and ground-truth.

$$DSC = \frac{2TP}{2TP + FP + FN} \tag{4}$$

where TP, FP and FN denote the true positive, false positive, and false negative predictions, respectively.

$$HD = \max\{\sup_{r\in\partial R} d_m(s, r), \sup_{s\in\partial S} d_m(r, s)\} \tag{5}$$

where ∂S and ∂R are the sets of the predicted tumor border voxels and the real tumor border voxels, and d_m is the minimum of the Euclidean distances.

[1] (https://ipp.cbica.upenn.edu/)

3.3 Experiment Results

We first conducted the ablation studies to assess the effect of each proposed components. Then we visualized the segmentation performance to further prove that the proposed method can obtain a promising segmentation result. Finally, we compare with the state-of-the-art methods.

Ablation Experiments of Our Proposed Method. We first conducted the ablation studies to prove the importance of the proposed components. We refer the baseline as the proposed method without dual attention fusion block and dual supervision strategy. Table 1 shows the comparison results. We can observe that the baseline achieves 76.8 and 8.7 in the terms of average Dice Score and average Hausdorff Distance, respectively. The proposed components can gradually improve the segmentation performance in each tumor region. The proposed method obtains 80.4 and 8.2 in the terms of average Dice Score and average Hausdorff Distance, respectively, which improved the baseline by 4.7% and 5.7% respectively. Figure 4 shows the visual comparison results of these methods, the green box highlights the mis-segmented regions. We can observed that our method can attribute to a promising segmentation result.

Table 1. Evaluation of our proposed method on BraTS 2019 training dataset, (1) Baseline (2) Baseline + Dual attention fusion (3) Baseline + Dual attention fusion + Spatial attention based supervision (4) Baseline + Dual attention fusion + Dual supervision strategy. WT, TC, ET denote whole tumor, tumor core and enhancing tumor, respectively, Avg denotes the average score across the three tumor regions, bold results denotes the best scores.

Methods	DSC (%)				HD (mm)			
	WT	TC	ET	Avg	WT	TC	ET	Avg
(1)	83.1	73.0	74.3	76.8	9.2	10.3	6.6	8.7
(2)	86.5	76.0	75.6	79.4	12.3	9.3	7.6	9.7
(3)	86.7	**76.7**	75.7	79.7	9.1	9.5	**6.3**	8.3
(4)	**88.7**	76.5	**75.9**	**80.4**	**7.9**	**8.8**	8.0	**8.2**

Comparison with the State-of-the-Art. We further compare our method with the existing state-of-the-art methods on BraTS 2019 dataset. The results are illustrated in Table 2. Starke et al. [11] used a multi-view segmentation network. Kim et al. [12] used a two-step segmentation network to achieve the segmentation. Amian et al. [13] introduced a multi-resolution 3D CNN for brain tumor segmentation. Compared with them, we can observe the proposed method can achieve a better segmentation performance, which achieves 79.3 and 7.3 in the terms of average Dice Score and Hausdorff Distance, respectively.

Effectiveness of the Dual Supervision Strategy. First, we selected an example to visualize the feature maps of the spatial attention based supervision in Fig. 5 (left part). We

Table 2. Comparison of different methods on BraTS 2019 validation dataset, bold results denotes the best scores.

Methods	DSC (%)				HD (mm)			
	WT	TC	ET	Avg	WT	TC	ET	Avg
Starke et al. [11]	85.1	71.0	71.0	75.7	8.9	10.3	**6.6**	8.6
Kim et al. [12]	87.6	76.4	67.2	77.1	14.1	11.6	8.8	11.5
Amian et al. [13]	86.0	77.0	71.0	78.0	8.4	11.5	6.9	8.9
Proposed	**88.2**	**77.1**	**72.7**	**79.3**	**5.7**	**9.0**	7.3	**7.3**

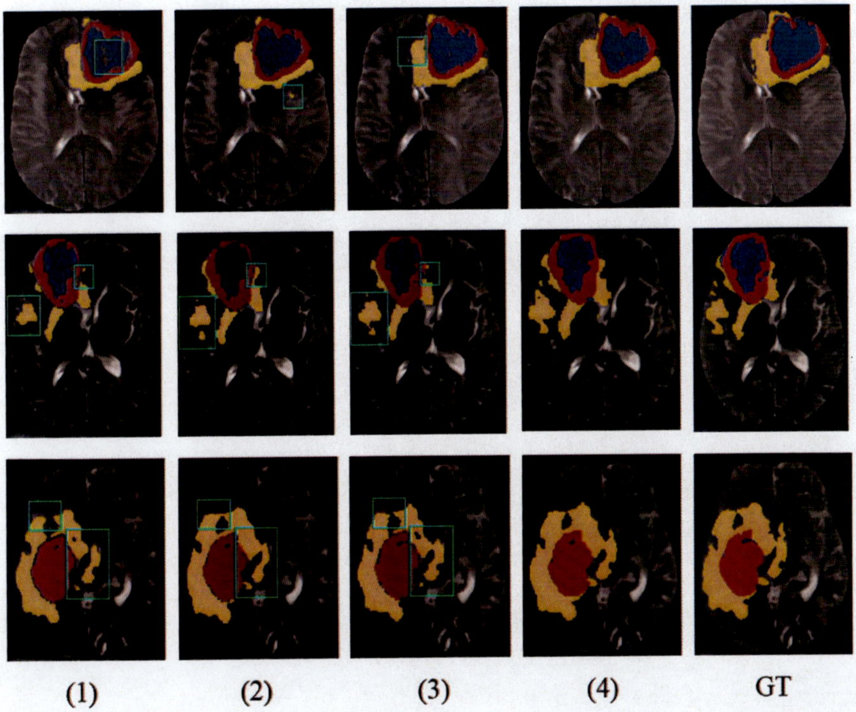

Fig. 4. The comparison results of different methods. (1) Baseline, (2) Baseline + dual fusion, (3) Baseline + dual fusion + spatial attention supervision, (4) Baseline + dual fusion + dual supervision strategy. Blue: necrotic and non-enhancing tumor, yellow: edema, red: enhancing tumor.

can observe that thanks to the spatial attention module, the network can extract the tumor related features. Therefore the multi-scale spatial information can be considered as a supervision to guide the network to achieve better segmentation performance. Then we visualize the reconstruction results in Fig. 5 (right part), it can be seen that the network has a good reconstruction result. We conclude that the proposed dual supervision strategy can enable the segmentation network to obtain a better result.

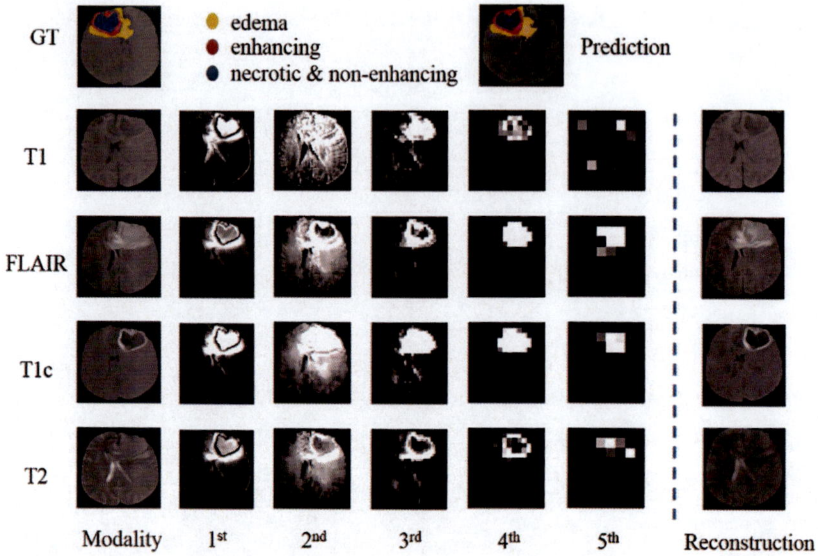

Fig. 5. Visualization of the feature maps. The first row: ground truth and the prediction result. The first column: input modalities, the next five columns: feature maps of spatial attention based supervision from different levels. The last column: reconstruction results.

4 Conclusion

In this work, we presented a dual supervision guided attentional network to do the multimodal brain tumor segmentation. The network consists of four encoders for feature extraction, one decoder for segmentation, and two auxiliary supervision paths. The proposed dual attention fusion block can emphasize the most discriminative features from different modalities. The dual supervision strategy can not only help the network focus on the ROIs but also help to regularize the shared encoders. The experiment results evaluated on BraTS 2019 proved the effectiveness of our method.

References

1. Zhou, T., Ruan, S., Canu, S.: A review: deep learning for medical image segmentation using multi-modality fusion. Array, 100004 (2019)
2. Kamnitsas, K., et al.: Ensembles of multiple models and architectures for robust brain tumour segmentation. In: Crimi, A., Bakas, S., Kuijf, H., Menze, B., Reyes, M. (eds.) Brainlesion: Glioma, Multiple Sclerosis, Stroke and Traumatic Brain Injuries: Third International Workshop, BrainLes 2017, Held in Conjunction with MICCAI 2017, Quebec City, QC, Canada, September 14, 2017, Revised Selected Papers, pp. 450–462. Springer , Cham (2018). https://doi.org/10.1007/978-3-319-75238-9_38
3. Myronenko, A.: 3D MRI brain tumor segmentation using autoencoder regularization. In: Crimi, A., Bakas, S., Kuijf, H., Keyvan, F., Reyes, M., van Walsum, T. (eds.) Brainlesion:

Glioma, Multiple Sclerosis, Stroke and Traumatic Brain Injuries: 4th International Workshop, BrainLes 2018, Held in Conjunction with MICCAI 2018, Granada, Spain, September 16, 2018, Revised Selected Papers, Part II, pp. 311–320. Springer, Cham (2019). https://doi.org/10.1007/978-3-030-11726-9_28
4. Isensee, F., Kickingereder, P., Wick, W., Bendszus, M., Maier-Hein, K.H.: No new-net. In: Crimi, A., Bakas, S., Kuijf, H., Keyvan, F., Reyes, M., van Walsum, T. (eds.) Brainlesion: Glioma, Multiple Sclerosis, Stroke and Traumatic Brain Injuries: 4th International Workshop, BrainLes 2018, Held in Conjunction with MICCAI 2018, Granada, Spain, September 16, 2018, Revised Selected Papers, Part II, pp. 234–244. Springer, Cham (2019). https://doi.org/10.1007/978-3-030-11726-9_21
5. Zhou, T., Ruan, S., Guo, Y., Canu, S.: A multi-modality fusion network based on attention mechanism for brain tumor segmentation. In: 2020 IEEE 17th International Symposium on Biomedical Imaging (ISBI), pp. 377–380. IEEE (2020)
6. Zhou, T., Canu, S., Vera, P., Ruan, S.: Brain tumor segmentation with missing modalities via latent multi-source correlation representation. In: Martel, A.L., et al. (eds.) MICCAI 2020. LNCS, vol. 12264, pp. 533–541. Springer, Cham (2020). https://doi.org/10.1007/978-3-030-59719-1_52
7. Ronneberger, O., Fischer, P., Brox, T.: U-net: convolutional networks for biomedical image segmentation. In: Navab, N., Hornegger, J., Wells, W.M., Frangi, A.F. (eds.) Medical Image Computing and Computer-Assisted Intervention – MICCAI 2015: 18th International Conference, Munich, Germany, October 5-9, 2015, Proceedings, Part III, pp. 234–241. Springer, Cham (2015). https://doi.org/10.1007/978-3-319-24574-4_28
8. Hu, J., Shen, L., Sun, G.: Squeeze-and-excitation networks. In: Proceedings of the IEEE Conference on Computer Vision and Pattern Recognition, pp. 7132–7141 (2018)
9. Roy, A.G., Navab, N., Wachinger, C.: Concurrent spatial and channel 'squeeze & excitation' in fully convolutional networks. In: Frangi, A.F., Schnabel, J.A., Davatzikos, C., Alberola-López, C., Fichtinger, G. (eds.) Medical Image Computing and Computer Assisted Intervention – MICCAI 2018: 21st International Conference, Granada, Spain, September 16–20, 2018, Proceedings, Part I, pp. 421–429. Springer, Heidelberg (2018). https://doi.org/10.1007/978-3-030-00928-1_48
10. Avants, B.B., Tustison, N., Song, G.: Advanced normalization tools (ants). Insight j, vol. 2, pp. 1–35 (2009)
11. Starke, S., Eckert, C., Zwanenburg, A., Speidel, S., Löck, S., Leger, S.: An integrative analysis of image segmentation and survival of brain tumour patients. In: Crimi, A., Bakas, S. (eds.) Brainlesion: Glioma, Multiple Sclerosis, Stroke and Traumatic Brain Injuries: 5th International Workshop, BrainLes 2019, Held in Conjunction with MICCAI 2019, Shenzhen, China, October 17, 2019, Revised Selected Papers, Part I, pp. 368–378. Springer, Cham (2020). https://doi.org/10.1007/978-3-030-46640-4_35
12. Kim, S., Luna, M., Chikontwe, P., Park, S.H.: Two-step u-nets for brain tumor segmentation and random forest with radiomics for survival time prediction. In: Crimi, A., Bakas, S. (eds.) Brainlesion: Glioma, Multiple Sclerosis, Stroke and Traumatic Brain Injuries: 5th International Workshop, BrainLes 2019, Held in Conjunction with MICCAI 2019, Shenzhen, China, October 17, 2019, Revised Selected Papers, Part I, pp. 200–209. Springer, Cham (2020). https://doi.org/10.1007/978-3-030-46640-4_19
13. Amian, M., Soltaninejad, M.: Multi-resolution 3D CNN for MRI brain tumor segmentation and survival prediction. In: Crimi, A., Bakas, S. (eds.) Brainlesion: Glioma, Multiple Sclerosis, Stroke and Traumatic Brain Injuries: 5th International Workshop, BrainLes 2019, Held in Conjunction with MICCAI 2019, Shenzhen, China, October 17, 2019, Revised Selected Papers, Part I, pp. 221–230. Springer, Cham (2020). https://doi.org/10.1007/978-3-030-46640-4_21

Three-Dimensional Image Reconstruction of Murine Heart Using Image Processing

Haowei Zhong[1], Cheng Huang[1], Jinrong Cui[1(✉)], and Wei Hu[2]

[1] College of Mathematics and Informatics, South China Agricultural University, Guangzhou 510642, China
[2] School of Physics and Astronomy, University of Manchester, Manchester M13 9PL, UK

Abstract. The key role of three-dimensional reconstructions in the analyses of medical imagery has gained more recognition over the past 20 years through many fields such as computer graphics and biological medicine. Specifically, lighting the role of isolated discrete mammalian cardiac tissues or organs typically involves a more accurate anatomical reconstruction procedure. To date, however, there has been no unified approach that could be extended to model establishments. This article seeks to amend these problems by introducing a new approach for studying the three-dimensional distribution of Pnmt+ cell-derived cells in isolated mouse hearts. Related data comes from Scientific Data that describes a new cardiomyocyte population which is a specific class of phenylethanolamine n-methyltransferase (Pnmt+) cell-derived cardiomyocytes (PdCMs). Rigid registration was implemented to match the raw sliced images of the murine heart using TrakEM2. Compared to previous reconstruction approaches, our methods have accomplished automated 3D reconstruction using image processing. The primary purpose of this paper is to propose an automatic image processing pipeline to recreate the 3D image of the murine heart, which prevents cell distribution distortion induced by handcrafted noise removal. The final 3D reconstructed exhibition was displayed by Paraview.

Keywords: 3D reconstruction · Murine heart · Image processing

1 Introduction

This typically involves the ability to recreate the multicellular system model [1], there is no question that such study is allowed by a thorough anatomical reconstruction. As computing technology advances exponentially, medical imaging and computer science are profoundly intertwined. The possibility of a very wide implementation lies in the use of 3D reconstruction technologies to restore the anatomical institutions and to track their distribution and function in the organ.

Reconstructing a variety of tissue slices in three dimensions (3D) is one of the most efficient means of displaying nearly all forms of tissue structures correctly and with great resolution, which was used extensively in the biological sciences. Full and continuous slices of tissue provide an important base for subsequent reconstruction. The

R. Su et al. (Eds.): MICAD 2021, LNEE 784, pp. 12–20, 2022.
https://doi.org/10.1007/978-981-16-3880-0_2

continuous slices should have constant, similarly remote, flat characteristics, without loss or deformation. Nevertheless, most tissue parts are prone to noise, contamination and incomplete staining. Manual sorting is typically used to process slices that require a great deal of time and effort to manage slices; because it is manual processing, the results after each processing may be different. To cope with these noises and emissions and to reconstruct the whole surface profile, we use digital imaging technologies for slice processing. The processed images are then reconstructed to show the dynamic three dimensional (3D) framework of biological tissue and can rotate the restored 3D model freely.

In this paper, we present a method for tissue slice batch processing and 3D rebuilding through images processed. Rigid registration (stiff rotation and translation) has been used to coordinate the images with TrakEM2 based on landmarks. Technique such as sampling [2], binarization, dilatation, compression, channel enhancement through MATLAB, slice images have been handled by digital image processing. After which, in a single VTK format file rebuilt by MATLAB software, the processed slices were reconstructed. Finally, the 3D model has been reconstructed using Paraview software (http://www.paraview.org/), for viewing purpose.

2 Related Work

In the previous study [3, 4], channelrhodopsin 2(ChR2) was introduced into the mouse gene that expressing the Phenylethanolamine N-methyltransferase(Pnmt) [5], which encode the enzyme responsible for transformation of noradrenaline to adrenaline. In this mouse model, it is convenient to identify a specific class of Pnmt-expressing neuroendocrine cells and their descendants. Furthermore, the $Pnmt^+$ cells derived cardiomyocytes are similar to routine mouse myocytes in electrical, morphological, and contractile properties. They use blued light to controls cardiac rhythm in the whole heart by optogenetic control technology. Optogenetics is the genetic approach for controlling cellular process with light. It provides spatiotemporal, quantitative and reversible control over biological signalling and metabolic processes, overcoming limitations of chemically inducible systems [6]. This new mouse model demonstrates the functional anatomy of cardiac myocytes by optogenetics. To find out the potential roles of PdCMs, then an anatomical reconstruction of this model was applied, using the dataset generated by experiment and calculation and this data set was published in Scientific Data.

Data sets have many advantages and unique characteristics. Firstly, the conditional expression of Pnmt-Cre/ChR2 promoted the tissue-specific expression of ChR2/TD tomato protein, and the ChR2/TD fluorescent tomato protein promotes the imaging. Secondly, a series of fixed tissue sections of Pnmt Cre/ChR2 mouse heart was imaged by wide-field deconvolution fluorescence microscope. This technique produces high-equality digital images, equivalent to high contrast and resolution confocal images, but with low fluorescence, and these images were assembled into two-dimensional coronal slice images [7]. These images were manually repaired to remove background noise and light, the manual repairment requires a certain degree of professional background, and most importantly, it is hard to recurrence and no operability. Then, a positive staining channel was defined in the previous study and so we continue to use that definition, 100 was added to the positive staining channel to mark the positive region.

3 Method

Firstly, the softWoRx [8] (Scientific Imaging, USA) was used to stitch raw frames that could capture fractional heart block sections; then the stitched images were tuned to the AutoContrarTool ImageJ [9], which increased the positive and negative areas to distinguish high contrast images. The high contrast images as shown in Fig. 1 are then physically inspected, stored as JPEG images (8-bits) and 48 of them are shown ready for restoration.

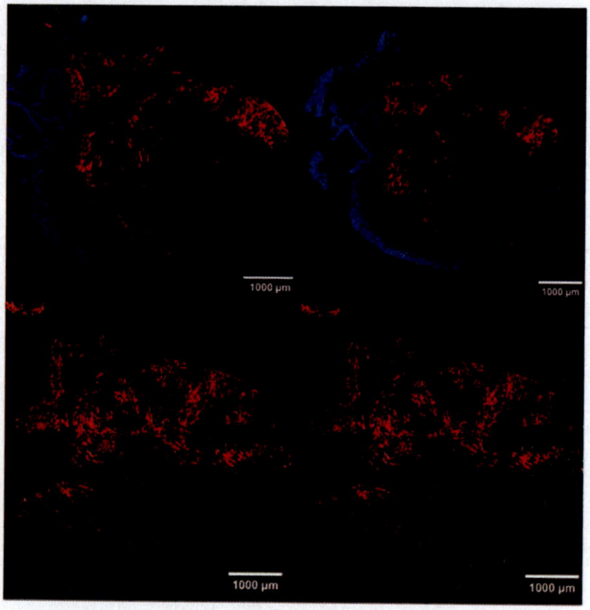

Fig. 1. High contrast image of murine heart

In order to minimize the size of the image and speed up the rendering of the image, the nearest neighbour interpolation has been used to scale the slices of the image to 0.2 to the original resolution. Subsequently, rigid registration (stiff translation and rotation, as shown in Fig. 2) was applied to such scaled image slices to match heart slices using TrakEM2 [10], an open source plugin in Fiji [11]. The specific method is to extend the scale of each image slice to same, and then change or flip the angle of the image slices to property position. In our method, the size and position of the initial part of the data set is used for rigid correction, and then the processed image is exported for subsequent reconstruction work.

After that, each heart slice picture was divided from the positive staining area and negative staining area where the positive spot area was defined as the channel area higher than 30. In the visualization of the image, the red region represents a positive staining area, and the blue area represents a negative staining area, the black area represents a non-tissue backdrop. At the same time, there are a lot of noises in the results as shown in Fig. 3.

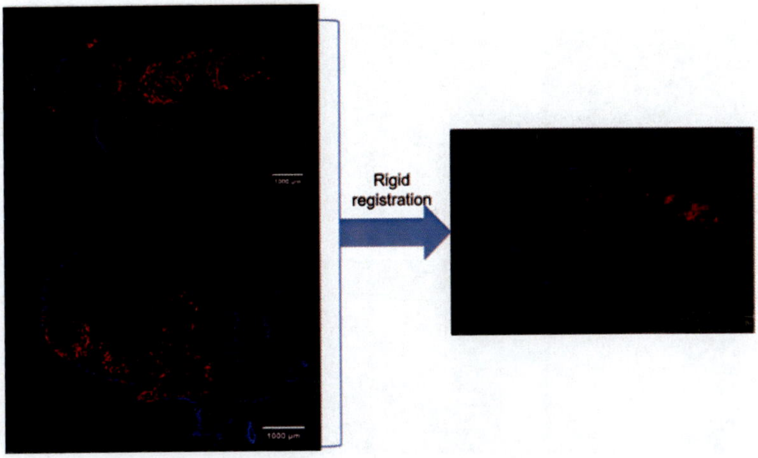

Fig. 2. Rigid rotation (stiff rotation and translation) was applied to murine heart slice images

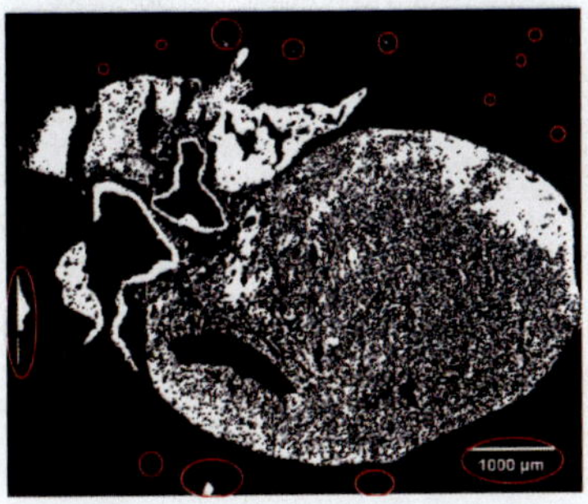

Fig. 3. Binary image of murine heart image which can find many noises around the heart.

We have transformed it into a gray-scale image using MATLAB [12] for the blue surface of each image that reflects the negative surface stain-scale. Following the surgery, a number of injuries arise due to the discontinuous coloring of the skin. Thereby, we inflate with 5x5 square structuring factor the blue area of the heart slice, and that is working well. Median filtering is a nonlinear technology that can efficiently eliminate noise on the basis of statistical sorting [13]. The fundamental principle of median filtering is that the value of a region is replaced by the median value of each point in a digital image, so that the pixel value surrounding it comes close to the actual value. In order to remove discrete noise, the grey image level is modified by reclassification through median filtering. The discrete, minor noises in the heart slice picture can be completely removed after this step. Nevertheless, there were still large noise blocks that could not be eliminated through median filtering in the blue region of murine heart slice images. Considering that what we need to maintain is the entire part of the heart as well as we have used inflate operation to eradicate heart image fracture, which means that within the heart contour a wide connected region was created and smaller connected regions outside the heart were formed. The smaller related regions are known to be the major

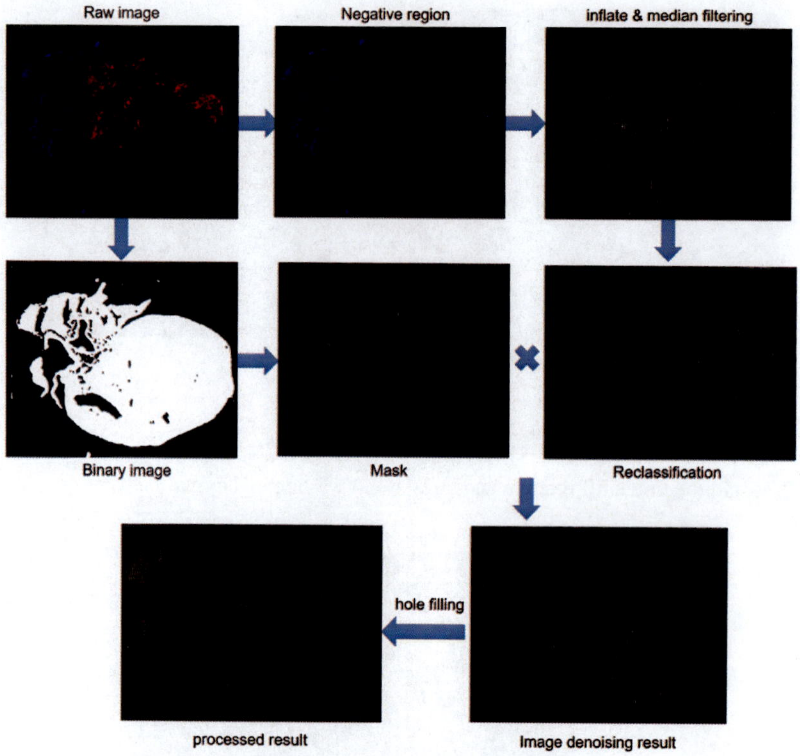

Fig. 4. The negative staining region image processing pipeline of 3D reconstruction based on murine heart slices images

noise blocks that cannot be removed by median filtering. We are attempting to create a filter for the shape of the heart to remove these noise blocks. The following are the basic steps: Firstly, the image is converted into a binary image for further mask fabrication. Secondly, the non eight connected regions and small areas will be removed, and a full heart contour picture will be obtained without missing the internal details of the heart, and the noise blocks outside the heart can be excluded. After this step, a binary heart contour mask can be obtained. Finally, to multiply the processed image, we use the binary mask of the heart, so we can delete the noise blocks outside the image of the heart contour. The whole process is shown in Fig. 4.

For the red area of each heart slice image, which reflects a positive staining region, the red area is a small part of the larger staining area, thus it is quite simple to handle. We wish to highlight the red regions because it is the positive staining area of murine heart slices. Therefore, the red channel of each heart slice image was added 200 to enhance the strength of the red region with a threshold of 30, and then it was sequentially converted into a gray scale image using MATLAB. After that operation, we enhance the gray level by adding 120 to those pixels which gray value over 50. Finally, the processed blue region image and red region image of murine heart slice image are superimposed to

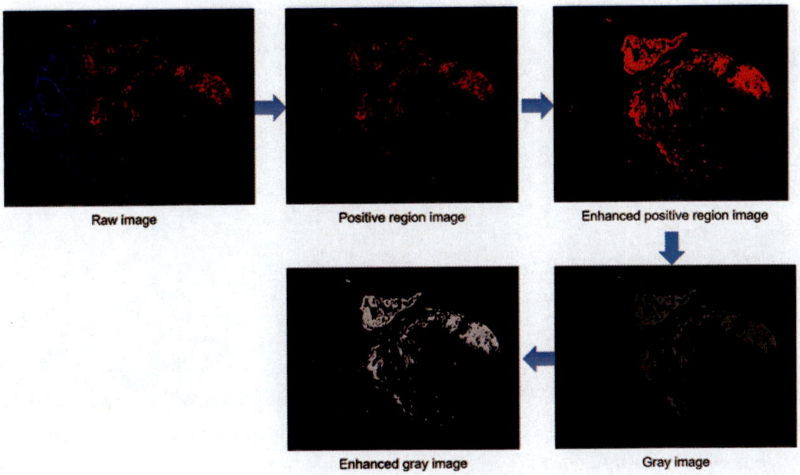

Fig. 5. The positive staining region image processing pipeline of 3D reconstruction based on murine heart slices images

obtain a new image. The conversion process is shown in Fig. 5. The original image will be used to next three-dimensional reconstruction.

The resulting data were then written to VTK data file using MATLAB for next visualization [14]. Then down-sampling was applied to VTK file to reduce the size of the file, which can facilitate fast visualization on typical office desk-top(with Inter(R) Core(TM) i5 CPU 8 GB RAM). Lastly, the resultant data were visualized in Paraview [15], an application for data processing and visualization. The image processing and visualization process is shown in Fig. 6, and the 3D visualization result of staining region is shown in Fig. 7.

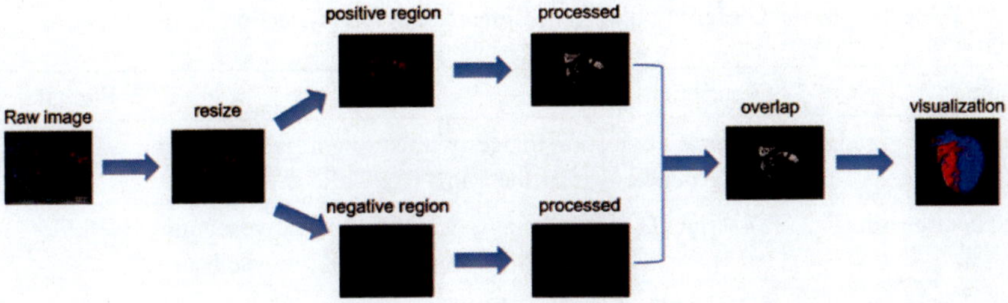

Fig. 6. The image processing pipeline of 3D reconstruction based on murine heart slices images

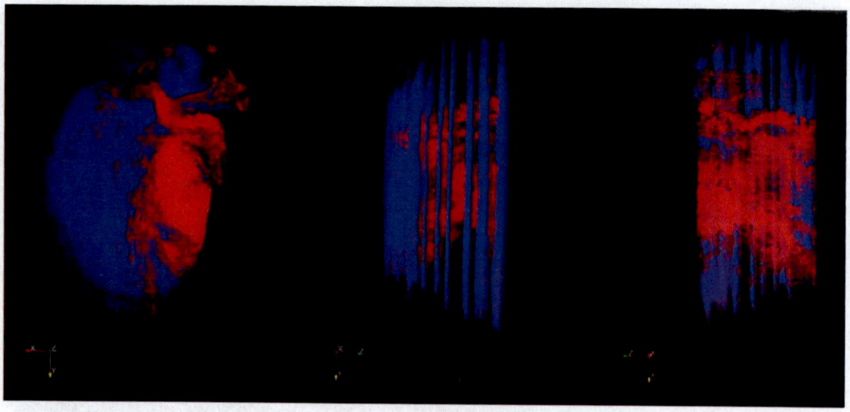

Fig. 7. 3D Reconstruction result of positive staining region and negative staining region of murine heart slice image in multiple views

4 Experimental Results

Compared with the previous reconstruction process, the traditional method needs to manually erase the noise and need a lot of manual inspection, which is not only inefficient, but also does not have repeatability. When facing a large amount of data to be processed, it needs to spend a lot of time. Our method uses digital image processing technology to reconstruct three-dimensional image slices of mouse heart, which reduce the cost and difficulty of processing. The raw data file, the VTK format file and the AVI format (as shown in Fig. 8) file of 3D reconstruction results of mouse heart are given below. The raw data is provided by Scientific Data (https://doi.org/10.6084/m9.figsh-are.c.3692131). The experimental results are listed in Table 1.

Table 1. The data description of three-dimensional reconstruction of mouse heart.

Name	Description	Format
Stitched raw image 1	27 serial 2D section images with strong negative staining background covering the Pnmt-Cre/ChR2 mouse heart	JPEG
Stitched raw image 2	27 serial 2D section images with weak negative staining background covering the Pnmt-Cre/ChR2 mouse heart	JPEG
Visualization	A VTK file containing the 3D reconstructed of the distribution of mouse heart. Data can be visualised using Paraview	VTL,PVSM
Reconstruction video	A Video show the reconstruction result	AVI

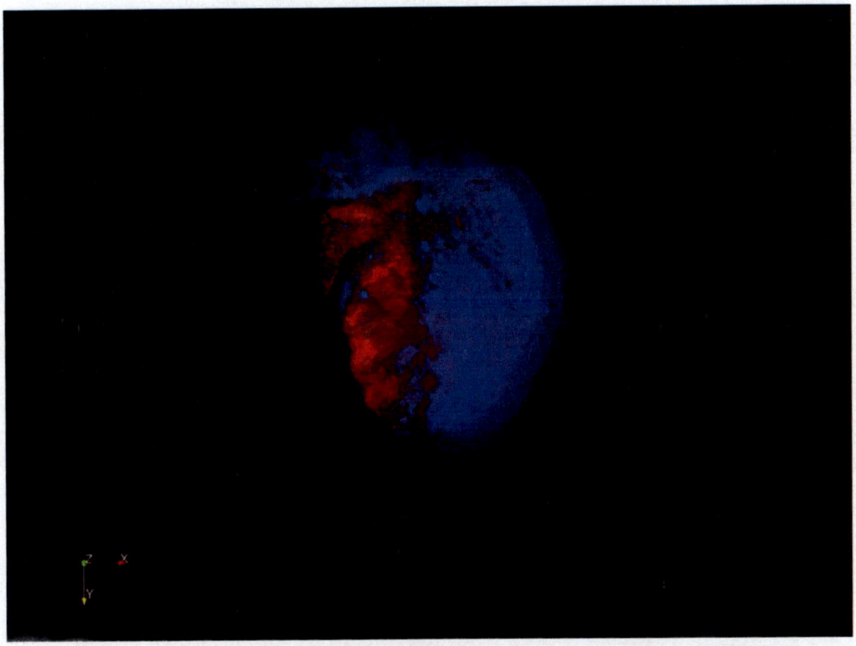

Fig. 8. The reconstruction visualization result of murine heart in Paraview

5 Conclusions

In this paper, we use digital image procession technology and MATLAB to realize the whole process from murine heart slice to three-dimension reconstruction. Compared with the previous reconstruction methods, our methods have achieved an automatic 3D reconstruction using image analysis. Previous methods need much handcrafted denoising and restoration, and may change the origin distribution of some critical cell-type. Our key insight is that providing an automated image processing pipeline to reconstruct 3D image of murine heart. However, there are still some deficiencies that need to be further improved. In the process of denoising by filter, some staining details in mouse heart slice images may disappear. Although the disappearance of staining details can be reduced by adjusting the size of the filter and other parameters, it may cause more noise and affect the 3D reconstruction effect of mouse heart.

References

1. Camelliti, P., Abou Al-Saud, S., Smolenski, R.T., et al.: Adult human heart slices are a multicellular system suitable for electrophysiological and pharmacological studies. J. Mol. Cell. Cardiol. **51**(3), 390–398 (2011)
2. Lin, W., Dong, L.: Adaptive downsampling to improve image compression at low bit rates. IEEE Trans. Image Process. **15**(9), 2513–2521 (2006)
3. Ni, H., et al.: Three-dimensional image reconstruction of distribution of Pnmt + cell-derived cells in murine heart. Sci. Data **4**, 170134 (2017). https://doi.org/10.1038/sdata.2017.134

4. Wang, Y., et al.: Optogenetic control of heart rhythm by selective stimulation of cardiomyocytes derived from Pnmt+ cells in murine heart. Sci. Rep. **7**, 40687 (2017). https://doi.org/10.1038/srep40687
5. Ruggiero, D.A., Ross, C.A., Anwar, M., et al.: Distribution of neurons containing phenylethanolamine N-methyltransferase in medulla and hypothalamus of rat. J. Comp. Neurol. **239**(2), 127–154 (1985)
6. Deisseroth, K.: Optogenetics. Nat. Methods **8**(1), 26–29 (2011). https://doi.org/10.1038/nmeth.f.324
7. Soulez, F., Denis, L., Tourneur, Y., et al.: Blind deconvolution of 3D data in wide field fluorescence microscopy. In: 2012 9th IEEE International Symposium on Biomedical Imaging (ISBI). Pp. 1735–1738. IEEE (2012)
8. SoftWoRx G E. Healthcare. http://incelldownload.gehealthcare.com/bin/download_data/softWoRx/7.00.SoftWoRx.htm
9. Abràmoff, M.D., Magalhães, P.J., Ram, S.J.: Image processing with ImageJ. Biophoton. Int. **11**(7), 36–42 (2004)
10. Cardona, A.: TrakEM2: an ImageJ-based program for morphological data mining and 3D modelling. In: Proceedings of the Image J User and Developer Conference (2006)
11. Schindelin, J., Arganda-Carreras, I., Frise, E., et al.: Fiji: an open-source platform for biological-image analysis. Nat. Methods **9**(7), 676–682 (2012)
12. Higham, D.J., Higham, N.J.: MATLAB guide. Society for Industrial and Applied Mathematics (2016)
13. Justusson, B.I.: Median filtering: Statistical properties. In: Justusson, B.I. (ed.) Two-Dimensional Digital Signal Prcessing II, 161–196. Springer, Heidelberg (1981). https://doi.org/10.1007/BFb0057597
14. Schroeder, W.J., Avila, L.S., Hoffman, W.: Visualizing with VTK: a tutorial. IEEE Comput. Graph. Appl. **20**(5), 20–27 (2000)
15. Ayachit, U.: The Paraview Guide: A Parallel Visualization Application. Kitware, Inc. (2015)

Identifying Melanoma in Lesion Images Using Cycle-Consistent Adversarial Networks-Based Data Augmentation

Mengjun Tao[1](✉) and Youwei Yan[2]

[1] New York University, New York, USA
[2] City University of Hong Kong, Hong Kong, China

Abstract. Early detection of melanoma is extremely important because melanoma is curable at the early stage. Due to the state-of-the-art performance of the Convolutional Neural Networks (CNNs), the CNNs have been widely used for the task. However, hand labeled data is not easily obtained in practical settings. In this paper, we firstly employ generative adversarial network (GAN) to artificially enlarge the dataset, which can generate fake data based on the generative confrontation network. Therefore, the problem of insufficient training samples in melanoma classification tasks has been alleviated. Second, CNNs is employed in our paper to automatically classification, which proved to be more effectively solve the problem of small discrimination between different categories. Based on the proposed method, the experimental results show that the use of deep learning technology can effectively improve the performance of the model in the melanoma classification task, with an average accuracy value of 94.5%, which is nearly 1.9% higher than the previous approaches.

Keywords: Cycle-consistent adversarial networks · Data augmentation · Melanoma · Images classification · Deep convolutional neural network

1 Introduction

It is widely Known that melanoma is one of the threatening skin cancer in the world, which is developed from normal moles and pigment spots on the skin. Despite the high mortality rate of this type disease, most of the patients can be cured at the early stage. With accurate early detection and recognition of melanoma images, it is curable for the most of the patients. Unfortunately, due to the short supply for experienced highly-trained dermatologists and professional equipment, the misdiagnosis rate of melanoma is very high, which lead to many death.

Therefore, the advanced computer assisted classification methods should be brought in to improve the accuracy of melanoma diagnosis. To address the problem, computer aided approaches have been applied to analyze dermoscopy

R. Su et al. (Eds.): MICAD 2021, LNEE 784, pp. 21–28, 2022.
https://doi.org/10.1007/978-981-16-3880-0_3

images [1]. For the traditional machine learning algorithms, the feature extraction was employed first and then these extracted features will be classified, which has been proved to be time-consuming and challenging. Recently, deep learning has been witnessed dramatically progress. The performance for melanoma classification has been improved dramatically, using deep learning methods [2,3]. Despite its advantage on images classification, traditional deep learning approach still has its limitations. During last several decades, the convolutional neural network (CNN) has been widely-used for melanoma classification, which has outperformed in the classification accuracy and performance. Despite its advantage, CNN is still facing some difficulties such as meeting unbalanced data, uneven quality image, and inconsistent image styles of pictures from different sources in reality. What's more, in the training process, the model tends to overly fit to the samples in the training set, which will result in poor generalization and uncertainty of the network. Data augmentation approaches are employed to avoid the overftting problem through enlarging the size of the training set to obtain abundant required melanoma images, which has turned out to be of the great help to improve the performance of the model.

In this paper, we employed a novel and powerful data augmentation technique called generative adversarial network (GAN) with the goal of improving classification accuracy. With proposed data augmentation method, the accuracy of automatic detection for malignant melanoma has been improved and the effectiveness and efficiency of the model have been optimized as well. We also conducted large number of the experiments and evaluation for the model, and the results have proved that the proposed data augmentation methods are excellent in improving the performance of the training model.

This paper is organized as follows. In Sect. 2, the related work is given, which describes the employed data augmentation methods called Generative adversarial network(GAN) and its variants. Section 3 provides a detailed description of methodology, and Sect. 4 gives the experimental results evaluated on the development dataset. Finally, Sect. 5 summarizes the paper and provides conclusions.

2 Related Work

2.1 Previous Study on Melanoma Image Classification

The previous study on the melanoma classification can be divided into three stages. At the first stage, manually features without using computer aided approach were analyzed. Although these traditional manual recognition methods can achieve a certain diagnostic effect, they are time-consuming and energy-consuming with low efficiency and high cost. And then at the second stage of the research, traditional machine learning methods using computer was introduced. The melanoma diagnosis classification system was built combining the powerful computing power with the manual analysis ability to reduce the misdiagnosis rate and improve the efficiency of diagnosis, which yield much experiences for melanoma classification. For example, at the stage of feature extraction, Celebi ME et al. [4] extracted relevant features such as shape, color and texture from images, using multi-features selection algorithm to sort the features and then inputs the top-ranked features into the support vector machine (SVM) for classification. In the classification and recognition phase, [5] used K-nearest neighbor model (KNN) for classification and recognition after extracting color and texture features. Despite its reference meaning, the traditional image classification method has poor performance on the tasks due to the fact that they depends too much on low-dimensional information such as color and texture of images for classification. At the third stage, deep learning approach is widely used in computer vision, and Convolutional Neural Network [6] is widely-employed as the basic deep learning method in melanoma detection. For example, the first proposed CNN is LeNet [7], then VGG [8], GoogleNet [9], ResNet [10], DenseNet [11], etc. These architecture has superiority in dealing with the tasks of image classification, target detection and natural language recognition.

2.2 Data Augmentation

The neural networks is prone to overfitting due to the lack of the data. In order to tackle this problem, the employment of data augmentation approaches are necessary. In general, data augmentation can be divided into two categories. The first category is the offline methods on dealing with smaller data sets including flipping, cropping [12], rotation, zoom deformation, translation, folding, and RGB transformation [13], the second category is data augmentation approaches including Augmix, mixup, cutmix, Generative Adversarial Nets [14]. Among them, Generative Adversarial Nets (GAN) is a novel model [15]. And it has been continuously improved to generate DCGAN [16], WGAN [17], PGGAN [18], CycleGAN [19], InfoGAN [20] and other new models used in the field of image natural language processing and even speech processing. Subsequently, introduction of the new activation function Selu makes the training more stable and perform excellent [21]. In this paper, we explored a novel Generative Adversarial Nets based on data augmentation method called CycleGAN. And we further explored its performance on enlarging the dataset and improving the generalization ability of the model so as to finally improve the classification accuracy.

3 Methodology

In deep learning method, to solve the problem of insufficient data, the data generation model should be built to generate the fake data which corresponds to the distribution of training data. In most cases, due to the restriction of the objective conditions, it is impossible to obtain more data unless to generate data from the raw data. Therefore, Generative adversarial networks are increasingly been used in data augmentation. In our paper, we employ deep convolutional generative adversarial networks known as CycleGAN to enlarge the dataset and discuss whether their melanoma classification performance can be improved.

3.1 GAN

GAN is a powerful generative model, which has outperformed in image generation, image editing, and characterization learning. Two important models are contained in the GAN model, including a generator and a discriminator. The function of discriminator is to discriminate whether a given image is real or fake, and the generator is used to generate images that look as if they are natural and real and even similar to the original data.

The main goal of GAN is to force the discriminator D to assist generator G to generate fake data similar to the real data distribution, where G and D are generally non-linear mapping functions. These functions are usually represented by network structures such as convolutional neural networks.

3.2 CycleGAN Image Transformation

Two generator networks and two discriminator networks are employed using the method of CycleGAN to realize the mutual mapping between two pictures X and Y. The generator G is defined to perform the mapping $X \rightarrow Y$ and the generator F performs the mapping $Y \rightarrow X$. The discriminator D_X is to distinguish whether the data comes from X or the generated F_Y . The discriminator D_Y is to distinguish whether the data comes from Yor the generated $G(x)$. CycleGAN also employs a cycle consistency loss [22], in which the picture X is mapped to Y and should be mapped back again at the same time. Finally, the loss of the original picture X and the picture mapped back is calculated, which is called the cycle consistency loss. The loss is trying to make $F(G(x)) \approx x$ and $G(F(y)) \approx y$. Figure 1 shows the structure of the network.

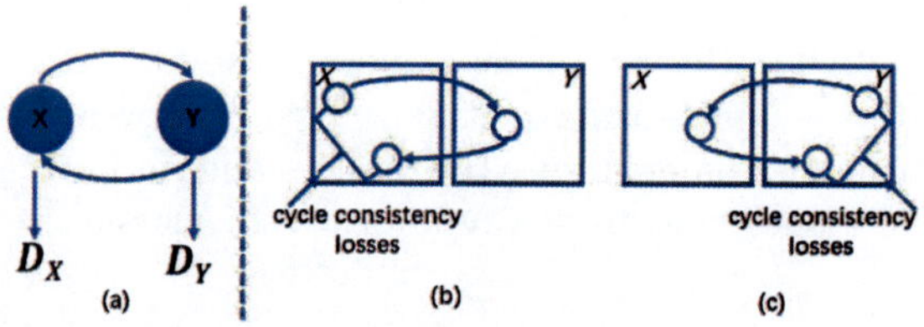

Fig. 1. The samples of the augmented dataset by using CycleGAN. In Fig. 1(a), G and F are the mapping functions, and D_X and D_Y are the corresponding discriminators, respectively; Fig. 1(b) and Fig. 1(c) are two cycle consistency losses.

The objective function of adversarial loss is maintained same with the original GAN, where the objective function of the mapping function G and the discriminator D_Y are defined by:

$$L_{GAN}(G, D_Y, X, Y) = E_{y \sim p_{data(y)}} [\log D_Y(y)] + E_{x \sim p_{data(x)}} [\log(1 - D_Y(G(x)))] \quad (1)$$

Similarly, we can define the objective function of the mapping function F and the discriminator D_X by:

$L_{GAN}(F, D_X, Y, X)$ where the cycle consistency loss directly calculates the norms of the picture mapped back and picture L1 in the original image:

$$L_{cyc}(G,F) = E_{x \sim p_{data(x)}} [\|F(G(x)) - x\|_1] + E_{y \sim p_{data(y)}} [\|G(F(y)) - y\|_1] \quad (2)$$

Here, the complete objective function is:

$$L(G,F,D_X,D_Y) = L_{GAN}(G,D_Y,X,Y) + L_{GAN}(F,D_X,X,Y)P + \lambda L_{cyc}(G,F) \quad (3)$$

where λ represents the importance of the two losses in the objective function.

3.3 Melanoma Detection Framework Based on Data Augmentation

In our study, a melanoma lesion screening framework based on data augmentation (CycleGAN) was designed for solving the binary classification problem of melanoma and non-melanoma to generate supplementary data using CycleGAN network. The framework of the algorithm includes: data augmentation module, preprocessing module and CNN-based image classification module. Figure 2 shows the framework for the whole approach.

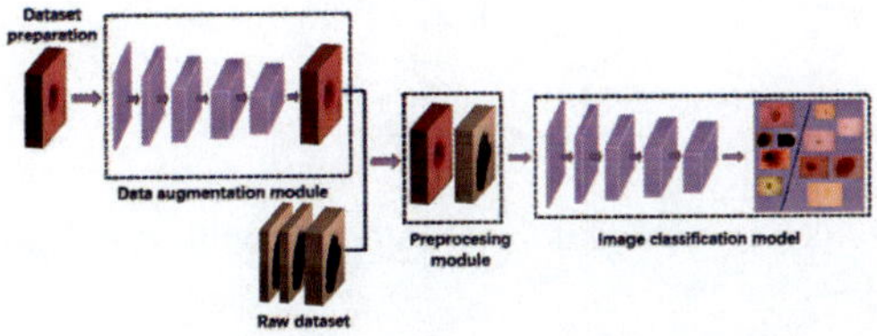

Fig. 2. Melanoma identification framework based on data augmentation.

First, the new immersive data is generated on the extracted data set using the generative adversarial network to generate, aiming to enlarge the dataset. Then, in the preprocessing stage, the supplementary data will be input in the extracted original data to generate new melanoma images dataset. Finally, the basic classification network will be trained to generate final classifier.

4 Experimental Results

4.1 Dataset

The dataset employed in our experiment for the melanoma classification task is provided by Kaggle competition. 33,126 training images and 10,980 test images are collected in the dataset. These images are all attached with corresponding patients information including sex, age approx, unique identifier, patient id, diagnosis and indicator of malignancy of imaged lesion.

4.2 Quantitative Comparisons Between Different Data Augmentation Methods

To make a fair comparison between different data augmentation approaches, we employ four widely-used augmentation approach in our experiment and EfficientNet is used as our the classification model. The experimental results are presented in this section. As can be seen from Fig. 3, it can be found that the CycleGAN data augmentation method is better than the other four data augmentation approaches, and the AUC reaches 0.945, which is significantly higher better other augmentation methods. Therefore, the extended data generated by CycleGAN can replace the real data to a certain extent, and it can obviously improve the training effect of the model.

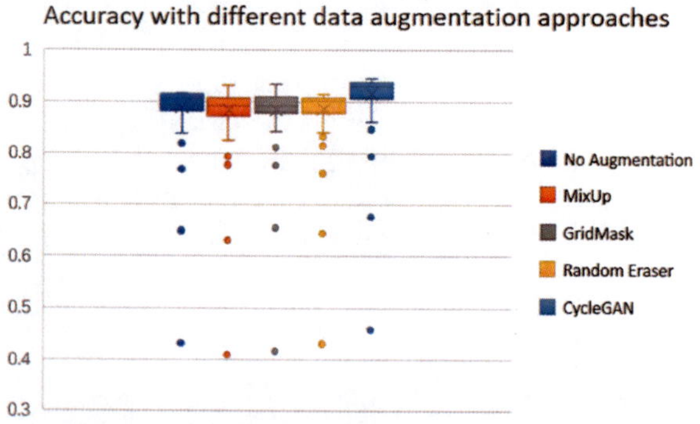

Fig. 3. Accuracy with different data augmentation approachess.

4.3 Quantitative Comparison Using Different Network Architectures

To further demonstrate the effectiveness of CycleGAN-based data augmentation, different neural network architectures are also tested, which include VGG, ResNet, Xception and EfficientNet. The experimental results are demonstrated in Table 1. It can be seen from Table 1 that, EfficientNet B1 has achieved better classification results compared to the other three networks, with accuracy reaching 0.945.

Table 1. Results of different network architectures.

Network architectures	ACC	ACU
VGG	0.891	0.822
ResNet50	0.913	0.863
Xception	0.926	0.881
EfficientNet B1	**0.945**	**0.923**

5 Conclusion

Melanoma image detection plays an important role in accurately identifying the disease for clinical diagnosis, while this task is challenging for many devoted researchers who have contributed to the previous study of the melanoma classification. Our study aim to explore a novel data augmentation strategy named CycleGAN based on deep learning approaches to tackle the problem. Extensive experiments have been employed to test the effectiveness of the strategy. The empirical findings in this study suggest that CycleGAN can alleviate the adverse effects of data imbalance on melanoma classification tasks to a certain extent. With regard to the research methods, some limitations need to be acknowledged. For the future work, we would like to further test our methods on the larger dataset to improve the classification accuracy.

References

1. Fleming, M.G., et al.: Techniques for a structural analysis of dermatoscopic imagery. Comput. Med. Imaging Graph. **22**(5), 375–389 (1998)
2. Hu, H., Luo, C., Guan, Q., Li, X., Chen, S., Zhou, Q.: A fast online multivariable identification method for greenhouse environment control problems. Neurocomputing **312**, 63–73 (2018)
3. Hu, H., Guan, Q., Chen, S., Ji, Z., Yao, L.: Detection and recognition for life state of cell cancer using two-stage cascade CNNs. IEEE/ACM Trans. Comput. Biol. Bioinform. (2017)
4. Celebi, M.E., et al.: A methodological approach to the classification of dermoscopy images. Comput. Med. Imaging Graph. **31**(6), 362–373 (2007)
5. Ballerini, L., Fisher, R.B., Aldridge, B., Rees, J.: A color and texture based hierarchical k-NN approach to the classification of non-melanoma skin lesions. In: Celebi, M., Schaefer, G. (eds.) Color Medical Image Analysis. Lecture Notes in Computational Vision and Biomechanics, pp. 63–86. Springer, Dordrecht (2013). https://doi.org/10.1007/978-94-007-5389-1_4
6. Acharya, U.R., Oh, S.L., Hagiwara, Y., Tan, J.H., Adeli, H.: Deep convolutional neural network for the automated detection and diagnosis of seizure using EEG signals. Comput. Biol. Med. **100**, 270–278 (2018)
7. LeCun, Y., Bottou, L., Bengio, Y., Haffner, P.: Gradient-based learning applied to document recognition. Proc. IEEE **86**(11), 2278–2324 (1998)
8. Simonyan, K., Zisserman, A.: Very deep convolutional networks for large-scale image recognition, arXiv preprint arXiv:1409.1556 (2014)

9. Szegedy, C., et al.: Going deeper with convolutions. In: Proceedings of the IEEE Conference on Computer Vision and Pattern Recognition, pp. 1–9 (2015)
10. He, K., Zhang, X., Ren, S., Sun, J.: Deep residual learning for image recognition. In: Proceedings of the IEEE Conference on Computer Vision and Pattern Recognition, pp. 770–778 (2016)
11. Huang, G., Liu, Z., Van Der Maaten, L., Weinberger, K.Q.: Densely connected convolutional networks. In: Proceedings of the IEEE Conference on Computer Vision and Pattern Recognition, pp. 4700–4708 (2017)
12. Zhong, Z., Zheng, L., Kang, G., Li, S., Yang, Y.: Random erasing data augmentation. In: AAAI, pp. 13 001–13 008 (2020)
13. Qu, H., Zhang, L., Wu, X., He, X., Hu, X., Wen, X.: Multiscale object detection in infrared streetscape images based on deep learning and instance level data augmentation. Appl. Sci. **9**(3), 565 (2019)
14. Antoniou, A., Storkey, A., Edwards, H.: Data augmentation generative adversarial networks, arXiv preprint arXiv:1711.04340 (2017)
15. Goodfellow, I., et al.: Generative adversarial nets. In: Advances in Neural Information Processing Systems, pp. 2672–2680 (2014)
16. Radford, A., Metz, L., Chintala, S.: Unsupervised representation learning with deep convolutional generative adversarial networks. arXiv preprint arXiv:1511.06434 (2015)
17. Arjovsky, M., Chintala, S., Bottou, L.: Wasserstein gan. arXiv preprint arXiv:1701.07875 (2017)
18. Karras, T., Aila, T., Laine, S., Lehtinen, J.: Progressive growing of gans for improved quality, stability, and variation. arXiv preprint arXiv:1710.10196 (2017)
19. Chu, C., Zhmoginov, A., Sandler, M.: Cyclegan, a master of steganography. arXiv preprint arXiv:1712.02950 (2017)
20. Chen, X., Duan, Y., Houthooft, R., Schulman, J., Sutskever, I., Abbeel, P.: Infogan: Interpretable representation learning by information maximizing generative adversarial nets. In: Advances in Neural Information Processing Systems, pp. 2172–2180 (2016)
21. Hoang, Q., Nguyen, T.D., Le, T., Phung, D.: MGAN: training generative adversarial nets with multiple generators. In: International Conference on Learning Representations (2018)
22. Zhou, T., Krahenbuhl, P., Aubry, M., Huang, Q., Efros, A.A.: Learning dense correspondence via 3d-guided cycle consistency. In: Proceedings of the IEEE Conference on Computer Vision and Pattern Recognition, pp. 117–126 (2016)

Ensembling Learning for Automated Detection of Diabetic Retinopathy

Yipeng Han[1], Mengjun Tao[2(✉)], and Xiaolu Zheng[3]

[1] University of New South Wales, Sydeny, Australia
[2] New York University, New York, USA
[3] Beihang University, Beijing, China

Abstract. It is widely known that diabetic retinopathy has become the main cause of irreversible vision loss among the working-age population world-widely. For clinical treatment, early and accurate identification of diabetic retinopathy using fundus image is a high-priority step, as early detection of diabetic retinopathy occurrence can be very helpful to prevent vision loss. Previous attempts for the detection task are based on the handcrafted-feature extraction and shallow architecture-based classifier (such as random forest, support vector machine). Recently, deep convolutional neural network (CNN) was successfully applied for the classification task. Despite sustainable efforts have been made, the task is still short of accuracy and time-consuming. In this paper, we propose an ensemble learning framework with the goal to improve the detection performance, using both handcrafted features and deep learning approaches. By leveraging the complementary information provided by handcrafted features and deep learning approaches, the ensemble learning framework is endowed with more discriminative power. Extensive experiments are conducted on the benchmark dataset, and the proposed framework provides superior performance, which demonstrated the effectiveness of proposed method.

Keywords: Medical image classification · Deep learning · Convolutional neural network · Ensemble learning

1 Introduction

The number of people having diabetic retinopathy has witnessed dramatic increasing over the last several decades, and diabetes increases the risk of many eye diseases, of which diabetic retinopathy is one of the most severe diseases [1]. Moreover, diabetic retinopathy is the leading cause of blindness among the working-age world widely. Early detection and routine eye examples can be helpful to prevent diabetic retinopathy and screening has become a high-priority healthcare service [2]. Although researchers have conducted sustainable efforts to improve the accuracy of automated diagnosis, th automatic analysis is still

R. Su et al. (Eds.): MICAD 2021, LNEE 784, pp. 29–36, 2022.
https://doi.org/10.1007/978-981-16-3880-0_4

short of robustness and accuracy. Currently, early detection of diabetic retinopathy is quite time-consuming and error-prone processing even for a well-trained optometrist or ophthalmologist. Nowadays, the fact that in the current medical system, there is limited medical staff and limited medical resources has greatly aggravated the handcrafted labor quantity. During the clarification process for retinal images, the automated system can significantly reduce the onerous consumption of manual labor and improve its selection efficiency for doctors to diagnosing diabetic retinopathy images from a huge number of images.

In our study, we focus on the automated classification of retinal images into based on the severe level. Indeed, dramatic progress has been made using image feature extraction and machine learning methods through previous efforts. Various features were used to classify the images, including hard exudates [3], red lesions [4], micro-aneurysms [5] and blood vessel detection [17]. Based on the handcrafted features, different shallow-architecture-based classifiers can be used to classify the images: such as sparse representation classifiers [18], linear discriminant analysis (LDA) [6], support vector machine (SVM) [7], k-nearest neighbors (KNN) algorithm [16]. Unfortunately, the manually-designed features cannot cover all the diabetic retinopathy symptoms in the images, and even it turned out massive time were wasted to diagnose the normal case due to the mistake and fraction case. Consequently, it constrained the practical applications of the diagnosing system.

Since the revolution of deep neural network, convolutional neural networks (CNNs) method has achieved tremendous progress to conduct classification tasks, whose variants have gradually been employed in its relative fields of computer vision, such as, object detection, image classification, object tracking, edge detection. Compared to manual-designed features, CNN can learn a hierarchy of features in classifying images using the automatic manner. The hierarchy method can conduct multi-tasks in higher layers: identify more complex features, translation, identify distortion features as well. CNN-based image classification method possesses higher accuracy. According to this assumption, CNN-based approach was used in many previous research for diabetic retinopathy detection [13–15]. Different CNN architectures have been proposed in last years. In this paper, we aim to employ the complementary information provided by handcrafted features and deep learning method. To that end, an novel ensemble learning is proposed in this paper, with the goal to improve the classification performance.

This paper is organized as follows: different CNN architectures and the ensemble learning framework is introduced in this Sect. 2. Section 3 presents the task definition and present the results for the quantitative comparison between different neural network architectures. The conclusion and future work are discussed in Sect. 4 (Fig. 1 and Table 1).

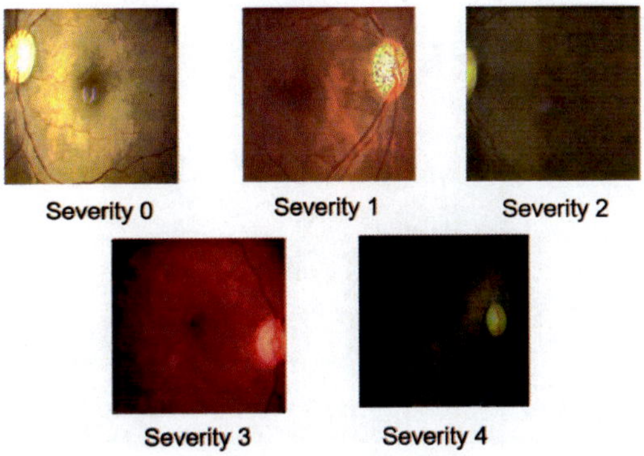

Fig. 1. Different severity level for diabetic retinopathy.

Table 1. The severity level of diabetic retinopathy.

Level ID	Severity level
0	No diabetic retinopathy
1	Mild diabetic retinopathy
2	Moderate diabetic retinopathy
3	Severe diabetic retinopathy
4	Proliferative diabetic retinopathy

2 Methodology

2.1 Ensemble Learning Framework

It is widely known that ensemble diverse classifiers can improve the accuracy and robustness for the classification task. However, the ensemble learning has been under-explored for the diabetic retinopathy detection task. In this paper, we propose a novel ensemble learning framework, leveraging the deep learning and handcrafted features, with the goal to improve accuracy and robustness of the detection task. Figure 2 shows the proposed ensemble learning framework used in our task, which is composed of two levels: feature extraction part and modeling part using gradient boosting trees. In our experiments, the first layers are composed of 3 different CNN architectures to build out-of-fold meta-features. The out-of-fold predicted probabilities of different deep convolutional neural networks will be concatenated to generate meta-features. Except for the deep learning-based meta features, we also employ the traditional handcrafted features (the details of handcrafted are given in the following part). For step 2, we employ the gradient tree boosting machine (GBM) for the detection task. LightGBM is used to implement the ensemble learning approaches [12].

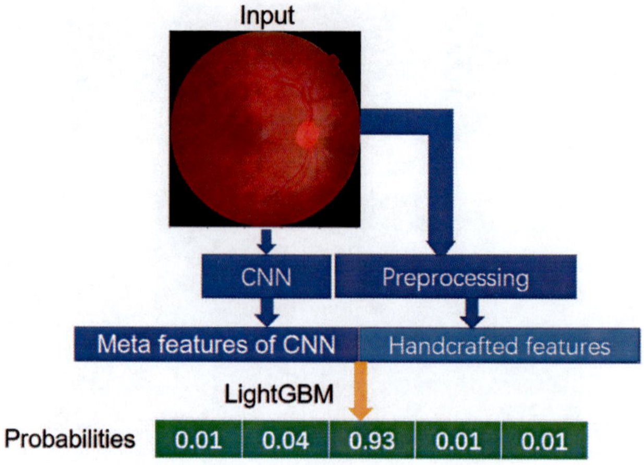

Fig. 2. Ensemble learning framework for automated detection of diabetic retinopathy. In the framework, both deep learning and handcrafted features are used for our task.

2.2 Deep Convolutional Networks Models

We employ three widely used convolutional network architectures, including VGGNet, Inception and ResNet, to build out-of-fold meta-features. The details of the CNN architectures are given in the following part.

VGGNet. VGGNet is characterized by its simplicity [11], using only 3×3 convolutional layers stacked on top of each other in increasing depth. VGGNet aims to increase the depth by reducing the size of receptive field. On the other hand, reducing volume size is handled by max pooling. Max-pooling is performed over a 2×2 pixel window, with a stride of 2. Two fully-connected layers, each with 4,096 nodes are then followed by a softmax classifier.

Inception. Inception model [10] originates from GoogLeNet [9]. One important property of the module is that it has a the bottleneck layer, which leads to massive reduction of the computation requirement. Inception model suggests to replace the fully-connected layers at the end with a simple global average pooling which averages out the channel values across the two dimension feature map, after the last convolutional layer, which drastically reduces the total number of parameters.

ResNet. ResNet [8] is a form of different architecture that relies on network-in-network architectures. The term network-in-network architecture refers to the set of blocks used to construct the network. A collection of micro-architecture building blocks (along with standard convolution, pooling, etc. layers) leads to the macro-architecture (i.e.,. the end network itself). ResNets uses a global average pooling followed by the classification layer. Through the changes mentioned,

ResNets were learned with network depth of as large as 152. It achieves better accuracy than VGGNet and GoogLeNet while being computationally more efficient than VGGNet.

2.3 Handcrafted Features

Different manual designed features have been tested in previous studies, to automatically detect diabetic retinopathy. Here, two different kinds of handcrafted features are implemented to demonstrate that the manual designed features can provide complementary information for deep learning.

- Blood vessels density Firstly, we convert the RGB image to its CMY representation, followed by morphological processing. After the morphological processing and histogram matching that increases its contrast, the resulting image is binary. To decrease the contamination of noise, dilation and erosion operations are conducted on the binary image. In the end, the density of white pixels (i.e., blood vessels) is computed.
- Hard exudates: During the early diagnose of diabetic retinopathy, hard exudates detection is an important characteristic. In our experiments, to detect hard exudates, we employed the threshold-based binarization approach for the CMY representation. Then, a dilation operation is employed to the processed image. In the end, an erosion operation is conducted, followed by the computing the density of hard exudates.

3 Experimental Results

3.1 Dataset

We employ a large set of high-resolution retina images taken under different imaging conditions, and the details of the dataset can be found in Kaggle website[1]. Both left and right field is employed for every subject. Images are labeled with a subject id as well as either left or right. Trained clinician has rated the presence of diabetic retinopathy in each image on a scale of 0 to 4, according to the following scale given in Table 2.

3.2 Implementation Details

In our experiments, the input sizes for different CNN architectures are kept same (as 224×224). It takes 8 h for the training process for different CNN architectures; however, the identification of diabetic retinopathy on test data can be almost real-time, which can be helpful in the clinical practice. The parameters of the CNN model are optimized with stochastic gradient descent. The cross-entropy was selected as the objective function. Moreover, an L2 weight decay penalty of 0.002 was employed in our model. The model is evaluated according to a four-fold cross-validation scheme. Finally, the overall quadratic weighted kappa is calculated by averaging the four per-fold accuracy.

[1] https://www.kaggle.com/c/aptos2019-blindness-detection/data.

3.3 Evaluation Metrics

The quadratic weighted kappa is used for the evaluation, which measures the agreement between two ratings. The quadratic weighted kappa is calculated between the scores assigned by the human rater and the predicted scores. In our piratical settings, the retina images have five possible ratings. Each retina image can be labeled by a tuple (e, e), which corresponds to its scores by Rater A (domain experts) and Rater B (predicted). The quadratic weighted kappa is calculated as follows. First, an N $\times$ N histogram matrix O is calculated, such that O corresponds to the number of images that received a rating i by A and a rating j by B. An N$\times$ N matrix of weights, w, is calculated based on the difference between raters' scores: an N$\times$N histogram matrix of expected ratings, E, is calculated, assuming that there is no correlation between rating scores. This is calculated as the outer product between each rater's histogram vector of ratings, normalized such that E and O have the same sum.

3.4 Quantitative Evaluation

We employ the classification performance for the quantitatively studies between different experiential settings.

In the experiment, we firstly employ different CNN architectures for the classification task so that the performance of the single deep model can be evaluated. The CNN architectures used here consists of VGGNet, Inception and ResNet. Moreover, the handcrafted features-based model is also used evaluated using the GBM model. In the end, we test the performance of our ensemble learning framework on this dataset. The quadratic weighted kappa obtained by different experiential settings are given in Table 2.

As can be seen from the table, deeper CNN a showed better performance as ResNet outperforms VGGNet and Inception. It is worthwhile to notice that handcrafted feature can provide satisfied performance, with a quadratic weighted kappa of 0.755. On the other hand, the proposed ensemble learning framework yields superior predictions in comparison with other approaches under the experimental conditions, which demonstrating its advantage in this particular task. It may also imply that the ensemble learning can employ the complementary information provided by handcrafted features and deep learning, which can be helpful to improve the accuracy for the detection task. In brief, the ensemble learning approach has high stability and good performance on this dataset.

Table 2. Performance comparison with different approaches.

Method	Quadratic weighted kappa
VGGNet	0.748
Inception	0.769
ResNet	0.784
Handcrafted features +GBM	0.755
Ensemble learning	0.803

4 Conclusion

It is widely known that ensemble learning has proven effective in many pattern recognition tasks. However, the ensemble learning is not fully explored for the diabetic retinopathy detection task in previous studies. In this paper, we proposed a novel ensemble learning framework for the detection task. A quantitative comparison is conducted between handcrafted feature-based method, deep learning approaches and our ensemble learning-based approaches. Experimental results demonstrate the effectiveness of our method. To the best knowledge of the authors, this is the first attempt of the ensemble learning which leveraging different deep learning and handcrafted features for the detection task. In our future work, we would like to test our framework on larger data set.

References

1. Mohan, V., Sandeep, S., Deepa, R., Shah, B., Varghese, C.: Epidemiology of type 2 diabetes: Indian scenario. Indian J. Med. Res. **125**(3), 217–30 (2007)
2. González-Gonzalo, C., et al.: Evaluation of a deep learning system for the joint automated detection of diabetic retinopathy and age-related macular degeneration. Acta Ophthalmologica (2019)
3. Hsu, W., Pallawala, P., Lee, M.L., Eong, K.-G.A.: The role of domain knowledge in the detection of retinal hard exudates. In: Proceedings of the 2001 IEEE Computer Society Conference on Computer Vision and Pattern Recognition. CVPR 2001, vol. 2, pp. II-II. IEEE (2001)
4. Larsen, M., et al.: Automated detection of fundus photographic red lesions in diabetic retinopathy. Invest. Ophthalmol. Vis. Sci. **44**(2), 761–766 (2003)
5. Spencer, T., Phillips, R.P., Sharp, P.F., Forrester, J.V.: Automated detection and quantification of microaneurysms in fluorescein angiograms. Graefe's Arch. Clin. Exp. Ophthalmol. **230**(1), 36–41 (1992). https://doi.org/10.1007/BF00166760
6. Kumar, D.K., Aliahmad, B., Hao, H.: Retinal vessel diameter measurement using unsupervised linear discriminant analysis. ISRN Ophthalmol. **2012** (2012)
7. Du, N., Li, Y.: Automated identification of diabetic retinopathy stages using support vector machine. Presented at the (2013)
8. He, K., Zhang, X., Ren, S., Sun, J.: Deep residual learning for image recognition. Presented at the (2016)

9. Zhong, Z., Jin, L., Xie, Z.: High performance offline handwritten Chinese character recognition using GoogLENet and directional feature maps. In: 2015 13th International Conference on Document Analysis and Recognition (ICDAR). IEEE, pp. 846–850 (2015)
10. Szegedy, C., Ioffe, S., Vanhoucke, V., Alemi, A.A.: Inception-v4, inception-resnet and the impact of residual connections on learning. Presented at the (2017)
11. Simonyan, K., Zisserman, A.: Very deep convolutional networks for large-scale image recognition. Presented at the (2014)
12. Ke, G., et al.: LightGBM: a highly efficient gradient boosting decision tree. Presented at the (2017)
13. Xu, K., Feng, D., Mi, H.: Deep convolutional neural network-based early automated detection of diabetic retinopathy using fundus image. Molecules **22**(12), 2054 (2017)
14. Lim, G., Lee, M.L., Hsu, W., Wong, T.Y.: Transformed representations for convolutional neural networks in diabetic retinopathy screening. Presented at the (2014)
15. Pratt, H., Coenen, F., Broadbent, D.M., Harding, S.P., Zheng, Y.: Convolutional neural networks for diabetic retinopathy. Procedia Comput. Sci. **90**, 200–205 (2016)
16. Roychowdhury, S., Koozekanani, D.D., Parhi, K.K.: Dream: diabetic retinopathy analysis using machine learning. IEEE J. Biomed. Health Inf. **18**(5), 1717–1728 (2013)
17. Faust, O., Acharya, R., Ng, E.Y.-K., Ng, K.-H., Suri, J.S.: Algorithms for the automated detection of diabetic retinopathy using digital fundus images: a review. J. Med. Syst. **36**(1), 145–157 (2012)
18. Zhang, B., Karray, F., Li, Q., Zhang, L.: Sparse representation classifier for microaneurysm detection and retinal blood vessel extraction. Inf. Sci. **200**, 78–90 (2012)

A Fully Automated End-to-End Process for Fluorescence Microscopy Images of Yeast Cells: From Segmentation to Detection and Classification

Asmaa Haja(✉) and Lambert R. B. Schomaker

Bernoulli Institute, University of Groningen, Groningen, The Netherlands
{a.haja,l.r.b.schomaker}@rug.nl

Abstract. In recent years, an enormous amount of fluorescence microscopy images were collected in high-throughput lab settings. Analyzing and extracting relevant information from all images in a short time is almost impossible. Detecting tiny individual cell compartments is one of many challenges faced by biologists. This paper aims at solving this problem by building an end-to-end process that employs methods from the deep learning field to automatically segment, detect and classify cell compartments of fluorescence microscopy images of yeast cells. With this intention we used Mask R-CNN to automatically segment and label a large amount of yeast cell data, and YOLOv4 to automatically detect and classify individual yeast cell compartments from these images. This fully automated end-to-end process is intended to be integrated into an interactive e-Science server in the PerICo (https://itn-perico.eu/home/) project, which can be used by biologists with minimized human effort in training and operation to complete their various classification tasks. In addition, we evaluated the detection and classification performance of state-of-the-art YOLOv4 on data from the NOP1pr-GFP-SWAT yeast-cell data library. Experimental results show that by dividing original images into 4 quadrants YOLOv4 outputs good detection and classification results with an F1-score of 98% in terms of accuracy and speed, which is optimally suited for the native resolution of the microscope and current GPU memory sizes. Although the application domain is optical microscopy in yeast cells, the method is also applicable to multiple-cell images in medical applications.

Keywords: Segmentation · Detection · Classification · Data augmentation · Convolutional neural network · Deep learning · Cross-validation · Cell microscopy · Organelles · Cell compartments

1 Introduction

The existence of modern microscopy facilitates the generation of high-throughput data: It is now possible to produce very large collections of microscopic images of cell samples in a short time. The enormous amount of data

R. Su et al. (Eds.): MICAD 2021, LNEE 784, pp. 37–46, 2022.
https://doi.org/10.1007/978-981-16-3880-0_5

opens the door for the biologists to study important and more complex aspects in their research field. However, one of many challenges they are recently facing is how to process such amount of data in a short time, extracting as much information as possible, as well as identifying biologically and clinically relevant diseases such as human diseases. Analyzing a huge volume of microscopy images by manually going though every image is a tedious task, can lead to fatigue and decision errors. Therefore, there is a desire to automatically process and analyse data in a high-throughput setting with minimized human effort in training and operation. Integrating techniques from the deep learning field of artificial intelligence seems to be a promising solution for this problem. Automatic detection and classification of details in microscopic images would dramatically speed up their research and contribute to their field of knowledge.

In this paper, our focus is on a specific problem in the field of biology, which is the automatic detection of individual-cell compartments in fluorescence microscopy images of yeast cells, notably organelle, as well as automatic specification of their type. In fact, the highlight of this paper is on the application of deep learning algorithms to biological data, i.e., images from optical cell microscopy. In this study we will not go into details to cover biological concepts.

Object detection and classification is one of the hottest topic in the deep learning field. Different approaches were developed for the detection, segmentation and classification of various cell types. In traditional approaches, each of these steps were implemented as separate algorithms. As an example, such approaches used morphology methods for detection [1,2], whereas new approaches use machine learning and/or deep learning methods to realize these steps in a more realistic manner. Notably, Convolutional Neural Networks (CNN) are able to realize the same functionality using end-to-end training [3,4], as opposed to meticulous design of a processing pipeline with individual processing stages. In [5], for instance, a morphological gray reconstruction based on a fuzzy cellular neural network is applied to detect white blood cells. Xipeng et al. [4] proposed a novel multi-scale fully CNNs approach for regression of a density map to detect both nuclei of pathology and microscopy images. Xie et al. [6] developed two convolutional regression networks to detect and count cells. Wang et al. [7] in 2016 combined two CNN for simultaneously detecting and classifying cells.

Although there are many specialised methods that are capable of detecting different types of cells, to the best of the authors knowledge there exists no generic system for detecting all kinds of cell compartment in an accurate and easy way. In this paper, we present a fully automated end-to-end process for yeast-cell data that is capable of solving various segmentation, detection and classification tasks. For that, we use Mask-RCNN [8] to automatically segment and label images from the input data, and YOLOv4 [9] to automatically detect and classify individual yeast cell compartments from these images. This end-to-end process is currently intended to be integrated into an interactive e-Science server in the PerICo[1] project. We also evaluate the detection and classification

[1] https://itn-perico.eu/home/.

performance of YOLOv4 on data from the NOP1pr-GFP-SWAT yeast-cell data library. We chose this particular algorithm because it is capable of detecting small objects, such as individual cell compartments, requiring a limited computation time. YOLO detects and classifies objects in only one stage, i.e., in one run.

The remainder of the paper is structured as follows: Sect. 2 presents the used data. In Sect. 3, our end-to-end process is introduced. Section 4 provides an overview of the our experimental design. The results of our study on the chosen dataset is presented in Sect. 5, while the last section concludes the paper and indicates the future works.

2 Data

To evaluate the end-to-end process we used publicly available fluorescence microscopy data from a library of yeast strains each expressing one protein under control of a constitutive promoter (NOP1) and fused to a Green Fluorescent Protein (GFP) at the N terminus (NOP1pr-GFP-SWAT library) [10]. This library contains annotated GFP and Bright Field (BF) yeast images of nearly 6000 strains each residing in a specific organelle in the cell. Overall, there were 18432 images from 16 well-plates, each consists of 1152 images for each channel with the dimension of 1344 x 1024 pixels. With respect to deep learning, each image is represented by a pre-defined class that describes the objects found in the image. Here, the classes are defined by the cell-compartments names.

Table 1 lists the classes that have more than 300 unique images. In Fig. 1, merging a BF and GFP channels of a random sample image is shown. The BF is shown on the left side of this Figure, while GFP channel is shown in the middle side of the Figure. The results of merging both channels are shown in green and grey colors in the right side of Fig. 1. We chose this particular data because individual cells are too small to detect, it contains overlapped and close cells, and it consists of different cell sizes and shapes as can be seen in this Figure.

Table 1. Number of unique images for cell compartments that have more than 300 images.

Name of cell compartments	# Unique images
ER (Endoplasmic Reticulum)	376
Cytosol & Nucleus	401
Mitochondria	461
Nucleus	660
Cytosol	1566

3 End-to-End Process

The main goal of this paper is to present the fully automated end-to-end segmentation, detection and classification process as well as to evaluate the individual-cell compartments detection performance of the state-of-the-art YOLOv4 model on fluorescence microscopy images. The traditional approach in the deep learning for carrying out any kind of task is to execute it in two phases: training- and testing phase. For that, the data will randomly be divided into two unmixed

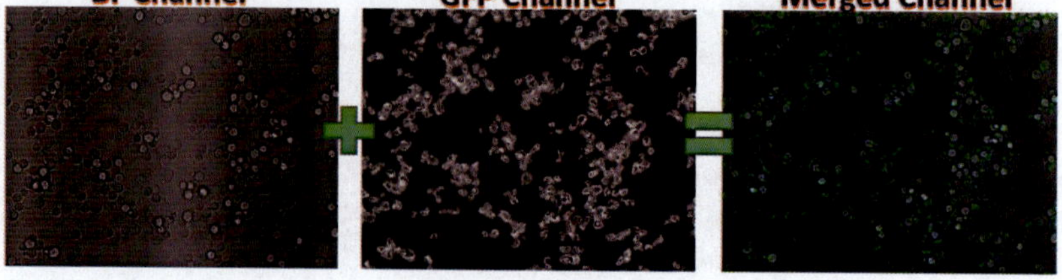

Fig. 1. Merging BF and GFP channels of a randomly selected image [Plate15 J9].

sets: train- and test sets, each contains the same amount of data for each class. In a training plus validation phase, we teach the model to detect individual-cell compartment by providing it with the different locations of almost all individual cells in the training images. In order to test the trained model, we provide it with test images that the model did not see before. In the end, the model is evaluated based on specific metrics that decide how well the model has learned the specific tasks, the detection and classification tasks in this case.

Every image in our data is characterized by a label (cell-compartment name). However, we are not only interested to know which type of cells can be found in the image but also the exact locations of each individual cell. One of many state-of-the-art solutions to automatically segment individual objects is the mask-RCNN model proposed in [8]. According to [11], a pre-trained mask-RCNN model can be used to segmented yeast cells without fine-tuning. We used their implementation to segment individual cells in our dataset. It is to be noticed that the segmentation is completed in an unsupervised manner, done on the bright-field channel and not on the GFP channel. For the detection and classification of the individual-cell compartments we use the state-of-the-art YOLOv4 model developed by Bochkovskiy, Wang and Liao [9]. The primary goal of their paper is to design a fast-operating object detector for production systems that is also optimized for parallel computations, and more importantly is that the training should be done on one single conventional GPU. In comparison to other existing state-of-the-art models, YOLOv4 outperforms them in term of speed, accuracy and performance [9]. Not only that but it seems a good candidate to use for detecting small objects seeing all modifications that were added to it, which are considered as a significant upgrade to its previous well-known versions. Therefore, we consider it as the best starting point for addressing the where and what question, i.e., detection and classification, in microscopic images.

Figure 2 shows the pipeline of the training phase. First, we use Mask-RCNN model to segment individual cells on each BF channel in the training set [segmentation step]. Simultaneously, we merge both BF and GFP channels for each image [pre-processing step]. With the purpose of training YOLOv4, we create specific YOLOv4 files from both the merged and the segmented images [post-processing step]. The last step in this phase would be to train YOLOv4 using both the created files and the merged images from the training set [training the model step]. In Fig. 3, a pipeline of the testing phase is presented. Similar to the training phase, we first need to merge both BF and GFP channels from the unseen images in the test set [pre-processing step]. We use these images to test the trained YOLOv4 model [testing the model step]. As a result, YOLOv4 yields files for each test image, where the predicted location of each individual cell is computed. We use these files to evaluate the performance of YOLOv4 [analysis step]. The results described by the segmentation outcome of the training images, the trained model parameters, and the outcome of the detection and classification of the trained model on the test images are presented to the user.

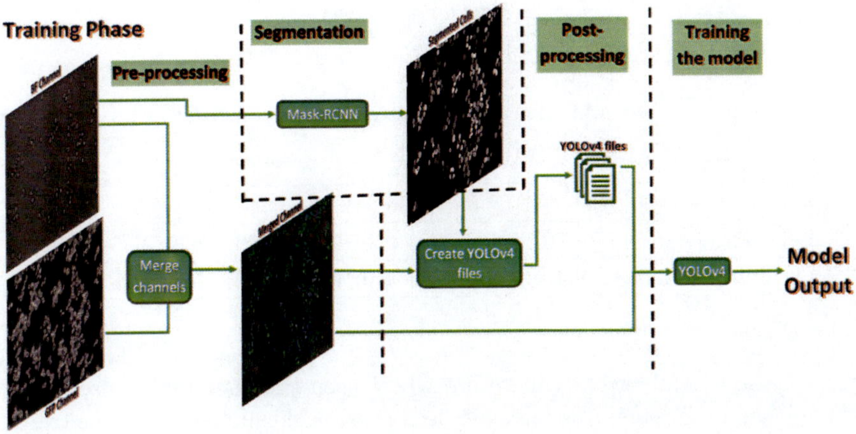

Fig. 2. Pipeline of the training phase.

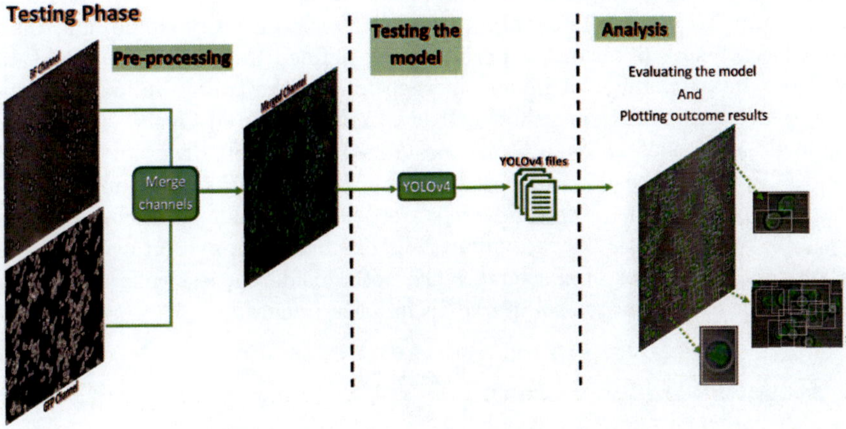

Fig. 3. Pipeline of the testing phase including analysis.

4 Experimental Design

In addition to building an end-to-end process for fluorescence microscopy images of yeast cells, this paper aims to evaluate the detection and classification performance of the state-of-the-art YOLOv4 algorithm on individual small objects.

Table 2. Experiment, image size, classes [ER, Mitochondria (M), Cytosol (C) and Nucleus (N)], number of images in train-, validation-, and test set.

# Experiment	Images size	Classes	# Train images	# Validation images	# Test images
Exp_1	1344 × 1024	M	≈990	≈110	≈270
Exp_2	1344 × 1024	ER, M	≈1620	≈180	≈450
Exp_3	1344 × 1024	ER, M, C, N	≈2980	≈330	≈912
Exp_4	672 × 512	M	≈3960	≈440	≈1110
Exp_5	672 × 512	ER, M	≈6480	≈720	≈1800
Exp_6	672 × 512	ER, M, C, N	≈12710	≈1410	≈3640

Table 3. Training time, mAP and average loss error [Time/mAP/avg loss] at the end of the training phase for each experiment.

	1-class	2-classes	4-classes
Full-size image	1h20/91%/15.02	2h30/91%/15.54	5h30/91%/14.54
Quadrants of image	0h40/94%/03.60	1h40/93%/03.45	2h50/93%/03.59

Here, we use five-fold cross validation, where each time one fold is used to test the model and the remaining folds are used to train the model. From the training set we randomly selected 10% of the train images to be used for validating the model during the training phase. We used the dataset introduced in Sect. 2 to evaluate YOLOv4. Based on the numbers of unique images shown in Table 1, we determine to assess the capability of YOLOv4 to classify single- and multi-class objects using 6 various experiments as defined in Table 2. In this Table, the approximate number of images in each fold in the train-, validate-and test sets for each experiment are shown. It is to note that YOLOv4 was trained on original images sizes (Exp_1, Exp_2 and Exp_3) versus quadrant of the images (Exp_4, Exp_5 and Exp_6). On average, 187k, 306k and 575k individual cells has been cropped for Exp_1, Exp_2 and Exp_3, respectively, while for Exp_4, Exp_5 and Exp_6, 173k, 284k and 539k individual cells has been cropped on average. Since the cells on the border of the images are not considered, less cells are cropped for quadrant of the images compared to full-size images.

5 Results and Discussion

This section presents and analyses the results obtained from 6 trained YOLOv4 models defined in Sect. 4. Each model describes one experiment and is obtained by employing the end-to-end process on the introduced dataset from Sect. 2. Table 3 reports the average training time, the average mAP[2] and the average loss error computed on the corresponding validation set for all folds. As it can be seen, the mAPs computed on quadrant of the images for all classification type

[2] Mean average precision.

Table 4. Test results for 5-fold cross validation on four classes for full-size images (left) and quadrant images (right).

Fold	Precision	Recall	F1	Accuracy	Fold	Precision	Recall	F1	Accuracy
0	0.989	0.989	0.989	0.989	0	0.980	0.980	0.980	0.980
1	0.984	0.984	0.984	0.984	1	0.974	0.974	0.974	0.974
2	0.987	0.986	0.987	0.986	2	0.978	0.978	0.978	0.978
3	0.984	0.984	0.984	0.984	3	0.973	0.973	0.973	0.973
4	0.978	0.978	0.980	0.980	4	0.965	0.965	0.965	0.965
AVG	**0.985**	**0.985**	**0.985**	**0.985**	AVG	**0.974**	**0.974**	**0.974**	**0.974**

(Exp_4, Exp_5 and Exp_6) are higher than the mAPs computed on full size of the original images (Exp_1, Exp_2 and Exp_3). This indicates that the detection on quadrant of the images works better than on the full-size image. Average loss error computed for quadrant of the images is around 3.5, which is way lower than for full-size images. This implies that the classification of quadrant of the images is better than on the complete images. Both of these observations suggest that YOLOv4 is able to detect and classify small objects best in native resolution, as opposed to a complete but subsampled image.

Table 4 reports the average precision, recall, F1-score and accuracy computed for each test fold for Exp_3 (left) and Exp_6 (right). The last row represents the average for all folds. Using the cross validation trick, it is evident that YOLOv4 is robust since its performance on various parts of the data is similar. Obviously, the outcomes of all these measures show that the classification of individual cells on full-size images is 1% better than on quadrant of the images. The reason for this is because less cells are detected on original image compared to quadrants of the image. This can be seen in the black circles in Fig. 4, where the left side of this Figure shows the detection of individual cells on the original image, and and right side shows the detection on each quadrant of the image. In addition, the labeling for each individual cell is not obtained from human experts but from the label class of the original image. A cell where the nucleus is seen more sharply than the ER should be called nucleus, even if the plate label is ER.

In Fig. 5, the detection results of randomly selected test images from Exp_6 are shown. It is apparent that all images have different brightness in their background, but this is not necessarily the general case in our dataset. The title of the images contains information about the plate number, position in the plate, cell compartment type, and cropped position from the original images. The latter can be TL, TR, BL, BR, which corresponds to top-left, top-right, bottom-left, and bottom-right, respectively. Clearly, YOLOv4 demonstrates good detection results on these images. It is also capable of detecting parts of cells found on the border of these images. However, the most remarkable result to emerge from the data is that the detection of the individual cells for ER, in contrast to other classes, has much lower accuracy. As it can be seen from bottom-left of Fig. 5, YOLOv4 fails to detect the tiny cells. According to biologists, ER in yeast always surrounds the nucleus. Therefore, differentiating it from a nuclear signal is not so easy. To demonstrate this, Table 5 represents the normalized confusion matrix

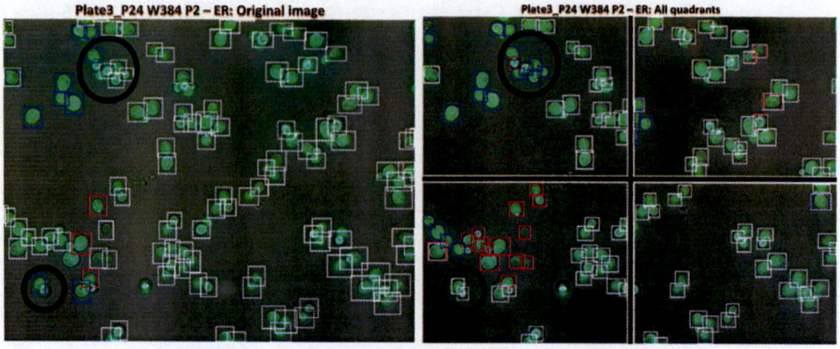

Fig. 4. Detection and classification results for an image [Plate3_P24] using both the complete, subsampled image and the native-resolution quadrants.

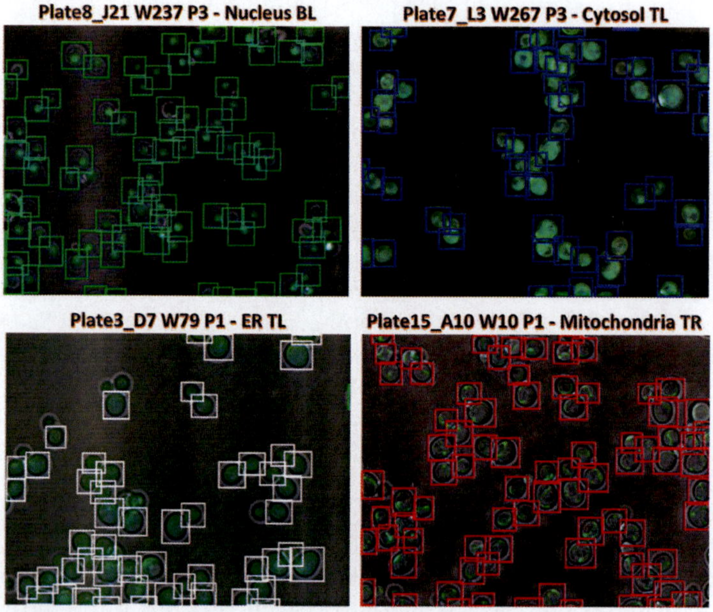

Fig. 5. Randomly selected test images for 4-classes [ER, Mitochondria, Cytosol and Nucleus] classification and by using only quadrant of the images.

of one fold of Exp_6. Here, we count the number of the true prediction and the negative prediction for all cell compartments. For example, for all ER images, we count the number of ER, Cytosol, Mitochondria and Nucleus predicted cell compartments, respectively. In this case, the latter three classes are considered the false prediction. Finally, we normalize all these four values, and show them in the first row of the normalized confusion matrix. From Table 5, it is noticeable that the classification for classes Nucleus and Mitochondria are the best with a 99% correct prediction, while the classification for ER is the worst with only 93%

correct individual cells prediction. The red text in Table 5 supports the previous assumption, since 3% of individual ER cells are predicted as Nucleus.

Table 5. Confusion matrix for one fold in Exp_6.

True	Predicted ER	Predicted C	Predicted M	Predicted N
ER	0.931	0.022	0.012	0.034
C	0.005	0.969	0.001	0.025
M	0.001	0.001	0.995	0.002
N	0.003	0.005	0.001	0.991

Further analysis shows that the classification results using majority vote of all quadrants to classify the whole plate are similar to using the majority to classify the full-size image. As previously mentioned, less cell compartments are detected when using full-size images as input for YOLOv4 (Exp_1, Exp_2 and Exp_3). Combining this result with the previous presented results, we deduce that the trick used to divide the images into 4 quadrants reveals better results when taking the training speed into account. Accordingly, the outcome of all parts of the images obtained from YOLOv4 can be combined and presented as one final result. All results shown in this section are presented to the user at the end of the testing phase of our end-to-end process.

6 Conclusion and Future Work

We presented our developed fully automated end-to-end process that employs methods from deep learning: Mask R-CNN for segmentation and YOLOv4 for detection and classification. This end-to-end system is designed for biologists, who are interested in performing any segmentation, detection or classification tasks with only a limited knowledge in the deep learning field. Although the application domain is optical microscopy in yeast cells, the method is also applicable to multiple-cell images in medical applications. Moreover, we evaluated the detection and classification performance of YOLOv4 on fluorescence microscopy images from the NOP1pr-GFP-SWAT library. We chose these images as they contain tiny cell compartments that are hard to detect. The results obtained from the last version of YOLO, YOLOv4, reveal its capability of detecting and classifying tiny objects. However, it has been shown that there is still a room for improvements. We showed that in term of accuracy and speed it is recommended to use the trick of dividing the original image into 4 quadrants, which is optimally suited for the native resolution of the microscope and current GPU memory sizes. Our approach also works for cell images with more than two channels. We are currently in the process of integrating this approach in a publicly available website that can also be used by external users in addition to PerICo users.

Acknowledgement. This project has received funding from the European Union's Horizon 2020 research and innovation programme under the Marie Skłodowska-Curie grant agreement No 812968. We thank Prof. Maya Schuldiner from Weizmann Institute of Science for providing us with their data as well as with her great collaboration with the authors. We also thank Tjaša Košir from University of Groningen for her supports and clear explanations.

References

1. Colin, J.G.A.C.F.A, Cisneros, M.T., Cervantes, J.G.A., Martinez, J.E.S., Debeir, O.: Detection of biological cells in phase-contrast microscopy images. In: Proceeding of the Fifth Mexican International Conference on Artificial Intelligent MICAI 2006 (2006)
2. Anoraganingrum, D.: Cell segmentation with median filter and mathematical morphology operation. In: Proceedings 10th International Conference on Image Analysis and Processing, pp. 1043–1046. IEEE (1999)
3. Dong, B., Shao, L., Da Costa, M., Bandmann, O., Frangi, A.F.: Deep learning for automatic cell detection in wide-field microscopy zebrafish images. In: 2015 IEEE 12th International Symposium on Biomedical Imaging (ISBI), pp. 772–776. IEEE (2015)
4. Pan, X., et al.: Cell detection in pathology and microscopy images with multi-scale fully convolutional neural networks. World Wide Web **21**(6), 1721–1743 (2018)
5. Shitong, W., Min, W.: A new detection algorithm (NDA) based on fuzzy cellular neural networks for white blood cell detection. IEEE Trans. Inf. Technol. Biomed. **10**(1), 5–10 (2006)
6. Xie, W., Noble, J.A., Zisserman, A.: Microscopy cell counting and detection with fully convolutional regression networks. Comput. Methods Biomech. Biomed. Eng. Imaging Vis. **6**(3), 283–292 (2018)
7. Wang, S., Yao, J., Xu, Z., Huang, J.: Subtype cell detection with an accelerated deep convolution neural network. In: International Conference on Medical Image Computing and Computer-Assisted Intervention, pp. 640–648. Springer (2016). https://doi.org/10.1007/978-3-319-46723-8_74
8. He, K., Gkioxari, G., Dollár, P., Girshick, R.: Mask R-CNN. In: Proceedings of the IEEE International Conference on Computer Vision, pp. 2961–2969 (2017)
9. Bochkovskiy, A., Wang, C.-Y., Liao, H.-Y.M.: Yolov4: optimal speed and accuracy of object detection. arXiv preprint arXiv:2004.10934 (2020)
10. Weill, U., et al.: Genome-wide swap-tag yeast libraries for proteome exploration. Nat. Methods **15**(8), 617–622 (2018)
11. Lu, A.X., Zarin, T., Hsu, I.S., Moses, A.M.: Yeastspotter: accurate and parameter-free web segmentation for microscopy images of yeast cells. Bioinformatics **35**(21), 4525–4527 (2019)

Glioblastoma Multiforme Patient Survival Prediction

Snehal Rajput[1(✉)], Rupal Agravat[2(✉)], Mohendra Roy[3(✉)], and Mehul S. Raval[2(✉)]

[1] Department of Information and Communication Technology, Department of Computer Science and Engineering, Pandit Deendayal Energy University, Gandhinagar, India
snehal.rphd19@sot.pdpu.ac.in

[2] School of Engineering and Applied Science, Ahmedabad University, Ahmedabad, India
rupal.agravat@iet.ahduni.edu.in,mehul.raval@ahduni.edu.in

[3] Pandit Deendayal Energy University, Gandhinagar, India
mohendra.roy@sot.pdpu.ac.in

Abstract. Glioblastoma Multiforme is a very aggressive type of brain tumor. Due to spatial and temporal intra-tissue inhomogeneity, location and the extent of the cancer tissue, it is difficult to detect and dissect the tumor regions. In this paper, we propose survival prognosis models using four regressors operating on handcrafted image-based and radiomics features. We hypothesize that the radiomics shape features have the highest correlation with survival prediction. The proposed approaches were assessed on the Brain Tumor Segmentation (BraTS-2020) challenge dataset. The highest accuracy of image features with random forest regressor approach was 51.5% for the training and 51.7% for the validation dataset. The gradient boosting regressor with shape features gave an accuracy of 91.5% and 62.1% on training and validation datasets respectively. It is better than the BraTS 2020 survival prediction challenge winners on the training and validation datasets. Our work shows that handcrafted features exhibit a strong correlation with survival prediction. The consensus based regressor with gradient boosting and radiomics shape features is the best combination for survival prediction.

Keywords: Brain tumor segmentation (BraTS 2020) · Glioblastoma · Survival prediction

1 Introduction

Glioblastoma multiforme (GBM) is the commonest type of primary malignant brain tumor. In the case of adults, glioblastoma makes up 60% of all brain tumors [1]. The World Health Organization (WHO) classified GBM as a grade IV type

All authors have contributed equally to this work.

R. Su et al. (Eds.): MICAD 2021, LNEE 784, pp. 47–58, 2022.
https://doi.org/10.1007/978-981-16-3880-0_6

of cancer due to its invasive and diffusive nature. Patients suffering from GBM have a poor prognosis, with a median survival rate of about ten months [1]. This is due to its aggressive nature, highly heterogeneous appearance, location, shape, and unpredictable response to therapy [2].

Magnetic Resonance Imaging (MRI) has been widely utilized to examine tumors due to its non-hazardousness, high contrast and superior resolution. Generally, manual segmentation of a tumor in MRI is time consuming and prone to subjective error. In this regards an automated segmentation method would be of enormous help to oncologists and clinicians. It can help in early diagnosis as well as in therapeutic strategy planning. In recent years, deep learning-based segmentation approaches have outperformed traditional state-of-the-art methods [3,4]. Segmentation delineates the brain tumor into Whole Tumor (WT), Enhancing Tumor (ET), and Tumor Core (TC). Handcrafted features extracted from these segments are used to classify the survival days of the patients.

There are many segmentation models available. Recently, Jiang et al. [5], in the BraTS 2019 challenge, proposed a two-stage asymmetry cascaded U-Net [2] structure. Each model is made up of a larger encoder in order to be able to extract more complex semantic features and a smaller decoder part for generating a segmentation map with a size identical to the input. Zhao et al. [3] proposed multiple methods to generate robust segmentation results. They grouped it into data processing, model devising, and optimization modules. Multiple methods are assimilated into each of these modules to enhance segmentation results. McKinley et al. [4] proposed a Densenet based U-Net architecture. Convolutions that were dilated were used to bring about an increase in the receptive field, which retains spatial information. The model was trained by combining label uncertainty loss, binary cross-entropy and focal loss. Dice scores on the BraTS-2019 validation dataset were 0.91(WT), 0.83(TC), 0.77(ET), and on the BraTS-2019 test dataset were 0.89(WT), 0.83(TC), 0.81(ET). Therefore, researchers seem to be favouring the U-Net based architecture for segmentation.

Once the tumor is segmented, features are extracted for overall survival prediction. Agravat et al. [6] used dense layers U-Net trained on the focal loss for segmentation. Next, age, statistical features and radiomic features train the Random Forest Regressor (RFR) for survival prediction and the obtained accuracy on the test dataset was 0.58. Wang et al. [7] used U-Net and U-Net ensembles with attention gates trained on soft dice scores and cross-entropy segmentation. For survival prediction, they proposed the following prognosis models: i) baseline model where only the age feature was used to train a linear regressor model. ii) Radiomic model where morphological and texture features were extracted from segmentation results. iii) Tumor invasiveness model, where relative invasiveness coefficient (RIC) and age feature train the support vector regressor model. The tumor invasive model was found best for survival prediction. The accuracy for survival prediction was 0.59 and 0.56 for BraTS-2019 validation and test dataset respectively. Feng et al. [8] used an ensemble of U-Net models. The models were trained on patches having brain pixels. The main advantage of using an ensemble method is that the network parameter need not be fine-tuned. Further, for OS prediction, volume and surface area features were extracted for each Region of Interest (ROIs) and age to train a linear regression model. The training and testing set accuracy was reported as 0.31 and 0.55 respectively on the BraTS-2019 datasets. Wang et al. [9] utilized a 3D U-Net-based model, and the training occurred in two phases using patching methods. The first phase included both brain and background pixels, whereas the second included only brain pixels. The dice score coefficient loss function was utilized to train the 3D U-Net model. Further for survival prediction, volume, surface area and age were used to train the ANN model. The training, validation, and testing accuracy of the models were 0.515, 0.448, and 0.551 respectively. Islam et al. [10] proposed a 3D U-Net architecture for segmentation, where attention blocks have been desegregated with the decoder modules. For survival prediction, various geometric, fractal, and histogram-based features were extracted to train multiple regressor models, i.e., support vector machine (SVM), multi-layer perceptron (MLP), random forest regressor (RFR), and eXtreme gradient Boosting (XGBOOST). The validation accuracies were: 0.329 for SVM, 0.414 for MLP, 0.356 for RFR and 0.429 for XGBOOST.

The proposed paper aims to establish the correlation between handcrafted features and overall survival prediction. Unlike the existing state-of-the-art methods used for survival prediction [6–9], the paper uses four predictors and two feature sets to establish their correlation with overall survival prediction of High Grade Glioma (HGG) patients. Shape features and gradient boosting regressors achieve better survival prediction accuracy than state-of-the-art methods. It establishes that shape features have a strong correlation with survival prediction. The organization of the remainder of the paper is as follows: The Brain Tumor Segmentation (BraTS) dataset is described in Sect. 2, survival prediction methods with four predictors and two feature sets are in Sect. 3, Sect. 4 contains results and discussions and finally the conclusion of the paper is in Sect. 5.

2 BraTS Dataset

Due to different standards and differences in the dataset, evaluating brain tumor segmentation methods objectively and predicting overall survival is a challenge. Nevertheless, for a comparison of different tumor segmentation and survival prediction techniques, the BraTS (brain tumor segmentation challenge) [11–14] has become a popular platform. Since the year 2018, there are three tasks that are included in this platform. The first task is the process of segmenting the brain tumor. The second task is predicting the overall survival (OS) and the third task is estimating the uncertainty for the predicted tumor sub-regions. The process of tumor segmentation involves delineating the tumor into three sub-regions, namely, the whole tumor, the tumor core, and the enhancing tumor. Specificity and sensitivity metrics as well as Dice score and Hausdorff Distance are used for evaluating performance.

The overall survival prediction task classifies survival days into the following categories: long-term survivors (>15 months), intermediate-survivors (between 10 and 15 months), and short-survivors (<10 months). Samples with resection status GTR (gross total resection) are used to rate the performance of the OS prediction. An accuracy metric is used for performance evaluation, whereas mean and median square error are used for postanalysis.

The BraTS 2020 training dataset includes 369 volumetric samples of high-grade glioma (HGG) and low-grade glioma (LGG) cases. It includes metadata of 236 samples such as age, survival days, and resection status for survival days prediction (Grosstotal Resection (GTR) = 119, Sub-total Resection (STR) = 10, and NA = 107). The validation dataset includes 125 sample images and metadata (age, survival days, and resection status) with 29 images having a GTR resection status. Each subject includes four MRI scans that are preoperative (T1-weighted, T1-CE, T2-weighted, and FLAIR) and manually annotated ground truth results. The annotations of ground truth include Necrotic and Non-Enhancing tumor core NCR/NET (label-1), Edema (label-2), Active Tumor (label-4), and 0 for everything else. The dataset has been pre-processed, i.e., all the scans are co-registered to the same anatomical structure, skull stripped and resampled to an isotropic resolution of $1 \times 1 \times 1\,\text{mm}^3$. The width, height, and depth of each sample are 240, 240, and 155 respectively.

3 Survival Prediction Methodology

We use the 3D U-Net model for brain tumor segmentation proposed by Isensee et al. [15]. This is the highest ranking and simple model in BraTS 2017. Like the U-Net [2], this model [15] comprises a contracting path to extract more feature information with increasing network depth. It has an expansion path to generate a segmentation mask with precise localization information and a skip connection for better feature reconstruction at every stage of the expansion path. In our work we have used the bias field correction, normalization, clipping maximum/minimum intensity to remove outliers, rescaled to [0, 1] and setting non-brain pixels to 0. The model was trained on a patch size of $128 \times 128 \times 128$, randomly generated from all the input MRI modalities. The obtained dice score on the BraTS 2020 validation dataset is 0.880(WT), 0.858(TC), 0.759(ET). The segmentation of tumor tissue of a validation sample is as shown in Fig. 1. The figures show a visual comparison of an input FLAIR image and a predicted image. The segmented parts are then used for survival prediction with the prognosis methods with 1) Image-based features, 2) Radiomics based features, and the following four predictors.

3.1 Predictors and Parameter Tuning

We have used four predictors and their parameter tuning in this paper. These are (1) Artificial Neural Network (ANN) [9,10], (2) Linear Regressor (LR) [7,8], (3) Gradient Boosting Regressor (GBR) [10], and (4) Random Forest Regressor (RFR) [6,10,15]. All these predictors were used by the top performing models in all recent BraTS challenges. These predictors deal with a small dataset and overfitting problems. The image-based prognosis method uses only seven features

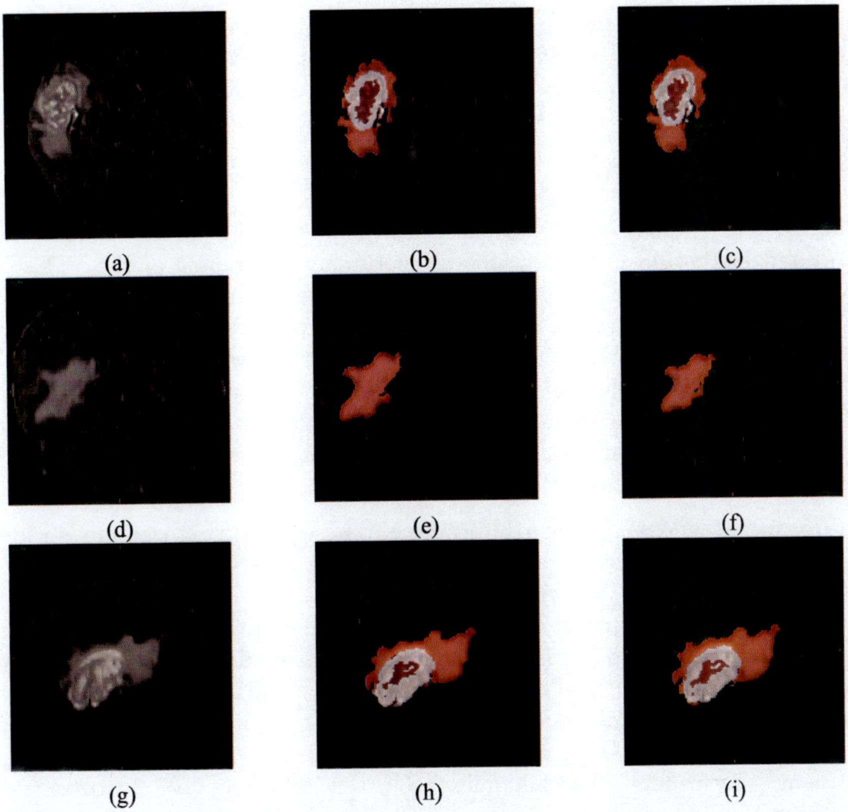

Fig. 1. Segmentation results of training set: (a) Axial FLAIR slice (b) Axial Ground truth (c) Axial Segmentation (d) Coronal FLAIR slice (e) Coronal Ground truth (f) Coronal Segmentation (g) Sagittal FLAIR slice (h) Sagittal Ground truth (i) Sagittal Segmentation, four color codes are: Brown for label-1(NCR/NET), white for label-4(Active Tumor), orange for label-2(Edema), black for label-0(back ground)

making it less vulnerable to overfitting. We retain default parameters for ANN and LR, while parameters for GBR and RFR are hyper-tuned using a grid search. We tuned the number of estimators, depth of the tree, sample split, and learning rate parameters for the GBR. In the case of the RFR, the number of estimators and the depth of the tree were hyper tuned. The predictors with radiomics features were also tuned.

For radiomics features it turns out that an ANN with five hidden layers was better compared to 2 or 3 hidden layers. Further, we tuned epochs, learning rate, number of neurons, and an optimizer for ANN. In the LR model, a search was also performed for the penalty term, the number of iterations, and upgrading of feature parameters using LASSO and a ridge regressor. We tuned the number of estimators, maximum depth, and learning rate for the GBR. In the RFR model, we tuned the number of estimators, maximum depth of the tree, minimum sample split, minimum samples in a leaf node, and maximum features parameters. Since the random forest and gradient boosting regressor work on ensemble-based learning, they are robust, efficient, and less prone to overfitting.

3.2 Prognosis Using Features

Image-Based Features [8,9]**.** Shape features extracted from the segmentation were used in the OS prediction. These features were volume of the WT, TC, and ET, surface area of the WT, TC, and ET, age. Since the tumor size was the decisive predicting factor for various cancer types, we extracted the volume and surface area of the WT, TC, and ET. The features were extracted from the segmentation maps and input images without any library dependency. Training with fewer features has the advantage that it limits the dimensions of feature space. Hence, the model did not overfit. However, we found saturation in the performance due to high bias in the model.

Radiomics Based Features [16]**.** Radiomics based feature extraction is widely used for disease diagnosis, classification, and survival prediction like lung cancer [17], breast cancer [18], and Alzheimer's disease [19]. Along with the size of the tumor, exploring the correlation of the other features with survival prediction is crucial to increase the performance of the predictor models. Radiomics features addresses this problem. It allows extracting various statistical, shape, intensity, and texture features from radiographic scans. Also, radiomics allow extracting features from many imaging techniques.

Using the package PyRadiomics [16], the following 107 features were extracted:

1. Shape features: Elongation, flatness, axis lengths, maximum diameter, mesh volume, sphericity, surface area, and surface volume ratio.
2. Gray level features: Gray-level size zone (GLSZ), Gray-level co-occurrence matrix (GLCM), Gray-level run-length matrix (GLRLM), Gray-level dependence matrix (GLDM), and Neighbouring gray-tone difference matrix (NGTDM).
3. First-order statistical features: Energy, entropy, minimum intensity value, maximum intensity value, mean, median, interquartile range, percentiles, absolute deviation, skewness, variance, kurtosis, and uniformity.

Radiomics features are typically multi-collinear and redundant [20]; hence the correlation between these features needs to be validated for specific real-world problems. We performed feature selection through recursive feature elimination (RFE) [21] to remove weaker features and avoid the curse of dimensionality. RFE is an example of backward feature elimination. With the given number of estimators, it selects principal features recursively from the feature set. It refits the model until the desired number of selected features is eventually reached. Out of 107 features, we selected 20 best ranking features.

In summary, the four predictors: ANN, RFR, LR, and GBR, are applied to: i) the seven image-based features, ii) 107 radiomics features, iii) 20 principal radiomics features, and iv) only shape radiomics features. Literature [6,15] also suggests dominance of shape features so we also used all predictors with only shape features for survival prediction. We trained the models with all the resection status (i.e., GTR, STR, and NA) given with the dataset to increase the database size and reduce overfitting.

4 Results and Discussions

Image-based feature prediction is derived from the BraTS 2019 dataset, and the BraTS 2020 dataset was used for radiomics based feature extraction. The results are shown in Tables 1, 2, 3 and 4. We have not participated in the BraTS 2020 challenge and do not have access to the test dataset. Therefore, results are derived on the training and validation datasets.

4.1 Image-Based Feature Prediction

We observe that the ensemble-based models, i.e., GBR and RFR, show a better performance on the training and validation dataset. Their consistency in the training and validation accuracy suggests that the model does not overfit.

Table 1. OS Performance comparison using image-based feature on training and validation BraTS-2019 dataset. MSE, medianSE, stdSE, and SpearmanR denote the mean square error, median square error, standard deviation squared error, and Spearman's ranking coefficient.

Dataset	Regressor	Accuracy	MSE	medianSE	stdSE	SpearmanR
Training	ANN	0.51	86148.10	21316	181346	0.48
	LR	0.49	87724.00	20736	183685	0.47
	GBR	0.52	63234.40	16900	126534	0.61
	RFR	0.52	63234.40	16900	126534	0.61
Validation	ANN	0.45	098312.70	39204	141392	0.24
	LR	0.52	100509.00	38809	141263	0.29
	GBR	0.52	102999.00	36481	152694	0.27
	RFR	0.52	102999.00	36481	152694	0.27

4.2 Radiomics Feature-Based Prediction

As mentioned, we extracted 107 radiomic features from the segmentation results of the BraTS 2020 images and fed them as input to four regressor models; ANN, LR, GBR, and RFR. It was observed that RFR gave the best results, and they are shown in Table 2. The other regressors performed poorly compared to RFR, and even the fine-tuning of the parameters did not improve the performance. The possible reasons are the redundant nature of radiomics [20], over complexity due to too many features and fewer training samples. Radiomics features are shallow and low-order image features, and unable to fully describe distinct image characteristics [22]. Also, when the number of observations is less for large extracted features, survival prediction is an ill-posed problem [20].

Table 2. OS performance evaluation using 107 radiomics features and Random Forest Regressor.

Dataset	Accuracy	MSE	medianSE	stdSE	SpearmanR
Training	0.479	079176.96	20702.21	169474.53	0.684
Validation	0.379	115424.30	28779.30	214028.11	0.138

It can be observed from Table 2 that the large feature set is unable to yield state-of-the-art accuracy results. Therefore, we reduced the feature set by applying recursive feature elimination to find the 20 most dominant features. Dominant features obtained using RFE are: age, amount of edema, elongation, maximum 2D diameter slice, sphericity, surface-volume ratio, minimum and maximum intensity, interquartile range, skewness, kurtosis, root mean absolute deviation, cluster prominence, cluster shade, inverse variance, coarseness, and dependence variance. We then applied four regressors on the dominant feature set, and performance has been noted in Table 3.

Table 3. OS performance comparison on 20 principal radiomics features.

Dataset	Regressor models	Accuracy	MSE	medianSE	stdSE	SpearmanR
Training	ANN	0.393	8.90E+12	2.46E+12	3.36E+13	0.125
	LR	0.462	96853.55	33279.52	190733.00	0.417
	GBR	0.923	17213.25	00000.00	074717.13	0.938
	RFR	0.744	31829.75	06077.32	075572.44	0.810
Validation	ANN	0.448	2.20E+20	3.46E+12	8.03E+20	0.290
	LR	0.483	2.73E+08	056167.55	9.86E+08	0.456
	GBR	0.414	255096.40	101995.06	420861.25	0.025
	RFR	0.448	098369.46	035521.48	126218.18	0.126

We observe that the linear regressor with regularisation outperforms all other regression models with the highest accuracy on the validation dataset. LR also provides similar accuracy for the training and validation datasets. The Spearman-R is also highest for LR. In contrast, RFR achieves the lowest mean square error (MSE) on the validation dataset.

Radiomic Shape Features Based Prediction. Reviewing the correlation between radiomics features and survival prediction, we found that radiomic shape features play a crucial role in survival prediction [6,15]. Shape features show significant statistical differences across ROIs [23]. Hence, shape features can capture tumor features related to genetic anomalies and profoundly impact survival prediction. We formulate the hypothesis that *shape features profoundly impact survival prediction.* In order to validate the hypothesis, we trained predictor models with the following shape features: the amount of necrotic, edema, enhancing tumor, the extent of the tumor, coordinates of tumor, elongation, flatness, axis lengths, 2D diameter row, 2D diameter column, 2 D diameter slice, maximum 3D diameter, mesh volume, sphericity, surface area, surface volume ratio, centroid of necrosis and age information. The performance of each predictor model has been noted in Table 4.

Table 4. OS performance comparison on BraTS-2020 dataset using radiomics shape features set.

Dataset	Predictor models	Accuracy	MSE	medianSE	stdSE	SpearmanR
Training	ANN	0.400	4.41E+11	7.15E+10	7.97E+11	0.149
	LR	0.470	89890.41	35160.09	162137.20	0.461
	GBR	0.915	31068.75	00000.00	150724.63	0.849
	RFR	0.615	62930.78	18562.88	130788.18	0.759
Validation	ANN	0.448	4.73E+11	2.14E+11	5.97E+11	0.149
	LR	0.414	087228.24	47820.00	111960.30	0.215
	GBR	0.621	141065.30	23528.48	236728.70	0.338
	RFR	0.448	109746.60	34689.29	200725.98	0.116

We observe that GBR and RFR have better performance. Specifically, the gradient boosting regressor outperforms all other regression models. In contrast, LR with regularization achieves the lowest mean square error (MSE) on the validation dataset.

4.3 Discussions

It has been observed that classical machine learning techniques performed better than the deep learning neural network-based models for survival prediction. Radiomics based approaches are well suited for survival prediction. Traditional regression algorithms have better interpretability than deep learning-based algorithms, they have fewer learnable parameters than CNN, and perform better with smaller sample data. A large sample dataset for training is crucial for direct regression from image modalities using CNN.

The predictors trained on the 107 radiomics features underperformed. The predictors modelled on the 20 principal features improved the performance. Further, to alleviate performance, we experimented and trained predictors on shape features and found a strong correlation with survival prediction. Shape features trained on the consensus model obtained state-of-the-art survival prediction accuracy. It was observed that the gradient boosting regressor model performed better than other classical algorithms because of: additive model, and with each tree built, the model becomes more expressive based on the ensemble learning model. The proposed GBR model is compared with the survival prediction challenge winners of BraTS 2020 and prediction accuracy for the state-of-the-art methods was obtained from the unranked leader board[1]. Performance comparison of the GBR model with top-ranking models has been noted in Table 5. It can be observed that shape-based features with the gradient boosting regressor outperform the best-ranking methods over the validation dataset.

Table 5. OS performance comparison with top-ranking models on the BraTS-2020 validation dataset.

Team name	Accuracy	MSE	medianSE	stdSE	SpearmanR
SCAN	0.414	098704.65	36100.00	152175.57	0.253
Redneucon	0.517	122515.76	70305.26	157673.99	0.134
VLB	0.379	093859.54	67348.26	102092.41	0.280
COMSATS-MIDL	0.483	105079.42	37004.93	146375.99	0.134
Proposed	**0.621**	141065.30	**23528.40**	236728.70	**0.338**

5 Conclusion

Predicting oncological outcomes is always very tricky due to multiple challenges from clinical and engineering perspectives. In this work, we have evaluated two feature sets over four predictors. We proposed the image-based and the radiomic based prognosis approaches for survival prediction. The image-based prognosis models performed well, but the performance saturates beyond a certain point because of fewer features, and models could not learn complexity. Similar observations are also made for the 107 radiomics features/20 principal features and the regressor combination. All above the combinations exhibited correlation with survival prediction. However, we recommend that shape based features with the gradient boosting regressor is the best combination for survival prediction. Comparing models, it was found that ensemble-based learning models became more useful for survival prediction because of their robustness. Whereas ANN converges speedily compared to classical models but due to lack of ample training samples, it overfits easily. With the availability of a large dataset and more clinical non-imaging information such as gender and treatment, survival prediction can be robust. It can further be applied to clinical practice.

[1] https://www.cbica.upenn.edu/BraTS20/lboardValidation.html.

References

1. Taylor, O.G., Brzozowski, J.S., Skelding, K.A.: Glioblastoma multiforme: an overview of emerging therapeutic targets. Front. Oncol. **9**, 963 (2019)
2. Ronneberger, O., Fischer, P., Brox, T.: U-net: convolutional networks for biomedical image segmentation. In: International Conference on Medical Image Computing and Computer-assisted Intervention, pp. 234–241. Springer (2015)
3. Zhao, Y.X., Zhang, Y.M., Liu, C.L.: Bag of tricks for 3D MRI brain tumor segmentation. In: International MICCAI Brainlesion Workshop, pp. 210–220. Springer (2019)
4. McKinley, R., Rebsamen, M., Meier, R., Wiest, R.: Triplanar ensemble of 3D-to-2D CNNs with label-uncertainty for brain tumor segmentation. In: International MICCAI Brainlesion Workshop, pp. 379–387. Springer (2019)
5. Jiang, Z., Ding, C., Liu, M., Tao, D.: Two-stage cascaded U-net: 1st place solution to brats challenge 2019 segmentation task. In: International MICCAI Brainlesion Workshop, pp. 231–241. Springer (2019)
6. Agravat, R.R., Raval, M.S.: Brain tumor segmentation and survival prediction. In: International MICCAI Brainlesion Workshop, pp. 338–348. Springer (2019)
7. Wang, S., Dai, C., Mo, Y., Angelini, E., Guo, Y., Bai, W.: Automatic brain tumour segmentation and biophysics-guided survival prediction. In: International MICCAI Brainlesion Workshop, pp. 61–72. Springer (2019)
8. Feng, X., Dou, Q., Tustison, N., Meyer, C.: Brain tumor segmentation with uncertainty estimation and overall survival prediction. In: International MICCAI Brainlesion Workshop, pp. 304–314. Springer (2019)
9. Wang, F., Jiang, R., Zheng, L., Meng, C., Biswal, B.: 3D U-net based brain tumor segmentation and survival days prediction. In: International MICCAI Brainlesion Workshop, pp. 131–141. Springer (2019)
10. Islam, M., Vibashan, V., Jose, V.J.M., Wijethilake, N., Utkarsh, U., Ren, H.: Brain tumor segmentation and survival prediction using 3D attention UNet. In: International MICCAI Brainlesion Workshop, pp. 262–272. Springer (2019)
11. Bakas, S., et al.: Advancing the cancer genome atlas glioma MRI collections with expert segmentation labels and radiomic features. Sci. Data **4**, 170117 (2017)
12. Bakas, S., et al.: Identifying the best machine learning algorithms for brain tumor segmentation, progression assessment, and overall survival prediction in the brats challenge. arXiv preprint arXiv:1811.02629 (2018)
13. Menze, B.H., et al.: The multimodal brain tumor image segmentation benchmark (brats). IEEE Trans. Med. Imaging **34**(10), 1993–2024 (2014)
14. Agravat, R., Raval, M.S.: 3D semantic segmentation of brain tumor for overall survival prediction. arXiv preprint arXiv:2008.11576 (2020)
15. Isensee, F., Kickingereder, P., Wick, W., Bendszus, M., Maier-Hein, K.H.: Brain tumor segmentation and radiomics survival prediction: contribution to the brats 2017 challenge. In: International MICCAI Brainlesion Workshop, pp. 287–297. Springer (2017)
16. Van Griethuysen, J.J., et al.: Computational radiomics system to decode the radiographic phenotype. Can. Res. **77**(21), e104–e107 (2017)
17. He, B., Zhao, W., Pi, J.Y., Han, D., Jiang, Y.M., Zhang, Z.G.: A biomarker basing on radiomics for the prediction of overall survival in non-small cell lung cancer patients. Respir. Res. **19**(1), 1–8 (2018)
18. Liu, C., et al.: Preoperative prediction of sentinel lymph node metastasis in breast cancer by radiomic signatures from dynamic contrast-enhanced MRI. J. Magn. Reson. Imaging **49**(1), 131–140 (2019)

19. Li, Y., Jiang, J., Lu, J., Jiang, J., Zhang, H., Zuo, C.: Radiomics: a novel feature extraction method for brain neuron degeneration disease using 18F-FDG pet imaging and its implementation for Alzheimer's disease and mild cognitive impairment. Ther. Adv. Neurol. Disord. **12**, 1756286419838682 (2019)
20. Weninger, L., Haarburger, C., Merhof, D.: Robustness of radiomics for survival prediction of brain tumor patients depending on resection status. Front. Comput. Neurosci. **13**, 73 (2019)
21. Pedregosa, F., et al.: Scikit-learn: machine learning in python. J. Mach. Learn. Res. **12**, 2825–2830 (2011)
22. Lao, J., et al.: A deep learning-based radiomics model for prediction of survival in glioblastoma multiforme. Sci. Rep. **7**(1), 1–8 (2017)
23. Chaddad, A., Desrosiers, C., Hassan, L., Tanougast, C.: A quantitative study of shape descriptors from glioblastoma multiforme phenotypes for predicting survival outcome. Br. J. Radiol. **89**(1068), 20160575 (2016)

Virtual Reality Application for Laparoscope in Clinical Surgery Based on Siamese Network and Census Transformation

Nannan Chong[1,2](✉), Yazhong Si[2], Wei Zhao[3], Qiushi Zhang[4], Boran Yin[1], and Yuehua Zhao[2]

[1] Tianjin University Renai College, Tianjin 301636, China
[2] Hebei University of Technology, Tianjin 300401, China
[3] Tianjin Academy of Traditional Chinese Medical Affiliated Hospital, Tianjin 300120, China
[4] Tianjin Hongqiao Hospital of Traditional Chinese Medicine, Tianjin 300132, China

Abstract. Virtual reality technology is now gradually being used in the field of clinical medicine. This paper presents a method of reconstruction abdominal tissue structure from laparoscope images and videos. The method is designed based on ORB-SLAM and introduced a two branch Siamese Network to extract more features for dense reconstruction. The contributions of this study are as follows: (i) We introduce a data augmentation thread to augment data and a dense reconstruction thread with GPU acceleration to get dense features without interruption of the original sparse reconstruction. (ii) We design an improved Census Transformation to reduces the effect of changes caused by camera gain and bias. For the outer point near the deep discontinuity, the robustness is improved. (iii) An experimental system was built to test the 3D reconstruction of liver, stomach, greater omentum and omental bursa from the public laparoscope datasets. (iv) Introducing the presented method to clinical surgery virtual reality system. This method achieved 1.2 ± 0.8 RMSE reconstruction accuracy in low time cost. Lens distortion has been considered to get more accurate feature detection and matching support for operation scenario application effectively. Compared with the current mainstream algorithm, it demonstrates the practicability and superiority of abdominal tissue images 3D reconstruction by laparoscope in clinical scenarios, such as surgical navigation, auxiliary diagnosis, surgery simulation, etc.

Keywords: Virtual Reality · Clinical Surgery · 3D Reconstruction · SLAM

1 Introduction

Laparoscopic surgery is a type of minimally invasive process which has shown great advantages when compared to the traditional methods, leading an inevitable trend in the development of the future operation method [1]. Laparoscopic greatly reduce trauma, surgical procedure and postoperative recovery, less painful intra-abdominal viscera to disrupt small, to avoid the air and dust in the air bacteria to stimulate and pollution of

R. Su et al. (Eds.): MICAD 2021, LNEE 784, pp. 59–70, 2022.
https://doi.org/10.1007/978-981-16-3880-0_7

the abdominal cavity the advantages and disadvantages of laparoscopic surgery. Laparoscopic surgery in the surgical instrument is through belly piercing holes into the abdominal cavity operation, small operation wound at the same time because of the surgical wound, light postoperative pain in patients with rapid recovery. The disadvantage is that the surgeon used a monitor to observe the abdominal picture during the operation, and the picture quality directly affects the completion of the operation. Therefore, for some complex surgeries and operations in relatively dangerous areas, some surgical difficulties and risks will be caused. Methods to produce a detailed reconstruction of objects or scenes from images and video have improved significantly over time. Introduce 3D reconstruction and virtual reality (VR) technology into the field of clinical medicine is of great benefit to surgical effect and medical training [2].

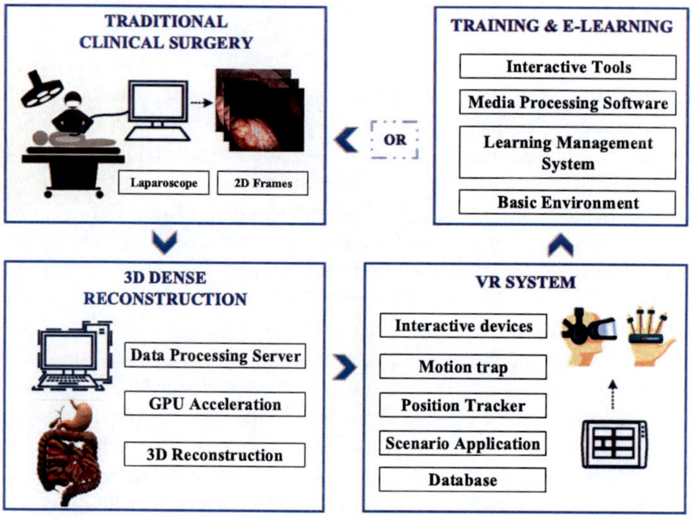

Fig. 1. Virtual reality application for laparoscope in clinical surgery

We focus on these problems mentioned above and made contributions as follows:

(i) A dense three dimensional (3D) reconstruction method from laparoscope images is designed based on ORB-SLAM, using a two branch Siamese Network to extract more features for dense reconstruction. We introduce a data pre-processing thread which contains data augmentation and evaluation of input frames to improved the quality of the depth and motion prediction from unmarked video.

(ii) We encode the global information to avoid semantic information lose and eliminate false matching. What's more, there's no need for memory vault or special architecture.

(iii) We extract ORB features and predict the camera's internal parameters based on the projection principle which is derived from Multi-Layer Perceptron (MLP) from the two dimensional (2D) frames, and introduce a dense reconstruction thread with GPU acceleration to get dense and live depth estimation without interruption of the original ORB-SLAM sparse reconstruction.
(iv) An experimental system was built to test the 3D reconstruction of liver, stomach, greater omentum and omental bursa computed from the public datasets and proved to achieve 1.2 ± 0.8 RMSE reconstruction accuracy in low time cost.
(v) We design a VR system based on the proposed 3D reconstruction method for clinical surgary and medial training.

The method has considered the lens distortion, which get more accurate feature detection and match to support for operation scenario application effectively. Compared with the current mainstream 3D reconstruction algorithm, we made tests and proved that this method has stronger practicability. What's more, the 3D reconstruction method can be further applied in the virtual reality of clinical medicine shown in Fig. 1.

2 Proposed Approach

A new method to reconstruct the 3D structure of abdominal tissues is described in this section.

2.1 Approach Overview

The method of 3d reconstruction of medical images by laparoscope based on contrastive learning and ORB-SLAM is presented as follows. Through encoding the global information and eliminating the ambiguity in mismatching, the system requires no more special architecture or memory bank. The data could be evaluated by a linear model of data augmentation such as random crops and color distortion [3]. In parallel with the traditional ORB-SLAM thread, we use a MLP projection/mapping and convolutional neural network to train and evaluate the density depth of 2D data. We outline the system architecture in Fig. 2. The proposed system consists of five threads, which expressed as Data Pre-Processing, Sparse Tracking, Sparse Reconstruction, Keyframe Cluster Selection and Dense Reconstruction.

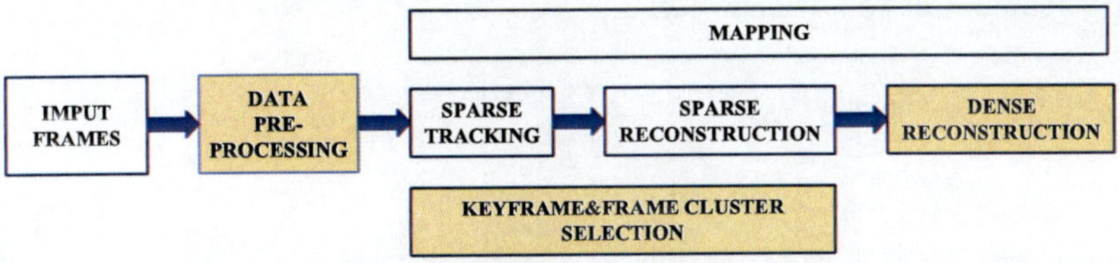

Fig. 2. 3D Reconstruction Network Architecture (The white box represents the original ORB-SLAM thread, and the yellow box represents our proposed optimization and the addition of a dense rebuild thread.)

2.2 Data Collection and Pre-processing

The data pre-processing is performed to estimate camera intrinsic parameters and to extract input images for SLAM. To increase the diversity of existing data and reduce the generalization error of the network, data augment technology was considered during the image analysis. Inspired by the recent contrastive learning, SimCLR algorithm, we introduced a new thread performing data augmentation based on a traditional ORB-SLAM architecture. Firstly, we applied two simple augmentations, random crop and color distortion, to the source image sequence in order to obtain good performance. The data decomposed into base layer and detail layer by a neural network base encoder and average filter. The data decomposed into low-rank and sparse parts by convex optimization. What's more, a visual saliency map is constructed on the basis of sparse features, and a weighted image is constructed to keep the spatial consistency between source image sequence and layers. The data augmentation pipeline is represented in Fig. 3.

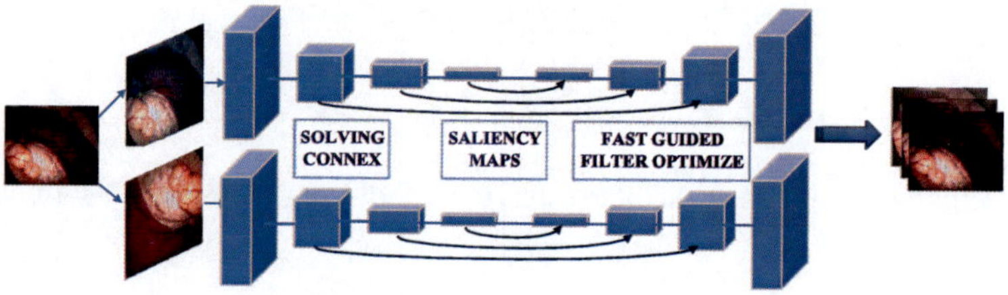

Fig. 3. Data pre-processing pipeline

- Random cropping and color distortion are performed on the input frame in the data augment module, in which the output is identified as i_m and i_n respectively. The network receives these two images as input.
- We use a MLP with one hidden layer and introduce a learnable nonlinear transformation representation and a contrast loss, the quality representation of learning is greatly improved.
- A contrastive loss function defined by a contrastive prediction task. Sequence i^+ defines as a positive sample which is same to i, whereas i^- defines as negative sample.

We optimize the following expectation,

$$\underset{i,i^+,i^-}{E}\left[-\log\left(\frac{\exp(f(i)^T f(i^+))}{\exp(f(i)^T f(i^+)) + \exp(f(i)^T f(i^-))}\right)\right] \quad (1)$$

If we have i positive samples and $N-1$ negative samples in a sequence, then the loss can be regarded as an N classification problem, which is actually a cross entropy, and this function is called InfoNCE in the comparative learning articles. In fact, minimizing the loss can maximize the lower bound of the mutual information of $f(i)$ and $f(i^+)$ and make them closer. Most importantly, there's no need for ground truth to extract the feature from the laparoscope images by self-supervised contrastive learning.

2.3 Traditional Sparse Tracking and Reconstruction

The traditional SLAM thread of sparse tracking thread is responsible for tracking the feature points of the laparoscope frames in real time, which is responsible for extracting the ORB feature points from each new image and comparing them with the latest keyframe to calculate the location of the feature points and roughly estimate the camera position. Local Bundle Adjustment (BA) [4] optimization achieves sparse reconstruction, including feature points and camera pose in local space, and is responsible for solving more detailed camera pose and feature point spatial position, which takes the responsible for visual odometry (VO).

2.4 Densification and Cluster BA

Estimate the depth of each pixel of a selected subset of key frames I_r in the dense reconstruction thread. A subset of key frame selected automatically to reduce the computation cost. The selection criteria are the current coverage of dense reconstruction in a given keyframe I_r, by setting it to 50%, and selecting densification if it less than 50%.

The pose of the frames in the cluster is imprecise because traditional sparse reconstruction does not perform any BA on them. Therefore, we accurately improve these gestures with a complete BA. Take advantage of the tracking features of ORB-SLAM and minimize (2) among all frames and keyframes (up to 15 keyframes). We selected those features that existed most commonly to keyframes I_r.

$$\arg\min_{T_i, I_j} \sum_{i,j} \rho_h(||i_{i,j} - \pi(T_i, I_j)||^2) \tag{2}$$

2.5 Keyframe's Depth Map Reconstruction

1) *The Variational Formulation*
   We use a variational energy minimization to get the inverse depth map estimation $\rho(u) : \Omega \rightarrow R$ for a keyframe I_r which is grayscale and denoted by $I_r : \Omega \rightarrow R$, where $\Omega \in R^2$ is the 2D image domain. Our energy is the sum of regularization term $R(u, \rho(u))$, and the weighted Census data term $C(u, \rho(u))$ with the form,

$$E(\rho) = \int_{\Omega} \{\lambda(u)C(u, \rho(u)) + R(u, \rho(u))\} du \tag{3}$$

$$\lambda(u) \triangleq \lambda\rho(u) \tag{4}$$

Where constant λ and spatially-varying non-convex weighting factor $\lambda(u)$ determine value of the data term of pixel u. Geometricall, the accuracy of depth estimation of the point far from the laporascopic is higher than that of the near point, because they have lower parallax. Using $\rho(u)$ to scale the weight and reduce the strength of distant points data term.

2) *Census Data Term*

Census transformation is a non-parametric transformation used for local stereo matching. The transformation process is simple and only uses addition and subtraction and xor operations [3]. Controlling the resource consumption of Census transformation is of great significance to the overall resource management and control of the stereo matching system. We used an improved Census transformation to calculate the matching cost. Meanwhile, the value of each pixel being weighted and averaged from itself and other pixels in the neighborhood. The specific method is as follows. The support window is used to scan every pixel in the image. The weighted average gray value of neighborhood pixels is used as the Census reference value in the support window. That means, the closer to the center, the pixel weight is higher, and the further away, the weight is lower.

We use the reference value calculation formula and the weight calculation formula as follows,

$$I_{\omega m} = \frac{1}{D}\sum_{p\in N} W_{pq} I_p \tag{5}$$

$$W_{pq} = e^{-(\omega_x+\omega_y)^2/\sigma^2} \tag{6}$$

where $I_{\omega m}$ denotes the reference value, I_p is the grayvalue of pixel p, the weight W_{pq} equals to the distance between the center pixel p and pixel q, D is the sum of weight of W_{pq}, s denotes the pixels in the supporting window, p, q is the index pixel respectively, ω_x, ω_y is the coordinate of pixel in the supporting window, σ is the standard deviation. We can calculate the bit string by Census transform,

$$C_{cen}(p) = \otimes_{p\in N'} \xi(I_{\omega m}, I_q) \tag{7}$$

$$\text{s.t} \quad \xi(x, y) = \begin{cases} 1, & x < y \\ 0, & else \end{cases} \tag{8}$$

where $\otimes$ denotes bitwise connect operation, N' is the neighborhood pixels in the supporting window, I_q is the neighborhood pixel values. The matching cost calculation model based on improved Census transformation follows,

$$C_{cen}(p, d) = \min\{\text{Ham min g}[c_{cen}(p), lc_{cen}(p-d), T_{cen}]\} \tag{9}$$

where $C_{cen}(p, d)$ is the matching cost computation of pixel p when the parallax value is d, T_{cen} is the cutoff value of improved Census transformation, Ham min g is the calculated Hamming distance, $C_{cen}(p)$ is the binary bit string corresponding to pixel p, $C_{cen}(p, d)$ is the binary bit string corresponding to pixel $p - d$.

3) *The Regularizer*
To make the reconstruction smooth and preserve depth discontinuities, we introduce a weighted Huber norm over the gradient of inverse depth image, the convex regularizer term descriped as

$$R(u, \rho(u)) = g(u)\|\nabla\rho(u)\|_{\in} \tag{10}$$

where $\in$ is a free parameter of Huber norm to reduce the effect of the undesired staircasing resultant from a pure TV. Parameter $\in$ depends on L^1 forming Total Variation (TV) or L^2 norm [5]. We use per-pixel weight $g(u)$ to keep the depth discontinuities at the edges of the image, and reference a free parameter ω in the reference keyframe I_r to reduce the regularization intensity of high-gradient pixels.

$$g(u) = \exp(-\omega\|\nabla I_r(u)\|_2) \tag{11}$$

4) *Initialization and Energy minimization*
In order to evaluate the keyframe, the 3D cost-volume method is used. The dimension of $M \times N \times \xi$, represents the image resolution of the frame I_r, where $M \times N$ is the number of points starting from the inverse depth ξ sampling ranging from $\rho_{\min}$ to $\rho_{\max}$. This cost quantity is calculated only once, and the initial depth map is estimated from the cost quantity by selecting $\rho(u)$ that minimize value (2) for each pixel u. To get a strong local minimum, we approximate the energy function with an auxiliary map $a : \Omega \rightarrow R$

$$E(\rho, a) = \int_{\Omega} \{\lambda(u)C(u, a(u)) + \frac{1}{2\theta}(\rho(u) - a(u))^2 + R(u, \rho(u))\}du \tag{12}$$

The coupling term $\frac{1}{2\theta}(\rho(u) - a(u))^2$ enforces $\rho(u)$ and $a(u)$ to be equal as $\theta \rightarrow 0$, at which point $E(\rho, a = 0) = E(\rho)$. The discretization level used for the cost volume construction impact the accuracy. As a result, we perform a single Newton step at each iteration to obtain a sub pixel accuracy.

2.6 Depth Maps Alignment of Keyframes

The computed depth map is combined into one coordinate system to obtain a globally consistent reconstruction, namely SLAM map coordinate system. We use the corresponding 3D points of traditional sparse SLAM points on the dense map as anchor points. Anchor points are used to keep the depth map aligned with the sparse SLAM map. As a result, any update to the SLAM map will result in a realignment of the dense map.

Each time BA refines the sparse points and keyframe pose which includes both rotation and translation, as well as scaling improvements that may cause failure of dense depth map alignment in SLAM map. Therefore, it is recommended to align each depth chart with a similarity transform.

2.7 VR System for Clinical Surgery and Medical Training

The VR virtual surgery system designed by us uses the previously designed 3D reconstruction method based on laparoscopy to build a virtual surgery simulation scene. Doctors, trainees and other intelligent systems perform surgical training, operation and planning in the scene with the help of virtual reality equipment. This system enables medical workers to immerse themselves in virtual scenes, learn the actual operation of various surgeries by using audio-visual perception, and simulate the clinical operation process. It can save the cost of training medical personnel, improve the training efficiency for the hospital and reduce the risk of mistakes in the practical operation of interns, which plays an important role in the medical education and the practical work of the hospital.

3 Result and Discussion

3.1 Benchmark Hardware and Compared Methods

The system is implemented using c++ and OpenCV, a desktop computer with 16 GB of RAM and an Intel(R) Core i7 CPU with 3.4 ghz GeForce RTX2070 GPU.Based on ground truth method (two leading dense three-dimensional methods [6, 7]), the accuracy of dense reconstruction is quantitatively evaluated.In addition, we compare the proposed system with one of the best multi-view stereo methods in the closest approach to SLAM, contemporary endoscope SLAM [7], LSD-SLAM [5], and [8], in which the camera attitude is calculated by SfM.

3.2 Quantitative Evaluation

We adopt two leading stereovision methods [6] and [7] intensive reconstruction as our gold standard for reconstruction.According to [9], the stereo imaging method of [8] is one of the endoscopic imaging methods with the best performance.

1) *Datasets*
   Four groups of laparoscope image sequences named as Sequence I II III and IV, from public Hamlyn [10] and anonymous videos offered by Tianjin Academy of Traditional Chinese Medical Affiliated Hospital and Tianjin Hongqiao Hospital of Traditional Chinese Medicine, are selected and shown in Fig. 4 which descriped as liver, greater omentum, stomach and omental bursa respectively.
   We used images from a monocular laparoscopic camera to reconstruct the scene. Figure 5 compares the point cloud of sparse and dense reconstruction of proposed method and algorithm [8] on different sequences. For evaluation, we used patients with CT data and compared with dense stereoscopic reconstruction method we proposed.
2) *Evaluation metrics*
   Reconstruction coverage per keyframe, stereo coverage metric, monocular scale recovery and averaged reconstruction error of algorithm [5–7] and proposed method are compared in Table 1 with four sequence, which is Sequence I to IV. Every

sequence we choose have varied α_1 and α_2 and submitted the reconstruction coverage, parallax and error calculated by different methods.The reconstructed coverage rate per keyframe is interpreted as the percentage of reconstructed pixels per keyframe.

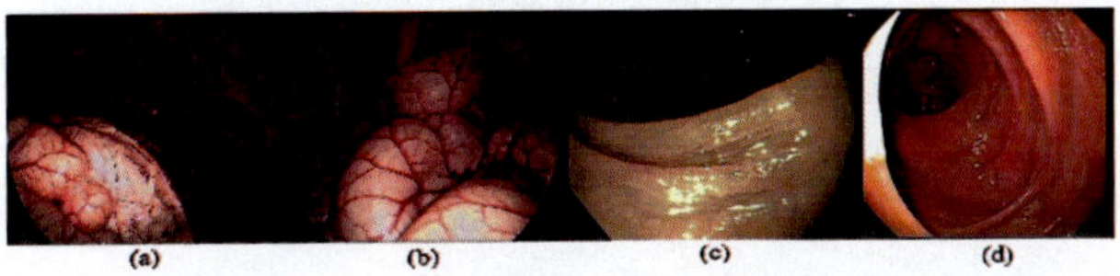

Fig. 4. Sample frames of liver, stomach, greater omentum and omental bursa sequences with smooth or strongly curved surfaces used from public Hamlyn, PhysioNet and hospitals. (c) (d) shows weak textures and (a) (b) have repetitive textures.

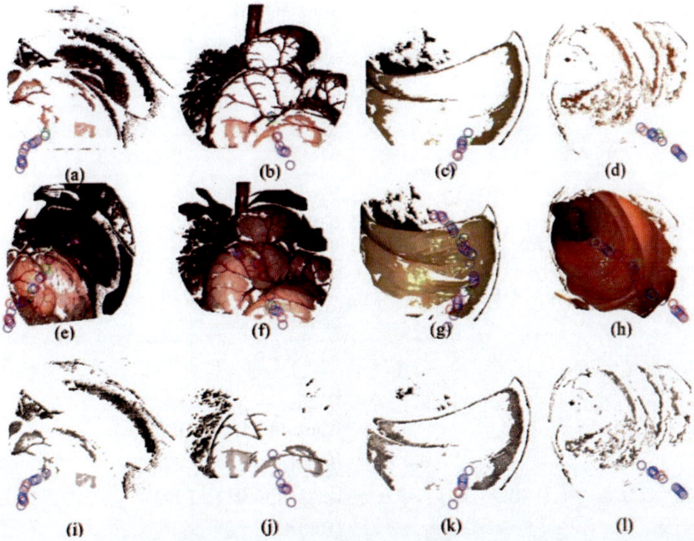

Fig. 5. Visualized as point cloud comparision of sparse(a-d) and dense(e-f) reconstruction of proposed method and algorithm (i-l) on different sequences. SLAM keyframes and points are colored in blue, and the selected keyfrmaes used for the dense reconstruction and frames cluster are colored in red.

We also calculate the root mean square error (RMSE). With the same or higher parallax by monocular cases, we achieve $\leqq 1.2 \pm 0.8$ RMSE. To all the pixels in all the key frames, we use our method and compared methods to estimate depth and measure the distance. We use two stereo approaches [6] and [7]. Our reconstruction is proportional (as with any monocular reconstruction method), so before the RMSE calculation, we use Least-Squares fitting to align by scale, where the initial hypothesis value is calculated using the robustness estimate of the Least Median of Squares. We report the use of RMSE

Table 1. Comparision of Evaluation metrics of different methods.

Sequence	I				Sequence	II			
Method	Proposed	[7]	[5]	[8]	Method	Proposed	[7]	[5]	[8]
Reconst. Coverage per KeyFrame /%	69	X	36	65	Reconst. Coverage per KeyFrame /%	52	1.1	29	47
Stereo coverage %	93	90	X	42	Stereo coverage %	88	84	76	38
Mono pllx /deg	12.3	6.4	X	6.7	Mono pllx /deg	8.9	8.9	X	14.2
Stereo pllx /deg	12.9				Stereo pllx /deg	7.2			
Avg. RMSE /mm	0.7	1	X	2.3	Avg. RMSE /mm	2.5	2.9	4.7	3.6
Avg. RMSE /mm	0.4	1.2	X	2.1	Avg. RMSE /mm	2.3	3.1	6.1	3.1
σ	0.2	0.2	X	0.2	σ	0.1	0.2	1.1	0.2
Sequence	III				Sequence	IV			
Method	Proposed	[7]	[5]	[8]	Method	Proposed	[7]	[5]	[8]
Reconst. Coverage per KeyFrame /%	48	1.6	15	44	Reconst. Coverage per KeyFrame /%	67	2.1	28	45
Stereo coverage %	89	80	8.5	34	Stereo coverage %	86	84	99	47
Mono pllx /deg	12.1	9.2	X	10.1	Mono pllx /deg	10.2	4.8	X	6.1
Stereo pllx /deg	11.9				Stereo pllx /deg	9.5			
Avg. RMSE /mm	0.7	0.9	2.1	3.6	Avg. RMSE (mm)	1.9	3.5	3.8	2.9
Avg. RMSE /mm	0.9	1.1	2.6	3.2	Avg. RMSE /mm	2.2	3.3	5.3	3.1
σ	0.1	0.1	1	0.3	σ	0.5	0.6	6	0.2

standard deviation (σ). In addition, the average reconstruction coverage and reconstruction error of [7] are due to strong respiration and failure due to excessive deformation due to the contractions of the touching surgical instrument. Parameter settings are shown in Table 2. Figure 6 shows the data increase (a - c) and reconstruction of sequence II (d - I) processing steps.

Table 2. Parameters settings.

α_1	α_2	θ^1	θ_{end}	λ	ω	ω_k	W
0.2	0.01	0.2	0.0005	0.5	0.01	8	19
$\beta_{\min}$	$\beta_{\max}$	ξ	$\in$	τ	T_g	T_h	T_{cen}
0.8	5	51	0.001	30	4.245	1	45

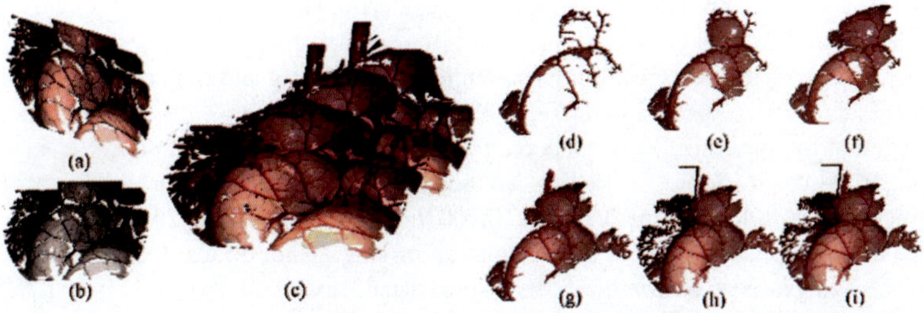

Fig. 6. Data Augment (a-c) and Reconstruction (d-i) processing of Sequence II by steps

4 Results and Discussion

In this paper, we propose a novel VR system, which can track the pose of laparoscope and reconstruct the 3D surface structure of internal organs according to the extracted image features. The high quality and dense reconstruction achieved by this method can be used in surgical scenes and medical training. More importantly, it uses a single monocular video input, without requiring any benchmarks or external trackers. Therefore, it can be easily extended on existing medical equipment. The method has been validated and evaluated on the sequence of abdominal tissues, showing robustness to different light changes and different scene textures. Finally, we designed a complete VR system that can be used for medical training and surgical navigation.

However, the method of this paper still has limitations. Due to the limited computing power devices (such as GPU), the processing efficiency is to be further improved. The time delay will also affect the user experience of VR system. In the future, we will optimize the algorithm to improve the reconstruction efficiency.

Acknowledgments. This work was supported by the Scientific Research Project of Tianjin Municipal Commission of Education (No. 2018KJ268).

References

1. Johnson, A.: Laparoscopic surgery. Lancet **349**(9061), 1323–1323 (1997)
2. Escalada-Hernandez, P., Soto Ruiz, N., San Martin-Rodriguez, L.: Design and evaluation of a prototype of augmented reality applied to medical devices. Int. J. Med. Inform. **128**, 87–92 (2019)

3. Chen, T., Kornblith, S., Norouzi, M., et al.: A simple framework for contrastive learning of visual representations (2020). arXiv:2002.05709
4. Wu, C., Agarwal, S., Curless, B., et al.: Multicore bundle adjustment, pp. 3057–3064 (2011)
5. Hadviger, A., Marković, I., Petrović, I.: Stereo dense depth tracking based on optical flow using frames and events. Adv. Robot. **35**, 1–12 (2020)
6. Chang, P.-L., Stoyanov, D., Davison, A. J., Edwards, P.E.: Real-time dense stereo reconstruction using convex optimisation with a cost-volume for image-guided robotic surgery. In: Mori, K., Sakuma, I., Sato, Y., Barillot, C., Navab, N. (eds.) Medical Image Computing and Computer-Assisted Intervention – MICCAI 2013. MICCAI 2013. Lecture Notes in Computer Science, vol. 8149, pp. 42–49 (2013). Springer, Berlin, Heidelberg. https://doi.org/10.1007/978-3-642-40811-3_6
7. Hirschmuller, H.: Stereo processing by semiglobal matching and mutual information. IEEE Trans. Pattern Anal. Mach. Intell. **30**(2), 328–341 (2008)
8. Langguth, F., Sunkavalli, K., Hadap, S., Goesele, M.: Shading-aware multi-view stereo. In: Leibe, B., Matas, J., Sebe, N., Welling, M. (eds.) ECCV 2016. LNCS, vol. 9907, pp. 469–485. Springer, Cham (2016). https://doi.org/10.1007/978-3-319-46487-9_29
9. Maier-Hein, L., et al.: Comparative validation of single-shot optical techniques for laparoscopic 3-D surface reconstruction. IEEE Trans. Med. Imag. **33**(10), 1913–1930 (2014)
10. Mountney, P., Stoyanov, D., Yang, G.Z.: Three-dimensional tissue deformation recovery and tracking. IEEE Signal Process. Mag. **27**(4), 14–24 (2010). http://hamlyn.doc.ic.ac.uk/vision/

Analyzing CT Scan Images Using Deep Transfer Learning for Patients with Covid-19 Disease

Mohammad Alodat(✉)

Sur University College, 440 411 Sur, Oman
Dr.maalodat@suc.edu.om

Abstract. The main aim of this research is to improve the experience of medical staff in recognizing three different lung diseases by making an analysis for chest Computed Tomography (CT) scan in the Sultanate of Oman. To facilitate differential diagnosis for patients with respiratory diseases; we used Deep transfer learning (DTL) from pre-trained network on ImageNet of convolutional neural networks (CNN) through using Fine-Tuning on Keras and TensorFlow 2.0 with tf.keras. The first purpose of the research is to Classify chest CT results either positive which means infected patients, with Covid-19, pneumonia viral or pneumonia bacterial. The other outcome is chest CT result is negative, so no-infection. The second purpose is improving the CNN architecture and to overcome its defects. The results of this study revealed that the best performance was chosen among five pre-trained network and it was ResNet50 model, which showed accuracy with (99%). After the chest CT image has been analyzed, we were able to match the actual diagnosis of the seven volunteer patients out of 8 (87.5%) the eighth patient (12.5%) was classified as covid-19 positive but actually the volunteer has no infection.

Keywords: Convolutional neural networks · Keras · Tensorflow · Deep transfer learning · Fine-tuning

1 Introduction

Coronaviruses are a large family of viruses that may cause illness in animals or humans [2]. One of the types of this family covid-19 and unknown before the outbreak began in Wuhan in December 2019 [3]. COVID-19 disease is threat worldwide and infectious disease because of its impact was on the individual's health, the economy of all countries [4]. Diagnosis of Covid-19 disease is time-consuming due to overlap, where the first symptoms are similar to flu-like and be similar in Computed Tomography (CT) images [5]. We turned to CT image instead of techniques X-ray due to provide low false positive rates, but it has a high cost [6], as shown in Fig. 1.

In the Sultanate of Oman, patients Infected with COVID-19 have been observed, and the community symptoms were divided as follows: 1) the common clinical symptoms as fever, fatigue, dyspnea, exhaustion and dry cough [7]. 2) Less common symptoms: Some patients may have pains in muscle, headache, conjunctivitis, Diarrhea, and losing a sense of taste or smell. 3) Rare symptoms: colds and digestive complaints, such as bowel

R. Su et al. (Eds.): MICAD 2021, LNEE 784, pp. 71–78, 2022.
https://doi.org/10.1007/978-981-16-3880-0_8

Fig. 1. The visualization Chest CT scan sample for COVID-19 disease.

movements, nausea, and vomiting. 4) The worst symptoms: it resembles symptoms of pneumonia and possibility of evolution to multiple organ dysfunction syndromes like kidney failure and even death [8]. 5) Chronic diseases as diabetes, cancer, heart problems blood pressure cardiovascular, kidney and lungs [9].

2 Methodology

Dataset was collected from eight patients, who has respiratory symptoms with different medical diagnosis. 8 participants were randomly chosen from different areas in the sultanate of Oman. Consent form taken and confidentiality of data was protected. Eligible participants have made Computed Tomography (CT) imaging to analyze and predict COVID-19. In order to gain a better insight dataset split into a training dataset and a validation dataset, which is known as cross-validation. To validate the model performance, we used a dataset that was extracted from training and validation. it was distributed as follows: Training 427/ Validation 143/ Test 55 images of non-infected patients, 492/164/9 images for patients with Covid-19 virus, 490/166/8 images for patients with pneumonia bacterial and 738/246/10 images for patients with pneumonia virus. Workflow was as the following: 1) Feature Extraction stage, Divided into two parts, a) Freeze all layers in model to avoid destroying any of the information during training. b) Add new trainable layers. 2) Fine-tuning stage, executed on the entire model, by unfreezing. 3) In both stages, a) run our dataset on the new model. b) Standardized the images by resizing them and using Data Augmentation to suite a neural network.

3 Tensor Flow and ImageNet

Tensor Flow and Keras are artificial neural network and open source software library for data flow [10, 11]. They ways to program deep learning models framework for high performance numerical computation. Keras was originally created and developed by Francois Chollet [12]. Tensor Flow developed by Google Brain Team in 2015 for internal use to google [13]. Google announced TensorFlow 2.0 in June 2019, they declared that Keras is high-level API of TensorFlow [13]. Francois stated that the first release of Keras 2.3.0, makes it in sync with tf.keras and final release of Keras which will support other backgrounds such as Theano. Keras' default backend was Theano until Keras started supporting TensorFlow became the default backend for Keras. Some researchers have used Transfer learning, to take the features learned on one problem, and take advantage of them on a, similar problem, such as team ImageNet, it is researchers and goal is to obtain image archive. The ImageNet Large Scale Visual Recognition Challenge (ILSVRC) allowed their models to be open source to test for image classification. Team ImageNet and ILSVRC an annual mutual competition between them hosted by the ImageNet team since 2010, where research teams test their computer vision algorithms for various visual recognition tasks [1, 15].

4 Convolutional Neural Networks

We had built Convolution Neural Networks (CNN) model that analyzes medical images and classify them based on Transfer Learning from pre-trained network [10]. CNN have internal layers, as follows: 1) Convolution layer leads to the production of Feature Map (activation map) by execute 32 filter (Feature Map), it is size 3×3. 2) Pooling layer leads to the production of pooled Feature Map by execute Max pooling, it is size 2×2, which called bottleneck layer. 3) Flatten layer leads to the production of first layer of full connection (ANN). CNN each layer contains multi-stage operation, as follows: a) Activation function Rectifier (ReLU) to allow only the positive values and makes all negative values to be zero. b) Filter (Feature Detector): is filters or weights, and this weight values have a spatial relationship. c) Training is updating the weight and biases by iterative optimization to learning rate. Learning rate mean amount of jumps equals 0.001, this technique is called the gradient descent optimizer. d) In this research, The last layer of full connection(ANN) have Soft-Max classifier and four neurons, where one neuron for negative which means is no-infection (normal), and three neuron for positive in cases of pneumonia virus, pneumonia bacterial and Covid-19 [16]. Drawbacks of CNN are that it needs more time to train, and more parameters to reach better recognition accuracy, which makes it more complicated.

5 Deep Transfer Learning (DTL)

CNN training network needs huge datasets and if get the data, it takes amount time to train the network. Overcome the shortcomings of the CNN model, we reuse learned feature maps (weights trained), and apply it to chest CT analysis, which called Deep Transfer Learning (DTL). DTL is Pre-trained network of Keras Applications of CNN canned architectures with weights, which also called an off-the-shelf. DTL accelerate the training because it does not re-training the network from scratch, Feature extraction with better precision and working with very small datasets [17]. we used in this paper to Feature Extraction, library Keras and TensorFlow 2.0 with tf.keras and using pre-trained network as Xception, ResNet50, ResNet, InceptionV3, MobileNetV2 models. We would build Deep Transfer Learning from five pre-trained networks of CNN to classify CT images, for feature extraction in steps, it is: The first step, a) we used input size (width = 75 × height = 75Xchannels = 3). b) Using Pre-loaded weights trained on ImageNet (by setting weights = 'imagenet'). c) Pre-loaded one of the five pre-trained network, that doesn't include the classification layers at the top, (by setting include_top = False). The second step, Freezing, freeze bottleneck layer which is last layer before the flatten operation in convolutional (by setting model.trainable = False). The third step, Fine-Tuning; Unfreezing with add layers during training and Using the weights that updated in the top layers (by setting model.trainable = True).

6 Result and Discussion

6.1 Performance Evaluation

As shown in Table 1, after fine tuning stage our model reaches 100% accuracy on the training and validation set in ResNet50 and Xception model. In freezing stage, the model nearly reaches 98, 97, 60% accuracy on the validation set in ResNet50, ResNet50V2 and Xception respectively. The Xception model almost similar as ResNet50, after Fine-Tuning stage, but it was excluded because the validation loss is much higher than the Test loss 4.670%, which indicate the presence of some overfitting.

Table 1. Accurate performance of deep learning transfer in Train, Validation and Test Sets.

Performance		Fine-Tuning			Freezing		
		Train	Validation	Test	Train	Validation	Test
ResNet50	Accuracy	1.000	1.000	0.660	1.000	0.981	0.678
	Loss	0.000	0.000	0.702	0.000	0.060	4.174
ResNet50V2	Accuracy	1.000	0.962	0.744	0.999	0.979	0.714
	Loss	0.000	0.312	3.102	0.002	0.111	3.705
Xception	Accuracy	1.000	1.000	0.662	0.613	0.604	0.545
	Loss	0.000	0.000	4.670	5.945	6.094	7.074
MobileNetV2	Accuracy	0.613	0.604	0.545	0.612	0.653	0.566
	Loss	5.959	6.094	7.074	5.969	5.344	6.791
VGG19	Accuracy	0.667	0.654	0.557	0.616	0.604	0.545
	Loss	5.118	5.315	5.998	5.902	6.094	7.074

The best performance among the five pre-trained networks models for CT analysis is ResNet50 model. The accuracy of MobileNetV2 model has the worst performance of precision = 0.058% correct predictions, as shown in Table 2.

Figure 2 shows a two-stage ResNet50V2 model 1) freezing stages: the learning curves of the training and validation accuracy/loss. 2) Fine-Tuning stage, as show in Fig. 3 a) Performance evaluation related to validation data by Confusion Matrix. Diagonal Elements represent the number of correct prediction, Other than that represent the number of the wrong prediction of the classification algorithm. As show Fig. 3 b) The Receiver Operating Characteristics (ROC) related to validation data in order to verify the ability to classify three lung diseases COVID-19, virus and bacterial in the CT images. As shown in Fig. 3 c) In the last few layers of fine tuning stage we were able to display vertical line with learning curves of cross-validation.

6.2 Classification of Diseases

We used the Pre-trained ResNet50 models with fine-tuned for Covid-19 disease recognition with who volunteer in the questionnaire, to distinguish between eight chest CT images. Diagnosis of volunteer patients in our model (ResNet50) for positive and negative cases, as follows two patients of Covid-19 disease and pneumonia virus, three patients of pneumonia bacterial, and one patient of no-infection, as shown as Fig. 4.

Our model, it is Pre-trained ResNet50 models with fine-tuned matched the actual diagnosis except for one patient who volunteered for the questionnaire did not have Covid-19 disease with the actual diagnosis, but it was not-infection.

7 Conclusion

We used Deep Transfer Learning (DTL) of ResNet50 Pre-trained network to Feature Extraction using two stages which are freezing and Fine-Tuning. It is more accurate, faster, takes a few lines of codes and very accessible. We used a very low learning rate, during training to avoid overfitting. Training performance proved the efficacy of the pre-trained CNNs fine-tuned in ResNet50 outperformed all pre-trained networks in Fine-tuning stage and has a better performance than freezing and CNN model. This model was able to classify respiratory diseases to improve the diagnostic performance and overcome workload through analyzing CT scan images, it's as accurate as 98%. Training performance evaluations indicate that the ResNet50 Network architectures not only built a CNN from scratch but able to reuse a pre-trained network to get much higher accuracy on our CT image in a few epochs and speeds up the training process. It contributes in detecting the complications, formulate rapid and accurate diagnosis, and therefore helps with early intervention to rescue high-risk patients. Furthermore, resources allocation will be managed appropriately and help junior radiologists and time saving. Future work includes, extending the CNN to three-dimensional data provided by CT volume scans.

Table 2. Comparison of the performance of the five models pre-trained network.

Confusion matrix		Covid-19	Normal	Bacterial	Virus	Total
ResNet50	Precision	1.000	1.000	1.000	0.960	0.990
	Recall	1.000	1.000	0.940	1.000	0.985
	F1-score	1.000	1.000	0.970	0.980	0.987
ResNet50V2	Precision	0.970	1.000	1.000	0.810	0.946
	Recall	1.000	1.000	0.630	1.000	0.908
	F1-score	0.980	1.000	0.770	0.900	0.914
Xception	Precision	0.000	0.000	0.000	0.340	0.086
	Recall	0.000	0.000	0.000	1.000	0.250
	F1-score	0.000	0.000	0.000	0.510	0.127
MobileNetV2	Precision	0.000	0.000	0.230	0.000	0.058
	Recall	0.000	0.000	1.000	0.000	0.250
	F1-score	0.000	0.000	0.380	0.000	0.094
VGG19	Precision	0.000	0.000	0.000	0.340	0.086
	Recall	0.000	0.000	0.000	1.000	0.250
	F1-score	0.000	0.000	0.000	0.510	0.127

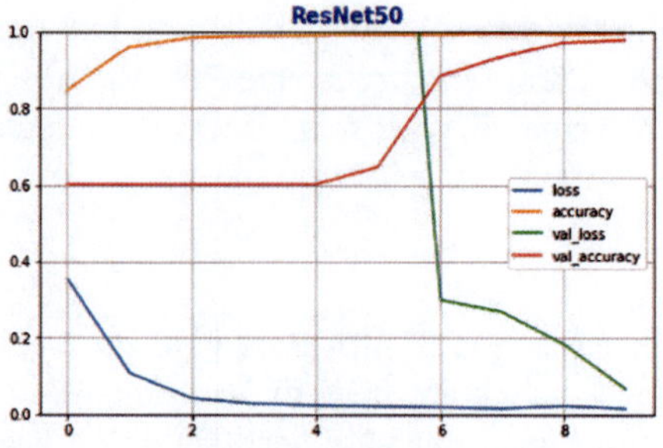

Loss and Accuracy Curves.

Fig. 2. Freezing stage; Evaluation results ResNet50 from pre-trained networks.

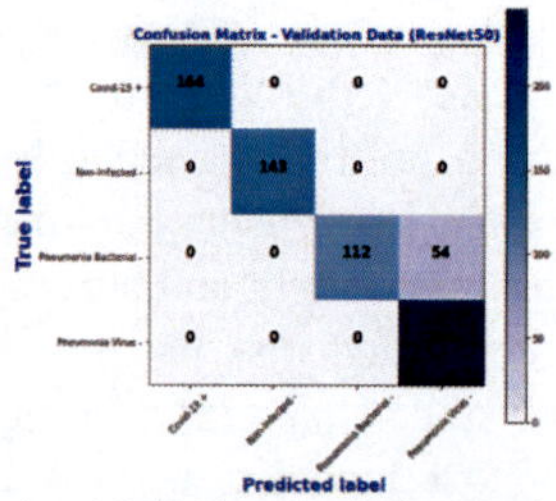

a) Multi-Class Confusion Matrix (4-Class confusion matrix)

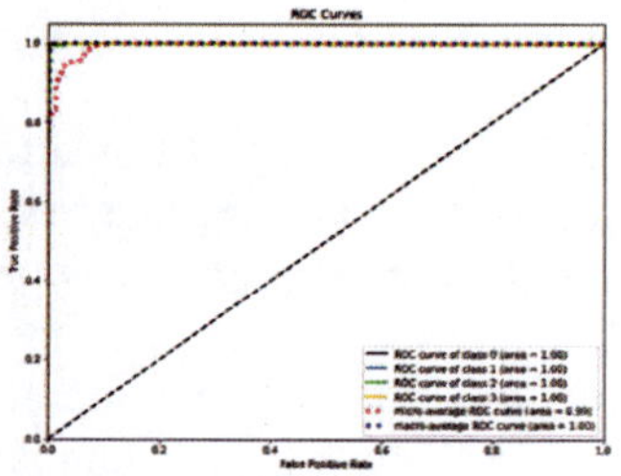

b) Roc Curves

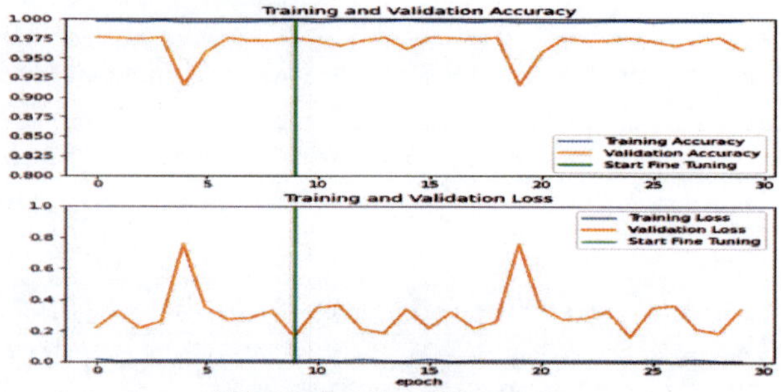

c) The Vertical Line of Fine-Tuning

Fig. 3. Fine-Tuning; Evaluation results ResNet50 from pre-trained networks.

8 Compliance with Ethical Standards

The author declares that there is No conflict of interest and no fund was obtained. Institution permission and Institution Review Board (IRB) was taken from Sur University College. Written informed consent was obtained from all individual participants included in the Study. The researcher explained the purpose, and the possible outcomes of the research. Participation was completely voluntary and participants were assured that they have rights to withdraw at any time throughout the study and non-participation would not have any detrimental effects in terms of the essential or regular professional issues or any penalty. Also participants were assured that their responses will be treated confidentially.

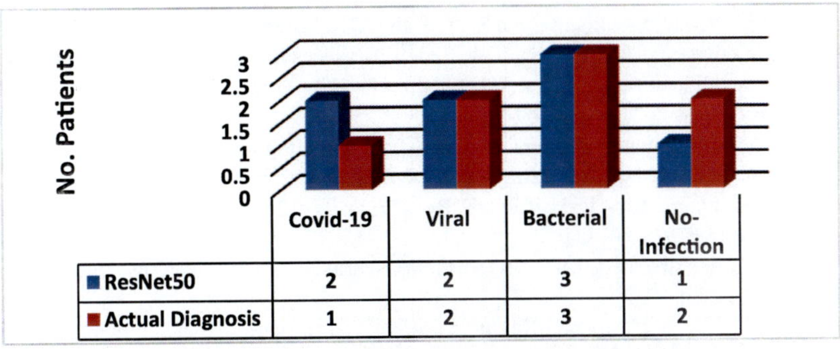

Fig. 4. Classification lung diseases using InceptionV3 and the actual diagnosis by CT scan.

Ethical Approval: This research paper contains a survey that was done by students' participants as per their ethical approval. "All procedures performed in studies involving human participants were in accordance with the ethical standards of the institutional and/or national research committee and with the 1964 Helsinki declaration and its later amendments or comparable ethical standards."

Acknowledgment. I would like to thank the management of Sur University College for the continued support and encouragement to conduct this research.

References

1. Shankar, V., et al.: Evaluating machine accuracy on imagenet. In: International Conference on Machine Learning, PMLR (2020)
2. Wang, L.-F., Anderson, D.E.: Viruses in bats and potential spillover to animals and humans. Curr. Opin. Virol. **34**, 79–89 (2019)
3. Riou, J., Althaus, C.L.: Pattern of early human-to-human transmission of Wuhan 2019 novel coronavirus (2019-nCoV), December 2019 to January 2020. Eurosurveillance **25**(4), 2000058 (2020)
4. Gao, Z., et al.: A systematic review of asymptomatic infections with COVID-19. J. Microbiol. Immunol. Infect. (2020).
5. Jha, S., et al.: Prevalence of flu-like symptoms and COVID-19 in healthcare workers from India. J. Assoc. Phys. India **68**(7), 27–29 (2020)
6. Zhang, J., et al.: Viral pneumonia screening on chest X-rays using confidence-aware anomaly detection. IEEE Trans. Med. Imaging **40**, 879–890 (2020)
7. Nami, M., et al.: The interrelation of neurological and psychological symptoms of COVID-19: risks and remedies. J. Clin. Med. **9**, 2624 (2020)
8. Yang, F., et al.: Analysis of 92 deceased patients with COVID-19. J. Med. Virol. **92**, 2511–2515 (2020)
9. Guo, W., et al.: Diabetes is a risk factor for the progression and prognosis of COVID-19. Diab./Metab. Res. Rev. **36**, e3319 (2020)
10. Alodat, M., Abdullah, I.: Surveillance rapid detection of signs of traffic services in real time. J. Telecommun. Electron. Comput. Eng. (JTEC) **10**(2–4), 193–196 (2018)

11. Alodat, M.: Predicting Student Final Score Using Deep Learning. In: Bhatia, S.K., Tiwari, S., Ruidan, S., Trivedi, M.C., Mishra, K.K. (eds.) Advances in Computer, Communication and Computational Sciences. AISC, vol. 1158, pp. 429–436. Springer, Singapore (2021). https://doi.org/10.1007/978-981-15-4409-5_39
12. Chollet, F.: Building autoencoders in keras. The Keras Blog (2016).
13. Nguyen, G., et al.: Machine learning and deep learning frameworks and libraries for large-scale data mining: a survey. Artif. Intell. Rev. **52**(1), 77–124 (2019). https://doi.org/10.1007/s10462-018-09679-z
14. Sarang, P.: Deep dive in tf. keras. In: Artificial Neural Networks with TensorFlow 2. Apress, Berkeley, CA, pp. 71–132
15. Russakovsky, O., et al.: ImagenNet large scale visual recognition challenge. Int. J. Comput. Visi. **115**(3), 211–252 (2015)
16. Sim, Y., et al.: Deep convolutional neural network–based software improves radiologist detection of malignant lung nodules on chest radiographs. Radiology **294**(1), 199–209 (2020)
17. Xie, M., et al.: Transfer learning from deep features for remote sensing and poverty mapping. In: Proceedings of the AAAI Conference on Artificial Intelligence, vol. 30, no. 1 (2016)

Geometrically Matched Multi-source Microscopic Image Synthesis Using Bidirectional Adversarial Networks

Jun Zhuang[1] and Dali Wang[2,3](✉)

[1] Indiana University-Purdue University Indianapolis, Indianapolis, IN 46202, USA
junz@iu.edu
[2] University of Tennessee, Knoxville, TN 37996, USA
dwang7@utk.edu
[3] Oak Ridge National Laboratory, PBox 2008, MS 6301, Oak Ridge, TN 37831, USA

Abstract. Microscopic images from multiple modalities can produce plentiful experimental information. In practice, biological or physical constraints under a given observation period may prevent researchers from acquiring enough microscopic scanning. Recent studies demonstrate that image synthesis is one of the popular approaches to release such constraints. Nonetheless, most existing synthesis approaches only translate images from the source domain to the target domain without solid geometric associations. To embrace this challenge, we propose an innovative model architecture, BANIS, to synthesize diversified microscopic images from multi-source domains with distinct geometric features. The experimental outcomes indicate that BANIS successfully synthesizes favorable image pairs on *C. elegans* microscopy embryonic images. To the best of our knowledge, BANIS is the first application to synthesize microscopic images that associate distinct spatial geometric features from multi-source domains.

Keywords: Cross domain synthesis · Bidirectional adversarial networks · Multi-source microscopic images · Geometric matching

1 Introduction

Multi-source observation, which observes the same objective from different sources, has been widely used in many different areas, such as biology and medical fields [2,5,6,8,12–14,16–21,23–27]. For example, microscopic imaging of cell nucleus and membrane separately, with different fluorescent materials, is one kind of multi-source observations.

Cross-domain synthesis [1,3,9,11,15] is one potential solution to augment multi-source observation. Given a source domain A, cross-domain synthesis aims at generating corresponding images of the same objective in a target domain B, or

This study is supported by an NIH research project grants (R01GM097576).

R. Su et al. (Eds.): MICAD 2021, LNEE 784, pp. 79–88, 2022.
https://doi.org/10.1007/978-981-16-3880-0_9

vice versa. According to [3], such synthesis can be divided into two main types, the registration-based [11,15] and the intensity-transformation-based methods [1,9]. The registration-based method assumes that images within both the source domain and the target domain are geometrically associated with each other. This method generates images from a co-registered set of images [15]. On the other hand, the intensity-transformation-based method does not fully rely on the geometric relationship. For example, multimodal is a deep learning approach for MRI image synthesis [1]. The model takes multi-source images as input from source contrasts and yields high-quality images in the target contrast. However, both types of methods mentioned above could not solve the issue that two domains come from different sources with quite different spatial features.

In this study, we propose a novel model, **B**idirectional **A**dversarial **N**etworks for microscopic **I**mage **S**ynthesis (**BANIS**), which uses bidirectional adversarial network to synthesize geometrically matched images from multiple domains. BANIS, to the best of our knowledge, is the first cross-domain synthesis application with multi-source images of entirely separated spatial patterns. In the experiment, we deploy our model to a set of microscopic images from *C. elegans* embryogenesis. The experimental results demonstrate that BANIS successfully synthesizes diversified, geometrically matched microscopic images and outperforms two baseline models.

Our contribution in this work can be summarized as follows:

- We propose a novel model, BANIS, to synthesize geometrically matched images from multiple domains. To the best of our knowledge, BANIS is the first cross-domain synthesis application with multi-source images of entirely separated spatial patterns.
- The experiments indicate that BANIS successfully synthesizes diversified, geometrically matched microscopic images and outperforms two baseline models. We will make the model source code and the *C. elegans* embryo microscopic dataset publicly available after the paper acceptance[1].

2 Methodology

2.1 Preliminary Background

The Generative Adversarial Network (GAN) is one of popular deep learning techniques for cross-domain synthesis [4,7]. Vanilla GAN [7] consists of two key components, a generator G and a discriminator D. Given a prior distribution Z as input, G maps a point $\mathbf{z} \sim Z$ from the latent space to the data space as $G(\mathbf{z})$. On the other hand, D attempts to distinguish an instance $\mathbf{x}$ from a synthetic instance $G(\mathbf{z})$, generated by G. The training process is set up as if G and D are playing a zero-sum game. On the one hand, G tries to generate the synthetic instances that are as close as possible to real instances. On the other hand, D distinguishes the synthetic instances from the real instances. After the model

[1] Our code is available on Github at: https://github.com/junzhuang-code/BANIS.

converges, both G and D reach a Nash equilibrium. At this point, G is able to generate instances which are very close to the real one. The objective function V of Vanilla GAN can be written as a summation of two Expectation values $\mathbb{E}$ as follows:

$$\min_{G} \max_{D} V(D, G) = \mathop{\mathbb{E}}_{\mathbf{x} \sim X} [\log D(\mathbf{x})] + \mathop{\mathbb{E}}_{\mathbf{z} \sim Z} [\log(1 - D(G(\mathbf{z})))] \tag{1}$$

where X and Z are the corresponding distribution that $\mathbf{x}$ and $\mathbf{z}$ are sampled from.

In cross-domain synthesis, however, many instances are unpaired between domains [28]. Zhu et al. [28] propose cycle-consistent loss to map the synthetic instances as close as possible to the original instances through the cycled generation, which is combined with two sets of generators and discriminators. The cycle-consistent loss function is described as follows:

$$L_{cyc}(G_A, G_B) = \mathop{\mathbb{E}}_{\mathbf{a} \sim A} [\| G_B(G_A(\mathbf{a})) - \mathbf{a} \|] + \mathop{\mathbb{E}}_{\mathbf{b} \sim B} [\| G_A(G_B(\mathbf{b})) - \mathbf{b} \|] \tag{2}$$

where $\mathbf{a}$ and $\mathbf{b}$ are instances from domain A and B.

2.2 Model Architecture

In this paper, we propose a novel model, Bidirectional Adversarial Networks for microscopic Image Synthesis (BANIS). As displayed in Fig. 1, BANIS contains two Pioneers P, two Successors S and two Coordinators C. The Pioneer is composed of a Generator G and a Discriminator D. The P is mainly responsible for pre-training in the warm-up stage to speed up the progress of synthesis. The Successor consists of an Encoder E and shares the Generator G with the Pioneer. The S uses its E to compress an input image into latent variables and then uses its G to reconstruct the new image from these latent variables. The Coordinator uses pixel-wise methods to preserve the geometric relationship between the images reconstructed by two Successors and the original observed images.

The training procedure of BANIS contains two stages. BANIS simultaneously takes the input images from domain A and domain B. On the warm-up stage, P_A and P_B are trained with given random uniform priors $\mathbf{z}$ and then respectively generate images A_{gen} and B_{gen}. Preliminary images start forming without geometric matching between these images. After the warm-up stage, both S and C join the training to enforce the geometrical relationship between these synthesized images. S_A and S_B learn prior knowledge from observed images, B and A, and reconstruct images with its pre-trained generators from the Pioneers. At the same time, C_A and C_B respectively reinforce the spatial similarity between observed images, B or A, and reconstructed images, B_{rec} and A_{rec}, separately. The model does not stop training until the geometric relationship between image pairs forms. After that, we decrease the learning rate of both S and C on subsequent training to improve the quality of synthesized images.

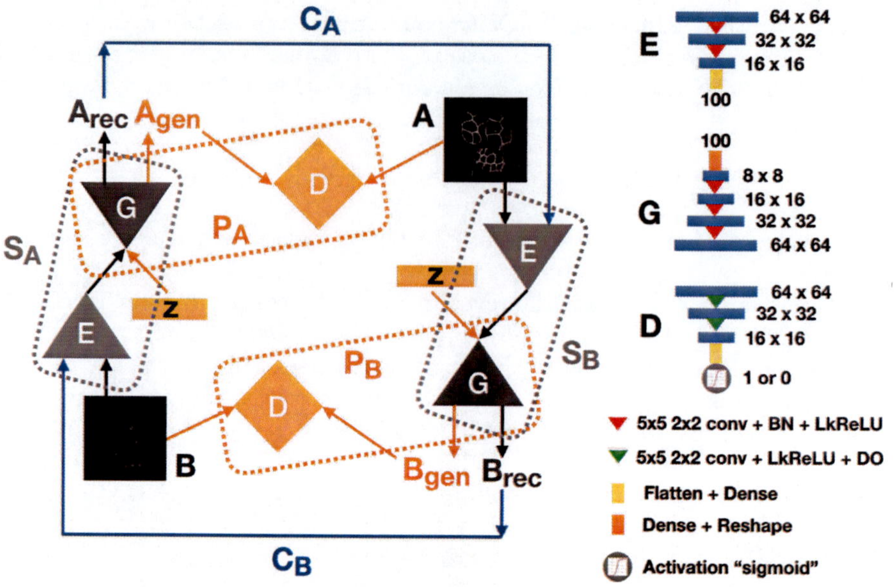

Fig. 1. Our model, BANIS, contains two Pioneers, two Successors, and two Coordinators. The Pioneer is composed of a generator G and a discriminator D. With random uniform priors $\mathbf{z}$ as inputs, P_A and P_B generate images A_{gen} or B_{gen}, respectively. The Successor consists of an encoder E and shares the generator G with the Pioneer. S_A and S_B learn the prior knowledge from observed images, B and A, and reconstruct new images A_{rec} or B_{rec}. By sequentially connecting two Successors, the Coordinators C_A and C_B are designed to reinforce the spatial similarity between the reconstructed images, B_{rec} and A_{rec}, and the observed images B and A, separately. The right side of Fig. 1 shows an exemplar architecture of E, G and D. The number indicates the size of network layer. For example, encoder E takes 64×64 image as input and outputs a 100-dimension vector of latent variables. 5×5 2×2 *conv* represents 2D convolutional layer with 5×5 kernel size and 2×2 strides. *BN*, *LkReLU* and *DO* stand for batch normalization layer, LeakyReLU activation layer, and dropout layer, respectively.

2.3 Loss Functions

BANIS uses three types of loss functions, Adversarial Loss, Identical Loss, and Pair-matched Loss, to help synthesize geometrically matched images.

Adversarial Loss [7] is employed to enforce the generated image A_{gen} or B_{gen}as similar as possible to the observed image A or B. The adversarial loss applies to the Pioneer in the whole training process. Given a random uniform prior, however, generated images don't preserve the spatial information between multiple source domains. Note that our model synthesizes the pair of images simultaneously. Thus, this loss applies to both domain A and domain B. Here we use the same denotation as Vanilla GAN.

$$L_{adv}(G, D) = \mathop{\mathbb{E}}_{\mathbf{x}\sim X}[\log D(\mathbf{x})] + \mathop{\mathbb{E}}_{\mathbf{z}\sim Z}[\log(1 - D(G(\mathbf{z})))] \quad (3)$$

Identical Loss applies to the Successor. To solve previous limitations, the Successor takes specific prior and attempts to reconstruct the images A_{rec} or B_{rec}. Note that the Pioneer helps speed up the synthesis in the warm-up stage. Pioneer's generator is shared with Successor. In other words, reconstructed images are expected to be as close as possible to both observed images A or B and generated images A_{gen} or B_{gen}. Identical loss ensures the quality of reconstructed images. In this paper, we use mean squared error (MSE) to measure the similarity.

$$\begin{aligned} L_{id}(S_A, S_B, G_A, G_B) = & \mathop{\mathbb{E}}_{\mathbf{b}\sim B,\mathbf{a}\sim A}[\|S_A(\mathbf{b}) - \mathbf{a}\|] + \mathop{\mathbb{E}}_{\mathbf{b}\sim B,\mathbf{z}\sim Z}[\|S_A(\mathbf{b}) - G_A(\mathbf{z})\|] + \\ & \mathop{\mathbb{E}}_{\mathbf{a}\sim A,\mathbf{b}\sim B}[\|S_B(\mathbf{a}) - \mathbf{b}\|] + \mathop{\mathbb{E}}_{\mathbf{a}\sim A,\mathbf{z}\sim Z}[\|S_B(\mathbf{a}) - G_B(\mathbf{z})\|] \end{aligned} \tag{4}$$

Pair-matched Loss applies to the Coordinator. This loss enforces the projection inside each Successor to ensure these two domains are spatially matched. The Coordinator sequentially connects these two Successors. C_A takes B as input and uses S_A and S_B sequentially to generate B_{rec}. Then it compares the new images with the observed image B. C_B operates similarly with observed image A. In other words, pair-matched loss helps preserve spatial information among two domains. In this paper, we also use MSE to measure the quality of the projection.

$$L_{pm}(C_A, C_B) = \mathop{\mathbb{E}}_{\mathbf{b}\sim B}[\|C_A(\mathbf{b}) - \mathbf{b}\|] + \mathop{\mathbb{E}}_{\mathbf{a}\sim A}[\|C_B(\mathbf{a}) - \mathbf{a}\|] \tag{5}$$

Algorithm 1: GEOMETRIC Matching Index (GMI)

Input: Testing set (A_{test}, B_{test}), Threshold TS

Initialize two counters, cnt_{total} and $cnt_{matched}$ as 0;
for *all* $(a^{\{i\}}, b^{\{i\}}) \in (A_{test}, B_{test})$ **do**
  $cnt_{total} \leftarrow cnt_{total} + 1$;
  $a^{\{i\}}_{rec}, b^{\{i\}}_{rec} = S_B(a^{\{i\}}), S_A(b^{\{i\}})$;
  $a^{\{i\}}_{bi}, b^{\{i\}}_{bi} = Bi(a^{\{i\}}_{rec}), Bi(b^{\{i\}}_{rec})$;
  $Dice_{AB} = DSC(a^{\{i\}}_{bi}, b^{\{i\}}_{bi})$;
  if $Dice_{AB} < TS$ **then**
    $cnt_{matched} \leftarrow cnt_{matched} + 1$;
  end
end
return $\frac{cnt_{matched}}{cnt_{total}}$.

2.4 Geometric Matching Index

Although the individual synthesized images come from different domains and have different geometric patterns, the pair of images should be geometrically matched. For example, in our microscopic data case, membranes and nucleus should be spatially matched without overlapping. For this purpose, we propose a new evaluation metric, Geometric Matching Index (GMI), to measure the quality of image synthesis. As the pseudo-code presented in Algorithm 1, GMI first extracts the binary masks from reconstructed image pairs and then measures their contours' overlapping by the Dice Similarity Coefficient (DSC) [29]. Less overlapping in our case means better matching. Given an overlapping threshold, GMI counts the number of well-matched image pairs whose DSC is lower than the given threshold and returns the percentage of these well-matched image pairs over the total number of reconstructed image pairs at the end.

3 Experiments

3.1 Dataset and Preprocessing

In this experiment, our model is evaluated on a set of *C. elegans* microscopy image dataset [22]. Each set contains 300 voxels, and each of them may contain one to three embryos. The scanner takes 75-second intervals on each voxel over the first 375 min of embryogenesis. We select 50 pseudo-3D voxels and each of them contains three embryos. Each voxel contains 30 slices at 1 µm vertical distance that covers the entire embryo(s). Each slice contains one 512 × 512 membrane image and one 512 × 512 nuclei image.

We use ImageJ to split these image stacks and pick the raw images from the middle 15 layers of each stake for our model experiments. We split the raw images into two 512 × 512 images, each contains membrane- or nuclei-only information. These 512 × 512 images are then converted to gray scale and denoised with a Gaussian filter. Then, we resized these images into 128 × 128 for a better computational efficiency. After that, we crop out a single embryo and generate smaller 64×64 images. Finally, we normalize the pixel value of the image between −1 and 1. 10% of images is used as a test set and the rest part is for training. Some samples of the 64 × 64 microscopic images are illustrated in Fig. 2.

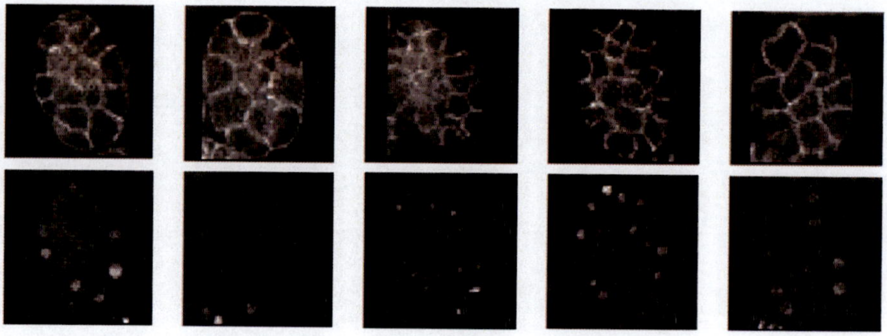

Fig. 2. Samples of the observed microscopic images

3.2 Model Parameters and Training

The shape of input images is $64 \times 64 \times 1$. The latent dimension for both random uniform prior and encoded prior is 100. Both D and P are trained with Adam optimizer. The initial learning rate for G_B is set as 1×10^{-5} and the learning rates for G_A, D_A and D_B are set as 2×10^{-5}. Both S and C are trained by Stochastic Gradient Descent (SGD) optimizer. Their initial learning rates are 1×10^{-4}. The batch size is empirically set as 128.

The model is trained with 17,000 epochs in the warm-up stage at the initial learning rate until adversarial the loss converges and the preliminary images start forming. After that, both S and C join the training for subsequent 13,000 epochs until both identical loss and pair-matched loss converge. To improve the quality of synthesized images, both S and C are trained with another 10,000 epochs at a new learning rate, which is decreased by 50%. The total model training with 40,000 epochs takes approximately 12.3 h on a Linux machine, which configured with 4 Intel Xeon central processing units (E5-1620 v4), 64-GB memory, and a 16-GB Nvidia GP104 graphical processing unit.

After the training, we evaluate the BANIS performance by calculating the GMIs of the entire synthesized dataset with different overlapping thresholds TS_{dsc}. A lower TS_{dsc} indicates a more strictly geometric matched is required.

3.3 Experimental Results

In this experiment, we first examine the performance of synthesis between BANIS and baselines. We select Cycle-GAN [28] and Auto-Encoder [10] as our baselines since BANIS is inspired by both of them. We train Cycle-GAN/Auto-Encoder to converge with 200/300 epochs, respectively. Rest experimental settings remain the same as BANIS. Figure 3 presents the synthesized images. BANIS can synthesize geometrically matched image pairs (the 1st and 2nd rows). These synthesized images have clear *C. elegan's* image features of membrane or nuclei and simultaneously preserve the geometric relationship between them. It is clear that these synthesized image pairs have very similar patterns shown in Fig. 2. On the contrary, the synthesized images from Cycle-GAN (the 3rd and 4th rows) couldn't preserve the geometric relationship as Cycle-GAN is only good at transferring the style or texture between two images with similar shapes. Auto-Encoder only generates fuzzy images with unclear contours (the 5th and 6th rows). What's worse, the nuclei are barely seen in some synthesized samples. We argue that partial information irreversibly gets loss in the encoding stage, which leads to this unsatisfied synthesis. Note that these images are slices and thus may not display all nuclei in one slice. These synthesized images demonstrate that BANIS achieves superior performance against two baselines.

We also evaluate the performance based on the aforementioned metric, GMI. We run each experiment five times and present the mean and standard deviation in Table 1. The outcome reveals that BANIS yields satisfied synthesized images under strict thresholds TS_{dsc} and outperforms the other two baselines across three different thresholds. Most (over 95%) images of the total image pairs

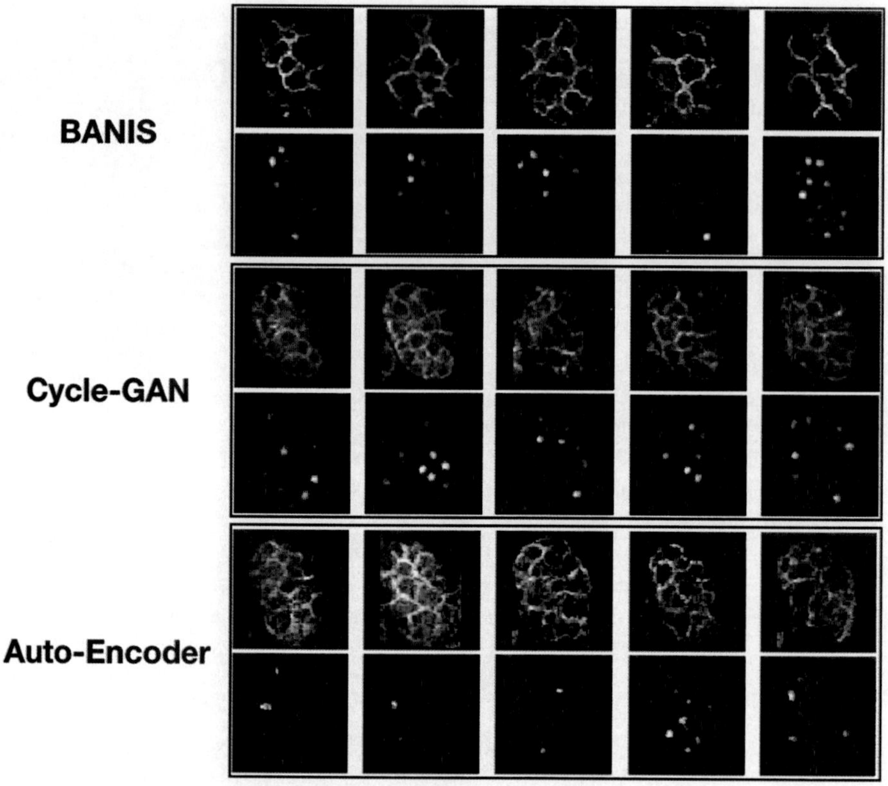

Fig. 3. Exemplar synthesized images from BANIS, Cycle-GAN, and Auto-Encoder

Table 1. Evaluation on the synthesized images By GMI

TS_{dsc} (%)	0.1	0.2	0.3
BANIS	75.26 (±0.65)	87.27 (±0.32)	95.39 (±0.11)
Cycle-GAN	69.04 (±0.48)	82.89 (±0.67)	90.14 (±0.28)
Auto-Encoder	71.48 (±1.21)	83.86 (±0.98)	90.91 (±0.51)

have an overlapping value less than 0.3. Even with a very restricted threshold requirement of 0.1 (that is less than 10% of overlapping between any two simultaneously synthesized images), the GMI of the total synthesized image pairs reaches 75.26%. We observe that Auto-Encoder achieves higher GMI, but it fails to synthesize nuclei images. We argue that this failure decreases the overlapping and thus increases GMI. Overall, GMI is a qualified metric to measure the geometrical matching relationship between two synthesized domains. However, it sometimes fails if other reasons weaken the overlapping as well.

4 Conclusion

In this study, we present an innovative model architecture, BANIS, to synthesize microscopic images from multiple domains. BANIS, to the best of our knowledge, is the first model that synthesizes geometrically matched images from multiple domains that exist entirely separated spatial patterns. The experiment using microscopic data from *C. elegan's* embryogenesis proves that our model can synthesize diversified and geometrically matched images that are as comparable as the observed microscopic images.

References

1. Chartsias, A., Joyce, T., Giuffrida, M.V., Tsaftaris, S.A.: Multimodal MR synthesis via modality-invariant latent representation. IEEE Trans. Med. Imaging **37**, 803–814 (2017)
2. Dai, M.Q., Zheng, W., Huang, Z., Yung, L.Y.L.: Aqueous phase synthesis of widely tunable photoluminescence emission CdtTe/CdS core/shell quantum dots under a totally ambient atmosphere. J. Mater. Chem. **22**, 16336–16345 (2012)
3. Dar, S.U., Yurt, M., Karacan, L., Erdem, A., Erdem, E., Çukur, T.: Image synthesis in multi-contrast MRI with conditional generative adversarial networks. IEEE Trans. Med. Imaging **38**, 2375–2388 (2019)
4. Donahue, J., Krähenbühl, P., Darrell, T.: Adversarial feature learning. arXiv preprint arXiv:1605.09782 (2016)
5. Femmam, S., Iles, A., Bessaid, A.: Optimizing magnetic resonance imaging reconstructions. Electron. Imaging Signal Process. J. SPIE Newsroom (2015)
6. Gao, L., Pan, H., Han, J., Xie, X., Zhang, Z., Zhai, X.: Corner detection and matching methods for brain medical image classification. In: 2016 IEEE International Conference on Bioinformatics and Biomedicine (BIBM). IEEE (2016)
7. Goodfellow, I., et al.: Generative adversarial nets. In: Advances in Neural Information Processing Systems, pp. 2672–2680 (2014)
8. Huo, Y., et al.: SynSeg-Net: synthetic segmentation without target modality ground truth. IEEE Trans. Med. Imaging **38**, 1016–1025 (2018)
9. Jog, A., Carass, A., Roy, S., Pham, D.L., Prince, J.L.: MR image synthesis by contrast learning on neighborhood ensembles. Med. Image Anal. **24**, 63–76 (2015)
10. Kingma, D.P., Welling, M.: Auto-encoding variational bayes. arXiv preprint arXiv:1312.6114 (2013)
11. Lee, J., Carass, A., Jog, A., Zhao, C., Prince, J.L.: Multi-atlas-based CT synthesis from conventional MRI with patch-based refinement for MRI-based radiotherapy planning. In: Medical Imaging 2017: Image Processing. International Society for Optics and Photonics (2017)
12. Liu, H., Cocea, M.: Granular computing-based approach of rule learning for binary classification. Granular Comput. **4**, 275–283 (2019)
13. Lu, C., Mandal, M.: Automated analysis and diagnosis of skin melanoma on whole slide histopathological images. Pattern Recogn. **48**, 2738–2750 (2015)
14. Meinel, L.A., Stolpen, A.H., Berbaum, K.S., Fajardo, L.L., Reinhardt, J.M.: Breast MRI lesion classification: improved performance of human readers with a backpropagation neural network computer-aided diagnosis (CAD) system. Journal of Magnetic Resonance Imaging: An Official Journal of the International Society for Magnetic Resonance in Medicine (2007)

15. Miller, M.I., Christensen, G.E., Amit, Y., Grenander, U.: Mathematical textbook of deformable neuroanatomies. Proceedings of the National Academy of Sciences (1993)
16. Mou, L., et al.: CS2-net: deep learning segmentation of curvilinear structures in medical imaging. Med. Image Anal. **67**, 101874 (2020)
17. Nie, D., et al.: Medical image synthesis with deep convolutional adversarial networks. IEEE Trans. Biomed. Eng. **65**, 2720–2730 (2018)
18. Parisi, L., RaviChandran, N., Lanzillotta, M.: Supervised machine learning for aiding diagnosis of knee osteoarthritis: a systematic review and meta-analysis (2020)
19. Peng, C., Pan, N., Xie, Z., Liu, L., Xiang, J., Liu, C.: Determination of bisphenol a by a gold nanoflower enhanced enzyme-linked immunosorbent assay. Anal. Lett. **49**, 1492–1501 (2016)
20. Su, R., Hu, Y.: Medical Imaging and Computer-Aided Diagnosis. Springer (2020)
21. Vakharia, V.N., et al.: The effect of vascular segmentation methods on stereotactic trajectory planning for drug-resistant focal epilepsy: a retrospective cohort study. World Neurosurg. X **4**, 100057 (2019)
22. Wang, D., Lu, Z., Xu, Y., Wang, Z., Santella, A., Bao, Z.: Cellular structure image classification with small targeted training samples. IEEE Access **7**, 148967–148974 (2019)
23. Wei, H., et al.: Precise targeting of the globus pallidus internus with quantitative susceptibility mapping for deep brain stimulation surgery. J. Neurosurg. **133**, 1605–1611 (2019)
24. Yuan, Y., Huang, W., Wang, X., Xu, H., Zuo, H., Su, R.: Automated accurate registration method between UAV image and google satellite map. Multimed. Tools Appl. **79**, 16573–16591 (2019)
25. Zamzmi, G., Rajaraman, S., Antani, S.: Accelerating super-resolution and visual task analysis in medical images. Appl. Sci. **10**, 4282 (2020)
26. Zhang, Y.D., Govindaraj, V.V., Tang, C., Zhu, W., Sun, J.: High performance multiple sclerosis classification by data augmentation and AlexNet transfer learning model. J. Med. Imaging Health Inform. **9**, 2012–2021 (2019)
27. Zhao, Y., Rada, L., Chen, K., Harding, S.P., Zheng, Y.: Automated vessel segmentation using infinite perimeter active contour model with hybrid region information with application to retinal images. IEEE Trans. Med. Imaging **34**, 1797–1807 (2015)
28. Zhu, J.Y., Park, T., Isola, P., Efros, A.A.: Unpaired image-to-image translation using cycle-consistent adversarial networks. In: Proceedings of the IEEE International Conference on Computer Vision, pp. 2223–2232 (2017)
29. Zhuang, J., Gao, M., Hasan, M.A.: Lighter U-net for segmenting white matter hyperintensities in MR images. In: Proceedings of the 16th EAI International Conference on Mobile and Ubiquitous Systems: Computing, Networking and Services (2019)

Color-Based Fusion of MRI Modalities for Brain Tumor Segmentation

Nachwa Aboubakr(✉), Mihaela Popova, and James L. Crowley

Univ. Grenoble Alpes, CNRS, Inria, Grenoble INP, LIG, 38000 Grenoble, France
{nachwa.aboubakr,mihaela.popova,james.crowley}@inria.fr

Abstract. Most attempts to provide automatic techniques to detect and locate suspected tumors in Magnetic Resonance images (MRI) concentrate on a single MRI modality. Radiologists typically use multiple MRI modalities for such tasks. In this paper, we report on experiments for automatic detection and segmentation of tumors in which multiple MRI modalities are encoded using classical color encodings. We investigate the use of 2D convolutional networks using a classic U-Net architecture.

Slice-by-slice MRI analysis for tumor detection is challenging because this task requires contextual information from 3D tissue structures. However, 3D convolutional networks are prohibitively expensive to train. To overcome this challenge, we extract a set of 2D images by projecting the 3D volume of MRI with maximum contrast. Multiple MRI modalities are then combined as independent colors to provide a color-encoded 2D image. We show experimentally that this led to better performance than slice-by-slice training while limiting the number of trainable parameters and the requirement for training data to a reasonable limit.

Keywords: Tumor segmentation · MRI · Modality fusion · Medical imaging

1 MRI Segmentation

Radiologists detect pathologies by visual inspection of X-rays, Computerized axial tomography (CAT) scans, and Magnetic Resonance Images (MRI). Unfortunately, competent diagnosis requires years of experience, and many common pathologies are misdiagnosed. MRI images, in particular, are difficult to interpret, as an accurate diagnosis can require adjustments to a number of parameters and the use of multiple MRI image modalities.

The automatic segmentation of MRI images offers a unique set of challenges. Pixels in each 2D image must be considered as part of a 3D volume as neighboring voxels provide contextual information that can be important for interpretation. This information can be lost when processing each slice independently. Approaches based on slice-by-slice segmentation of pathologies tend to ignore this information. On the other hand, 3D convolutional neural networks used for direct 3D segmentation require training large models as well as a considerable computational power and training data to converge. One possible approach to overcome this limitation is to transform the MRI 3D volume into 2D

R. Su et al. (Eds.): MICAD 2021, LNEE 784, pp. 89–97, 2022.
https://doi.org/10.1007/978-981-16-3880-0_10

images using projections or slices at various angles [1, 2, 13]. However, different MRI modalities provide different information. Radiologists use multiple modalities when manually segment pathologies in MRI images.

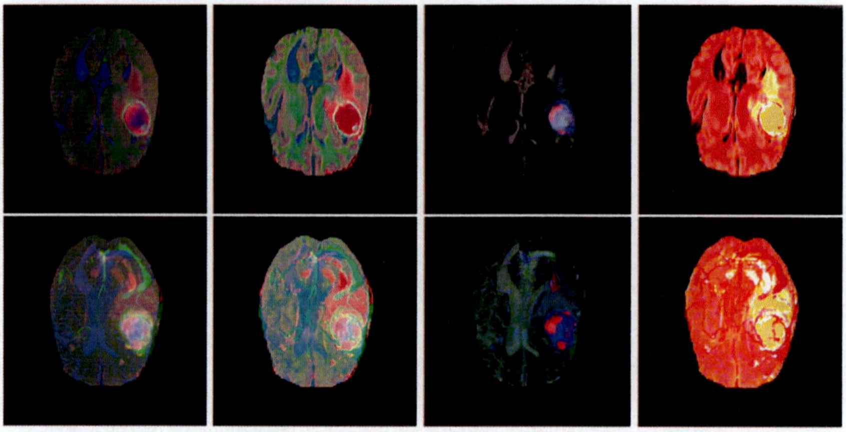

(a) RGB (b) XYZ (c) HSV (d) LAB

Fig. 1. Color-based fusion of MRI modalities. First row is slice-by-slice fusion. Second row is fusion of the Maximum Intensity Images of each modality. The fused modalities are (Flair, T1GD and T2) on different color-space channels, respectively.

Traditionally, radiologists use classical segmentation methods to segment different MRI modalities using techniques such as thresholding, region growing, edge detection, K-means [8, 15, 18]. With the rapid advances of artificial neural networks, a variety of MRI segmentation methods have been demonstrated to provide very promising tools to help radiologists. These approaches take an MRI image and produce a segmented image on areas of interest. Such approaches either process the whole 3D volume at once as in 3D U-Net [5] or they treat the MRI image slice-by-slice where each slice is processed independently. In some cases, slice-by-slice analysis is followed by intra-slice processing in a form of recurrent neural networks as in [3, 7, 14]. Approaches that treat the image slice-by-slice can be more affordable in terms of model size and number of parameters than approaches that treat the whole image at once. However, this generally comes at the cost of a reduction of performance.

Most work on automatic MRI segmentation either rely on a single MRI modality or consider each modality separately. To overcome the limitations of 2D approaches, several works have investigated ideas to transform the 3D MRI volume into 2D while keeping some kind of contextual information. These techniques include the use of multiple planes from different angles of an MRI image [6, 9, 13]. In addition, some recent works have investigated the use of MRI image projections from 3D to 2D using statistical measures such as Maximum Intensity Projection (MIP) [1, 2]. Few works have investigated the effect fusion of different medical imaging modalities. In [4], (CT, PET and MRI) images are color-fused which make them visually appealing and offer an accurate representation of the source images, and thus improving the diagnosis.

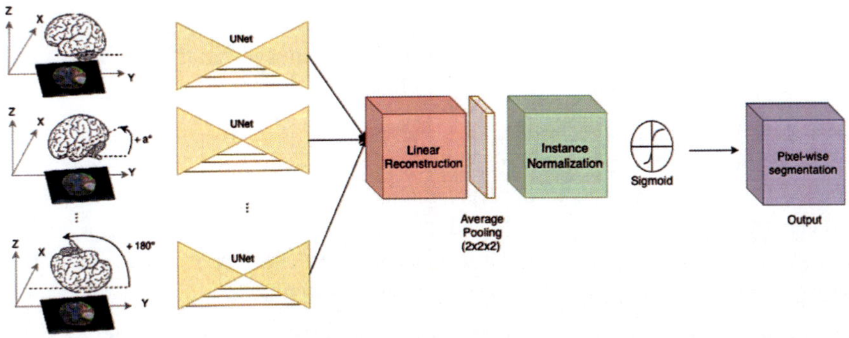

Fig. 2. Our model architecture. The input is a color-fused image of MRI modalities projected with Maximum Intensity projection. The 3D MRI image is rotated with "a" degrees. These projected images are input to a standard 2D U-Net. After that, the segmentation volume is reconstructed from the decoded U-Net output. After that, the segmentation volume is passed through refinement and normalization operations before producing the final pixel-wise segmentation.

In this paper, we investigate the use of multiple MRI modalities for the automatic segmentation process, and examine the trade-off between computational cost and segmentation quality for different MRI modalities. To fuse MRI modalities, we encode each modality on a color channel and use encoded images as input for the automatic segmentation. We study the effect of using 2D projected images of the MRI volume instead of using the whole volume to minimize computational cost while preserving performance. We investigate an alternative approach for overcoming the limitations of 2D approaches by using Maximum Intensity projection of MRI volumes while exploiting information presence in different modalities by fusing them in color spaces.

2 Fusion of MRI Modalities

Different MRI modalities are employed for clinical diagnosis. These modalities include T1-weighted MRI (T1), T1 with contrast enhancement such as Gadolinium ions (T1GD), T2-weighted MRI (T2) and FLuid-Attenuated Inversion Recovery (FLAIR). Different MRI modalities show different information about the pathology. T1 shows healthy tissues with high intensity and the pathology with low intensity, T2 images represent pathology with high intensity. In T1GD images, the tumor border can be easily distinguished by the bright signal of the accumulated contrast agent in the active cell region of the tumor tissue. In FLAIR images, signal of water molecules is suppressed which helps in distinguishing edema region [10].

To exploit the knowledge that exists in different MRI modalities, we study the fusion of MRI modalities using a color space for brain tumor segmentation. We compare modality fusion using different color-space. These include RGB, XYZ, HSV and LAB. For the XYZ space; Y is the luminance, Z is quasi-equal to blue in RGB and X is the mix of three colors RGB, HSV is a color space that combines Hue, Saturation, and Values from different modalities and LAB is composed of L the luminance, A is a color value between green and red and B is a color value between blue and yellow. Of these spaces,

RGB offers a linear fusion of the different modalities. The fusion with the other modalities is computed using color-space transformation formulas that transforms the fused image from the corresponding color space to RGB.

Model Structure. Our model architecture is shown in Fig. 2. The base model is a standard U-Net model randomly initialized. The model receives fused 2D projected images extracted from MRI volumes of different modalities. The output of U-Net is used for 3D reconstruction of the images followed with a denoising layer. For training, we use a joint loss function of Dice loss and Cross-Entropy Loss, each contribute equally to the final loss. The implementation code of our method is available.[1]

Preprocessing. We extract multiple Maximum Intensity Images (MIP) from the 3D volume of MRI by rotating the volume from 0° to 180° around the axial plane with a steps and then project the resulting volume on the axial plane. We fuse MIPs from different modalities using a specific color-space. The resulted set of 2D images are used for training. We take color-fused MIPs of each angle and pass it to our model.

Linear Reconstruction. We use linear reconstruction to form a 3D tensor from 2D activation maps. Starting from an empty 3D tensor that matches the size of the 3D output mask, we add the first activation map to all the slices of the tensor. Then, we rotate the reconstruction tensor to match the angle of the new projection image, and we add the values of that projection to the resulted tensor from the previous computation. A voxel value in the result tensor is defined as the sum over the corresponding 2D projected values. This is repeated until all projections are added to the reconstruction tensor. Then the tensor is rotated one last time so that it goes to its original state.

Denoising. The linear reconstruction process produces artifacts and thus, the reconstructed volume needs denoising. The denoising process involves an average pooling layer with a kernel of $(2 \times 2 \times 2)$. This is followed by an instance normalization layer and activated by a Sigmoid function to output the final predicted mask of the pathology.

3 Experimental Evaluation

For our experiments we used the BRATS 2017 dataset from the MICCAI Medical Imaging Decathlon [17, 19]. This dataset set provides Magnetic resonance images for the segmentation of brain tumor. The dataset contains four MRI modalities: Flair, T1, T1 with Gadolinium (T1GD), and T2. During our experiments, we use a fusion of Flair, T1GD and T2. The tumor/pathology has the highest intensity in T2 and Flair. In T1GD, the active part of the tumor has the highest intensity. We exclude T1 from our experiments since the pathology response to T1 modality has the lowest intensity which is incompatible with Maximum intensity projection.

The dataset provides labels for Edema, enhanced tumor, Non-enhanced tumor and Background. We consider for our experiments two classes only: The pathology which includes enhanced and non-enhanced tumor, and the background class which includes edema and background labels. For the evaluation of our experiments, we use four metrics: Dice score, Intersection over Union (IoU), Precision and Recall.

[1] https://github.com/Nachwa/Color-MRI-Seg.

3.1 Comparison with 2D/3D U-Nets

We compared our model with three already established models that can give us a good idea how well fusion and projections work in comparison with standard slice based or 3D image techniques. We compared with 3D U-Net with instance normalization and leaky ReLU which segments the whole 3D image [11]. Another method that we use for comparison is 2D U-Net [16] which segments each slice from the volume separately without taking into account the relationship between the slices. The third method that we used for comparison is 2.5D U-Net which takes a group of slices together for segmentation. When considering our method and these methods, we wanted to find a network that provided good quality of segmentation and does not need too many resources so that it can be used in real situation.

From Table 1, we found that 3D U-Net is performing the best for segmenting brain tumor in MRI. Our network placed second in terms of the quality of the segmentation after 3D U-Net. Our model outperforms, 2D U-Net which operates on slice by slice basis for the segmentation. Our model also outperforms both Proj U-Net and 2.5D U-Net which consider relations between slices either by using maximum intensity projections or using skip connections respectively. These results show that our model take advantage of the multi-modality fusion in addition of the intensity projection. Note that we report results of Proj U-Net using other modalities in Table 3 (top).

Table 1. Segmentation results of our model compared to other competitive techniques. 3D U-Net and 2.5D U-Net results are reported in [11] and [12] respectively while the results of the other models are implemented. The best result in bold and the second best is underlined.

Model	Dice	Precision	Recall	# Param
2D U-Net [16]	61.63	59.39	65.91	17M
Proj U-Net [1]	64.22	72.79	59.64	17M
2.5D U-Net [12]	64.98	62.86	67.26	–
3D U-Net [11]	**85.81**	**91.00**	**83.12**	51M
Ours	<u>79.20</u>	<u>79.06</u>	<u>80.94</u>	17M

In terms of parameters 3D U-Net requires a high number of parameters to tune with 51 million. On the other hand, both our method and 2D U-Net require only 17 million parameters to tune. Following these experiments, we found that our proposed network provides a good balance between quality of segmentation and the training parameters needed.

3.2 Comparison with a Single Modality

In order to compare the differences in the quality of segmentation using a single modality and fusion of modalities, we compared the fusion of T1 with Gadolinium (T1GD), T2, Flair using RGB, XYZ, HSV and LAB color spaces. During these experiments, we have chosen against using T1 modality, because we use Maximum Intensity Projections and the pathology there has the lowest intensity while the healthy tissue has the highest intensity, so in that projection nothing significant can be observed in T1.

Comparing only the results for single modality, we can note that segmenting T1GD as input achieved the best results. This is likely the consequence of using the contrasting agent which highlights the active part of the tumor and could be used in finding easily the boundary between the healthy tissue and the pathology which is a very important part in projection-based segmentation. On the other hand, the results for T2 and Flair alone are not as good, because on those images in addition to the pathology, the edema (swelling caused by the pathology) can also be seen with higher intensity than the healthy tissue and finding the boundary there would be more difficult.

From Table 2, we found that fusing the modalities in a color space makes a great difference in the quality of the segmentation. The use modalities fusion shows more details about different parts of the pathology. From our sample fusion images in Fig. 1, we can see that the fusion in the HSV color space is visually more apparent than the other examples; in particular, we can notice that blood vessels in T1 with Gadolinium do not show in the image and the difference between the active tumor and the tumor core can be spotted easily.

Table 2. Tumor segmentation results of our model on different modalities. First rows are the results of each modality alone. Last rows are the results of fusing these modalities in corresponding color spaces.

Modality	Dice	IoU	Precision	Recall
T1GD	72.50	60.56	77.78	72.08
T2	63.80	51.81	70.59	63.68
FLAIR	66.07	50.97	64.77	70.58
RGB	76.46	65.17	79.39	78.34
XYZ	76.00	62.92	**81.41**	73.36
HSV	**79.20**	**67.04**	79.06	**80.94**
LAB	78.10	65.59	77.51	80.38

From the Table 2, we can see similar conclusion, fusion with HSV color-space outperforms the other color-spaces. RGB has an advantage over the other color spaces as it does not need any additional computation, so we can directly stack the projections of different modalities after normalization. For simplicity, we use RGB fusion for the rest of our experiments.

Table 3. Ablation study shows the effect of our model structure choices. Method A (Proj U-Net) is implemented as described in [1]. Method D is our proposed model.

Method		Dice	IoU	Precision	Recall
A	With T2	52.15	40.81	57.68	56.59
A	With T1GD	52.92	39.86	64.68	48.52
A	With FLAIR	64.22	49.73	72.79	59.64
B	A + RGB color fusion	72.23	58.32	74.93	72.20
C	B + Leaky ReLU	72.43	58.79	77.04	71.25
D	C + Instance norm	**76.46**	**65.17**	**79.39**	**78.34**
E	2D-UNet + RGB fusion	67.09	55.69	64.83	70.35

3.3 Ablation Study

In this section, we discuss our choice of the activation function and the normalization layer. In the related works [1, 2] they used ReLU as activation function and for normalization they choose Batch normalization.

When the activation function is ReLU, all negative values are reassigned to 0 while all positive values stay the same. The assigned of all negative values to 0 can lead to the vanishing gradient problem which can subsequently stop the network from training. One solution for this problem is to use leaky ReLU. For all negative values, leaky ReLU assigns them to the result of the multiplication of the value with 0.1 which removes the problem of neuron reaching 0 and dying. Thus, we wanted to experiment if changing the activation function would improve the segmentation. The results from this experiment can be found in Table 3 (Row C) and we found that leaky ReLU improves the segmentation.

When working with medical dataset, we can expect that the pathology class would have less samples than the background, because the background contains the background of the medical image and the healthy tissue. In batch normalization, all images in the batch would be normalized together and, in our network, that would mean that all images from one patient are normalized together. Instance normalization normalizes each projection on its own. From Table 3 (Row D), we found that Instance normalization can significantly improve the segmentation of the pathology in all reported metrics.

We also compared the use of projected images against using the MRI all slices directly. Using maximum intensity projected images, the preprocessing time is 0.2 s for one patient, and additional half a second for the inference segmentation of the 3D image. On the other hand, segmentation using slice-by-slice MRI is 15 times more costly. Although, training slice by slice uses more data and takes more processing time, it does not improve the quality of the segmentation. From the results in Table 3 (Row E), we can notice that Modality fusion can improve the performance of standard slice-by-slice

2D-UNet with about 6 points. However, the use maximum intensity projection with the linear reconstruction improves the quality of the segmentation by about 10% over 2D-UNets.

4 Conclusion

In this paper, we investigate the fusion of Maximum intensity projected (MIP) images of MRI modalities using color spaces. We use MIP images of the MRI volume at different angles to minimize the processing time. We then color-fuse these projected on the RGB color space. In addition, we compare the performance of our model to 3D, 2.5D, and 2D U-Nets and show that our pipeline architecture provides a trade-off between performance and computational cost. We found that the use of modality fusion in a color space can improve the segmentation quality and the training time while preserving similar number of training parameters as 2D U-Net.

References

1. Angermann, C., Haltmeier, M.: Random 2.5D U-net for fully 3D segmentation. In: Liao, H., et al. (eds.) MLMECH/CVII-STENT -2019. LNCS, vol. 11794, pp. 158–166. Springer, Cham (2019). https://doi.org/10.1007/978-3-030-33327-0_19
2. Angermann, C., Haltmeier, M., Steiger, R., Pereverzyev Jr, S., Gizewski, E.: Projection-based 2.5D u-net architecture for fast volumetric segmentation. arXiv preprint arXiv:1902.00347 (2019)
3. Alom, Md.Z., Hasan, M., Yakopcic, C., Taha, T.M., Asari, V.K.: Recurrent residual convolutional neural network based on U-Net (R2U-Net) for medical image segmentation. arXiv preprint arXiv:1802.06955 (2018)
4. Baum, K.G., et al.: Techniques for fusion of multimodal images: application to breast imaging. In: 2006 International Conference on Image Processing, pp. 2521–2524. IEEE (2006)
5. Çiçek, Ö., Abdulkadir, A., Lienkamp, S., Brox, T., Ronneberger, O.: 3D U-Net: learning dense volumetric segmentation from sparse annotation. In: Ourselin, S., Joskowicz, L., Sabuncu, M.R., Unal, G., Wells, W. (eds.) MICCAI 2016. LNCS, vol. 9901, pp. 424–432. Springer, Cham (2016). https://doi.org/10.1007/978-3-319-46723-8_49
6. Chung, S., Gan, K., Achuthan, A., Mandava, R.: Liver tumor segmentation using triplanar convolutional neural network: A pilot study. In: Adzhar, Md.., Zawawi, S.S., Teoh, N.B., Abdullah, M.I., Sazali, S.M. (eds.) 10th International Conference on Robotics, Vision, Signal Processing and Power Applications. LNEE, vol. 547, pp. 607–614. Springer, Singapore (2019). https://doi.org/10.1007/978-981-13-6447-1_77
7. Chen, J., Yang, L., Zhang, Y., Alber, M., Chen, D.Z.: Combining fully convolutional and recurrent neural networks for 3D biomedical image segmentation. In: Advances in Neural Information Processing Systems, pp. 3036–3044 (2016)
8. Efford, N.: Digital Image Processing: A Practical Introduction Using Java. Addison-Wesley Longman Publishing Co., Inc., Boston (2000)
9. Haque, H., Hashimoto, M., Uetake, N., Jin-zaki, M.: Semantic segmentation of thigh muscle using 2.5D deep learning network trained with limited datasets. arXiv:1911.09249 (2019)
10. Işın, A., Direkoğlu, C., Şah, M.: Review of MRI-based brain tumor image segmentation using deep learning methods. Procedia Comput. Sci. **102**, 317–324 (2016)
11. Isensee, F., Petersen, J., Kohl, S.A., Jäger, P.F., Maier-Hein, K.H.: nnU-Net: Breaking the spell on successful medical image segmentation. arXiv:1904.08128 (2019)

12. Johansen, J.S., Pedersen, M.A.: Medical image segmentation: a general u-net architecture and novel capsule network approaches. Master's thesis, NTNU (2019)
13. Perslev, M., Dam, E., Pai, A., Igel, C.: One network to segment them all: a general, lightweight system for accurate 3D medical image segmentation. In: Shen, Dinggang, et al. (eds.) MICCAI 2019. LNCS, vol. 11765, pp. 30–38. Springer, Cham (2019). https://doi.org/10.1007/978-3-030-32245-8_4
14. Poudel, R., Lamata, P., Montana, G.: Recurrent fully convolutional neural networks for multi-slice MRI cardiac segmentation. In: Zuluaga, M.A., Bhatia, K., Kainz, B., Moghari, M.H., Pace, D.F. (eds.) RAMBO/HVSMR -2016. LNCS, vol. 10129, pp. 83–94. Springer, Cham (2017). https://doi.org/10.1007/978-3-319-52280-7_8
15. Pal, N., Pal, S.: A review on image segmentation techniques. Pattern Recognit. **26**(9), 1277–1294 (1993)
16. Ronneberger, O., Fischer, P., Brox, T.: U-Net: convolutional networks for biomedical image segmentation. In: Navab, N., Hornegger, J., Wells, W.M., Frangi, A.F. (eds.) MICCAI 2015. LNCS, vol. 9351, pp. 234–241. Springer, Cham (2015). https://doi.org/10.1007/978-3-319-24574-4_28
17. Simpson, A.L., et al.: A large annotated medical image dataset for the development and evaluation of segmentation algorithms. arXiv:1902.09063 (2019)
18. Song, Y., Yan, H.: Image segmentation algorithms overview. arXiv:1707.02051 (2017)
19. Bakas, S., Akbari, H., Sotiras, A., Bilello, M., Rozycki, M., Kirby, J.S., et al.: Advancing the cancer genome atlas glioma MRI collections with expert segmentation labels and radiomic features. Nat. Sci. Data **4**, 170117 (2017). https://doi.org/10.1038/sdata.2017.117

Quantification of Epicardial Adipose Tissue in Low-Dose Computed Tomography Images

Mikhail Goncharov[1(✉)], Valeria Chernina[2], Maxim Pisov[1], Victor Gombolevskiy[2], Sergey Morozov[2], and Mikhail Belyaev[1]

[1] Skolkovo Institute of Science and Technology, Moscow, Russia
m.belyaev@skoltech.ru

[2] Research and Practical Clinical Center for Diagnostics and Telemedicine Technologies of the Moscow Health Care Department, Moscow, Russia

Abstract. The total volume of Epicardial Adipose Tissue (EAT) is a well-known independent early marker of coronary heart disease. Though several deep learning methods were proposed for CT-based EAT volume estimation with promising results recently, automatic EAT quantification on screening Low-Dose CT (LDCT) has not been studied. We first systematically investigate a deep-learning-based approach for EAT quantification on challenging noisy LDCT images using a large dataset consisting of 493 LDCT and 154 CT studies from 569 subjects. Our results demonstrate that (1) 3D U-net precisely segment the pericardium interior region (Dice score 0.95 ± 0.00); (2) postprocessing based on narrow 1-mm Gaussian filter does not require adjustments of EAT Hounsfield interval and leads to accurate estimation of EAT volume (Pearson's R 0.96 ± 0.01) comparing to CT-based manual EAT assessment for the same subjects.

Keywords: Epicardial fat · Low-dose CT · Deep learning

1 Introduction

Coronary heart disease (CHD) remains the leading cause of death and disability worldwide [8]. The primary pathological process leading to the development of CHD is coronary artery atherosclerosis, an inflammatory disease associated with lipid deposits in the vascular walls [1]. According to the results of the Multi-Ethnic Study of Atherosclerosis (MESA), the amount of adipose tissue surrounding the heart - pericardial adipose tissue - is an independent predictor of CHD [4]. Pericardial adipose tissue includes epicardial adipose tissue (EAT) located inside the pericardial contour and paracardial adipose tissue located outside and adjacent to the pericardium.

For a long time, CHD is asymptomatic and manifests at late stages with myocardial infarction or sudden death, so it is crucial to determine disease predictors even before the symptoms appear. The primary approach to addressing

R. Su et al. (Eds.): MICAD 2021, LNEE 784, pp. 98–107, 2022.
https://doi.org/10.1007/978-981-16-3880-0_11

this issue is the organization of mass preventive examinations. Since "large-scale screening" excludes the use of invasive diagnostic methods due to labor intensity, high cost, and risks of complications, the possibilities of noninvasive diagnostic techniques have attracted wide attention from the scientific community. EAT can be assessed by echocardiography (EchoCG), computed tomography (CT), and magnetic resonance imaging (MRI). EchoCG is not an optimal method to quantify EAT because of low reproducibility [9]. Cardiac MRI is an expensive and time-consuming procedure [5]. Traditionally, EAT is assessed by CT scan triggered by an electrocardiogram (ECG) with or without intravenous contrast agent [15]; non-ECG CT scan can also be used for EAT quantification as a reliable and reproducible predictor for CHD [17].

Recently, several deep-learning-based methods were proposed for EAT quantification for non-ECG-triggered CT scans. The majority of works consist of two steps: (1) pericardium delineation or segmentation of Pericardium Interior Region (PIR) segmentation followed by (2) estimation of EAT mask by simple thresholding of Hounsfield Units (HU). Also, a simple median filter is used for CT to suppress noise before thresholding in many works. A comprehensive approach with two convolutional neural networks was proposed in [2] and later replaced by a single multitask network in [3], subsequent work of the same authors. In both works, EAT quantification perfectly correlated with manual estimation (Pearson's R was 0.97). At the same time, a simpler 3D U-Net with attention was successfully used in [7] where authors reported Dice score 0.85 ± 0.05 for a small training sample of 40 subjects.

However, standard CT is associated with high radiation exposure and can not be used for screening. At the same time, as EAT reflects early signs of the disease, an automatic tool for a screening examination such as low-dose chest CT (LDCT) is required. To date, there have been only a few studies demonstrating the possibility of using non-ECG-gated low-dose chest CT for EAT volumetry [11, 19]. However, these studies use labor- and time-consuming semi-automatic techniques, which complicates their implementation within clinical settings. The previously described automatic technique had been validated only for standard ECG-gated CT, not used for screening [2]. Finally, despite substantial progress in researching CT-oriented methods, automatic LDCT-based EAT volumetry in screening patients remains highly relevant.

From the technical point of view, LDCT is much noisier than CT, and this difference may affect both abovementioned steps of the pipeline

1. Worse quality of images may result in deterioration of pericardium detection or PIR segmentation quality.
2. Presence of noise may make EAT mask estimation via thresholding more challenging. Besides, the difference in scanning protocol may result in a systematic shift of HU intensities, as was shown for EAT quantification in [12] where a modified upper HU threshold showed the best match with CT-based estimations.

We aim to study both effects systematically to validate the deep learning-based method's applicability for automatic estimation of EAT volume on LDCT.

Our contributions are as follows. **(1)** We first developed and tested a pipeline for EAT quantification in LDCT. **(2)** We show that a simple 3D Unet achieves the excellent quality of PIR segmentation approaching expert's variability. **(3)** We studied several post-processing approaches and identified that (a) popular median filtering results in a systematic shift of intensities and (b) a Gaussian filter with the standard EAT HU-range provides an excellent EAT estimation with Pearson's R 0.96 ± 0.01 comparing to CT-based manual EAT assessment for the same subjects.

2 Data

Our data includes standard-dose chest CT and LDCT; the latter images were collected within a lung cancer screening pilot [16]; the radiation dose for all cases is less than one mSv. Scanning with both CT types was performed on Toshiba Aquilion 64 (Canon medical systems, Japan), with a rotation time of 0.5 sec, slice thickness 1 mm, and convolution kernel (FC07, FC51). The main differences between CT and LDCT protocols were (1) voltage: 120 kV vs. 135 kV, (2) X-ray tube current: automatic tube modulation vs. up to 25 mA, and (3) radiation dose: 7–8 mSv vs. less than 1 mSv.

Some CT and LDCT images (see details below) were annotated in an in-house tool conceptually close to the methodology described in [13]. Ten radiologists annotated CT and LDCT images by drawing pericardium contours on axial slices with the help of inter-slice interpolation. At least two readers annotated every study.

We use four datasets to conduct computational experiments; see more details of its usage in Sect. 3.

- *Labeled-LDCT.* 415 annotated LDCT studies. The main training dataset.
- *Labeled-CT.* 76 annotated chest CT studies. An auxiliary dataset to compare pericardium interior segmentation quality for CT and LDCT images.
- *Unlabeled-Paired.* 57 non annotated pairs CT-LDCT; each pair consists of CT study and LDCT study collected from the same subject with no more than 60 days between studies. The primary dataset for experimenting with the second pipeline step - different postprocessing approaches.
- *Labeled-Paired.* 21 annotated pairs CT-LDCT prepared using the same approach as *Unlabeled-Paired.* Hold-out dataset designated exclusively for testing of final models.

Patients cohorts were selected carefully to guarantee zero intersections between datasets and avoid possible data leaks.

3 Experimental Setup

As discussed in Sect. 1, the authors of [2,3] split their method for estimating EAT volume in thoracic CT images into two following consecutive steps.

1. Segmentation of the interior region of the pericardium via CNN.
2. Postprocessing, which includes applying median filter with a 3×3 kernel size to each axial slice of the CT image and calculating the volume of the EAT thresholded as voxels inside pericardium with intensity in range $[l, u] = [-190, -30]$HU. We refer to this postprocessing step as *Median-Thresholding* (l, u).

We aim to adapt and validate this two-step approach in LDCT images. Therefore, we design our experiments as follows.

- First, we train and validate a CNN for PIR segmentation in both low-dose and full-dose CT images. As we show in Sect. 4, this network followed by *Median-Thresholding* $(-190, -30)$ successfully quantifies EAT volume in full-dose CT images. We describe details in Sect. 3.1.
- Then, we use the trained CNN to delineate pericardiums in both low-dose and full-dose CT images from the *Unlabeled-Paired* dataset. For each patient, we quantify EAT inside the predicted pericardium in the full-dose CT image using *Median-Thresholding* $(-190, -30)$. Taking these volumes as ground truth, we calibrate postprocessing step for estimating EAT volumes in the low-dose CT images. See details in Sect. 3.2.
- Finally, we test the CNN followed by the calibrated postprocessing in low-dose CT images from the *Labeled-Paired* dataset. As a ground truth we take EAT volumes calculated in full-dose CT images using manually annotated pericardiums and *Median-Thresholding* $(-190, -30)$.

3.1 Pericardium Interior Region Segmentation

Our network for segmentation of PIR has a 3D U-Net [18] architecture which is a de facto standard for medical image segmentation. We replace plain convolutional layers with residual blocks [6]. In upsampling branch of U-Net, we also replace transposed convolutions with simple trilinear interpolation.

We split all the images from *Labeled-CT* and *Labeled-LDCT* using 5-fold cross-validation in a stratified by dose (low or full) manner. For each split we train a single network on both low-dose and full-dose images. As mentioned in Sect. 2, patients in *Labeled-CT* and *Labeled-LDCT* datasets are unique and do not intersect with each other and with patients from *Unlabeled-Paired* and *Labeled-Paired* datasets. Therefore, training setup excludes overfitting to the validation and test sets.

Before feeding thoracic CT images to the network, we preprocess them in the following steps. First, we crop each axial CT slice to the bounding box of the pixels with intensities greater than -500 HU, which is in fact the body bounding box. Then, we trilinearly interpolate the cropped 3D image, such that resulting image has a $2 \times 2 \times 3$ mm^3 voxel spacing. Finally, we clip intensities to a $[-200, 200]$ HU window and scale them to the $[0, 1]$ range.

We train the network for 15k batches of size 3 using Adam optimizer [10] with default parameters and a learning rate of $3 \cdot 10^{-4}$. As a loss function we use a sum of binary cross entropy and dice loss [14] weighted by 0.1.

To assess the quality of pericardium prediction we calculate the average Dice scores between the network's predictions and the ground truth PIR masks, separately for low-dose and full-dose images, in each validation fold. In Sect. 4.1 we report the mean value and standard deviation of these Dice scores along 5 folds. Also, for each image, we calculate the average Dice score between multiple ground truth masks annotated by different radiologists. In Sect. 4.1 we report the mean values of these inter-rater Dice scores on the *Labeled-CT* and *Labeled-LDCT* datasets as a strong baseline for predictions' Dice scores.

Also, we assess the quality of EAT volume estimation in full-dose CT images using network's pericardium predictions and *Median-Thresholding* $(-190, -30)$. As a ground truth we use EAT volumes calculated using annotated ground truth pericardiums and *Median-Thresholding* $(-190, -30)$. As quality metrics we calculate mean absolute errors, and Pearson's correlation between predicted and ground truth volumes in each validation fold. In Sect. 4.1 we report the mean values and the standard deviations of these metrics along 5 folds. Also, we report the inter-rater mean absolute errors for the ground truth volumes in *Labeled-CT* dataset.

3.2 Postprocessing Calibration for LDCT

A postprocessing step takes a CT image and the PIR mask as inputs and aims to assign 1 to fat voxels inside pericardium, and 0 to other voxels. After that, EAT volume is calculated as a sum of positive voxels' volumes.

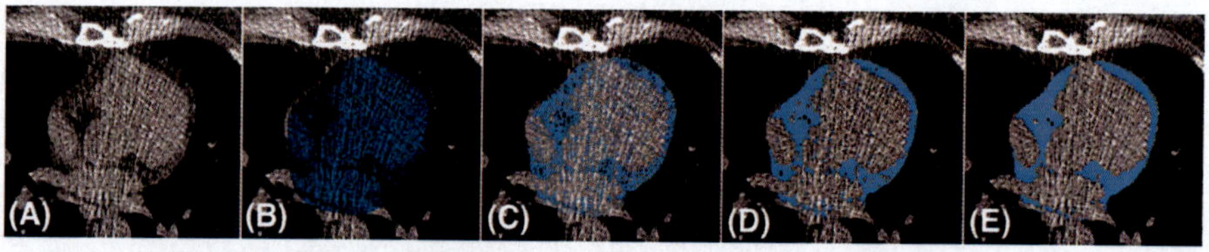

Fig. 1. From left to right: (A) - a patch of an axial low-dose CT slice containing the heart; (B) - the PIR mask predicted via 3D U-Net; (C), (D), and (E) - the fat voxels inside pericardium obtained via *Naïve-Thresholding* $(-190, -30)$, *Median-Thresholding* $(-190, -30)$, and *Gaussian-Thresholding* $(-190, -30, \sigma = 1 \text{ mm})$, correspondingly.

The most straightforward approach for postprocessing is to exclude voxels with the original CT intensity beyond range $[l, u]$ from the PIR. We refer to this approach as *Naïve-Thresholding* (l, u). However, it results in errors due to noise in CT images, especially low-dose CT images (see Fig. 1(C)). Therefore, in [2,3] authors apply *Median-Thresholding* $(-190, -30)$ as an attempt to eliminate noise effect. We take this approach as a gold standard for full-dose CT images, however, in Sect. 4 we show that it yields poor quality in low-dose CT images. Therefore, we need to adjust the postprocessing step for LDCT. In addition to *Naïve-Thresholding* (l, u) and *Median-Thresholding* (l, u) we also validate the

Gaussian-Thresholding (l, u, σ), which is applying the gaussian filtering with scale σ to the CT image, followed by thresholding voxels inside pericardium to $[l, u]$ range. The simple way to adjust all three aforementioned approaches is to calibrate the parameters (l, u).

To compare different approaches for postprocessing in LDCT, we use the *Unlabeled-Paired* dataset. We predict the PIR masks in both full-dose and low-dose image for each patient using the network described in Sect. 3.1. Then we apply *Median-Thresholding* $(-190, -30)$ to the PIR predictions in full-dose CT images and take the resulting volumes as a ground truth for each patient. After that, we apply *Naïve-Thresholding* (l, u), *Median-Thresholding* (l, u), and *Gaussian-Thresholding* (l, u, σ) for $\sigma \in \{1, 3\}$ mm, for $(l, u) \in \{-300, -290, \dots, -110, -100\} \times \{-70, -65, \dots, -15, -10\}$HU to the PIR predictions in LDCT images. For each postprocessing setup we calculate the mean absolute errors between the resulting volumes and the ground truth volumes. Thus, we choose the best setup for postprocessing in LDCT images to fit the ground truth volumes predicted in the corresponding CT images. The results of this calibration are described in Sect. 4.

3.3 EAT Quantification in LDCT

The proposed method for EAT volume estimation in LDCT images consists of PIR segmentation using the network described in Sect. 3.1 and the calibrated postprocessing described in Sect. 3.2.

To finally assess the quality of this method we use the *Labeled-Paired* dataset. For each patient we predict the EAT volume in LDCT image and calculate the ground truth EAT folume in full-dose CT image using the ground truth pericardium annotation and *Median-Thresholding* $(-190, -30)$, following [2,3]. In Sect. 4 we report the mean absolute error and Pearson's correlation between the predicted and ground truth volumes. Also, we report the inter-rater mean absolute errors for the ground truth volumes, as a strong baseline for the quality of EAT volume estimation in the *Labeled-Paired* dataset.

4 Results

4.1 Pericardium Interior Region Segmentation

In Table 1, we report the quality metrics for PIR segmentation in low-dose and full-dose CT images via the network described in Sect. 3.1. As seen, the quality in low-dose CT is as good as quality in full-dose CT. Also we show that the network's error achieves the inter-rater variability.

Also, in the first row of Table 2, we report the quality metrics for the EAT volume estimation in full-dose CT images via the network followed by *Median-Thresholding* $(-190, -30)$. Despite that volume prediction error substantially exceeds the inter-rater volume estimation, we obtained the same mean Pearson's R of 0.97 as authors of [3], and conclude that estimation of EAT volume in full-dose CT images is reliable.

Table 1. Pericardium interior region segmentation Dice scores. We used 5-fold cross-validation for the proposed approach; the numbers are presented as *mean (std)*. Inter-rater variability estimation is based on multiple annotations per image.

Dataset	Proposed	Inter-rater
Labeled-ULDCT	0.95(0.00)	0.95
Labeled-CT	0.95(0.00)	0.96

4.2 Postprocessing Calibration for LDCT

The mean absolute errors between predicted EAT volumes in low-dose and full-dose CT images for the same patients from *Unlabeled-Paired* dataset, for different LDCT-postprocessing setups, are shown in Fig. 2.

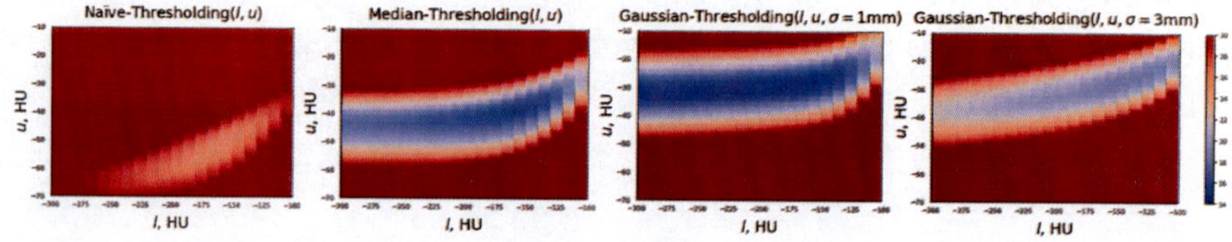

Fig. 2. The mean absolute errors maps on the grid of (l, v) values for the different postprocessing setups. Mean absolute errors are shown by color; colorbar values are given in milliliters.

Gaussian-Thresholding $(l, u, \sigma = 1$ mm) allows to achieve an optimal mean absolute error of 14.54 ml, when setting $(l, u) = (-170, -29)$, while setting the standard fat attenuation range $(l, u) = (-190, -30)$ yields mean absolute error of 14.58 ml. *Median-Thresholding* (l, u) yields the optimal mean absolute error of 15.54 ml, when setting $(l, u) = (-160, -39)$, which significantly differs from the standard range.

Both these optimums are comparable with the error between the unknown true and the predicted, taken as ground truth, EAT volumes in the CT image. Therefore, we cannot conclude that gaussian filtering allows to estimate the EAT volume in LDCT more accurately then median filtering. However, we give preference to the *Gaussian-Thresholding* $(-190, -30, \sigma = 1$ mm) postprocessing, because it achieves the optimal error, while keeping the standard thresholds for the fat voxels.

4.3 EAT Quantification in LDCT

In the second row of the Table 2 we report the quality metrics for the EAT volume estimation via the network, described in Sect. 3.1, followed by *Gaussian-Thresholding* $(-190, -30, \sigma = 1$ mm) postprocessing, chosen as a result of the calibration, described in Sect. 3.2 and Sect. 4.2. As seen, the proposed method achieves the same quality in low-dose CT and full-dose CT images.

Table 2. Epicardial Adipose Tissue quantification metrics. We report Mean Absolute Error (MAE) in milliliters, Pearson's R, and mean Bias between the predicted and the average manually estimated EAT volumes, as well as mean absolute error between multiple manually estimated volumes. The numbers are presented as *mean (std)*. The first row contains the metrics calculated using the 5-fold cross-validation on *Labeled-CT* dataset. The second row compares the network followed by *Gaussian-Thresholding* $(-190, -30, \sigma = 1$ mm) as a model for EAT quantification in LDCTs versus manual estimations in corresponding CTs from the *Labeled-Paired* dataset.

Dataset	EAT volume MAE, ml		Pearson's R	Bias, ml
	Proposed	Inter-rater		
Labeled-CT	14.45(3.14)	9.84	0.97(0.02)	−0.12(6.0)
Labeled-Paired	13.73(0.96)	7.6	0.96(0.01)	2.26(2.46)

5 Discussion

We studied automatic EAT quantification on LDCT images using a large database with more than 500 subjects. Despite poor image quality due to ultra-low dose (less than 1 ms), the proposed combination of classical 3D U-net and postprocessing achieves excellent results. The quality of automatic EAT quantification is almost equal to that for CTs images (Pearson's R 0.96 ± 0.01 and 0.97 ± 0.02 correspondingly). A slightly higher std for CTs can be explained by a much smaller number of full dose studies in the training set (415 vs 76). The obtained scores are aligned with findings in other studeis, e.g. see a large multicenter study [3] where Pearson's R 0.974 was reported.

Another interesting finding shows that a popular postprocessing approach based on the median filter may lead to a systematic shift in HU range of EAT voxels, whereas a Gaussian filter yields better results even within the standard $[-190, -30]$ range. It is important to note that this outcome depends on a particular LDCT protocol and may not be generalized to other protocols (for example, with voltage reduced to 100 kV).

Despite the high quality of the solution, the mean absolute error of our LDCT-based estimation is higher than inter-rater variability on CTs collected from the same subjects (14.45 ± 3.14 and 7.6, correspondingly). Due to several limitations of our study, we can not identify the key contributing factors. Among these limitations, we highlight the interval up to 60 days between the collection of CT and LDCT images for subjects from *Labeled Paired* which could result in systematic differences not related to change in CT dose.

Acknowledgments. This research was supported by the Russian Science Foundation grant 20-71-10134. Computational experiments were powered by Zhores, a super computer at Skolkovo Institute of Science and Technology [20].

References

1. Ambrose, J.A., Singh, M.: Pathophysiology of coronary artery disease leading to acute coronary syndromes. F1000prime reports 7 (2015)
2. Commandeur, F., et al.: Deep learning for quantification of epicardial and thoracic adipose tissue from non-contrast CT. IEEE Trans. Med. Imaging **37**(8), 1835–1846 (2018)
3. Commandeur, F., et al.: Fully automated CT quantification of epicardial adipose tissue by deep learning: a multicenter study. Radiol.: Artif. Intell. **1**(6), e190045 (2019)
4. Ding, J., et al.: The association of pericardial fat with incident coronary heart disease: the multi-ethnic study of atherosclerosis (MESA). Am. J. Clin. Nutr. **90**(3), 499–504 (2009)
5. Flüchter, S., et al.: Volumetric assessment of epicardial adipose tissue with cardiovascular magnetic resonance imaging. Obesity **15**(4), 870–878 (2007)
6. He, K., Zhang, X., Ren, S., Sun, J.: Deep residual learning for image recognition. In: Proceedings of the IEEE Conference on Computer Vision and Pattern Recognition, pp. 770–778 (2016)
7. He, X., et al.: Automatic epicardial fat segmentation in cardiac CT imaging using 3D deep attention U-Net. In: Medical Imaging 2020: Image Processing. vol. 11313, p. 113132D. International Society for Optics and Photonics (2020)
8. Khan, M.A., et al.: Global epidemiology of ischemic heart disease: results from the global burden of disease study. Cureus **12**(7) (2020)
9. Kim, B.J., et al.: Relationship of echocardiographic epicardial fat thickness and epicardial fat volume by computed tomography with coronary artery calcification: data from the Caesar study. Arch. Med. Res. **48**(4), 352–359 (2017)
10. Kingma, D.P., Ba, J.: Adam: a method for stochastic optimization. arXiv preprint arXiv:1412.6980 (2014)
11. Lee, K.C., Yong, H.S., Lee, J., Kang, E.Y., Na, J.O.: Is the epicardial adipose tissue area on non-ECG gated low-dose chest CT useful for predicting coronary atherosclerosis in an asymptomatic population considered for lung cancer screening? Eur. Radiol. **29**(2), 932–940 (2019)
12. Marwan, M., et al.: Quantification of epicardial adipose tissue by cardiac CT: influence of acquisition parameters and contrast enhancement. Eur. J. Radiol. **121**, 108732 (2019)
13. Militello, C., et al.: A semi-automatic approach for epicardial adipose tissue segmentation and quantification on cardiac CT scans. Comput. Biol. Med. **114**, 103424 (2019)
14. Milletari, F., Navab, N., Ahmadi, S.A.: V-net: fully convolutional neural networks for volumetric medical image segmentation. In: 2016 Fourth International Conference on 3D Vision (3DV), pp. 565–571. IEEE (2016)
15. Miyazawa, I., et al.: Change in pericardial fat volume and cardiovascular risk factors in a general population of Japanese men. Circul. J. CJ-18 (2018)
16. Morozov, S., et al.: Moscow screening: lung cancer screening with low-dose computed tomography. Problemy sotsial'noi gigieny, zdravookhraneniia i istorii meditsiny **27**(Special Issue), 630–636 (2019)
17. Nagayama, Y., et al.: Epicardial fat volume measured on nongated chest CT is a predictor of coronary artery disease. Eur. Radiol. **29**(7), 3638–3646 (2019)
18. Ronneberger, O., Fischer, P., Brox, T.: U-net: convolutional networks for biomedical image segmentation. In: International Conference on Medical Image Computing and Computer-Assisted Intervention, pp. 234–241. Springer (2015)

19. Simon-Yarza, I., Viteri-Ramírez, G., Saiz-Mendiguren, R., Slon-Roblero, P.J., Paramo, M., Bastarrika, G.: Feasibility of epicardial adipose tissue quantification in non-ECG-gated low-radiation-dose CT: comparison with prospectively ECG-gated cardiac CT. Acta Radiol. **53**(5), 536–540 (2012)
20. Zacharov, I., et al.: 'Zhores'-petaflops supercomputer for data-driven modeling, machine learning and artificial intelligence installed in Skolkovo institute of science and technology. Open Eng. **9**(1), 512–520 (2019)

Modulated Rotating Orthogonal Polarization Parametric Imaging, A Preliminary Study

Bozhi Liu[1], Jichuan Xiong[1], Juan Liu[1], Heng Zhang[1], Bin Xu[1], Lianping Hou[2], John H. Marsh[2], and Xuefeng Liu[1](✉)

[1] School of Electronic and Optical Engineering, Nanjing University of Science and Technology, 200 Xiaolingwei, Nanjing 210094, China

[2] James Watt School of Engineering, University of Glasgow, Glasgow G12 8QQ, UK

Abstract. We propose a new microscopic imaging technique in which the polarization angles of illumination light and a polarizer in front of the imaging sensor oriented orthogonally to the illumination polarization are rotated synchronously. A series of images of cervical cells was recorded under different illumination polarization angles and an algorithm was used to fit the pixel intensity variations of the images. A reconstruction method was employed to map the anisotropic properties of cervical cells in the form of a set of polarization parameters. Analysis of the images of the cervical cells and comparison with traditional methods indicate that this technique provides higher contrast and sensitivity.

Keywords: Orthogonal polarization · Polarization parameter · Cervical cell

1 Introduction

Orthogonal polarization imaging is a useful method for imaging superficial tissues such as microcirculation [1, 2]. Orthogonal polarization imaging uses linearly polarized light to illuminate the tissue and captures images through a linear polarizer that is oriented in the orthogonal polarization state. It prevents surface-reflected light and polarization-maintaining light from contributing to the recorded image [1–4]. This method can create high-contrast microvascular images and can be implemented in a small optical probe for clinical diagnosis. An improved technique called rotating orthogonal polarization difference imaging was subsequently introduced [5]. In this technique an orthogonal polarization image is captured and then the angles of the two polarizers are exchanged to obtain a second image. The images are processed to give a normalized orthogonal polarization difference image [(first − second)/(first + second)] that is free from surface reflection and sensitive to the polarization properties of the underlying tissue. This technique has been applied to image the tendon and results indicate that it has potential for analyzing the alignment of collagen. However, this approach does not provide direct quantification of the polarization properties. It has been found that modulating the polarization in the imaging system is usually beneficial in extracting quantitative parameters [6–9].

B. Liu and J. Xiong—Have contributed equally to this work.

R. Su et al. (Eds.): MICAD 2021, LNEE 784, pp. 108–115, 2022.
https://doi.org/10.1007/978-981-16-3880-0_12

In this paper, we present a new technique, namely modulated rotating orthogonal polarization parametric imaging, which utilizes the advantages of orthogonal polarization imaging and polarization modulation to generate higher contrast and signal-to-noise ratio images that can be used to quantify the polarization properties of a sample. The technique is based on a conventional orthogonal polarization imaging system but the illumination and detection polarization angles are rotated synchronously in defined steps over a range of 180°. Each corresponding pixel of the images recorded under different angles is fitted to an analytical function based on the Jones matrix to reconstruct a set of polarization parametric images. Experiments on cervical cells have been conducted and the results show that this technique can improve the contrast and resolution. This suggests that it is useful for characterizing superficial tissues in clinical diagnosis.

2 Experiment Setup and Data Processing

The system uses a conventional microscopic light path (Olympus BX51) with additional motorized rotating polarizers. The polarization of the incident light is modulated accurately with a rotating polarizer and reflected light from the sample is filtered through another synchronously rotating polarizer which is oriented orthogonally to the illumination polarizer. The motors and CCD camera are controlled by a computer, so the polarizers are rotated and images are recorded automatically during the process of image acquisition.

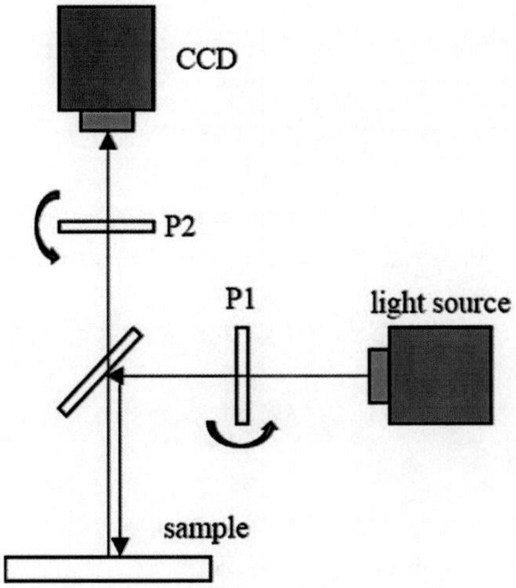

Fig. 1. Schematic of the experimental setup

As shown in Fig. 1, illumination light with a central wavelength of 532 nm is propagated through a linear polarizer P1, reflected by a beam-splitter and used to illuminate the sample. Surface reflected or polarization-maintaining light is rejected while multiple-scattered light passes through the linear polarizer that is always oriented in the orthogonal polarization state. Two orthogonally oriented linear polarizers P1 and P2 are driven by motors to rotate synchronously in angular steps of (π/N) and then the CCD camera (Basler acA2040-35gm) records an image for each step. The image size is 2448 × 2050 pixels and each pixel represents an area of 3.45 μm × 3.45 μm. The process is repeated n times over a range of π radians and N images are recorded.

First, consider the linear birefringence. When the two polarizers are rotated continuously, the intensity of the output light changes periodically. The Jones matrix of the elements in the optical path can be written as,

$$E_{out} = G_{P2} G_S G_{P1} E_{in} \tag{1}$$

$$G_{P1} E_{in} = \begin{pmatrix} \cos\theta \\ \sin\theta \end{pmatrix} \tag{2}$$

$$G_S = \begin{pmatrix} \cos\varphi & -\sin\varphi \\ \sin\varphi & \cos\varphi \end{pmatrix} \begin{pmatrix} 1 & 0 \\ 0 & e^{i\delta} \end{pmatrix} \begin{pmatrix} \cos\varphi & \sin\varphi \\ -\sin\varphi & \cos\varphi \end{pmatrix} \tag{3}$$

$$G_{P2} = \begin{pmatrix} \cos^2\left(\theta + \frac{\pi}{2}\right) & \frac{1}{2}\sin\left[2\left(\theta + \frac{\pi}{2}\right)\right] \\ \frac{1}{2}\sin\left[2\left(\theta + \frac{\pi}{2}\right)\right] & \sin^2\left(\theta + \frac{\pi}{2}\right) \end{pmatrix} \tag{4}$$

where θ is the angle of the polarizer P1. The sample is treated as a waveplate with δ as the phase retardance between the x and y components and φ as the rotation angle of the polarization ellipse. G_{P1}, G_{P2}, and G_{sample} are the Jones matrices of the polarizer P1, P2 and the sample respectively. E_{in} and E_{out} are the electric fields of light from the source and that incident on the CCD.

The intensity of the light incident on the CCD can be expressed as

$$I = E_{out} E_{out}^* = \frac{1}{2}\sin^2\left(\frac{\delta}{2}\right)(1 - \cos 4\varphi \cos 4\theta - \sin 4\varphi \sin 4\theta) \tag{5}$$

For the recorded images at certain limited number of angles θ_i in the experiment, the intensity also follows the expression in Eq. 6, only the variation is discrete,

$$I_i = k_0 + k_1 \cos 4\theta_i + k_2 \sin 4\theta_i \tag{6}$$

$$k_0 = \frac{1}{2}\sin^2\left(\frac{\delta}{2}\right),\ k_1 = -\frac{1}{2}\sin^2\left(\frac{\delta}{2}\right)\cos 4\varphi,\ k_2 = -\frac{1}{2}\sin^2\left(\frac{\delta}{2}\right)\sin 4\varphi \tag{7}$$

Second, consider the dichroism. The difference of absorptivity in different polarization directions introduces a component,

$$I_{D_i} = D\cos(2(\theta_i - \varphi_D)) = k_3 \cos 2\theta_i + k_4 \sin 2\theta_i \tag{8}$$

Here, φ_D represents the orientation of the dichroism, which means that the absorptivity is the lowest in this direction.

Finally, the intensity should follow the expression in Eq. 9,

$$I_i = k_0 + k_1 \cos 4\theta_i + k_2 \sin 4\theta_i + k_3 \cos 2\theta_i + k_4 \sin 2\theta_i \tag{9}$$

The coefficients k_i are calculated from

$$\begin{aligned} &k_0 = \sum_1^N I_i \frac{1}{N},\ k_1 = \sum_1^N I_i \frac{2}{N} \cos 4\theta_i,\ k_2 = \sum_1^N I_i \frac{2}{N} \sin 4\theta_i, \\ &k_3 = \sum_1^N I_i \frac{2}{N} \cos 2\theta_i,\ k_4 = \sum_1^N I_i \frac{2}{N} \sin 2\theta_i \end{aligned} \tag{10}$$

then the polarization parameters of the sample are calculated from

$$\cos\delta = 1 - 4k_0,\ \varphi = \frac{1}{4}\tan^{-1}\left(\frac{k_2}{k_1}\right),\ \varphi_D = \frac{1}{2}\tan^{-1}\left(\frac{k_4}{k_3}\right) \tag{11}$$

Expressions for calculating these parameters are retained in each of the corresponding pixels of the CCD and a series of parametric images can be formed with them, enables the polarization properties of the sample to be quantified.

During the measurement, the recorded images were first normalized before reconstruction. A new image $I_i'(x, y)$ was calculated for each recorded raw image $I_i(x, y)$,

$$I_i'(x, y) = \frac{I_i(x, y)}{\frac{2}{N}\sum_1^N I_i(x, y)} \tag{12}$$

This technique is compatible with the conventional orthogonal polarization imaging method because the recorded images at each rotation angle of the polarizers are equivalent to those of orthogonal polarization images, while any two pairs of images at different rotation angles θ and $\theta + 90°$ taken by this method can be used to create results of orthogonal polarization difference imaging.

3 Results and Discussion

As shown in Fig. 2, in reflection images using a conventional microscope, we can only observe the surface shape of the cervical cell because of the cell membrane. The inner structures, such as the endoplasmic reticulum composed of cytoplasm distributed outside the nucleus, can only observed in transmission imaging results as stripe net patterns. Also, it is difficult to observe the structure of the nucleus in either transmission or reflection.

The polarization parameter images cos δ, φ and φ_D of the same cervical cell were taken using the system described in Fig. 1. In this experiment, a 100× objective was used and 12 images were recorded ($N = 12$, $\Delta\theta = 15°$). The polarization parameter images cos δ, φ are shown in Fig. 3. For comparison, the polarization parameter images φ_D and orthogonal polarization difference image processed from the same set of raw data are shown in Fig. 4. They are all significantly different from reflection imaging results by conventional microscope.

Figures 3(a) and (b) are the polarization parameter images cos δ and φ, which are free from surface reflections and sensitive to the polarization properties of the sample. The cos δ parametric image provides more detail of the anisotropic optical property

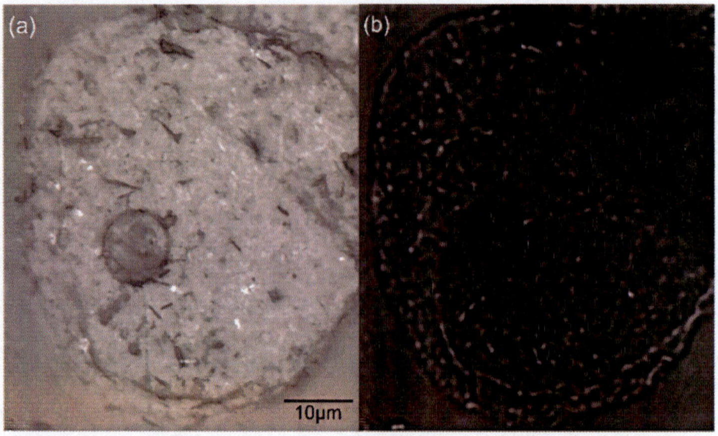

Fig. 2. (a) Reflection imaging results and (b) transmission imaging results by conventional microscope. Scale bar, 10 μm.

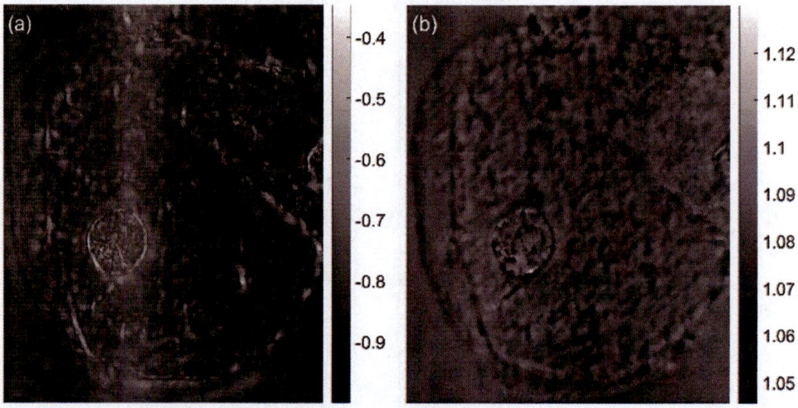

Fig. 3. (a) The polarization parameter image of cos δ; (b) the polarization parameter image of φ. Color bar, the range of value of different polarization parameters.

inside the cell with patterns corresponding to details of the endoplasmic reticulum in the transmission imaging result, which can help in determining the distribution of the cytoplasm in the cell. The edges of the nucleus in the cos δ parametric images are sharper than in other images, i.e. φ in Fig. 3(b) and conventional microscope images in Fig. 2, because the cos δ parameter image is not affected by initial polarization direction of the polarizers; photons back-scattered by nucleolemma are mainly collected and lead to different optical phase retardance from nearby areas.

Figure 4(a) is the orthogonal polarization difference image, which was calculated from the first and seventh images ($\Delta\theta = 90°$), i.e. $[(I_1 - I_7)/(I_1 + I_7)]$. Figure 4(b) is the φ_D parametric image, which is similar to Fig. 4(a), demonstrating that the φ_D parametric images also correspond to dichroism [5]. However, the initial polarization state of the polarizers will affect the orthogonal polarization difference image greatly, as the results

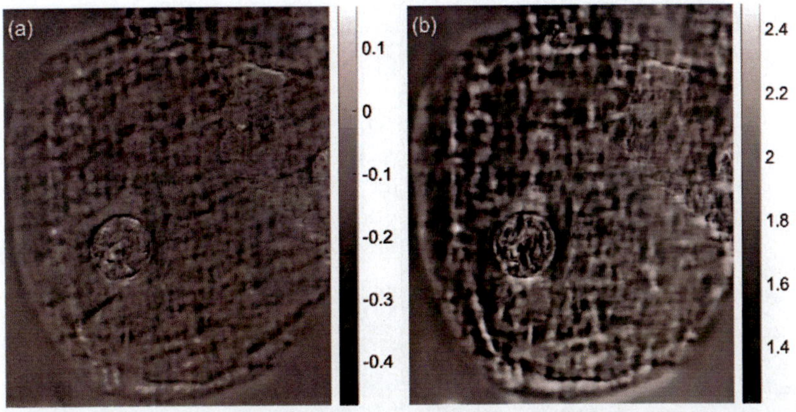

Fig. 4. (a) The orthogonal polarization difference image; (b) the polarization parameter images of φ_D. Color bar, the range of value of different polarization parameters.

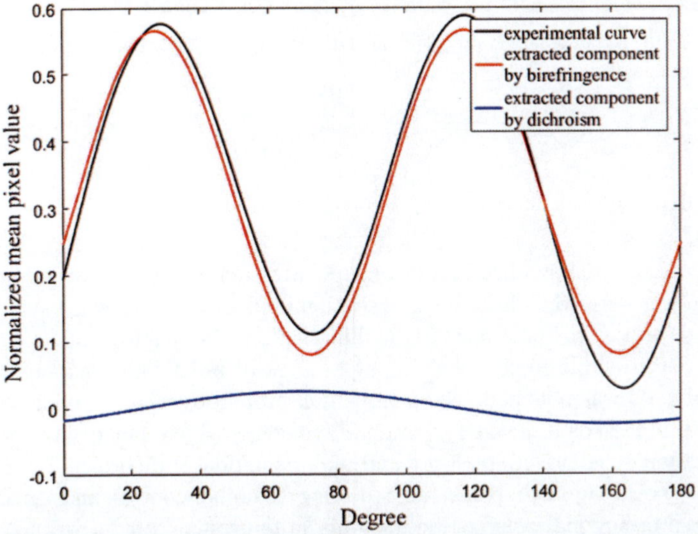

Fig. 5. The curves of normalized mean pixel value of raw images, and separated components caused by birefringence and dichroism which are used to calculate different polarization parameters

for different initial states are quite different. In our method, all the recorded images are used in the calculation; as is shown in Fig. 5, the phase of the component in the light intensity curve caused by dichroism of the sample is used to determine the orientation of the dichroism. Compared with the orthogonal polarization difference image which only uses two images with random initial states, the influence of the initial polarization direction of polarizer on the φ_D parameter image is far smaller. Besides, the φ_D parameter image has higher contrast and lower noise. The φ_D parameter image is believed to be related to the alignment of the fibrous structure, which can be used to map endoplasmic reticulum composed of cytoplasm inside the cell [5, 10].

The nucleus areas of the cells are compared in Fig. 6, using different imaging methods. In general, modulated rotating orthogonal polarization parametric imaging has significant advantages over traditional methods. This is due to the elimination of surface-reflections by the orthogonal polarizers and the polarization properties that are recovered as a result of rotating the modulation of the illumination polarization states.

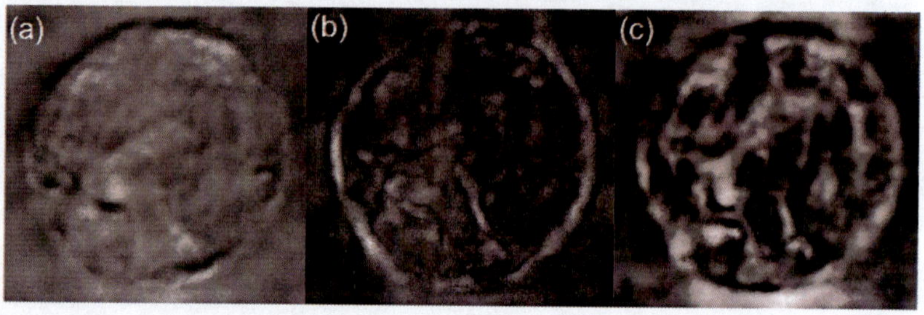

Fig. 6. (a) Orthogonal polarization difference image (b) cos δ parametric image and (c) φ_D parametric image of the nucleus, respectively.

4 Conclusion

We have developed a modulated orthogonal polarization parametric imaging technique. A function was derived to describe the variation in pixel intensity when synchronously rotating two orthogonal polarizers in the illumination and imaging optical path. By fitting each corresponding pixel of the images, a set of polarization parametric images of cervical cells was obtained. The polarization properties of the cervical cell can be retrieved from the cos δ, φ and φ_D parametric images, which quantify the phase retardance, rotation of polarization ellipse and the orientation of dichroism by the sample. The results show that the proposed method achieves higher contrast and sensitivity than conventional orthogonal polarization imaging. In future work, the performance of this method will be investigated comprehensively and utilized for imaging other cells and tissues.

Acknowledgement. This work was supported by the National Key Scientific Instruments and Equipment Development Project under Grant No. 61827814, Natural Science Foundation of Beijing Municipality under Grant No. Z190018, the Fundamental Research Funds for the Central Universities under Grant No. 30920010011 the Postdoctoral Foundation of Jiangsu Province under Grant No. 2020Z331, and the Ministry of Education collaborative project B17023. The authors would like to acknowledge support from the UK Engineering and Physical Sciences Research Council (Grant EP/R042578/1).

References

1. Groner, W., et al.: Orthogonal polarization spectral imaging: a new method for study of the microcirculation. Nat. Med. **5**, 1209–1212 (1999)
2. Černý, V., Turek, Z., Pařízková, R.: Orthogonal polarization spectral imaging. Physiol. Res. **56**, 141–147 (2007)
3. Morgan, S.P., Stockford, I.M.: Surface-reflection elimination in polarization imaging of superficial tissue. Opt. Lett. **28**, 114–116 (2003)
4. Zhu, Q., Stockford, I., Crowe, J., Morgan, S.: Experimental and theoretical evaluation of rotating orthogonal polarization imaging. J. Biomed. Opt. **14**(3), 034006 (2009). https://doi.org/10.1117/1.3130268
5. Morgan, S.P., Zhu, Q., Stockford, I.M., Crowe, J.A.: Rotating orthogonal polarization imaging. Optics Lett. **33**, 1503–1505 (2008)
6. Oldenbourg, R.: Polarized light microscopy: principles and practice. Cold Spring Harbor Protoc. **2013**, pdb-top078600 (2013)
7. Kaminsky, W., Claborn, K., Kahr, B.: Polarimetric imaging of crystals. Chem. Soc. Rev. **33**, 514–525 (2004)
8. Liao, R., Zeng, N., Jiang, X., Li, D., Yun, T., He, Y., Ma, H.: Rotating linear polarization imaging technique for anisotropic tissues. J. Biomed. Opt. **15**, 036014 (2010)
9. Ullah, K., Liu, X., Habib, M., Shen, Z.: Subwavelength far field imaging of nanoparticles with parametric indirect microscopic imaging. ACS Photonics **5**, 1388–1397 (2018)
10. Beach, D., Bustamante, C., Wells, K., Foucar, K.: Differential polarization imaging. III. Theory confirmation. Patterns of polymerization of hemoglobin S in red blood sickle cells. Biophys. J. **52**, 947–954 (1987)

Evaluating Mobile Tele-radiology Performance for the Task of Analyzing Lung Lesions on CT Images

Omer Kaya[1] (✉), Ezgi Kara[2], Ibrahim Inan[3], Erkan Kara[5], Miray Matur[4], and Albert Guvenis[2]

[1] Faculty of Medicine, Department of Radiology, Cukurova University, Adana, Turkey
[2] Institute of Biomedical Engineering, Bogazici University, Istanbul, Turkey
albert.guvenis@ieee.org
[3] Department of Radiology, Biruni University Hospital, Istanbul, Turkey
[4] Electrical and Electronics Engineering, Bogazici University, Istanbul, Turkey
miray.matur@boun.edu.tr
[5] Faculty of Medicine, Mustafa Kemal University, Hatay, Turkey

Abstract. The accurate detection of lung lesions as well as the precise measurement of their sizes on Computed Tomography (CT) images is known to be crucial for the response to therapy assessment of cancer patients. The goal of this study is to investigate the feasibility of using mobile tele-radiology for this task in order to improve efficiency in radiology. Lung CT Images were obtained from The Cancer Imaging Archive (TCIA). The Bland-Altman analysis method was used to compare and assess conventional radiology and mobile radiology based lesion size measurements. Percentage of correctly detected lesions at the right image locations was also recorded. Sizes of 183 lung lesions between 5 and 52 mm in CT images were measured by two experienced radiologists. Bland-Altman plots were drawn, and limits of agreements (LOA) were determined as 0.025 and 0.975 percentiles (−1.00, 0.00), (−1.39, 0.00). For lesions of 10 mm and higher, these intervals were found to be much smaller than the decision interval (−30% and + 20%) recommended by the RECIST 1.1 criteria. In average, observers accurately detected 98.2% of the total 271 lesions on the medical monitor, while they detected 92.8% of the nodules on the iPhone.

In conclusion, mobile tele-radiology can be a feasible alternative for the accurate measurement of lung lesions on CT images. A higher resolution display technology such as iPad may be preferred in order to detect new small <5 mm lesions more accurately. Further studies are needed to confirm these results with more mobile technologies and types of lesions.

Keywords: Lung CT · Lung lesions · Lesion size measurement · Tumor burden measurement · Measurement uncertainties · Tele-radiology · Bland-Altman method · Non-parametric method

R. Su et al. (Eds.): MICAD 2021, LNEE 784, pp. 116–123, 2022.
https://doi.org/10.1007/978-981-16-3880-0_13

1 Introduction

The accurate and precise measurement of lung lesions on Computed Tomography (CT) images is a challenging issue in cancer management [1]. Measurement guidelines have been developed for interpreting lung CT images used in cancer screening studies [2]. Lung lesion size measurement at the baseline CT image is necessary in assessing the likelihood of malignancy and in determining the algorithms to be used for follow-up. Changes in consecutive scans may indicate malignancy.

Lesion size determination on CT images is also required for assessing response to therapy [3]. Guidelines are in constant revision as new knowledge and needs emerge [4]. Lesion size is most commonly measured manually using electronic calipers, with the long and perpendicular short-axis being measured on two-dimensional images.

The different causes of uncertainties in lesion size measurement have been investigated and discussed in the literature [5, 6]. Uncertainties in technical factors are discussed and it is suggested that different image reconstructions may be necessary for visual and automated analysis. In [6], it was found that inter-observer variability can be substantial. The reproducibility with different observers has been found to be very low and therefore one recommendation has been for the consecutive measurements to be conducted by the same radiologist. Other uncertainties are related to imaging parameters such as imaging system hardware, software and image acquisition parameters, image display monitors and ambient light conditions. Patient motion has also been mentioned in the literature. However, to our knowledge, the effect of mobile tele-radiology on measurement uncertainty has not been addressed before. This may have a significant impact on decisions made in clinical practice.

The use of portable displays in tele-medicine practices is becoming increasingly important [7, 8]. Tele-radiology in particular has been shown to be feasible and is being used to increase healthcare efficiency. Recently a number of portable technologies such as laptops, tablets and smart phones have been evaluated for their suitability for tele-radiology [9]. It has also been pointed out that these technologies started to make a major impact in global health where cooperation between distant medical centers may become possible due to these advances in communication and portable technologies [10].

Motivated by these developments and the emerging needs of efficiency, our objective was to investigate the achievable performance in mobile tele-radiology using an iPhone in comparison with traditional radiology. The problem was considered primarily in the context of assessing the response to therapy using lung CT images. The findings may have important consequences in decision making when the initial radiologist is not available at the imaging site.

2 Materials and Methods

2.1 Patient Image Data

Data were imported from The Cancer Imaging Archive TCIA [11]. Details on CT scans can be found on the web site. TCIA is a service which anonymizes and stores a repository of acquired images of cancer patients available for research. Supporting data related to images such as patient outcomes, treatment details, TCIA collections are managed by

Washington University in St. Louis. Within TCIA, the LIDC-IDRI database contains diagnostic and lung cancer screening thoracic computed tomography (CT) scans with marked-up annotated lesions. 271 lesions between 3 and 51 mm were assembled. Of those, lesions less than 5 mm are often ill-defined on CT scans and have not been considered for measurement experiments. Overall 183 lesions were considered for the measurement studies. Images were obtained using different CT scanners, technique factors and slice thicknesses as described in [12, 13].

2.2 Experimental Design

The experiment was designed following the conditions established in [9]. The reading environment outside the reading room (<50 lx) was not uniform so that real-world conditions could be simulated. The measurements have been conducted by two radiologists from Ceyhan State Hospital, Adana and Biruni University Hospital, Istanbul. Radiant Digital Imaging and Communications in Medicine (DICOM) Viewer Version 4.1.16 was utilized to examine lung CT images on the Viewsonic VA2410-mh model DICOM calibrated PACS monitor. The monitor was of 1559 cm^2 size, made with LCD technology and had 1920 × 1080 image resolution.

A mobile DICOM viewer named Medfilm was used on the iPhone 6S model smartphone. The phone screen was of 60.9 cm^2 size, made with LCD technology, had 750 × 1334 image resolution and 16:9 aspect ratio (~326 ppi density). The iPhone was not DICOM calibrated. The technical specifications of the displays are summarized in Table 1. The images were shown in random order to two radiologists with at least seven years of experience. Data were produced by the radiologists who evaluated the images on each display with a time interval of three weeks. No time restriction was specified. The radiologists marked the detected lesions and their coordinates and measured their size.

Table 1. Technical specifications of displays

Specification	Viewsonic VA2410-mh	iPhone 6S
Monitor size	23.8 in.	4.7 in.
Technology	IPS technology TFT LCD	IPS technology LCD
Resolution	1920 × 1080	1334 × 750
Aspect ratio	16:9	16:9
Brightness	250 cd/m^2	500 cd/m^2
Contrast ratio	1000:1 (Typ)	1400:1 (Typ)

2.3 Statistical Analysis

The Bland-Altman method was used to analyze the results [14, 15]. An example analysis can be found in [15], where lung lesion size measurements in ultra-low-dose CT were compared to low dose CT by using two observers. Normality of data was assessed by using the Shapiro Wilk test as well as visually by inspecting the histograms. The limits of agreements (LOA) were defined as 0.025 and 0.975 percentiles. Variances were compared using the non-parametric squared ranks test. Excel 2013/16 and StatsDirect (version 16) were used for the statistical analysis.

3 Results

Measurement results are tabulated in Table 2. Shapiro Wilk normality test yielded $p < 0.0001$ for all four difference data for 183 lesions. Percentiles were therefore used for computing LOA's. The Bland-Altman plots can be seen in Fig. 2 (Fig. 1).

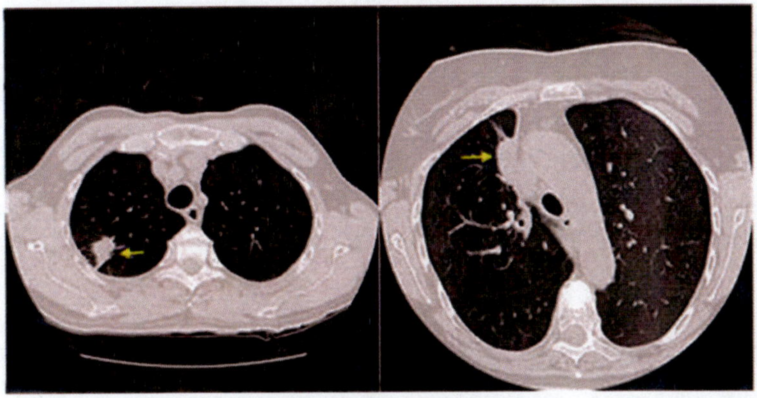

Fig. 1. Examples of lung CT scans and lesions[11].

Table 2. Statistics obtained from measurements (mm).

Differences	Mean	Standard Deviation (SD)	Median	Lower LOA[a]	Upper LOA	Length of Interval	Variance tests (p)[b]
PMM-O1	0.68	0.41	1.00	0.00	1.00	1.00	1–2 0.65 1–3 < 0.0001 1–4 < 0.0001
PMM-O2	0.67	0.39	0.70	0.00	1.39	1.39	2–3 < 0.0001 2–4 < 0.0001
O1O2-MM	−0.16	0.59	−0.10	−1.00	1.00	2.00	3–4 0.03
O1O2-P	−0.17	0.70	0.00	−1.50	1.00	2.50	-

LOA, Limits of Agreement; SD, Standard Deviation.
[a]Using 0.025 and 0.975 percentiles.
[b]p values based on the non-parametric squared ranks test. The unit is mm N = 183.

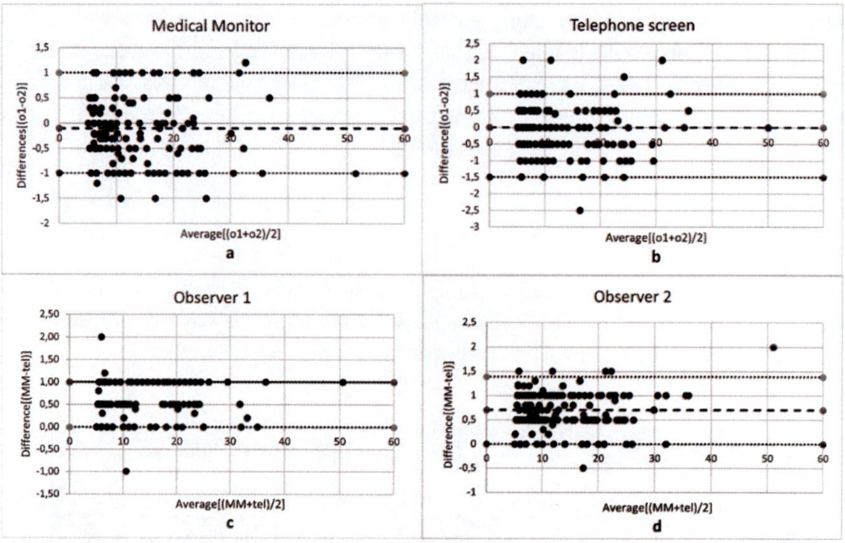

Fig. 2. Bland-Altman plots for the four measurement differences. a) Difference of observer readings for the iPhone b) Difference of observer readings for the medical monitor c) Difference of readings between displays for observer 1 d) Difference of readings between displays for observer 2. All values are in mm.

Observers accurately detected 98.2% of the 271 lesions on the medical monitor, while they detected 92.8% of the nodules on the iPhone. The undetected lesions were all under 5 mm.

4 Discussion

In this study, the performance of mobile tele-radiology using an iPhone for measuring lung lesion sizes has been investigated. Bland-Altman plots have been used to assess the agreement between measurements obtained in a radiology reading room and in a tele-radiology setting. Table 2 demonstrates that there is a small offset in the difference between the types of measurements. The bias between the two observer readings was found negligible for both displays. Standard deviations of differences between technologies and between observers can also be found in the same table. LOA's were calculated using percentiles. Nonparametric statistical tests were conducted for comparing variances. Several observations can be made based on these results:

1. The uncertainties and the bias do not seem to change significantly with tumor size within the chosen range.
2. For a lesion of 10 mm and higher, these uncertainty intervals for two readers (1, 1.39 mm) are quite smaller than the (−30%, 20%) or 5 mm interval for deciding stable disease (SD by the RECIST criteria for both readers [3, 16]. When considering typically larger lesions or the sum of several lesions, the decision interval becomes even higher such as 25 mm for a sum of 50 mm.

3. The standard deviations of errors and LOA intervals due to the difference between observers are higher than the standard deviations of errors and LOA intervals produced due to the difference in technologies for single observers (0.59 and 0.70 versus 0.41 and 0.39, $p < 0.001$ using the non-parametric squared ranks test) or LOA of 2–2.5 mm versus LOA of 1 and 1.39 mm extent). This implies that with each one observer, the use of iPhone (versus the use of the medical monitor) was found to produce less uncertainty than the one produced by two observers using a standard medical monitor. These results extend previous findings [5] that uncertainties produced by multiple observers can be larger compared to other measurement uncertainties.
4. The standard deviation of errors due to the difference between observers is somehow lower (by about 15%) for the medical monitor.
5. The bias due to change in technologies should be corrected when making measurements in order to obtain more accurate results.
6. Results show that in average, observers accurately detected 98.2% of the 271 lesions on the medical monitor, while they detected 92.8% of the nodules on the iPhone. This implies that the iPhone may present difficulties in detecting new small (<5 mm) lesions. A previous study on iPad in [17] had shown that lesion detectability can be satisfactory for these small lesions. Therefore, this study may prompt the use of larger and higher-resolution technologies such as an iPad for detecting these lesions.
7. The results obtained using two observers on the same technology show that for a minimally acceptable lesion of 10 mm and higher, LOA's (2, 2.50) mm are slightly closer to the (−30%, 20%) decision interval of 5 mm recommended by the RECIST criteria [3, 16]. This confirms the previously stated conclusion that readings by multiple observers consecutively are not recommended in assessing lung lesions [5].

To the best of our knowledge, this study is the first one to assess mobile tele-radiology for lesion measurement purposes using lung CT images. The previous study mentioned above [17] had shown that iPad is adequate for detecting these lesions. The two studies can indicate that mobile tele-radiology may be feasible.

The findings presented in this study may be important for consecutive readings of the same patient's images when the initial radiologist is not available. Tele-radiology can be seen as a practical solution to the shortage of radiologists in hospitals. Based on the above given findings, in these cases, it may be preferable to have the same radiologist perform the reading using a portable display outside the hospital rather than to have another radiologist perform that reading using a medical monitor.

This work provides a suspicion and early evidence that an even a non-DICOM portable display may produce a smaller uncertainty than the one potentially caused by multi-observer reading. DICOM calibration and the use of better/larger portable displays such as tablets can be expected to further reinforce these conclusions. In particular, tablets may enhance the detectability of small lesions.

Further studies, therefore can be beneficial with a higher number of radiologists and different types of medical displays, DICOM viewer software programs and types of portable displays which may greatly change from hospital to hospital.

5 Conclusions

In conclusion, mobile tele-radiology can be a potentially feasible alternative for the accurate measurement of lung lesions on CT images when needed. However, due to lower lesion detectability on the iPhone, a higher resolution display technology than iPhone such as an iPad may be necessary in order to detect new small <5 mm lesions accurately. Initial results also suggest that subsequent readings by the same radiologist with mobile tele-radiology may produce less uncertainty than readings by different observers on a medical monitor. These findings may have an important impact on decisions related to the use of mobile tele-radiology that aim to improve departmental efficiency. Further studies are needed to extend these results to other mobile technologies.

Acknowledgements. The authors acknowledge the National Cancer Institute and the Foundation for the National Institutes of Health, and their critical role in the creation of the free publicly available LIDC/IDRI Database used in this study.

References

1. Bankier, A.A., MacMahon, H., Goo, J.M., Rubin, G.D., Schaefer-Prokop, C.M., Naidich, D.P.: Recommendations for measuring pulmonary nodules at CT: a statement from the Fleischner Society. Radiology **285**(2), 584–600 (2017)
2. American College of Radiology. Lung CT Screening Reporting and Data System (Lung-RADS) (2014). http://www.acr.org/Quality-Safety/Resources/LungRADS. Accessed 20 May 2020
3. Lathrop, K., Kaklamani, V.: The response evaluation criteria in solid tumors (RECIST). In: Badve, S., Kumar, G.L. (eds.) Predictive Biomarkers in Oncology, pp. 501–511. Springer, Cham (2019). https://doi.org/10.1007/978-3-319-95228-4_46
4. Kuhl, C.K.: RECIST needs revision: a wake-up call for radiologists. Radiology **292**(1) (2019)
5. Yoon, S.H., Kim, K.W., Goo, J.M., Kim, D.W., Hahn, S.: Observer variability in RECIST-based tumor burden measurements: a meta-analysis. Eur. J. Cancer **53**, 5–15 (2016)
6. Dinkel, J., Khalilzadeh, O., Hintze, C., Fabel, M., Puderbach, M., Eichinger, M., et al.: Inter-observer reproducibility of semi-automatic tumor diameter measurement and volumetric analysis in patients with lung cancer. Lung Cancer **82**(1), 76–82 (2013)
7. Mendel, J., Lee, J.T., Dhiman, N., Swanson, J.A.: Humanitarian teleradiology. Curr. Radiol. Rep. **7**(6), 17 (2019)
8. Nicholas, J.L.: Technology-mediated education in global radiology: opportunities and challenges. Curr. Radiol. Rep. **7**(5), 1–6 (2019). https://doi.org/10.1007/s40134-019-0323-y
9. John, S., Poh, A.C., Lim, T.C., Chan, E.H.: The iPad tablet computer for mobile on-call radiology diagnosis? Auditing discrepancy in CT and MRI reporting. J. Digit. Imaging **25**(5), 628–634 (2012)
10. Krupinski, E.: Tele-radiology: current perspectives. Rep. Med. Imaging **7**(1), 5–14 (2014)
11. Armato, S.G., III: Data from LIDC-IDRI. The Cancer Imaging Archive (2015). https://doi.org/10.7937/K9/TCIA.2015.LO9QL9SX
12. Armato, S.G., 3rd., et al.: The lung image database consortium (LIDC) and image database resource initiative (IDRI): a completed reference database of lung nodules on CT scans. Med. Phys. **38**, 915–931 (2011). https://doi.org/10.1118/1.3528204

13. Clark, K., et al.: The cancer imaging archive (TCIA): maintaining and operating a public information repository. J. Digit. Imaging **26**(6), 1045–1057 (2013). https://doi.org/10.1007/s10278-013-9622-7
14. Bland, J.M., Altman, D.G.: Statistical methods for assessing agreement between two methods of clinical measurement. Int. J. Nurs. Stud. **47**(8), 931–936 (2010)
15. Sui, X., Meinel, F.G., Song, W., Xu, X., Wang, Z., Wang, Y., et al.: Detection and size measurements of pulmonary nodules in ultra-low-dose CT with iterative reconstruction compared to low dose CT. Eur. J. Radiol. **85**(3), 564–570 (2016)
16. Nishino, M.: New response evaluation criteria in solid tumors (RECIST) guidelines for advanced non–small cell lung cancer: comparison with original RECIST and impact on assessment of tumor response to targeted therapy. Am. J. Roentgenol. **195**(3), W221-8 (2010)
17. Faggioni, L., Neri, E., Sbragia, P., Angeli, S., Angeli, S., Bartolozzi, C.: Chest CT and the iPad2®: preliminary 2D assessment of pulmonary nodules. Presented at RSNA, 29 November 2011

Learning Transferable Features for Diagnosis of Breast Cancer from Histopathological Images

Maisun Mohamed Al Zorgani(✉), Irfan Mehmood, and Hassan Ugail

Faculty of Engineering Informatics, School of Media, Design and Technology, University of Bradford, Bradford, UK
M.M.S.AlZoragani@bradford.ac.uk

Abstract. Nowadays, there is no argument that deep learning algorithms provide impressive results in many applications of medical image analysis. However, data scarcity problem and its consequences are challenges in implementation of deep learning for the digital histopathology domain. Deep transfer learning is one of the possible solutions for these challenges. The method of off-the-shelf features extraction from pre-trained convolutional neural networks (CNNs) is one of the common deep transfer learning approaches. The architecture of deep CNNs has a significant role in the choice of the optimal learning transferable features to adopt for classifying the cancerous histopathological image. In this study, we have investigated three pre-trained CNNs on ImageNet dataset; ResNet-50, DenseNet-201 and ShuffleNet models for classifying the Breast Cancer Histopathology (BACH) Challenge 2018 dataset. The extracted deep features from these three models were utilised to train two machine learning classifiers; namely, the K-Nearest Neighbour (KNN) and Support Vector Machine (SVM) to classify the breast cancer grades. Four grades of breast cancer were presented in the BACH challenge dataset; these grades namely normal tissue, benign tumour, in-situ carcinoma and invasive carcinoma. The performance of the target classifiers was evaluated. Our experimental results showed that the extracted off-the-shelf features from DenseNet-201 model provide the best predictive accuracy using both SVM and KNN classifiers. They yielded the image-wise classification accuracy of 93.75% and 88.75% for SVM and KNN classifiers, respectively. These results indicate the high robustness of our proposed framework.

Keywords: Breast cancer · Deep transfer learning · Machine learning classifier · Histopathological image classification

1 Introduction

There are evidences that the breast cancer is higher death rates than other cancers that affecting women [1–3]. However, the diagnosis of breast cancer in the

R. Su et al. (Eds.): MICAD 2021, LNEE 784, pp. 124–133, 2022.
https://doi.org/10.1007/978-981-16-3880-0_14

early stages can improve the treatment as well increase patient survival rate [4]. Recently, the Hematoxylin and Eosin (H&E) stained samples of the breast tissue biopsy are inspected by using Whole Slide Imaging (WSI) scanners to determine any change in tissue. Coincided with the increasing use of WSI scanners for digitizing the histopathological slides, it becomes necessary to develop the conventional Computer-Aided Diagnosis (CAD) techniques for enhancing diagnostic efficiency as well as reducing diagnostic time and cost. The CAD techniques are aimed to assist the histopathologists with some of the tedious and laborious routine tasks. Hence, utilising CAD technique is reduced their workload and avoided the inter-observer variation among histopathologists that produces from manual extraction of specific visual features of tumour. This, in turn, results in better assessment outcomes and improved patient experience.

In the last few years, deep learning-based CAD systems have achieved impressive results in the several applications of histopathological image analysis. Whereas employing of such systems optimizes the diagnostic performance of cancer. The performance of traditional machine learning methods relies heavily on hand-crafted features, which can be greatly affected by the human bias. Furthermore, the field in-depth knowledge for the classification is necessary to select the useful features. In the hand-crafted techniques, the low-level features are only extracted from images. Whereas in deep learning techniques, the high-level abstract features are extracted automatically from images in a standardised way [5,6]. Hence, they deliver unbiased outcomes for dataset images [7]. The CNNs are type of the neural network architectures and the most popular in deep learning field. The CNNs have the ability to extract the hierarchy features of the image through their multiple layers [6]. These features can be learned hierarchically at multiple levels from lower to higher through network architecture. Multi-level abstraction makes the CNNs well suited for discovering the complex structures within high-dimensional data, such as WSI [7,8].

Although deep CNNs have achieved successfully performance in the digital histopathology domain, they have some unique challenges in their employment. They require the vast amount of labeled training images to learn their deep features. Currently, these labeled images are not being available; this is because pathologists consume a long time to collect them as well need the expertise to label them[7]. In contrast, training the CNNs by small amounts of training images leads to over-fitting and poorly generation of features [6]. The over-fitting is considered as a critical case when the training images have the high appearance variance, which is usually common in the histopathological images [7,8]. Furthermore, training CNNs from scratch consumes long time as well needs extensive memory resources and high computational cost.

The rest of paper is organized as; the related works is provided in Sect. 2. The methodology is explained in Sect. 3. The Experimental results are presented in Sect. 4. Lastly, Sect. 5 concludes the paper.

2 Related Works

This section reviews some of the works that participated in contest The Grand Challenge on Breast Cancer Histology (BACH) images, which is coordinated with the 15th International Conference on Image Analysis and Recognition (ICIAR 2018) [9]. There are two main parts were proposed in this challenge. The first part goal was to classifying H&E stained breast histophathological images into four classes: Normal tissue, benign tumor, in-situ carcinoma and invasive carcinoma. On the other hand, the second part goal was to segmenting the pixel-wise labeling WSIs. More information on the BACH Challenge Dataset can be found in the paper was published by Aresta et al. [10]. In this paper, we work on the first part, which composed 400 images with the same size (2048 × 1536 pixels) as well each of the four classes contains 100 labelled images.

Most of the proposed deep learning-based techniques are divided into two categories. One is based on deep transfer learning approaches to tackle the annotated training images scarcity challenge more effectively. The researchers in [11–16], fine-tuned the pre-trained CNNs as classifiers to identify the four grades of breast cancer histopathological images in the ICIAR 2018 dataset. Golatkar et al. [11] fed the fine-tuned Inception-V3 model by overlapping patches extracted from the original images, then got the final classification accuracy using majority voting. Gue et al. [12] fine-tuned two pre-trained GooLeNet models, then employed bagging technique, patch voting, hierarchy voting and merge module to improve the performance. Nawaz et al. [13] fed the fine-tuned AlexNet model by non-overlapping patches extracted from the original images. In the same way, Ferreira et al. [14] fine-tuned the Inception ResNet-V2 model, Mahbod et al. [15], fine-tuned ResNet architectures and Kwok [16] fine-tuned four Inception-Resnet-v2 as the classifiers.

The other proposed works [17–21] utilised the pre-trained CNNs as feature extractors, and then the extracted deep features were used to train the different classifiers to classify the four grades of breast cancer histopathological images in the ICIAR 2018 dataset. Cao et al. [17] combined the extracted deep features from six feature extractors to train the random forest classifier. Awan et al. [18], used the extracted deep features from ResNet-50 to train SVM classifiers, and then employed the majority-voting algorithm for final classification. Vang et al. [19] employed Inception- V3 model to generate the patch predictions which fed the ensemble classifiers. In recent years, Yan et al. [20] fine-tuned Inception-V3 model, and then extracted the patch feature vectors to fed Bidirectional Long Short-Term Memory network. Similarly, Kassani et al. [21] combined the extracted deep features from five feature extractors into single feature vector, which were used to trained their target classifier.

In this study, ResNet-50 [22], DenseNet-169 [23] and ShuffleNet [24] networks are employed as features extractors to tackle the lack of training images issue in ICIAR 2018 dataset; the SVM and KNN classifiers are utilised to identify the four classes of breast cancer histopathological images. Both classifiers are trained on the deep features that have been extracted from feature maps for global average pooling layer of three features extractors. Then, the predictive performance of different classifiers is compared.

3 Methodology

In this section, a brief explanation of the proposed framework is presented. Our framework architecture is based on off the-shelf feature extractors to extract the deep features, which then utilise to train the machine learning classifiers for predicting of breast cancer grades in ICIAR 2018 dataset.

3.1 Stain Normalisation Techniques

The stain normalisation of histopathological images is the first step to reduce the color variation and standardise the H&E stained images. Therefore, we stain normalise histopathological images of ICIAR 2018 dataset as described in [25]. Khan et al. [25] introduced the non-linear mapping approach to normalize of the H&E stain in breast histopathological images by using Image-Specific Color Deconvolution method. The difficulties we faced in an implementation of this technique is the choice of reference image. There is a stain normalisation toolbox [26] for many of the current techniques for histological images in the Warwick University website.

3.2 Data Augmentation

The optimum performance of CNNs depends on the amount of training images. As the ICIAR 2018 dataset is a small, hence the image augmentation technique is essential step to increase the training images number. In this paper, we have rotated the training images with angle of 180 degree, and then flipped them horizontally and vertically. As for the patches, we have rotated with angles of 90, 180, 270 degree and flipped in both directions. This is for purpose of enlarge the training images size without affecting on the quality of input images [27,28] as well as to avoid over-fitting problems [29] and features poorly generation.

3.3 Choice of Off The-Shelf Feature Extractors

Choice of the appropriate feature extractors for specific application is an essential step. In this work, we have investigated three pre-trained CNNs trained on ImageNet dataset [30]; Reset-50, DenseNet-201 and ShuffleNet models. ResNet (Residual Network) architecture uses skip connections to reduce the effect of vanishing gradient problem significantly. DenseNet architecture utilise the skip connections from each layer to the succeeding layers that promote reusing the features through entirety of the network. Whereas ShuffleNet architecture utilises the channel shuffle operation to overcome the consequences of using the group convolutions.

3.4 Proposed Framework Architecture

The proposed framework comprises of three models as illustrated in the Fig. 1.

- **Patch Model:** In this model, we divide each original image into twelve non-overlapping patches, each patch has a size of 512 × 512 pixels. We label these patches according to the main image label. We chose the patch size based on the image size (2048 × 1536 pixels), in which the partitions cover the whole input image to guarantee that the proposed model can learn the different features of images. Whereas, these features describe the overall tissue architecture and distinguish between classes. The proposed extractors are fed by these patches to extract the deep feature vectors from an average global layer. These vectors represent the local features of images and are utilised to train the target classifiers, which produce four-dimensional probability vector for each patch.
- **Global Model:** In this model, the proposed extractors are fed by the original images to extract the deep feature vectors from an average global layer. Whereas, these vectors represent the global features of images and are used to train the target classifiers, which produce four-dimensional probability vector for each image.
- **Hierarchy Voting Module:** In this module, the patch-level voting are placed after the patch model to select the specific prediction vector with highest probability. Whereas the global-level voting are placed at the end in our framework to get the final classification.

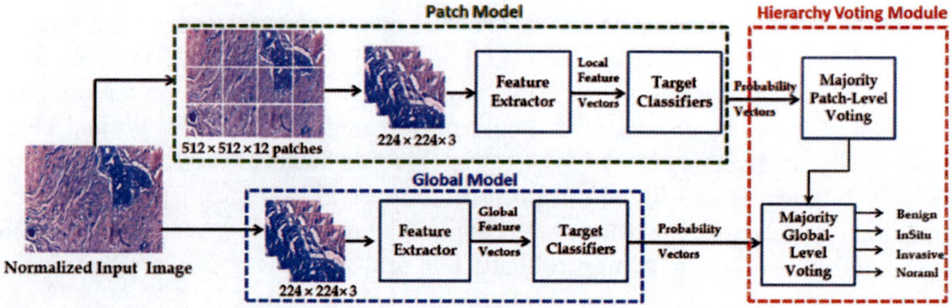

Fig. 1. Proposed framework architecture of image-wise classification. Feature extractor unit represents one of the three investigated CNNs; Reset-50, DenseNet-201 or ShuffleNet. Target Classifiers unit represents both KNN and SVM classifiers, which produces four-element probability vectors and each element represents probability of each class.

4 The Experiments and Their Results

Three experiments are carried out using ICIAR 2018 dataset images. In each experiment, one of the three CNN models is employed as feature extractor.

The deep feature vectors are extracted from the average global layers of ResNet-50 ($1 \times 1 \times 2048$), DenseNet-201($1 \times 1 \times 192$) and shuffleNet($1 \times 1 \times 544$) models. Subsequently, these vectors are utilised to train both target classifiers to identify the four classes of breast cancer. The experiments are implemented in MATLAB R2020a on a desktop computer has a CPU with a 3.60-GHz Intel®, Core-i7-7700, 16-GB RAM, and NVIDIA GeForce GTX 1070 GPU.

For patch model, the feature extractors are fed by a total number of 4800 patches, and then resized into ($224 \times 224 \times 3$) according to the input layer size of ResNet-50, DenseNet or ShuffleNet model. After that, the patches are divided into training 80% (3840 patches), and testing 20% (960 patches). Next, training patches are augmented. Then, they are ready to train the both target classifiers.

Similarly for global model, the feature extractors are fed by the original images, resized according to the input layer size for the three models. After that, the images are divided randomly into training set 80% (320 images) and testing set 20% (80 images). Next, training images are augmented. Then, they are ready to train both target classifiers.

For SVM classifier, we have employed an Error-Correcting Output Codes (ECOC) framework to classify four-class model. ECOC is a commonly used function to model a multi-class classification problem. We have assigned One-versus-one coding design of ECOC function. Escalera et al. [31] have demonstrated that ECOC function could improve the classification accuracy, even compared to the other multi-class models.

The 4×4 confusion matrices are utilised to represent prediction results of the four breast cancer grades in ICIAR 2018 dataset. The matrices are shown in Fig. 2, they composed on four rows and four columns representing number of classes, i.e. Benign, Insitu, Invasive and Normal. The results of target classifiers performance with different feature extractors are reported in the Table 1. The standard metrics (accuracy and recall) are used to evaluate the performance of different deep classifiers. These terms have derived from the confusion matrices and formulated in Eqs. 1 and 2 for multi-class classification, as in [32]. It can be seen from Table 1 that SVM classifier with DenseNet extractor is achieved the highest accuracy rate with 93.75%. In general, the accuracy rates of both classifiers that trained on the extracted features from DeseNet model are better than the other models.

$$Accuracy = \frac{1}{4}\sum_{i=1}^{L}\frac{tp_i + tn_i}{tp_i + fn_i + fp_i + tn_i}, \tag{1}$$

$$Recall = \frac{1}{4}\sum_{i=1}^{L}\frac{tp_i}{tp_i + fn_i}, \tag{2}$$

where tp_i is true positive for i^{th} class (i.e. correctly prediction to the class), fp_i is false positive for i^{th} class (i.e. wrongly prediction to the class), fn_i is false negative for i^{th} class (i.e. missed prediction to the class), tn_i is true negative for i^{th} class (i.e. correctly prediction not belong to the class).

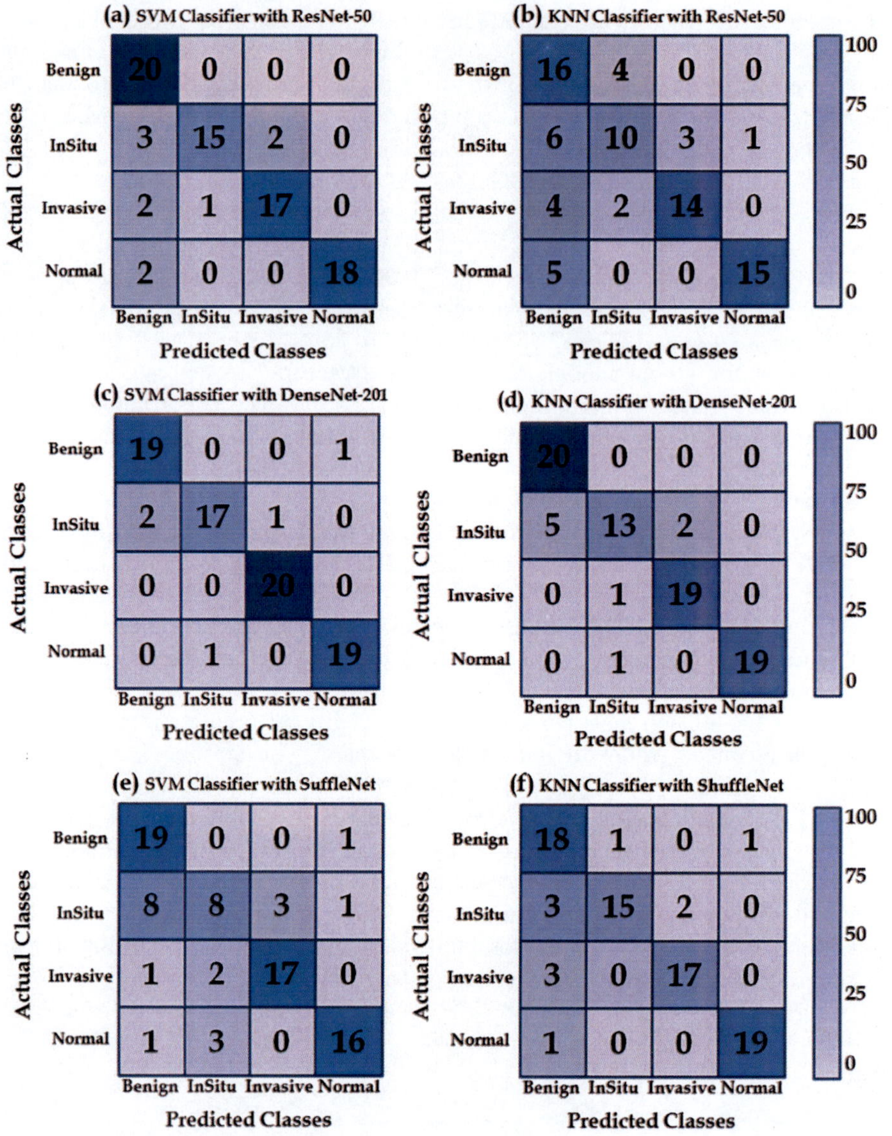

Fig. 2. Confusion matrices of the obtained prediction results using SVM and KNN classifiers.

By comparing the obtained results from our experiments with some of the previous works is reported in Table 2. It can be observed from Table 2 that the result of DenseNet architecture with SVM is the highest classification accuracy of 93.75%. While the result of DenseNet with KNN is an acceptable compared to the other results. It is 88.75% an accuracy rate. These results confirm that our method in term of classification accuracy outperforms the other methods that used the same dataset images.

Table 1. The standard metrics of target classifiers with different feature extractors

CNNs	ResNet50		DenseNet201		ShuffleNet	
	SVM	KNN	SVM	KNN	SVM	KNN
Accuracy (%)	68.75	87.50	**93.75**	88.75	70.00	86.25
Recall	0.7255	0.8932	**0.9379**	0.8929	0.7524	0.8756

Table 2. Performance comparison of the proposed framework with other methods

Methods	Accuracy (%)
[16]	79.00
[13]	81.25
[18]	83.00
[11]	85.00
[17]	87.10
[19]	87.50
[12]	87.50
[15]	88.50
Proposed DenseNet with KNN	88.75
[14]	90.00
[20]	91.30
[21]	92.50
Proposed DenseNet with SVM	**93.75**

5 Conclusion

In this study, we have investigated three off-the-shelf feature extractors to overcome the automated multi-classification challenges of breast cancer using histopathological image analysis. The off-the-shelf feature extractors are ResNet-50, DenseNet-201 and ShuffleNet models. We leveraged the generalization property that makes the extracted deep features have transferable to other applications [7]. The extracted deep features from the global average layer of feature extractors have been used to train both target classifiers. Therefore, generalizability property is especially useful when dataset is small and not enough for training the CNN from scratch, as in the ICIAR 2018 challenge dataset. From comparing the predictive performance of target classifiers, it is observed that the extracted deep features from DenseNet architecture are learned better than the other two architectures. Target classifiers that trained on these features outperform the other in terms of classification accuracy. Whereas, the SVM and KNN classifiers yield the classification accuracy of 93.75% and 88.75%, respectively.

Acknowledgements. The authors thank Dr. Aya Al Kabariti for her cooperation in illustrate some information on the histopathological images. She is Ph.D. student in Institute of Cancer Therapeutics, University of Bradford, Bradford, UK.

References

1. Bray, F., Ferlay, J., Soerjomataram, I., Siegel, R.L., Torre, L.A., Jemal, A.: Global cancer statistics 2018: GLOBOCAN estimates of incidence and mortality worldwide for 36 cancers in 185 countries. CA: Cancer J. Cli. **68**, 394–424 (2018)
2. Siegel, R.L., Miller, K.D., Jemal, A.: Cancer statistics, 2016. CA: A Cancer J. Clin. **66**, 7–30 (2016)
3. Ma, J., Jemal, A.: Breast cancer statistics. In: Breast Cancer Metastasis and Drug Resistance, pp. 1–18. Springer (2013)
4. Miller, K.D., et al.: Cancer treatment and survivorship statistics, CA: a cancer. J. Clin. **66**, 271–289 (2016)
5. Yosinski, J., Clune, J., Bengio, Y., Lipson, H.: How transferable are features in deep neural networks? In: Advances Neural Information Processing System, pp. 3320–3328 (2014)
6. Litjens, G., et al.: A survey on deep learning in medical image analysis. Med. Image Anal. **42**, 60–88 (2017)
7. Ravishankar, H., Sudhakar, P., Venkataramani, R., Thiruvenkadam, P., Babu, N., Vaidya, V.: Understanding the mechanisms of deep transfer learning for medical image. In: Deep Learning for Medical Applications, pp. 188–196. Springer (2016)
8. Bayramoglu, N., Heikkilä, J.: Transfer learning for cell nuclei classification in histopathology images. In: European Conference on Computer Vision, pp. 532–539. Springer (2016)
9. ICIAR 2018 Grand Challenge on Breast Cancer Histology (BACH) images. https://iciar2018-challenge.grand-challenge.org/. Accessed 23 Nov 2020
10. Aresta, G., et al.: Bach: grand challenge on breast cancer histology images. Med. Image Anal. **56**, 122–139 (2019)
11. Golatkar, A., Anand, D., Sethi, A.: Classification of breast cancer histology using deep learning. In: Proceedings of ICIAR 2018, pp. 837–844. Springer (2018)
12. Guo, Y., Dong, H., Song, F., Zhu, C., Liu, J.: Breast cancer histology image classification based on deep neural networks. In: Proceedings of ICIAR 2018, pp. 827–836. Springer (2018)
13. Nawaz, W., Ahmed, S., Tahir, A., Khan, H.A.: Classification of breast cancer histology images using AlexNet. In: Proceedings of ICIAR 2018, pp. 869–876. Springer (2018)
14. Ferreira, C., et al.: Classification of breast cancer histology images through transfer learning using a pre-trained inception Resnet V2. In: Proceedings of ICIAR 2018, pp. 763–770 (2018)
15. Mahbod, A., Ellinger, I., Ecker, R., Smedby, Ö., Wang, C.: Breast cancer histological image classification using fine-tuned deep network fusion. In: Proceedings of ICIAR 2018, pp. 75–762. Springer (2018)

16. Kwok, S.: Multiclass classification of breast cancer in whole-slide images. In: Proceedings of ICIAR 2018, Springer, pp. 931–940 (2018)
17. Cao, H., Bernard, S., Heutte, L., Sabourin, R.: Improve the performance of transfer learning without fine-tuning using dissimilarity-based multi-view learning for breast cancer histology images. In: Proceedings of ICIAR 2018, pp. 779–787. Springer (2018)
18. Awan, R., Koohbanani, N.A., Shaban, M., Lisowska, A., Rajpoot, N.: Context-aware learning using transferable features for classification of breast cancer histology images. In: Proceedings of ICIAR 2018, pp. 788–795. Springer (2018)
19. Vang, Y.S., Chen, Z., Xie, X.: Deep learning framework for multi-class breast cancer histology image classification. In: Proceedings of ICIAR 2018, pp. 91–92. Springer (2018)
20. Yan, R., et al.: Breast cancer histopathological image classification using a hybrid deep neural network. Methods **173**, 52–60 (2020)
21. Kassani, S., Kassani, P., Wesolowski, M., Schneider, K., Deters, R.: Breast cancer diagnosis with transfer learning and global pooling. In: Proceedings of ICTC 2019, IEEE, pp. 519–524 (2019)
22. He, K., Zhang, X., Ren, S., Sun, J.: Deep residual learning for image recognition. In: Proceedings of the IEEE Conference on Computer Vision and Pattern Recognition, Las Vegas, NV, USA, pp. 770–778 (2016)
23. Huang, G., Liu, Z., Van Der Maaten, L., Weinberger, K.: Densely connected convolutional networks. In: Proceedings of the IEEE Conference on Computer Vision and Pattern Recognition, pp. 4700–4708 (2017)
24. Zhang, X., Zhou, X., Lin, M., Sun, J. ShuffleNet: an extremely efficient convolutional neural network for mobile devices. In: Proceedings of the IEEE Conference on Computer Vision and Pattern Recognition, pp. 6848–6856 (2018)
25. Khan, A.M., Rajpoot, N., Treanor, D., Magee, D.A.: Nonlinear mapping approach to stain normalization in digital histopathology images using image-specific color deconvolution. IEEE Trans. Bio. Eng. **61**, 1729–1738 (2014)
26. Stain Normalisation Toolbox. https://warwick.ac.uk/fac/sci/dcs/research/tia/software/sntoolbox/. Accessed 12 Dec 2020
27. Mikołajczyk, A., Grochowski, M.: Data augmentation for improving deep learning in image classification problem. In: 2018 International Interdisciplinary PhD Workshop (IIPhDW), pp. 117–122 (2018)
28. Cireşan, D.C., Giusti, A., Gambardella, L.M., Schmidhuber, J.: Mitosis detection in breast cancer histology images with deep neural networks. In: International Conference on Medical Image Computing, pp. 411–418 (2013)
29. Shorten, C., Khoshgoftaar, T.M.: A survey on image data augmentation for deep learning. J. Big Data **6**(1), 60 (2019)
30. Russakovsky, O., et al.: ImageNet large scale visual recognition challenge. Int. J. Comput. Vis. **115**, 211–252 (2015)
31. Escalera, S., Pujol, O., Radeva, P.: Separability of ternary codes for sparse designs of error-correcting output codes. Pattern Recogn. Lett. **30**, 285–297 (2009)
32. Sokolova, M., Lapalme, G.: A systematic analysis of performance measures for classification tasks. J. Info. Pro. Manag. **45**, 427–437 (2009)

Improving Topology Consistency of Retinal Vessel Segmentation via a Double U-Net with Asymmetric Convolution

Xiaomin Li and Gengsheng Chen(✉)

State Key Laboratory of ASIC and System, Fudan University, No. 825 Zhangheng Road, Shanghai 201203, People's Republic of China
gschen@fudan.edu.cn

Abstract. Retinal vessel segmentation (RVS) plays a significant role in the diagnosis of ocular diseases, like diabetic retinopathy and glaucoma disease. However, many works have neglected keeping the topology consistency of the vascular segmentation, which is more crucial for the clinical diagnosis system. In this paper, we propose a double U-shape network to tackle this problem. The first U-Net architecture is DAS-UNet. With the help of the dense connectivity and the parallel atrous convolution (PAC) block, DAS-UNet can exploit various receptive fields to segment retinal vessel accurately. Through salient computing block (SCB), it can focus more on responsive regions and suppress uncorrelated regions. In addition, we add an auxiliary U-Net which adopts asymmetric convolutions to strengthen the kernel skeleton and correct the connectivity incoherence of retinal vessels. By exploiting the weighted Binary Cross Entropy loss (BCE loss), the double U-shape network can segment retinal vessels more accurately and improve the topological consistency of the segmented vessels. We tested the proposed network for accurate RVS task on DRIVE benchmark, which achieved the SOTA performance with a better segmentation results in terms of topology.

Keywords: Retinal vessel segmentation · Double U-Net · Asymmetric convolution · Topology consistency

1 Introduction

Retinal fundus assessment has been widely used in the diagnosis of ocular diseases such as diabetic retinopathy and glaucoma disease. However, manual segmentation requires experienced clinicians a large volume of time, bringing about low efficiency and high subjectivity. Therefore developing an automate diagnosis system based on computer vision methods can largely improve the efficacy of clinical diagnosis.

Retinal vessel segmentation (RVS) denotes a semantic segmentation task of labeling each pixel with its corresponding class, vessel or non-vessel regions. In recent years, deep neural networks (DNNs) have demonstrated near-radiologist performance in sematic segmentation tasks. Especially, the encoder-decoder structure, like U-Net [1] and its variants, provides a widely used framework for optic fundus assessment. Based on

R. Su et al. (Eds.): MICAD 2021, LNEE 784, pp. 134–144, 2022.
https://doi.org/10.1007/978-981-16-3880-0_15

the U-shape path of U-Net, coarse-to-fine information can be effectively incorporated to generate accurate segmentation results. In addition, feature propagation also gets improved via the skip connections of U-Net, which is especially suitable for medical image tasks with limited training samples.

However, the encoder-decoder structure is far from being flawless. Detailed information of retinal vessels has not been fully exploited because of its consecutive down-sampling operations in the contracting path. As a result, the accuracy of retinal vessel segmentation is degraded considerably. Several pioneer works tried to tackle this problem by designing more elaborate architectures. Zhang et al. [2] added a guided filter in the expanding path to transfer structural information and to reduce the negative influence of non-vessel regions. Xu et al. [3] used semantic aggregation blocks to extracted multi-scale features for an accurate retinal vessel segmentation. The above methods focused more on local information. To take global information into account, Wang et al. [4] proposed a non-local UNet based on the self-attention mechanism, using global aggregation blocks to capture long term dependencies instead of a very deep network. Zhang proposed a STD-UNet [5] to learn structural and textural information in a more rational way, which improved the performance significantly and excluded the human bias as far as possible. However, all their efforts tended to design more complicated architectures, by either introducing new sub-modules or by using different kinds of connections, which limited both the efficiency and effectiveness.

On the other hand, current DNN-based RVS methods are normally trained with pixel-level loss. For instance, the Binary Cross Entropy loss (BCE loss) is calculated by comparing the pixels between the predicted segmentation result and the ground truth, which treats all image pixels with equal importance. However, as the non-vessel region occupies more pixels than the vessel region, the pixel-level loss inclines to omit capillary vessel pixels occasionally.

Furthermore, retinal vessel varies largely in size. Capillary vessels may only occupy several pixels and main vessels may occupy dozens of pixels. The diameter imbalance increases the difficulty for segmenting retinal vessel accurately.

These studies mentioned above indicate that the whole vessel tree segmentation still remains a challenging task. Moreover, the segmented vessel tree often contains topological errors such as broken vessels and under-segmentation vessels. Consequently, more constraints are added during the training process, such as the local saliency loss [6], the boundary and entropy driven loss [7] and the topology ranking (TR) loss [8]. For instance, the topology ranking loss in TR-GAN can improve the topological connectivity of the segmented vessels by ranking the generated masks. These peer works indicate that adding more constraints to the loss function can improve the vascular topology effectively (Fig. 1).

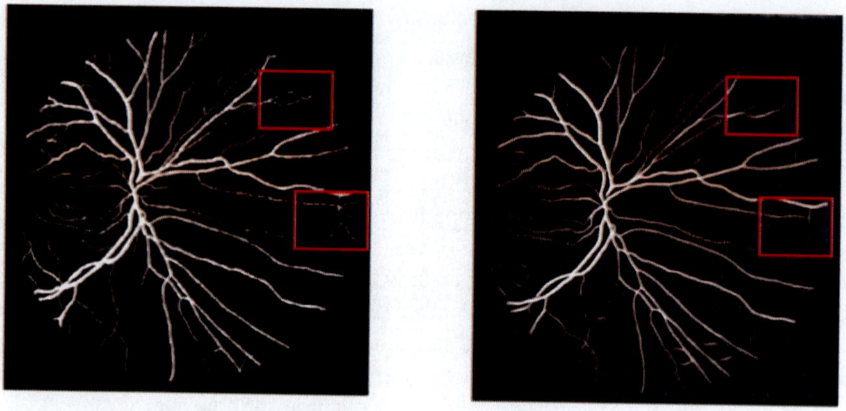

Fig. 1. Retinal vessel images and the corresponding topological errors.

In this paper, a double U-shape network combining two U-Net architectures is proposed. The first network is an improved U-Net architecture called DAS-UNet for an accurate retinal vessel segmentation. While using DAS-UNet as the backbone, another U-Net architecture employing asymmetric convolutions is added to elevate the topology consistency. This new double U-shape network can strengthen the kernel skeleton while at the same time helps to correct the connectivity incoherence.

The contributions of this work can be summarized as follows.

1) We design a double U-shape network which is capable of improving the topological consistency of the retinal vessel. The first DAS-UNet extracts multi-level features for accurate retinal vessel segmentation. The auxiliary AC-UNet focuses more on the weights of the kernel skeleton in order to strengthen the connectivity of retinal vessels.
2) We use the weighted BCE loss in the training process, which can combine the information extracted by the two architectures effectively to get the segmentation map with a better topological consistency.
3) We test the double U-shape network for retinal vessel segmentation task on DRIVE benchmark. The results demonstrated a better vascular continuity than the methods investigated in peer works.

2 Double U-Net for Retinal Vessel Segmentation

As illustrated in Fig. 2, the proposed Double U-shape network (Double U-Net) is comprised of two U-shape architectures. The first network (DAS-UNet) serves as the segmentation backbone. The second network (AC-UNet) is a traditional U-Net replacing all the convolution operation with asymmetric convolutions.

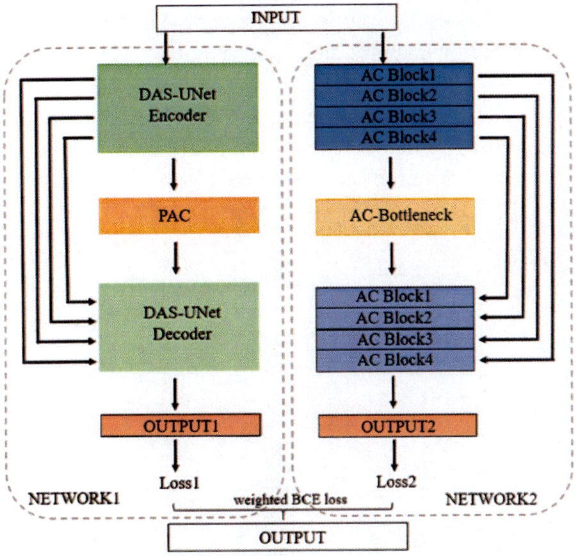

Fig. 2. The diagram of the proposed Double U-shape network.

2.1 Dense Atrous U-Net with Salient Computing

The design of DAS-UNet aims to extract multi-scale features of retinal vessels, thus we can segment main and capillary vessels simultaneously. As illustrated in Fig. 3, the proposed DAS-UNet uses U-Net as its backbone, improved by adding three major components: dense connectivity, parallel atrous convolution block and salient computing block.

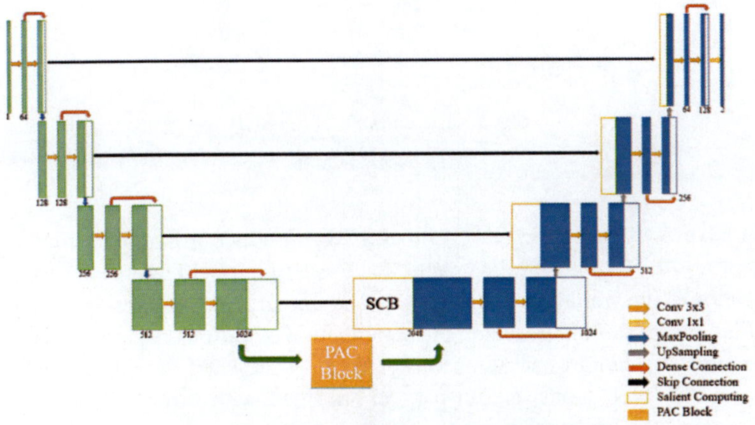

Fig. 3. The architecture of the DAS-UNet.

Dense Connectivity. Dense Convolutional Network (DenseNet) [9] connects the feature maps of all the preceding layers to their subsequent layers in order to ensure the information propagation. Motivated by DenseNet, we utilize dense connections to enhance feature propagation. The skip connections in DAS-UNet can assist the expanding path by feature reuse. By utilizing the benefits of both skip connections and dense connections, DAS-UNet can maximize the use of extracted features to generate elaborate retinal vessel tree.

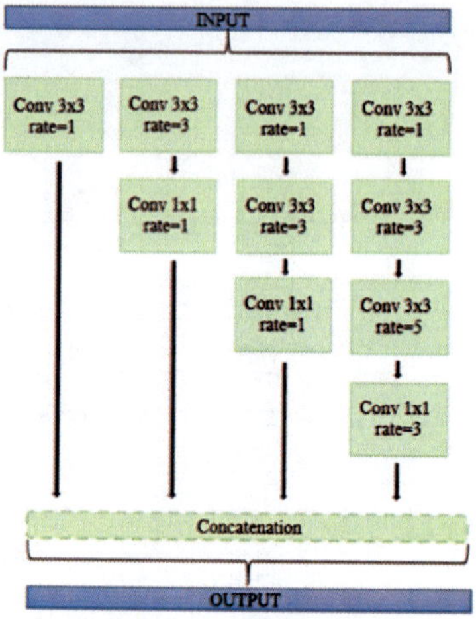

Fig. 4. The diagram of the PAC Block.

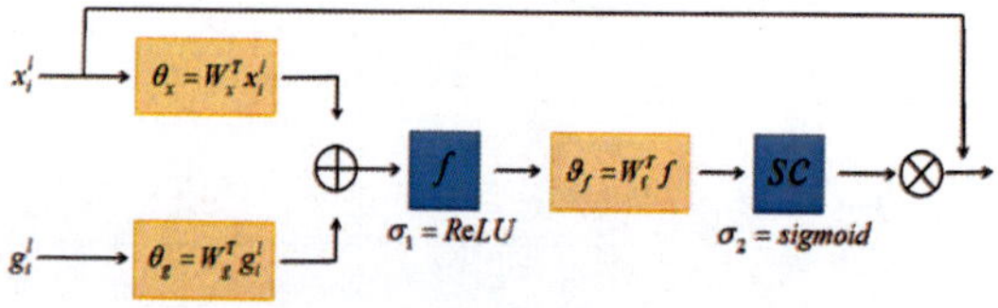

Fig. 5. The diagram of the SCB.

Parallel Atrous Convolution (PAC) Block. We introduce a parallel atrous convolution block to utilize multi-level semantic features. As global features are vital for the identification of the whole vascular structure and fine-grained features are indispensable for detailed segmentation. Based on the combination of various receptive fields, we can extract multi-level features simultaneously. Figure 4 indicates the diagram of our PAC Block. The PAC block consists four parallel branches, with various dilated rate ranges from 1 to 3 and 5. The outputs of the extracting path are fed into the PAC block to incorporate multi-level semantic features. Hence, we can get global and fine-grained features of retinal vessels by concatenating these branches on channels.

Salient Computing Block (SCB). In this study, highlighting responsive regions and suppressing uncorrelated activations are realized by introducing a salient computing block. The salient computing block is laid before the channel-wise concatenation in the expanding path. For illustration, the output of SCB can be expressed as follows:

$$\theta_x = W_x^T x_i^l \tag{1}$$

$$\theta_g = W_g^T g_i^l \tag{2}$$

$$f = \sigma_1(\theta_x + \theta_g) \tag{3}$$

$$\theta_f = W_f^T f \tag{4}$$

$$salient\_coefficient = \sigma_2 \theta_f \tag{5}$$

where x_i^l represents feature maps extracted from level l in the contracting path and g_i^l indicates the information extracted from the expanding path. The focus region f mainly depends on the contextual information of the two layers mentioned before. After the sigmoid activation, we can get the salient coefficient of the focus region f. As presented in Fig. 5, each pixel before concatenation has been weighted by the salient coefficient. Therefore, the output of SCB contains information from input feature maps and up-sampling feature maps, and its magnitude indicates the relevant significance of spatial pixels.

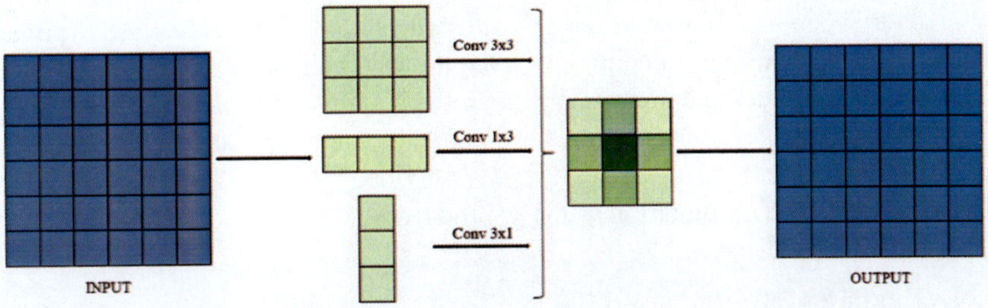

Fig. 6. The diagram of the ACB.

2.2 Asymmetric Convolution Module

The representative power of the convolution filter with a fixed size changes according to the position, which is observed in ACNet [10]. To be precise, the weights on the central cross position usually have a larger set of magnitude, which have a greater influence on the accuracy. The affiliation of 1D convolution kernels onto the central cross position can make the filter more powerful.

Hence, we replace all the convolution filters in the auxiliary AC-UNet with the asymmetric convolution block (ACB). As shown in Fig. 6, ACB comprises three layers with 3x3, 1x3 and 3x1 kernels concretely, and the output of each kernel are summed up. The advantage of ACB is that it can enrich the feature space and enhance the representative power of the traditional convolution filter without introducing any hyper-parameters during the training process.

2.3 Weighted Binary Cross Entropy Loss

We implement a weighted Binary Cross Entropy loss to exploit the information extracted from the double U-shape network effectively. DAS-UNet is capable of incorporating multi-level features and producing more accurate segmentation results, whose loss function is labeled as $loss_1$. AC-UNet works as an auxiliary network to improve the topological consistency, whose loss function is labeled as $loss_2$. The total loss function is expressed as:

$$l_{total} = \alpha loss_1 + \beta loss_2 \tag{6}$$

Where α and β represent the weights of the two networks. We have explored various combinations of weights, and setting $[\alpha, \beta] = [0.8, 0.2]$ achieves the best segmentation results.

3 Experiment

3.1 Dataset

We conduct the test of retinal vessel segmentation task on the public DRIVE [11] dataset. DRIVE dataset contains 40 fundus images with a resolution of 565×584. All the images are provided with pixel-level annotations from the Dutch diabetic retinopathy program, where 7 of them contain pathology. The dataset is equally split into 10 training images and 10 test images. For the training dataset, each image is provided with one manual annotation. For the test dataset, each image is provided with two annotations. We both utilize the first expert's annotation as the ground truth.

3.2 Evaluation Metrics

We evaluate the proposed method by calculating 4 widely used metrics for the performance of RVS task, including accuracy (Acc), sensitivity (Sen), specificity (Spe) and the area under curve (AUC).

True Positive (TP) indicates the annotated vessel regions which are segmented as vessel pixels and False Negative (FN) denotes those which are mis-classified as non-vessel pixels. In a similar way, True Negative (TN) means the annotated non-vessel regions are segmented as non-vessel pixels and False Positive (FP) denotes those which are mis-classified as vessel pixels. Thus, the evaluation metrics can be calculated as follows:

$$\text{Acc} = \frac{TP + TN}{TP + TN + FP + FN} \tag{7}$$

$$\text{Sen} = \frac{TP}{TP + FN} \tag{8}$$

$$\text{Spe} = \frac{TN}{TN + FP} \tag{9}$$

In order to evaluate the topology quality of retinal vessels, we use the metrics which are first used for road extraction [12]. Evaluation metrics are computed in the following way:

1) Sample two points which lie both on the ground truth and on the retinal vessel segmentation map randomly.
2) Calculate the length between the two points and check whether the two paths have the same length.
3) If such path does not exist, the prediction is classified as infeasible (INF). If the two paths have the same length, the prediction is classified as correct (COR), otherwise it is classified as a wrong path.

It stands to reason that more correct paths and less infeasible paths indicate a better topological coherence on the segmented retinal vessels.

3.3 Ablation Study

Compared with the baseline U-Net architecture, DAS-UNet can achieve a better segmentation result. Table 1 illustrates the performance of DAS-UNet, Sen = 0.7899, Spe = 0.9916, Acc = 0.9563, and AUC = 0.9796 respectively.

It is notable that the segmentation results of DAS-UNet are more similar to the ground truth, as depicted in Fig. 7. It has a cleaner segmentation map with less fake vessels in the background. We finally get the vessel tree with both main and capillary vessels, which is more suitable for accurate retinal vessel segmentation.

Table 1. Ablation study of DAS-UNet.

Architecture	Sen	Spe	Acc	AUC
UNet	0.7565	0.9823	0.9517	0.9757
UNet + DC	0.7520	0.9879	0.9536	0.9774
UNet + DC + PAC	0.7549	0.9912	0.9552	0.9785
UNet + DC + PAC + SCB	0.7899	0.9916	0.9563	0.9796

3.4 Comparison Results

We also compare the proposed double U-shape network with other leading methods. Ara et al. [12] improved the encoder-decoder structure by stacking a variational auto-encoder

(VAE) to improve the topological consistence of retinal vessels. Xu et al. [13] designed a semantics-guided network in a recursive way, which can enhance the connectivity whit no extra parameters. To the best of our knowledge, they are the only two works which study the topological consistency of retinal vessels.

The results are listed in Table 2. We can see that our double U-shape network can achieve a decrease of INF to 17.6%, and an increases of COR to 68.4%. The results indicate that the proposed double U-shape network achieves the best performance on the topological consistency of retinal vessel segmentation, which outperforms the other 2 leading methods by 11.5% and 9.8% respectively. Finally, we demonstrate examples of our double U-shape network with a better topological structure, as presented in Fig. 7.

Table 2. Comparison with other leading methods.

Methods	Year	AUC	Sen	Spe	INF	COR
Oliveira et al. [14]	2018	**0.982**	0.804	0.980	0.437	0.489
Ara et al. [12]	2019	0.979	0.897	0.953	0.291	0.612
Xu et al. [3]	2020	0.980	0.795	**0.981**	0.539	0.387
Xu et al. [13]	2020	0.981	0.912	0.947	0.274	0.633
Proposed	2021	0.979	**0.951**	0.907	**0.176**	**0.684**

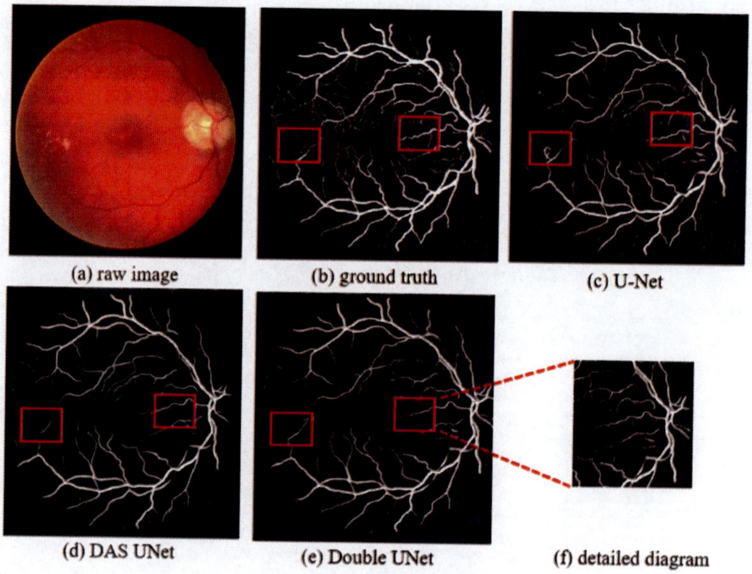

Fig. 7. Comparison results on DRIVE dataset.

4 Conclusion

In this paper, we analyze the limitations of clinical RVS task and propose a double U-shape network to improve the topology consistence. The first network (DAS-UNet) is a dense-atrous U-Net with salient computing, which can extract multi-level features for accurate retinal vessel segmentation. The second network (AC-UNet) is a traditional U-Net with asymmetric convolutions, which is capable of strengthening the kernel skeleton and correcting the connectivity incoherence of retinal vessels. Experiment results conveys that the proposed double U-shape network can achieve a better topology coherence by predicting more correct paths and less infeasible paths without degrading the overall accuracy.

In the future, we will investigate how to accelerate the computing and speed up the inference time, make it more suitable for clinical diagnosis of ocular disease.

References

1. Ronneberger, O., Fischer, P., Brox, T.: U-Net: convolutional networks for biomedical image segmentation. In: Navab, N., Hornegger, J., Wells, W.M., Frangi, A.F. (eds.) MICCAI 2015. LNCS, vol. 9351, pp. 234–241. Springer, Cham (2015). https://doi.org/10.1007/978-3-319-24574-4_28
2. Zhang, S., et al.: Attention guided network for retinal image segmentation. In: Shen, D., et al. (eds.) MICCAI 2019. LNCS, vol. 11764, pp. 797–805. Springer, Cham (2019). https://doi.org/10.1007/978-3-030-32239-7_88
3. Xu, R., Ye, X., Jiang, G., Liu, T., Tanaka, S.: Vessel segmentation via a semantics and multi-scale aggregation network. In: International Conference on Acoustics, Speech and Signal Processing (ICASSP), pp. 1085–1089 (2020)
4. Wang, Z., Zou, N., Shen, D., Ji, S.: Non-local U-Nets for biomedical image segmentation. In: AAAI Conference on Artificial Intelligence, pp. 6315–6322 (2020)
5. Zhang, S., Fu, H., Xu, Y., Liu, Y., Tan, M.: Retinal image segmentation with a structure-texture demixing network. In: Martel, A.L., et al. (eds.) MICCAI 2020. LNCS, vol. 12265, pp. 765–774. Springer, Cham (2020). https://doi.org/10.1007/978-3-030-59722-1_74
6. Mahapatra, D.: Retinal vasculature segmentation using local saliency maps and generative adversarial networks for image super resolution. In: Medical Image Computing and Computer-Assisted Intervention (MICCAI), pp. 242–250 (2017)
7. Wang, S., Yu, L., Li, K., Yang, X., Fu, C.-W., Heng, P.-A.: Boundary and entropy-driven adversarial learning for fundus image segmentation. In: Shen, D., et al. (eds.) MICCAI 2019. LNCS, vol. 11764, pp. 102–110. Springer, Cham (2019). https://doi.org/10.1007/978-3-030-32239-7_12
8. Chen, W., et al.: TR-GAN: topology ranking GAN with triplet loss for retinal artery/vein classification. In: Martel, A.L., et al. (eds.) MICCAI 2020. LNCS, vol. 12265, pp. 616–625. Springer, Cham (2020). https://doi.org/10.1007/978-3-030-59722-1_59
9. Huang, G., Liu, Z., Van Der Maaten, L.: Densely connected convolutional networks. In: Computer Vision and Pattern Recognition (CVPR), pp. 2261–2269 (2017)
10. Ding, X., Guo, Y., Din, G.: ACNet: strengthening the kernel skeletons for powerful CNN via asymmetric convolution blocks. In: International Conference on Computer Vision (ICCV), pp. 1911–1920 (2019)
11. Staal, J., Abramoff, M.D., Niemeijer, M.: Ridge-based vessel segmentation in color images of the retina. Trans. Med. Imaging (TMI) **23**(4), 501–509 (2004)

12. Araújo, R.J., Cardoso, J.S., Oliveira, H.P.: A deep learning design for improving topology coherence in blood vessel segmentation. In: Shen, D., et al. (eds.) MICCAI 2019. LNCS, vol. 11764, pp. 93–101. Springer, Cham (2019). https://doi.org/10.1007/978-3-030-32239-7_11
13. Xu, R., Liu, T., Ye, X., Lin, L., Chen, Y.-W.: Boosting connectivity in retinal vessel segmentation via a recursive semantics-guided network. In: Martel, A.L., et al. (eds.) MICCAI 2020. LNCS, vol. 12265, pp. 786–795. Springer, Cham (2020). https://doi.org/10.1007/978-3-030-59722-1_76
14. Oliveira, A., Pereira, S., Silva, C.A.: Retinal vessel segmentation based on fully convolutional neural networks. Expert Syst. Appl. **112**, 229–242 (2018)

The CT Liver Image Segmentation Based on RTV and GMM

Yueqin Dun[1(✉)] and Yu Kong[2]

[1] School of Electrical Engineering, University of Jinan, Jinan, Shandong, China
cse_dunyq@ujn.edu.cn
[2] Shandong Medical College, 5460 Erhuananlu, Jinan, Shandong, China
kongy@sdmcjn.edu.cn

Abstract. The accurate medical image segmentation can help doctors to improve disease diagnosis and treatment. How to achieve the accurate segmentation results depends on the image preprocessing and segmentation algorithm. Traditional filtering methods can erase the noise of the image, but the contrast of the boundaries between different tissues is also weakened at the same time. While the Relative Total Variation method can better filter out the noise and keep the contrast of the boundaries, which plays an important role for improving the accuracy of the threshold segmentation. The Gaussian mixture model is used to segment the CT liver images based on the Gaussian filter and the RTV filter, respectively. The experiment results are compared, and it is verified that the segmentation result based on Gaussian filter is much better than that based on Relative Total Variation filter.

Keywords: Image segmentation · Relative total variation · Gaussian mixture model

1 Introduction

With the explosive growth of the number of medical images, medical image processing technology plays a more and more important role in the field of medical disease diagnosis and treatment. As a main branch of medical research, medical image segmentation has extensive research and application value, such as clinical diagnosis, pathological analysis, surgical planning, computer-assisted surgery and other medical research.

The research and application fields of medical image segmentation are mainly focus on the following five aspects: (1) Extracting the interest region for medical image analysis and recognition. Such as medical image registration and fusion of different forms or sources, quantitative measurement of anatomical structure, movement tracking and synchronization of organs, etc. (2) Measuring the size or volume of human organs, tissues or lesions. Quantitative measurement and analysis of relevant imaging before and after treatment will help doctors to diagnose, follow up or revise the treatment plan for patients; (3) Three-dimensional reconstruction and visualization of medical images. This is helpful not only to the formulation and simulation of a surgical plan, but also

R. Su et al. (Eds.): MICAD 2021, LNEE 784, pp. 145–152, 2022.
https://doi.org/10.1007/978-981-16-3880-0_16

to the reference of anatomical teaching and the three-dimensional positioning in radiotherapy plan. (4) Data compression and transmission on the premise of keeping the key information. It is of great value to realize the efficient transmission of medical images in telemedicine. (5) The research of content-based medical image database retrieval. Medical image data can be accessed and searched in semantic sense by establishing medical image database.

In fact, the medical image segmentation is the process of dividing a medical image into several textures, areas, local statistical features or spectral features according to some similar features of a medical image, such as, brightness, color, texture, area, shape, local statistical feature or spectral feature. And it is also the process of dividing a medical image into a number of disjoint "connected" and "connected" regions. The related features show consistency or similarity in the same region, while the related features will appear obvious differences in different regions, that is to say, there is some discontinuity in the pixels on the boundary between different regions. Generally speaking, there exists at least one region containing the interest object in the meaningful image segmentation result.

The abdominal organs of patients are always overlap each other, disorderly and vary from person to person, and the medical CT images usually have these main characteristics: (1) low contrast; (2) the variability of tissue features; (3) the fuzziness of boundaries between different tissues or between tissues and lesions; (4) the complexity of the distribution of fine structures, such as, blood vessels, nerves, etc. Therefore, it is a difficulty for researchers to accurately segment the CT liver image due to the complex structure of organs and tissues in the abdominal cavity. In addition, another factor related to the segmentation accuracy is the noise of the medical CT image, which is caused by operator or equipment in the process of shooting the image, which always leads to the blurred edge of the target object in CT image. In order to solve the problem, scholars have made a lot of efforts to improve the segmentation accuracy, and a variety of algorithms emerged. According to the segmentation principle, Yu Kong divided these algorithms into three main categories: the principle based on plane shape (model), t boundary curve and image pixel (voxel), respectively [1].

Generally, the CT liver image will be preprocessed by removing the noise from the image before segmenting. The traditional filtering methods not only can erase the noise, but also weak the contrast of the boundary at the same time. According to the complex characteristics of abdominal CT liver images, we propose a new filtering method based on Relative Total Variation method, which can better filter out the noise from the CT liver image and keep the boundary of different tissues at the same time. Then, the threshold method based on Gaussian mixture finite model is used to segment the denoised image.

2 Threshold Segmentation Method

The threshold segmentation method based on the gray value of image pixels is one kind of the various methods of image segmentation. The basic principle is to make full use of the difference of the gray level between the background and the actual object. Firstly, perform the distribution processing of image pixels according to this difference; then transform the distribution to gray level and divide it into multiple gray levels; and finally determine a threshold T to distinguish these differences. So, any point (x, y) in the image is called an object point if f(x, y) > T. Otherwise, this point will be called a back spot. That is to say, the segmented image can be expressed as the following g(x, y) [2].

$$g(x, y) = \begin{cases} 1 \; f(x, y) > T \\ 0 \; f(x, y) \leq T \end{cases}$$

The key problem of threshold segmentation is how to obtain an optimal threshold T. At present, the Gaussian mixture model segmentation algorithm is a better way than other methods to obtain the threshold T. However, the threshold segmentation method is very sensitive to the noise of image. In addition to the signal noise in liver CT image, the texture and complexity of the liver will also affect the segmentation result. Therefore, the common denoising methods can't obtain good segmentation result. So, the total variation filter is used for the preprocessing of CT images in this paper.

3 Relative Total Variation for Image Denoising

The Gaussian filter is a common method used to denoise, it is a linear filtering method. It is relatively simple, but the denoising effect is not satisfactory. In 1992, Rudin proposed a total variation model [3], which denoises the image by getting the minimum value of the total variation energy function expressed as Eq. (1). This method can effectively keep the boundary information of the image while denoising, and the image is clearer after denoising.

$$min\, J(f) = \int_p \frac{\lambda}{2}(f - I_0)^2 + |\nabla f| dp \tag{1}$$

The corresponding discrete form of Eq. (1) is as follow.

$$min\, J(f) = \sum\nolimits_p \frac{\lambda}{2}(f - I_0)^2 + \sum\nolimits_p |\nabla f| dp \tag{2}$$

where

$$\sum\nolimits_p |\nabla f| dp = \sum\nolimits_p |f_x| + |f_y| \tag{3}$$

f is the image to be sought, I_0 is the original image, and $\lambda > 0$ is the control parameter.

The total variation model is an active research topic in the field of image restoration. Bayram and Kamasak provided a Directional Total Variation (DTV) model for image denoising in a specified direction [4]. Hua Zhang and Yuanquan Wang proposed the Edge Adaptive Directional Total Variation (EADTV) method [5], which introduced a spatially varying parameter to enable total variation to deal with multiple dominant directions. However, the direction of the texture in the CT liver image is not fixed, and the meaningful boundaries in the image are fused with the texture units. Belongs to the "structure + texture" picture. Though without removing the texture, the human visual system is fully capable of understanding these images. But for image segmentation, the whole structure of the image cannot be acquired because of the texture and the noise. Li Xu put forward the Relative Total Variation (RTV) method [6] by considering two types of variation, the inherent variation and relative total variation, to extract the main structures. At the same time, this RTV model can effectively decompose the structure information and texture in the image, and it does not need to care whether the texture is regular or symmetrical. Taking into account the obvious difference between the total variation caused by the noise in image and the variation caused by the boundary in the image, the RTV model modifies the Eq. (2) to the following Eq. (4).

$$min\, J(f) = \sum_p (f - I_0)^2 + \lambda \cdot \left(\frac{D_x(p)}{L_x(p) + \varepsilon} + \frac{D_y(p)}{L_y(p) + \varepsilon} \right) \tag{4}$$

Where,

$$D_x(p) = \sum_{q \in R(\Omega)} g_{p,q} \cdot \left| (f_x)_q \right|$$

$$D_y(p) = \sum_{q \in R(\Omega)} g_{p,q} \cdot \left| (f_y)_q \right|$$

$$L_x(p) = \left| \sum_{q \in R(\Omega)} g_{p,q} \cdot (f_x)_q \right|$$

$$L_y(p) = \left| \sum_{q \in R(\Omega)} g_{p,q} \cdot (f_y)_q \right|$$

q is all the pixels in a square region with p as the center, and g is the following Gaussian kernel function.

$$g_{p,q} \propto e^{-\frac{(x_p - x_q)^2 + (y_p - y_q)^2}{2\sigma^2}}$$

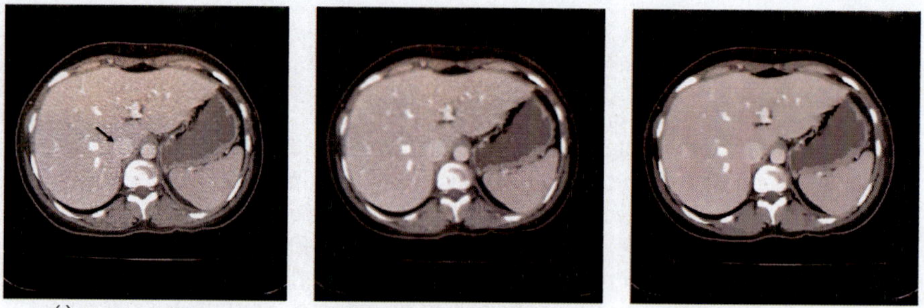

(a) Original CT image (b) Gaussian filter CT image (c) RTV filter CT image

Fig. 1. The original CT image of the liver and filtered images

Figure 1(a) shows an original CT section of the abdominal cavity. In this image, the inferior vena cava, the circular organ pointed by the arrow, is closely attached to the liver. It is difficult to segment accurately. Figure 1(b) gives the results after Gaussian filtering and Fig. 1(c) shows the result after RTV filtering. According to the filtering effect, the boundary of the inferior vena cava in Fig. 1(c) seems to be more obvious than that in Fig. 1(b).

4 Gaussian Mixture Model Segmentation

The image gray histogram reflects the frequency of a certain gray value in the image, and it can also be regarded as the estimation of the gray probability density of the image. If the image contains a large difference between the target region and the background region, and there is a certain difference in gray between the background region and the target region, then the gray histogram of the image shows a double peak-valley shape, one of the two peaks corresponds to the target, and the other peak corresponds to the grayscale of the background. For complex images, especially medical images, it is generally multi-peak. The image segmentation can be solved by regarding the multi-peak characteristic of the histogram as the superposition of multiple distributions. The mixture model can just be used to represent the probability model of the superposition of multiple distributions in the global distribution. In other words, the mixture model represents the probability distribution of the observed data in the population, which is a mixed distribution composed of K sub-distributions. The mixture model does not require the observed data to provide information about the sub-distribution to calculate the probability of the observed data in the overall distribution. Gaussian Mixture Model (GMM) is a common and effective mixture model due to the good mathematical properties and the good computational performance of the Gaussian distribution. Gaussian mixture model can be regarded as a model composed of K single Gaussian models [7]. For the gray histogram, a single Gaussian distribution obeys the following probability density function.

$$P(x|\theta) = \frac{1}{\sqrt{2\pi\sigma^2}} e^{-\frac{(x-\mu)^2}{2\sigma^2}}$$

The Log-Likelihood function of the Gaussian mixture model is expressed as Eq. (5).

$$logL(\theta) = \sum_{j=1}^{N} logP(x_j|\theta) = \sum_{j=1}^{N} log\left(\sum_{k=1}^{K} \alpha_k \varphi(x|\theta_k)\right) \quad (5)$$

$\theta = (\mu_k, \sigma_k, \alpha_k)$ is the expectation, variance and probability of each sub-model.
x_j represents the observation data, $j = 1, 2, \cdots, N$.
k is the number of sub-Gaussian model, $k = 1, 2, \cdots, K$.
α_k is the probability belonging to the kth sub-model, $\alpha_k \geq 0$, $\sum_{k=1}^{K} \alpha_k = 1$.
$\varphi(x|\theta_k)$ is the Gaussian distribution density function of the kth sub-model, here $\theta_k = (\mu_k, \sigma_k^2)$.

The parameters in Eq. (5) can be calculated by applying the following Algorithm 1.

Algorithm.1 EM algorithm for calculating GMM parameters

1. Initialization parameters
2. E-step：Calculate the possibility of each x_j coming from the sub-model k, based on the current parameters.

$$\gamma_{jk} = \frac{\alpha_k \varphi(x_j|\theta_k)}{\sum_{k=1}^{K} \alpha_k \varphi(x_j|\theta_k)}, j = 1,2,\cdots,N; k = 1,2,\cdots,K$$

γ_{jk} represents the probability that the x_j belongs to the kth sub-model.

3. M-step：Calculate the model parameters of the new iteration.

$$\mu_k = \frac{\sum_{j=1}^{N}(\gamma_{jk}x_j)}{\sum_{j=1}^{N}\gamma_{jk}}, k = 1,2,\cdots,K$$

$$\sigma_k = \frac{\sum_{j=1}^{N}\gamma_{jk}(x_j - \mu_k)^2}{\sum_{j=1}^{N}\gamma_{jk}}, k = 1,2,\cdots,K$$

$$\alpha_k = \frac{\sum_{j=1}^{N}\gamma_{jk}}{N}, k = 1,2,\cdots,K$$

4. Repeat the E-step and M-step until all the parameters converge.

5 Segmentation Results and Conclusions

The CT slice in Fig. 1 is segmented by GMM. Figure 2 shows the result of GMM segmentation of Fig. 1(b). Figure 3 shows the result of GMM segmentation of Fig. 1(c). Compared with Fig. 2(a) and Fig. 3(a), we find that although the shape of the image is similar, the peak height of histogram statistics has a significant difference. Every peak in Fig. 3(a) is almost twice as high as that in Fig. 2(a). Figure 3(a) shows that the gray statistical value of the liver in Fig. 1(c) is more than 5000, while Fig. 2(a) shows that the gray statistical value of the liver in Fig. 1(b) is less than 3000. This significant difference makes the threshold of the Fig. 3(a) more accurate than that of the Fig. 2(a) when the threshold is calculated in following GMM, which is shown as Fig. 3(b) and Fig. 2(b), respectively. The threshold range shown in Fig. 3(b) is 193–215, while that shown in Fig. 2(b) is 187–221. The difference between the upper and lower bounds of the two threshold ranges happens to be the key to accurate segmentation. Figure 3(c) and Fig. 2(c) are the segmentation results of Fig. 1(a) based on the two segmentation threshold ranges shown as Fig. 3(b) and Fig. 2(b), respectively. We combine the boundaries of Fig. 3(c) and Fig. 2(c) with Fig. 1(a) to get Fig. 3(d) and Fig. 2(d), respectively. Figure 2(d) does not separate inferior vena cava from the liver, and the inferior vena cava is misclassified into the liver. It is clear that Fig. 3(d) is correct and better than Fig. 2(d).

From Fig. 1(a) we can see that there is no gap between inferior vena cava and liver, and the difference in gray value is very small, so this kind of segmentation has always been a difficult point in image segmentation. If Gaussian filtering is used, the sharpness of the boundary will be weakened and the gray values with smaller differences will become closer. Therefore, the distribution of grayscale values is more dispersed. After we use RTV filtering, the inner of the inferior vena cava gray difference becomes smaller, but the boundary is not affected in any way. Therefore, the pixel gray distribution of the whole image is more concentrated.

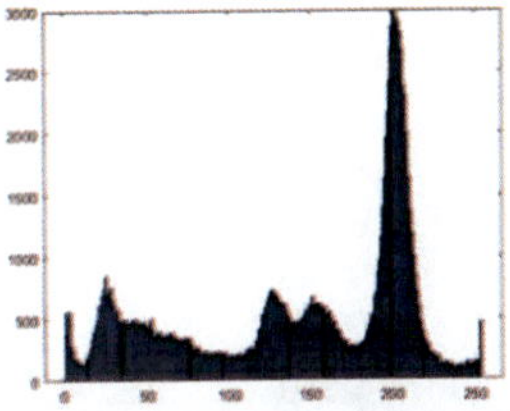

(a)The grayscale histogram of Fig.1.(b)

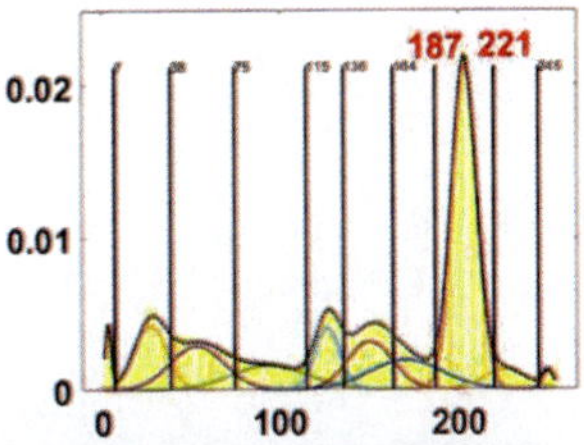

(b)GMM segmentation threshold of Fig.2.(a)

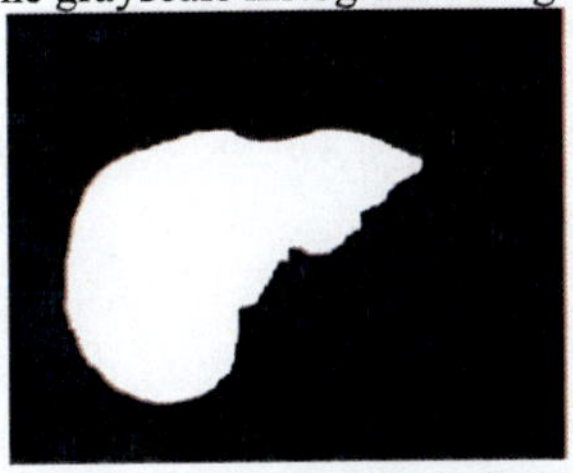

(c)The segmentation result of Fig.1.(b) according to the threshold of Fig.2.(b)

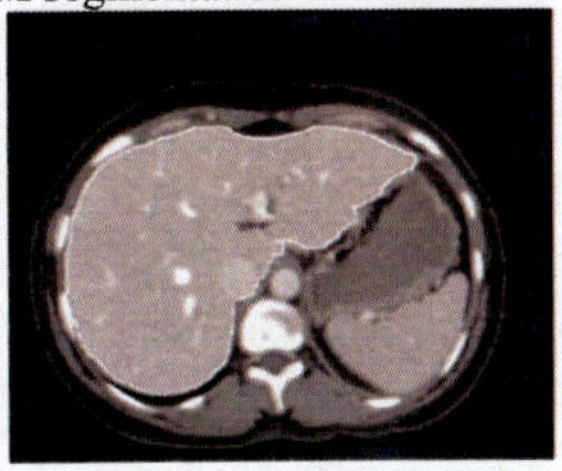

(d)The combination result of Fig.1.(a) and the contour of Fig.2.(c)

Fig. 2. The segmentation result of Fig. 1 with GMM based on the Gaussian filter

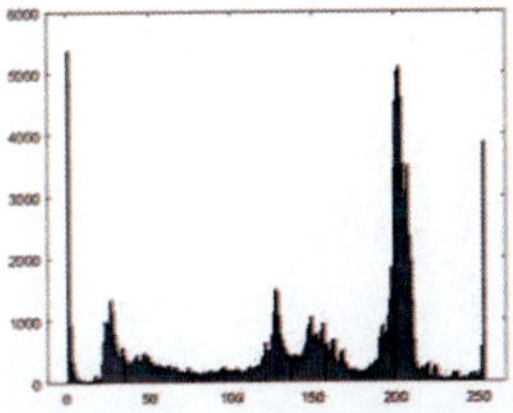

(a)The grayscale histogram of Fig.1.(c)

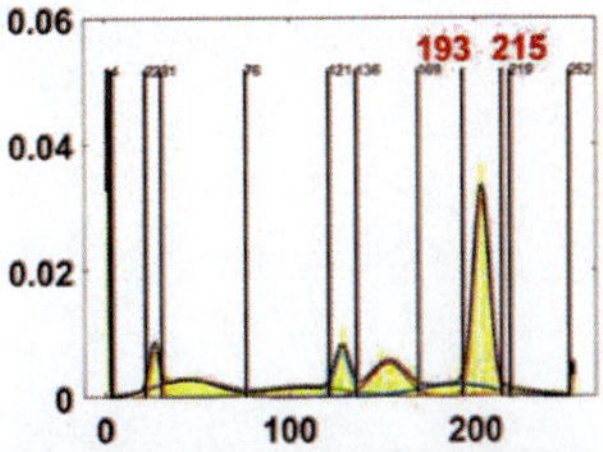

(b)GMM segmentation threshold of Fig.3.(a)

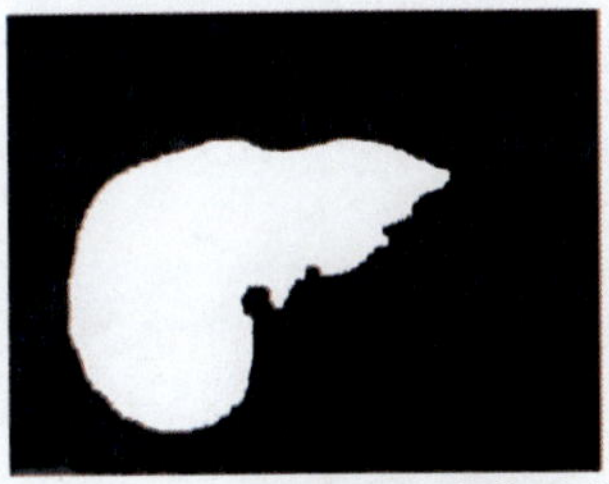

(c)The segmentation result of Fig.1.(c) according to the threshold of Fig.3.(b)

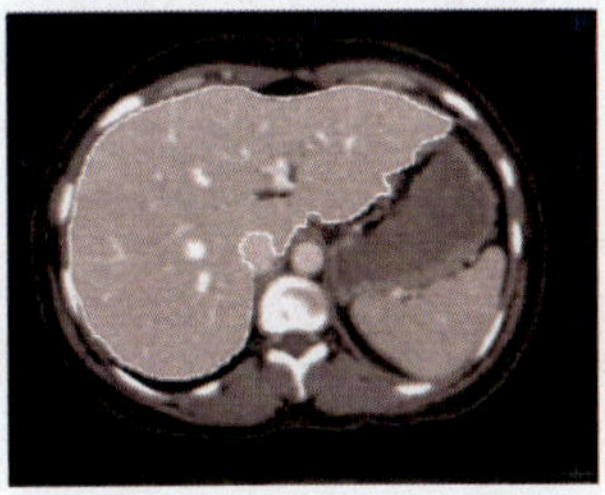

(d)The combination result of Fig.1.(a) and the contour of Fig.3.(c)

Fig. 3. The segmentation result of Fig. 1 with GMM based on the RTV filter

The above experimental results verify that the segmentation result of the CT liver image by using GMM based on RTV filter is obviously better than that based on Gaussian filtering. And this method also can be used in MRI and Ultrasonic Image post-processing to improve the accuracy of image segmentation.

References

1. Kong, Y., et al.: A novel classification method of medical image segmentation algorithm. In: Su, R., Liu, H., Su, R., Liu, H. (eds.) Proceeding of 2020 International Conference on Medical Imaging and Computer-Aided Diagnosis (MICAD 2020), pp. 107–115. Springer, Singapore (2020)
2. Gonzalez, R.C., Bayram, I.: Digital Image Processing, 4th edn. Pearson Education, Inc., New Jersey (2018)
3. Rudin, L.I., Osher, S., Fatemi, E.: Nonlinear total variation based noise removal algorithms. Phys. D **60**(1–4), 259–268 (1992)
4. Bayram, I., Kamasak, M.E.: Directional total variation. IEEE Signal Process. Lett. **19**(12), 781–784 (2012)
5. Zhang, H., Wang, Y.: Edge adaptive directional total variation. J. Eng. (Stevenage, Engl.) **2013**(11), 61–62 (2013)
6. Xu, L., et al.: Structure extraction from texture via relative total variation. ACM Trans. Graph. **31**(6), 1–10 (2012)
7. Reynolds, D.: Gaussian mixture models. In: Li, S.Z., Jain, A. (eds.) Encyclopedia of Biometrics, pp. 659–663. Springer US, Boston (2009)

Automated Gland Detection in Colorectal Histopathological Images

Maisun Mohamed Al Zorgani(✉), Irfan Mehmood, and Hassan Ugail

School of Media, Design and Technology, Faculty of Engineering and Informatics, University of Bradford, Bradford, UK
M.M.S.AlZoragani@bradford.ac.uk

Abstract. Clinical morphological analysis of histopathological specimens is a successful manner for diagnosing benign and malignant diseases. Analysis of glandular architecture is a major challenge for colon histopathologists as a result of the difficulty of identifying morphological structures in glandular malignant tumours due to the distortion of glands boundaries, furthermore the variation in the appearance of staining specimens. For reliable analysis of colon specimens, several deep learning methods have exhibited encouraging performance in the glands automatic segmentation despite the challenges. In the histopathology field, the vast number of annotation images for training the deep learning algorithms is the major challenge. In this work, we propose a trainable Convolutional Neural Network (CNN) from end to end for detecting the glands automatically. More specifically, the Modified Res-U-Net is employed for segmenting the colorectal glands in Haematoxylin and Eosin (H&E) stained images for challenging Gland Segmentation (GlaS) dataset. The proposed Res-U-Net outperformed the prior methods that utilise U-Net architecture on the images of the GlaS dataset.

Keywords: Histopathological image analysis · Colorectal adenocarcinoma · Colon gland semantic segmentation · Deep learning

1 Introduction

In the analysis of histopathological images, the glands segmentation is an essential process, and is among the major criteria for grading and staging the colorectal adenocarcinoma cancer [1]. In clinical practice, pathologists segment the glands manually, so this routine is tedious, tiresome and time-consuming, furthermore, the inter-observer diagnosis variation among them. As well it depends heavily on the experience of pathologists [1,2]. To tackle the challenges mentioned above, these tasks will be done automatically to help the pathologists on a precise assessment of the glands morphologies in colon cancer.

The recent developments in digital whole slide imaging (WSI) scanners have transformed the field of histopathology. Therefore, most of the routines pathologist tasks are digitized. Thus, the advancing of Computer-Aided Diagnosis

R. Su et al. (Eds.): MICAD 2021, LNEE 784, pp. 153–162, 2022.
https://doi.org/10.1007/978-981-16-3880-0_17

(CAD) methods is necessitated. Such methods aim to assist pathologists in some laborious routine tasks. In traditional CAD methods, most of the researches have focused on hand-craft features. The problem of such methods is the difficulty of choosing the optimal features. In the past few years, several deep learning algorithms have emerged and been employed in the field of histopathology analysis. These algorithms have the ability to automatically extract deep features from images and are thus more effective than traditional methods [1]. However, the development of CADs that build on deep learning algorithms (Deep-CAD) is suffering from the lack of the annotated images amount that is needed for training such algorithms [1,2]. So in this work, we present a Deep-CAD method to segment the glands automatically in colorectal histopathological images.

We have organized this paper as; Sect. 2 displayed an overview of the relevant works; Sect. 3 described the proposed data and method briefly in this work; Sect. 4 presented in detail the experiment and its results. The last section provided a summary of the paper.

2 Related Works

This section is reviewed some of the proposed models for segmenting the glands in colorectal histopathological images of the GlaS dataset. Starting from [3,4], Sirinukunwattana et al. utilised the colour and texture features to classify the candidate glands into binary classes (gland or non-gland). In [3], the authors have combined Markov Chain with Monte Carlo in Reversible Jumping for generating the polygonal contour for candidate glands, while in [4], the authors have generated the structure maps of candidate glands by computing the scattering coefficients based on texture features, then utilised these maps to feed CNN for detecting tumour cells in histopathological images. Subsequently, they have released the Warwick QU challenge dataset for segmenting of glands automatically, so it is known as Gland Segmentation (GlaS) challenge dataset [5]. The contest was held in 2015 at the 18th International Conference on Medical Image Computing and Computer-Assisted Intervention (MICCAI 2015).

Since GlaS challenge contest [5], several models [6–13] have been carried out by using CNNs for solving the glands segmentation issue in GlaS dataset images and preventing the merge of neighbouring gland structures. Some researchers employed handcrafted features for training deep networks [6–8]. The others [9–13] investigated trainable end-to-end fully convolutional networks (FCNs) [14] for mapping images directly to their gland segmentation maps. Chen et al. [9] proposed two frameworks, CUMedVision1 (the 5th model in GlaS contest) is based on FCN for representing the multi-level features of the gland object masks. Whereas, CUMedVision2 (the winning model in GlaS contest) is a deep contour-aware network based on FCN for combining both glands foreground maps and glands boundary maps to generate glands maps simultaneously. The authors in [11] utilised a Loss-Function with penalty terms to obtain the smooth gland boundary with the correct label hierarchy. The authors in [12] proposed FCN architecture with forked channels for incorporating boundary maps into their architecture; the output maps of the different convolutional layers were employed to feed the side channels for predicting gland boundary maps and finally, these maps were combined to estimate the gland maps.

While other researchers [13,15,16] leveraging U-Net [17] architecture, which is a deep learning network based on a modified FCN model and combines the context information of lower layers and the semantic information of higher layers through skip connection for improving the performance of image segmentation. Ronneberger et al. [17] presented trainable end-to-end U-Net for segmenting the biomedical images semantically. Freiburg team [13] (team participating in the contest) proposed two deep models based on U-Net for generating the binary segmentation maps (background and glands). More recently, Graham et al. [15] have proposed MILD-net model which based on U-Net architecture for incorporating the low-level features at each decoder block. Binder et al. [16] have contributed two Dense-U-Net models; one for segmenting the glands directly and the other for segmenting the stroma to predict glands. Both models are U-Net architecture based on the pre-trained DenseNet [18] model as encoder network.

In this work, we proposed a modified Res-U-Net model based on U-Net architecture for detecting the glands in GlaS dataset images. The encoder portion of the proposed model utilise the pre-trained ResNet-50 network [19] on the ImageNet [20] dataset. So, the ResNet-50 network here acts as the feature extractor.

3 Data and Method

3.1 The Warwick-QU Dataset Image

We have trained and tested our proposed methodology on the images of Warwick-QU dataset. The dataset was acquired from the University Hospitals Coventry and Warwickshire NHS Trust, Coventry, United Kingdom. The dataset histopathology images were derived from sixteen H&E stained WSIs of stages T3 or T4 colorectal adenocarcinoma of human clinical samples. In colon cancer, T3 stage refers to expand the tumour into the bowel wall, whereas T4 through the bowel wall. WSIs were scanned with a pixel resolution of 0.620 μm/pixel to visualize a complete slide on a screen at 20$\times$ objective magnification. The images together with their ground truth of glands were annotated by the trained histopathologists. A total of 165 images is divided into 85 images for training and 80 images for testing. Furthermore, the testing images are split into two sets: Test-A is sixteen images for off-line evaluation, and Test-B is twenty images for an on-site evaluation. For more information, Sirinukunwattana et al. [13] have published a research paper about the GlaS challenge dataset.

3.2 Pre-processing Image Dataset

In this section, we have pre-processed dataset images into three steps as follows:

- **Stain Normalisation**, to reduce the variations of H&E stain in the appearance of images, we stained normalise the histopathological images of GlaS dataset as described in [21]. The stain normalisation toolbox [22] for several techniques is found on the Warwick University website.
- **Image Size Standardization**, to standardize the size of images in the GlaS dataset, we resized the images and their respective ground truth masks into $512 \times 512 \times 3$ pixels.
- **Glands Aggregation**, we grouped the 30 original gland classes into one class as well as background, as described in [23]. Figure 1 shows examples of the GlaS dataset images from different grades with glands annotated and their ground truth after grouped the classes.
- **Data Augmentation**, we augmented the training images of GlaS dataset by rotated them with angles of 90, 180 and 270 degrees and then flipped in the horizontal and vertical direction. This is to enlarge the training images size without affecting the quality of input images [24] and avoid the over-fitting problems [25] and the features poorly generation.

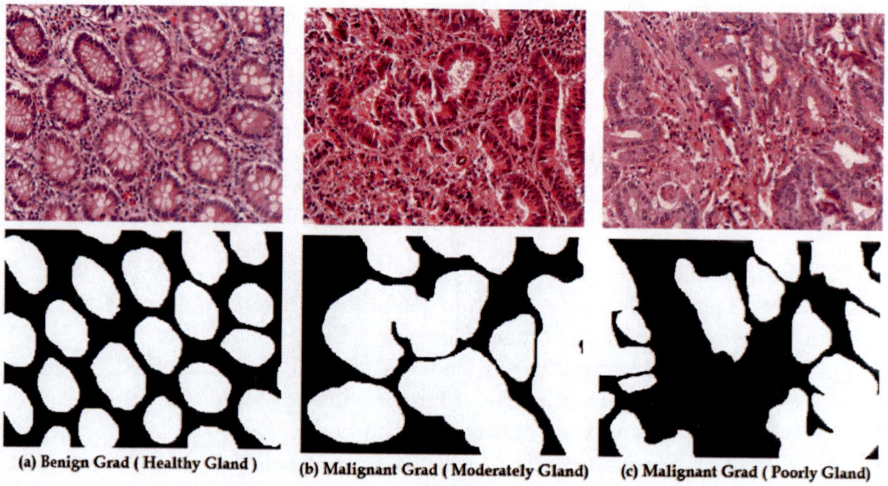

Fig. 1. Example of the GlaS dataset images; upper row: the original images; Bottom row: corresponding ground truth: (**a**) shows a healthy tissue, (**b**) shows a moderately differentiated tumour and (**c**) shows a poorly differentiated tumour

3.3 Evaluation Metrics

The performance of our proposed method was evaluated according to four criteria: Accuracy (Acc), F1-Score, Intersection over Union (IoU), and Dice coefficient (Dice Coef.). These criteria use the following standard metrics; tp (true positive) is the number of the correctly predicted glands that intersect with their corresponding in ground truth; fn (false negative) is the number of the true glands in ground truth that is neglected by the proposed method; otherwise is fp (false positive) which represents the number of the predicted glands that wrongly predicted as glands by the proposed method.

Performance Accuracy. This criterion is used Accuracy metric to measure a network's ability to segment. It is formulated as;

$$Acc. = \frac{tn + tp}{fp + tp + fn + tn} \tag{1}$$

Detection Accuracy. This criterion is used F1-Score metric for measuring the detection accuracy of glands individually. It is formulated as;

$$F1 - Score = \frac{2 \times Precision \times Recall}{Recall + Precision} \tag{2}$$

where

$$Precision = \frac{tp}{tp + fp}, and\ Recall = \frac{tp}{tp + fn}$$

From the above two equations, Precision ratio indicates the total detected glands that are really glands; Recall ratio indicates the total reference glands that are actually detected.

Shape Similarity. This criterion is used Jaccard similarity coefficient and also known as IoU for comparing the similarities between the glands in the original images and the predicted images at the pixel level. It is calculated as;

$$Jaccard(IoU) = \frac{tp}{tp + fp + fn} \tag{3}$$

Segmentation Accuracy. This criterion is also known as Volume-Based Accuracy. It is used Dice Coefficient for measuring the similarity between glands in the original and predicted images at object level. It is calculated as;

$$DiceCoef. = \frac{2|G \cap S|}{|G| + |S|} \tag{4}$$

Where |.| points out the number of elements in a target set. G is a pixel set that belonging to the gland of ground truth and S is a pixel set that belonging to the segmented gland of the predicted image. It is used to measure similarity between G and S and produces scores between 0 and 1, whereas 0 points out no overlap between gland sets and 1 point out a perfect match between gland sets.

3.4 Proposed Model

The proposed Res-U-Net model is shown in Fig. 2, which is composed of an encoder portion and a decoder portion.

- **Encoder Portion:** it is employed for down-sampling of the feature maps and is comprised of an input layer, convolutional layer, a Batch Normalization (BN) layer, a Rectified Linear Unit (ReLU) layer, MaxPooling layer and followed by four residual units. The first residual unit is composed of three blocks with nine convolutional layers. The second residual unit consists of four blocks with twelve convolutional layers. The third residual unit includes six blocks with eighteen convolutional layers. The fourth residual unit contains three blocks with nine convolutional layers. The default parameters were transferred from the residual units of the pre-trained Res-Net-50 model.
- **Decoder Portion:** it contains three concatenate blocks, five up-sampling units, a segmentation unit, and an output unit. Each up-sampling unit contains one 1×1 convolution filter and an up-sampling ($2\times$) block to double the size of the feature maps as well as halve the number of feature channels. The segmentation layer comprises a 1×1 convolution filter and a sigmoid activation layer to map results of segmentation for binary classification (Gland or Non-Gland). The concatenate blocks were implemented between the output of residual block for encoder portion and the output of up-sampling ($2\times$) block for decoder portion for the fusion of multi-scale features.

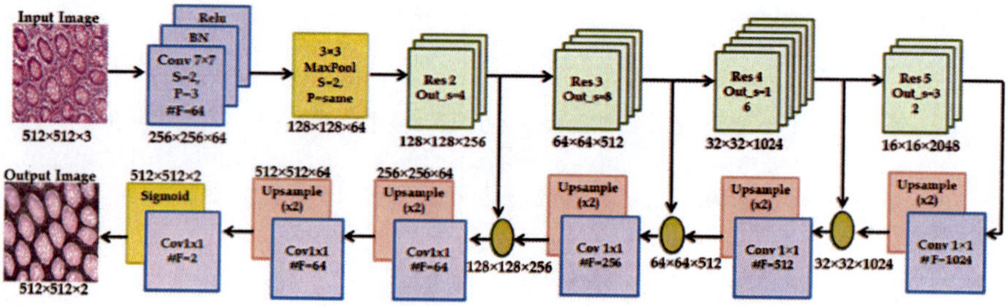

Fig. 2. Shows the proposed Res-U-Net architecture, Whereas the abbreviated terms "CONV" represents the convolution block; BN represents Batch Normalization layer; ReLU represents the Rectified Linear Unit layer; "#F" represents the filter number; "S" represents the stride; "P" represents padding.

4 The Experiment and Its Results

The experiment was carried out by using GlaS dataset images. It was implemented in MATLAB R2020a framework on a desktop computer that has a 3.60-GHz Intel® Core-i7 CPU, NVIDIA GeForce GTX 1070 GPU and 32 GB RAM. To set up our model, we fine-tuned the ResNet-50 model as encoder and set Stochastic Gradient Descent (SGD) with Momentum to 0.90, Max-Epochs is 120. We started running the program with Learning Rate (LR) equal to 0.001 and decreased after each update. For the training procedure, we divide the augmented training images randomly into 80% for training and 20% for validation.

The weights of the encoder portion were initialised by the weights of the pre-trained ResNet-50 model. Analysis of the obtained results in Fig. 3 indicates that our model is gaining convergence during the first 70 epochs in the training stage and the accuracy rate was approximately steady and the error falls slowly from the 80th epoch. We represented the obtained prediction results from the experiment by 2×2 normalised confusion matrices. These matrices were constructed on two rows and two columns: gland and non-gland representing the classes. These 2×2 normalized confusion matrices are shown in Fig. 4. The obtained prediction results for our proposed model were summarized in Table 1. Whereas we calculated the standard metrics of accuracy, precision, recall, F1-Score and IoU by substituting into the 1, 2, 3 and 4 equations, respectively. Whereas example of the visual experiment result is shown in Fig. 5.

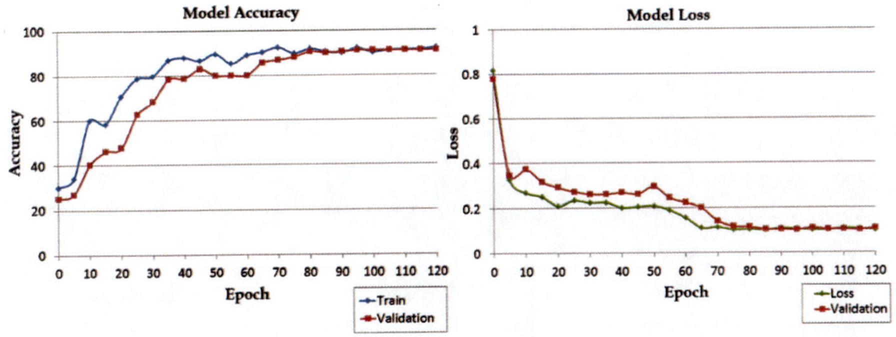

Fig. 3. Visualization of the progress of training, loss and validation over the training time for the proposed Res-U-Net model.

Table 1. Standard metrics of our proposed model

GlaS dataset	Standard metrics				
	Accuracy	Recall	Precision	F_1-Score	IoU
Test A	0.9192	0.9427	0.8993	0.9201	0.8520
Test B	0.8962	0.8697	0.9423	0.9046	0.8258

The comparative analysis of the obtained results from our proposed model against some other models that used the same dataset images is reported in Table 2. By comparing the results in Table 2, we derive that the proposed Res-U-Net model outperforms all of them on Test-B test set. Whereas it got a good result on Test-A test set. At pixel-level, it achieved F-score values; 0.913 and 0.881 on Test-A and Test-B test sets, respectively. At object detection level, it achieved Dice index values; 0.911 and 0.871 on Test-A and Test-B test sets, respectively.

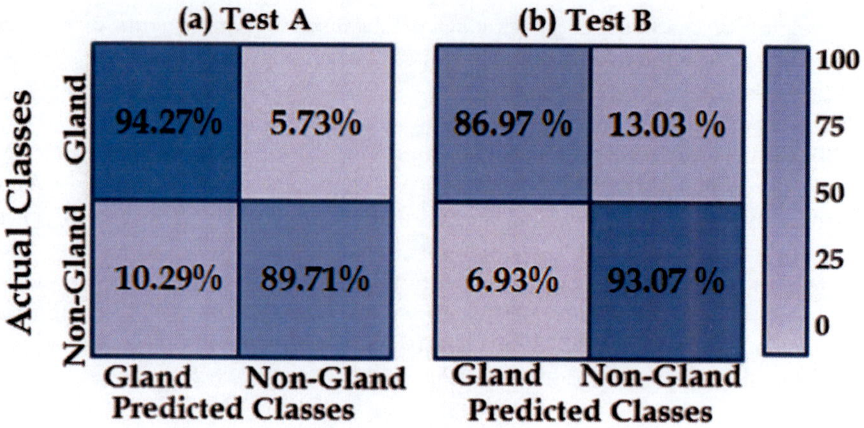

Fig. 4. Normalized confusion matrices for the proposed model.

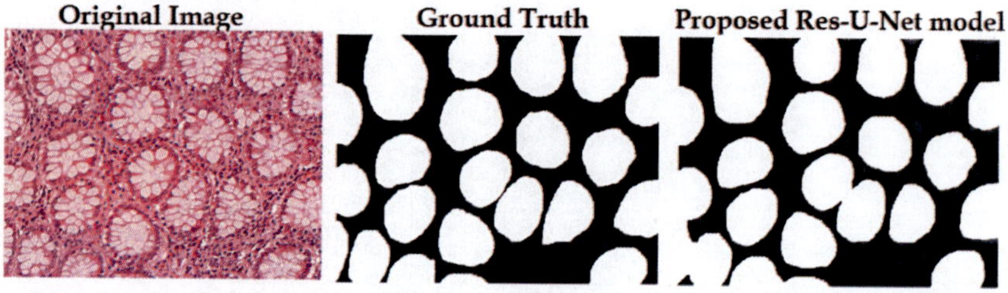

Fig. 5. Example on the visual results of gland segmentation on the GLaS dataset.

Table 2. Comparative analysis of different models on GlaS challenge dataset.

Deep model	F1 score		Obj. dice	
	Test A	Test B	Test A	Test B
MILD-Net	**0.914**	0.844	**0.913**	0.836
Xu et al.	0.893	0.843	0.908	0.833
CUMedVision1	0.868	0.769	0.867	0.800
CUMedVision2	0.912	0.716	0.897	0.781
Freiburg1	0.834	0.605	0.875	0.783
Freiburg2	0.870	0.695	0.876	0.786
Proposed Res-U-Net	0.913	**0.881**	0.911	**0.871**

5 Conclusion

For this study, We explored Res-U-Net architecture as a model for segmenting the glands at the semantic level in histopathological colorectal adenocarcinoma images. We also leveraged of deep transfer learning strategy to tackle the lack of GlaS dataset images. More specifically, we transferred the deep ResNet-50 model as the backbone encoder in the proposed Res-U-Net architecture. From the obtained results in our experiment, it is observed that transferring a deep pre-trained encoder model can considerably reduce the time consumption and the resources required for training from scratch. The significance of the proposed model is based on segmenting the glands at the semantic level in GlaS dataset images, different from other models that are based on segmenting the glands at the instance level on the same dataset. Therefore, it helps the pathologists to distinguish between histological glandular structures whether it is adenocarcinoma or not, specifically in the case of significant variation in the appearance of the glandular structures. The proposed approach was compared against the gland segmentation approaches that were developed using GlaS dataset images. As a result, the proposed model exhibits significant potential for gland detection in histopathological images.

References

1. Litjens, G., et al.: A survey on deep learning in medical image analysis. Med. Image Anal. **42**, 60–88 (2017)
2. Deng, S., et al.: Deep learning in digital pathology image analysis: a survey. Front. Med. 1–18 (2020)
3. Sirinukunwattana, K., Snead, D.R., Rajpoot, N.M.: A stochastic polygons model for glandular structures in colon histology images. IEEE Trans. Med. Imaging **34**(11), 2366–2378 (2015)
4. Sirinukunwattana, K., Snead, D.R., Rajpoot, N.M.: A novel texture descriptor for detection of glandular structures in colon histology images. In: Medical Imaging 2015: Digital Pathology, vol. 9420, p. 94200S (2015)
5. GLaS, 2015. GlaS@MICCAI'2015: gland segmentation challenge contest (2015). www2.warwick.ac.uk/fac/sci/dcs/research/tia/glascontest. Accessed 13 June 2020
6. Li, W., Manivannan, S., Akbar, S., Zhang, J., Trucco, E., McKenna, S.J.: Gland segmentation in colon histology images using hand-crafted features and convolutional neural networks. In: Proceedings of the 13th International Symposium on Biomedical Imaging (ISBI), pp. 1405–1408. IEEE (2016)
7. Manivannan, S., Li, W., Zhang, J., Trucco, E., McKenna, S.J.: Structure prediction for gland segmentation with hand-crafted and deep convolutional features. IEEE Trans. Med. Imaging **37**, 210–221 (2017)
8. Rezaei, S., et al.: Gland segmentation in histopathology images using deep networks and handcrafted features. In: EMBC, pp. 1031–1034. IEEE (2019)
9. Chen, H., Qi, X., Yu, L., Dou, Q., Qin, J., Heng, P.-A.: DCAN: deep contour-aware networks for object instance segmentation from histology images. Med. Image Anal. **36**, 135–146 (2017)
10. Yang, L., Zhang, Y., Chen, J., Zhang, S., Chen, D.Z.: Suggestive annotation: a deep active learning framework for biomedical image segmentation. In: Medical Image Computing and Computer-Assisted Intervention, pp. 399–407. Springer (2017)
11. BenTaieb, A., Hamarneh, G.: Topology aware fully convolutional networks for histology gland segmentation. In: Medical Image Computing and Computer-Assisted Intervention, pp. 460–468. Springer (2016)

12. Xu, Y., et al.: Gland instance segmentation by deep multichannel side supervision. In: Medical Image Computing and Computer-Assisted Intervention, pp. 496–504. Springer (2016)
13. Sirinukunwattana, K., et al.: Gland segmentation in colon histology images: the glas challenge contest. Med. Image Anal. **35**, 489–502 (2016)
14. Long, J., Shelhamer, E., Darrell, T.: Fully convolutional networks for semantic segmentation. In: IEEE Conference on Computer Vision and Pattern Recognition, pp. 3431–3440 (2015)
15. Graham, S., et al.: MILD-Net: minimal information loss dilated network for gland instance segmentation in colon histology images. Med. Image Anal. **52**, 199–211 (2019)
16. Binder, T., Tantaoui, E.M., Pati, P., Catena, R., Set-Aghayan, A., Gabrani, M.: Multi-organ gland segmentation using deep learning. Front. Med. **6**, 173 (2019)
17. Ronneberger, O., Fischer, P., Brox, T.: U-Net: convolutional networks for biomedical image segmentation. In: Medical Image Computing and Computer-Assisted Intervention (MICCAI 2015), vol. 931, pp. 234–241 (2015)
18. Huang, G., Liu, Z., Van Der Maaten, L., Weinberger, K.: Densely connected convolutional networks. In: IEEE Conference on Computer Vision and Pattern Recognition, pp. 4700–4708 (2017)
19. He, K., Zhang, X., Ren, S., Sun, J.: Deep residual learning for image recognition. In: Proceedings of the IEEE Conference on Computer Vision and Pattern Recognition (CVPR), pp. 770–778 (2016)
20. Russakovsky, O., et al.: ImageNet large scale visual recognition challenge. Int. J. Comput. Vis. **115**, 211–252 (2015)
21. Khan, A.M., Rajpoot, N., Treanor, D., Magee, D.A.: Nonlinear mapping approach to stain normalization in digital histopathology images using image-specific color deconvolution. IEEE Trans. Bio. Eng. **61**, 1729–1738 (2014)
22. Stain Normalisation Toolbox. https://warwick.ac.uk/fac/sci/dcs/research/tia/software/sntoolbox/. Accessed 12 Dec 2020
23. Badrinarayanan, V., Kendall, A., Cipolla, R.: SegNet: a deep convolutional encoder-decoder architecture for image segmentation. IEEE Trans. Pattern Anal. Mach. Intell. **39**, 2481–2495 (2017)
24. Mikołajczyk, A., Grochowski, M.: Data augmentation for improving deep learning in image classification problem. In: 2018 International Interdisciplinary Ph.D. Workshop (IIPhDW), pp. 117–122 (2018)
25. Shorten, C., Khoshgoftaar, T.M.. A survey on image data augmentation for deep learning. J. Big Data **6**, 60 (2019)

Ultrasonic Image Segmentation Algorithm of Thyroid Nodules Based on DPCNN

Deng Xiangyu(✉), Zhang Huan, and Yang Yahan

College of Physics and Electronic Engineering, Northwest Normal University, Lanzhou 730070, Gansu, China

Abstract. The segmentation of ultrasound images of thyroid nodules is a key technology for computer-aided diagnosis of thyroid. How to achieve precise segmentation of nodules has always been a hot issue in the field of medical image segmentation. To solve the problem that the traditional models are sensitive to the background area when segmenting ultrasound images with low contrast, we propose an ultrasonic image segmentation algorithm for thyroid nodules based on pulse coupled neural network with direct current component (DPCNN) in this paper. Firstly, the algorithm performs rough location of suspicious region on the optimal segmentation image output by DPCNN iteration, and uses the comprehensive judgment criteria of the maximum variance and covariance of the local region to determine the lesion area. On this basis, the nodule image is segmented based on DPCNN according to the gray features of the nodule image, so as to realize the precise segmentation of the thyroid nodule area. The experimental results show that this algorithm can effectively achieve the accurate segmentation of thyroid nodule area and has good robustness.

Keywords: Pulse coupled neural network · Rough localization of nodules · Method of regional expansion · Maximum covariance · Precise segmentation of nodules

1 Introduction

Thyroid gland is a very important endocrine gland in the human body, which regulates human function and metabolism by producing thyroxine. Thyroid nodules are local masses formed by thyroid lesions and structural abnormalities [1]. According to global epidemiological statistics, the incidence of thyroid-related diseases is increasing year by year, and the incidence of thyroid cancer ranks first in endocrine tumors. Ultrasound examination is the most extensive way to detect and diagnose thyroid diseases. It can quickly and accurately locate the position of thyroid nodules and find small lesions and blood flow. Therefore, in order to achieve effective diagnosis and treatment of thyroid nodules, it is first necessary to accurately segment the thyroid nodules [2]. However, due to the low resolution of ultrasonic images and the complex surrounding thyroid tissues, the ultrasound image segmentation of thyroid nodules is extremely challenging.

In order to achieve effective segmentation of thyroid nodules, scholars at home and abroad continue to innovate and propose many classic segmentation algorithms

R. Su et al. (Eds.): MICAD 2021, LNEE 784, pp. 163–174, 2022.
https://doi.org/10.1007/978-981-16-3880-0_18

of thyroid images, such as: Gabriel et al. [3] proposes a method for segmentation of thyroid images based on texture according to the texture characteristics of thyroid nodules; Iakovidis et al. [4] proposed a variable background active contour model based on the level set method, which uses variable background regions to reduce the influence of uneven grayscale distribution of ultrasound images of thyroid nodules on the segmentation results; Chang et al. [5] proposed a decision tree algorithm for adaptive segmentation of possible lesion areas; Koundal et al. [6] proposed a fully automatic thyroid image segmentation method based on intuitionistic fuzzy C-means clustering. This method combined intuitionistic fuzzy clustering with active contour to eliminate manual intervention and effectively segment multiple nodular nodes in an image. However, this method did not consider spatial information and was easily affected by noise. Ma et al. [7] proposed a thyroid nodule segmentation algorithm based on deep convolutional neural network based on two-dimensional ultrasound images. Prabal et al. [8] uses two-dimensional active contour models to achieve segmentation of thyroid images; Binny et al. [9] proposed a mean shift clustering algorithm for ultrasonic image speckle noise filtering and segmentation, which suppresses speckle noise by enhancing the contrast and improves the quality and information content of thyroid ultrasonic images. However, the algorithm has a large number of iterations and time complexity is too high.

2 DPCNN Model and Its Characteristics

Pulse Coupled Neural Network (PCNN) is an artificial neural network based on the signal conduction characteristics of mammalian visual cortex neurons proposed by Eckhorn et al. [10]. It has been widely used in image segmentation, edge detection, thinning, recognition and other processing. For example, Guo et al. [11] proposed an improved simplified PCNN model based on saliency for target segmentation. This model has obvious advantages in segmentation accuracy and algorithm robustness, and does not require any training; Zhou et al. [12] aimed at the shortcomings of PCNN network parameters that need to be manually adjusted for different images, and proposed a method to improve the automatic edge detection of color images of the PCNN model, but it takes more time to process the image, which limits the model's real-time Application in the environment. This paper adopts the improved PCNN model proposed in the previous research results [13], which adds a direct current component D to the modulation subsystem, so the model is named DPCNN in this paper, and its neuron structure is shown in Fig. 1.

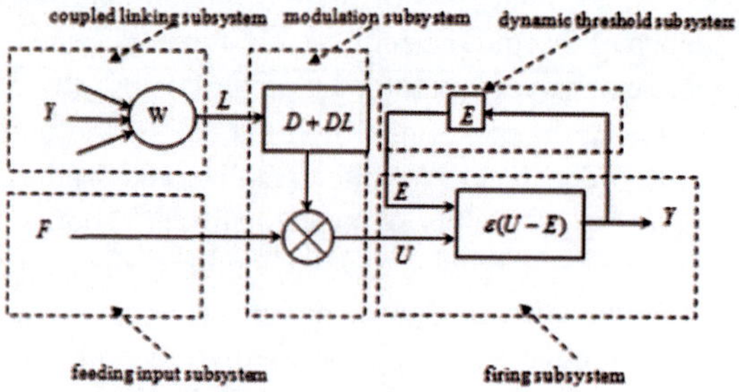

Fig. 1. Pulse coupled neuron mode.

In the neuron model shown in Fig. 1, each subsystem can be described as a discrete system, and the basic mathematical model of the neuron can be expressed as Eq. (1) to Eq. (4).

$$F_{ij}(n) = S_{ij} \tag{1}$$

$$U_{ij}(n) = F_{ij}(n)[\mathrm{D} + \mathrm{D}\sum W_{ijkl}Y_{ijkl}(n-1)] \tag{2}$$

$$E_{ij}(n) = e^{-a_E}E_{ij}(n-1) + V_E Y_{ij}(n-1) \tag{3}$$

$$Y_{ij}(n) = \varepsilon[U_{ij}(n) - E_{ij}(n)] \tag{4}$$

Where, S_{ij} is the gray value of the neuron at pixel (i, j); $F_{ij}(n)$ represents the feedback input item of the neuron; $U_{ij}(n)$ is an internal activity item; k, l represents the 8 neighborhoods corresponding to the center pixel; W_{ijkl} is the connection weight matrix of center pixel and neighborhood pixel. When W_{ijkl} is set in a weak coupling mode, Eq. (2) can be analogized to an amplitude modulation system; $E_{ij}(n)$ is the dynamic threshold of the neuron; a_E and V_E respectively represent the iterative decay time constant and the connection weight amplification coefficient of the dynamic threshold subsystem; $Y_{ij}(n)$ represents the ignition state of the (i, j) pixel in the nth iteration; D is the carrier amplitude, and the value of D has an influence on the pulse transmission speed. The larger D is, the slower the pulse transmission speed will be, and the smoother the segmentation process will be when it is used in thyroid nodule images. Therefore, in order to achieve an ideal segmentation effect for thyroid nodule images, we set the value of D as 25 and other parameters as

$$a_E = 0.0001,\ V_E = S_{\max},\ \boldsymbol{W} = \begin{bmatrix} 0.5/\mathrm{D} & 1/\mathrm{D} & 0.5/\mathrm{D} \\ 1/\mathrm{D} & 1 & 1/\mathrm{D} \\ 0.5/\mathrm{D} & 1/\mathrm{D} & 0.5/\mathrm{D} \end{bmatrix}$$

3 Coarse Segmentation of Thyroid Nodules Based on DPCNN

Ultrasound images of thyroid nodules often have low contrast and uneven grayscale distribution. It is difficult to achieve the ideal effect if it is directly segmented. Therefore, first use DPCNN to coarsely segment the thyroid image. By analyzing the relationship between the contrast of the thyroid nodule image and the iterative entropy of DPCNN, the optimal segmentation image that covers the prominent local details in the gland as much as possible is selected. Part of the iterative output of the thyroid image DPCNN is shown in Fig. 2.

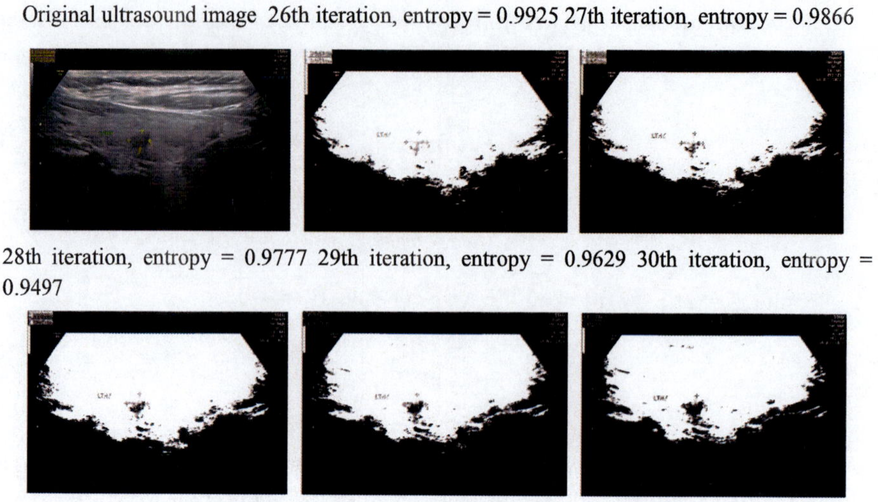

Fig. 2. Partial DPCNN iterative output of thyroid ultrasound image.

It can be seen from Fig. 2 that in the 26th iteration, the local area of the nodule is under-segmented. With the increase of the number of iterations of DPCNN, its detailed information gradually appeared, but the nodular region and non-nodular region showed partial adhesion phenomenon. Therefore, the 28th iteration of the thyroid ultrasound image is selected as the optimal segmentation image for subsequent coarse positioning of the lesion area.

In order to obtain the contour of the target region, the optimal iterative image is reversed, and then the connected domain is filtered. Through a large number of experiments, it is found that in the thyroid segmentation image, the row, column and column-to-row ratio of the connected domain of the nodule area meet certain constraints, as shown in Eq. (5).

$$\begin{cases} 18 < h < 95 \\ 38 < l < 210 \\ \frac{l}{h} < 2.5 \end{cases} \tag{5}$$

Where, h, l, $\frac{l}{h}$ respectively represent the row width, column width and the ratio of column width to row width of the connected domain. Connected domains satisfying the above conditions are retained, and the rest are filtered out. According to the above constraints, the connected domain is filtered out of the coarse segmented image, and the effect is shown in Fig. 3.

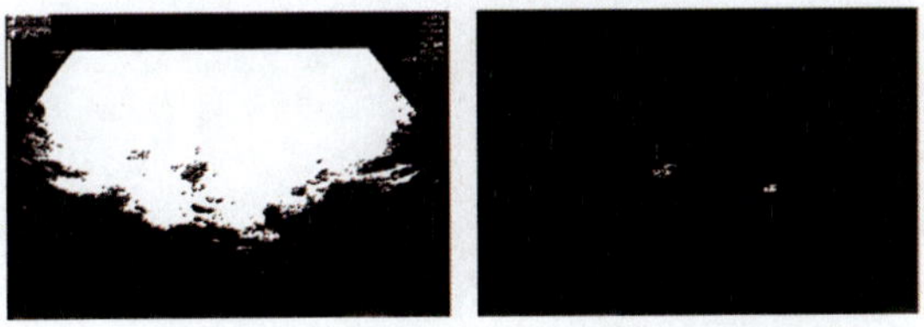

(a) (b)

Fig. 3. The effect of filtering out connected domains. (a) thyroid rough segmentation image; (b) connected domain filter image.

4 Coarse Localization of Nodules Based on Regional Expansion Method

As shown in Fig. 3(b), It can be seen that after DPCNN rough segmentation, connected domain filtering and other operations of thyroid ultrasound images, there may be non-nodular regions. In order to display the detailed information more completely, this article first corresponds to each connected domain in Fig. 3(b) to the corresponding area of the original gray-scale image, and then uses the center of the connected domain as the reference and takes 5 pixels is the length, and 1 pixel is the step length, expand up, down, left and right respectively, and finally get the complete target area. Where, Eq. (6) to Eq. (9) are the algorithm of right-expanding.

$$m_r = \frac{r_{max} + r_{min}}{2} \tag{6}$$

$$m_c = \frac{c_{max} + c_{min}}{2} \tag{7}$$

$$h(m_r, k) = \frac{1}{5}\sum_{k=i}^{i+4} \text{image}(m_r, m_c + k) \qquad (i = 0, 1, \ldots, (c-4)) \tag{8}$$

$$P = p(m_r, k) - p(m_r, k-1) \qquad (i = 0, 1, \ldots, (c-4)) \tag{9}$$

where, (m_r, m_c) is the coordinate of the center point of the connected domain, c is the column width of the original image, r_{max}, r_{min} and c_{max}, c_{min} respectively represent the largest row, smallest row, largest column and smallest column of the connected domain, $h(m_r, t_{k+i})$ represents the average gray value of the 5 pixel area during the expansion process, every time the average gray value of 5 coordinate points is calculated, the column coordinates will increase by 1 to the right, and k represents the number of increments of the ordinate. P represents the difference of the average gray value of the two expansion regions before and after. Because the tissue density and gray value of different regions are different, if $P > \sigma$, the expansion stops. Similarly, the connected domain is expanded in the three directions of up, down and left in the same way, so as to complete the expansion and location of the suspicious region in the original gray image. Figure 4 is the result of regional expansion based on the two connected domains in Fig. 3(b).

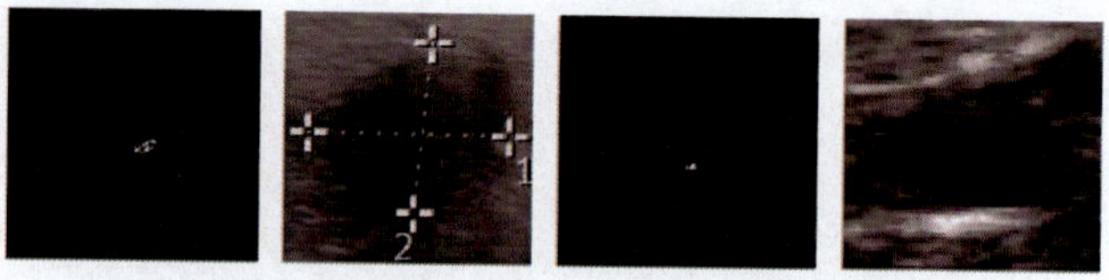

Fig. 4. Connected domains and regions expansion effect.

When performing regional expansion, x usually takes an empirical value of 0.2 to get a better expansion effect. In order to exclude the non-nodular area, this paper combines variance and covariance to construct a comprehensive judgment criterion based on maximum variance and covariance to determine the lesion area. First of all, the variance of the standard template and the suspicious area are calculated respectively, and then calculate the covariance between the standard template and the suspicious area. If the covariance is positive, and its value is greater, the probability of being a nodular area is greater. If the covariance is small or negative, it is an irrelevant area. The specific steps of the comprehensive judgment criterion are as follows:

(1) First, select 50 thyroid images that have been diagnosed and marked by professional doctors from the ultrasound image database. In the lesion area manually marked by the doctor, the neighborhood with pixels of $M \times N$ is selected as the calibration area (in this paper, $M = N = 9$), and the variance of the pixel gray value in the calibration area is calculated. Define the average gray value of the corresponding pixels of all selected images in the calibration area as the standard area, and the average of all variances as the standard deviation.
(2) After the region expansion method is used to expand each suspect region, the suspicious area of the same size as the standard area is selected, and the variance of the suspicious area and the covariance between the suspicious area and the standard area are calculated. The quantitative calculation formula is shown in Eqs. (10)–(14).

$$\eta_R = \frac{1}{MN}\sum_{k=1}^{MN}(R_k - \mu_R)^2 \tag{10}$$

$$\eta_X = \frac{1}{MN}\sum_{k=1}^{MN}(X_k - \mu_X)^2 \tag{11}$$

$$C_{R,X} = \frac{1}{MN}\sum_{k=1}^{MN}(R_k - \mu_R)(X_k - \mu_X) \tag{12}$$

$$g = \eta_R + 2C_{R,X} \tag{13}$$

$$s = \log_2 \frac{R_{\max} - R_{\min}}{X_{\max} - X_{\min}} \tag{14}$$

Where, R and X are standard regions and suspect regions; μ_R and μ_X, η_R and η_X respectively represent the mean value and variance of the corresponding area,

R_{max}, R_{min} and X_{max}, X_{min} are the maximum and minimum gray values of the corresponding area. Based on the above quantitative features, we construct an index that can reflect the similarity of gray features of the two regions: The regional variance descriptor g and the regional difference descriptor s. According to the characteristics of thyroid ultrasound images with low contrast and large difference in gray values, the logarithmic function is used in Eq. (14) to enlarge the ratio results, If $g \geq \frac{1}{2}\eta_R$ and $s \leq 1$, it is judged as a thyroid lesion area. The experimental results are shown in Table 1.

Table 1. Judgment of thyroid lesion area

The suspicious area	Regional variance descriptor G	Regional difference descriptor S	Whether it is a nodule
Suspicious Zone 1	43.8205	0.52083	√
Suspicious Zone 2	11.7711	1.1375	×

As can be seen from Table 1, G = 43.8205 and S = 0.52083 of suspicious region 1 are judged as nodular region. G = 11.7711 and S = 1.1375 of suspicious region 2 were determined to be non-nodular region. The coarse location image of nodules determined by the above algorithm is shown in Fig. 5.

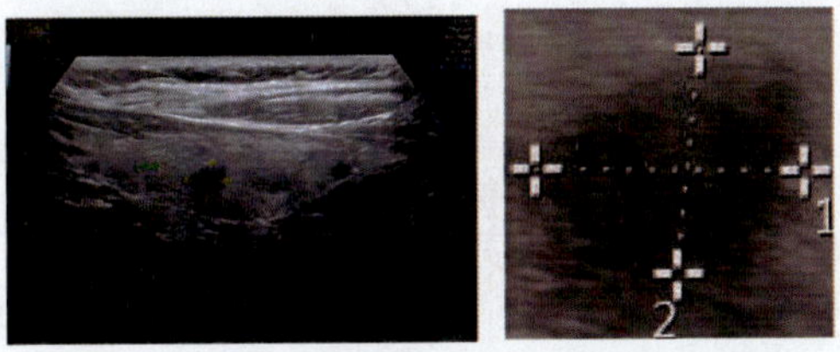

(a) (b)

Fig. 5. Rough localization of thyroid nodule. (a) original ultrasound image; (b) image of nodule area.

Figure 5(b) shows the nodular region determined by the above algorithm. It can be seen that the algorithm of maximum variance and covariance of the local region can accurately screen out the lesion region by relying on the local information of the image, excluding the irrelevant areas.

5 Accurate Segmentation of Nodule Coarse Positioning Image

The ultrasound image of thyroid nodules processed in this paper is a gray-scaled image. Due to the low contrast between the nodule and the background area in the gray-scaled image, therefore, in this paper, the coarse positioning image of the thyroid nodule is divided into different sub-blocks, and then each sub-block is iteratively output by DPCNN. The optimal iteration output of each sub-block is combined to obtain the precise segmentation map of thyroid nodule.

According to the analysis of the mathematical coupling characteristics of the DPCNN model, combined with the influence of the value of D on the segmentation of thyroid nodules, the value of D is set to 1. Figure 6 shows the optimal DPCNN segmentation of the Block image. It can be seen from the DPCNN segmentation results of the block image that the image after the block segmentation process can effectively reduce the influence of the background area, avoiding. The problem of large error rate caused by segmentation of the whole image is solved.

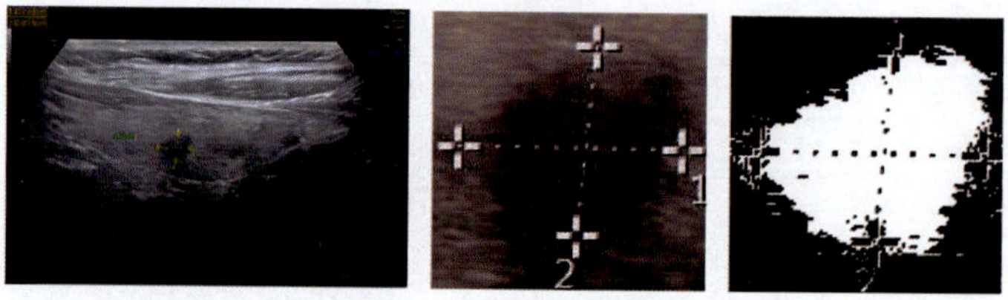

Fig. 6. DPCNN segmentation of block image.

6 Experimental Results and Analysis

In order to further verify the effectiveness and accuracy of the proposed algorithm for segmentation of ultrasound images of thyroid nodules, this paper randomly selects three original thyroid ultrasound images with different contrast and boundary clarity for experimental explanation, as shown in Fig. 7. Figure 8 is a rough location image corresponding to the thyroid nodule in Fig. 7. The experimental results obtained by the algorithm in this paper are compared with the OTSU algorithm, histogram threshold segmentation, the traditional PCNN algorithm and the segmentation results of the literature [14]. The segmentation effect is shown in Fig. 9.

As can be seen from Fig. 8(a), the boundary of the lower part of the thyroid nodule is not clear, and the image has over-segmentation phenomenon when the OTSU algorithm and the PCNN algorithm segment it. When the histogram threshold is used for segmentation, the local area is adhered to the background area. In literature [14], the lower part of thyroid nodule was not segmented when it was segmented. In Fig. 8(b), the contrast between the upper half of the thyroid nodule and the background area is low, and the local grayscale distribution is uneven. When OTSU algorithm, histogram threshold algorithm and traditional PCNN algorithm segment the thyroid nodule, the upper part is not segmented. In literature [14], there is the problem of incomplete edge in the segmentation of thyroid nodule. In Fig. 8(c), the contrast between the thyroid nodule area and the background area is relatively high. There is a small area with higher brightness in the nodule area. When the OTSU algorithm, histogram threshold algorithm and PCNN algorithm segment the thyroid nodule, there is adhesion between the nodule area and the non-nodule area. While ensuring the accuracy of the segmentation results, the algorithm in this paper can also achieve a good segmentation effect for thyroid nodules with unclear boundaries and low contrast, and the detailed information of the image is relatively complete.

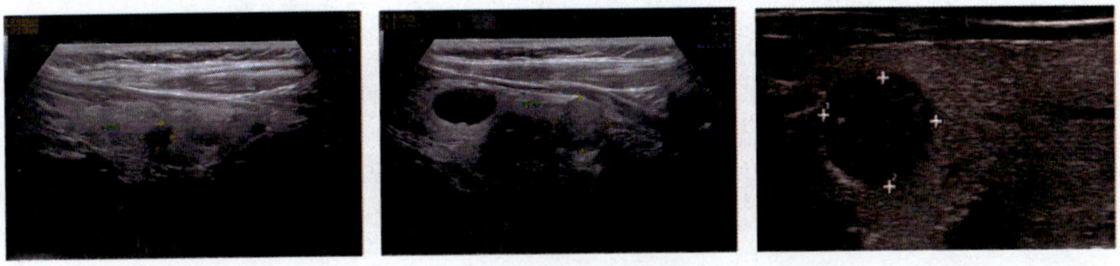

(a) (b) (c)

Fig. 7. Original ultrasound images of thyroid nodule. (a) Original image 1; (b) original image 2; (c) original image 3.

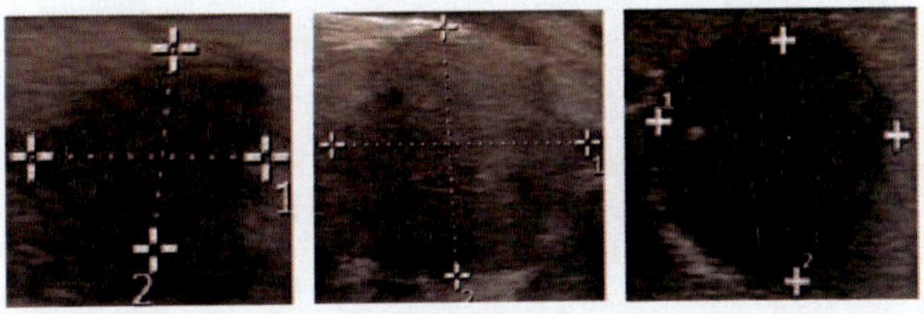

(a) (b) (c)

Fig. 8. Rough localization images of thyroid nodule. (a) Thyroid nodule 1; (b) thyroid nodule 2; (c) thyroid nodule 3.

In order to make a quantitative analysis of the above experimental results, this paper took the results of manual segmentation by doctors as the benchmark diagram, as shown in Fig. 10. The segmentation performance of the five models was quantified by means of MSE, PSNR and comprehensive evaluation index F1-Measure. The experimental results were shown in Table 2.

It can be seen from Table 2 that compared with the other four algorithms, the f1 value of the algorithm in this paper is 0.9469 and the peak signal-to-noise ratio is 38.8719. The f1 value and peak signal-to-noise ratio of the algorithm in this paper are the highest among the five algorithms, and the mean square error is the lowest among the five algorithms. Each objective evaluation index is optimal, which shows that the algorithm in this paper has obvious advantages in edge processing and highlighting details of thyroid nodule images, and its effectiveness and robustness are better than the other four algorithms.

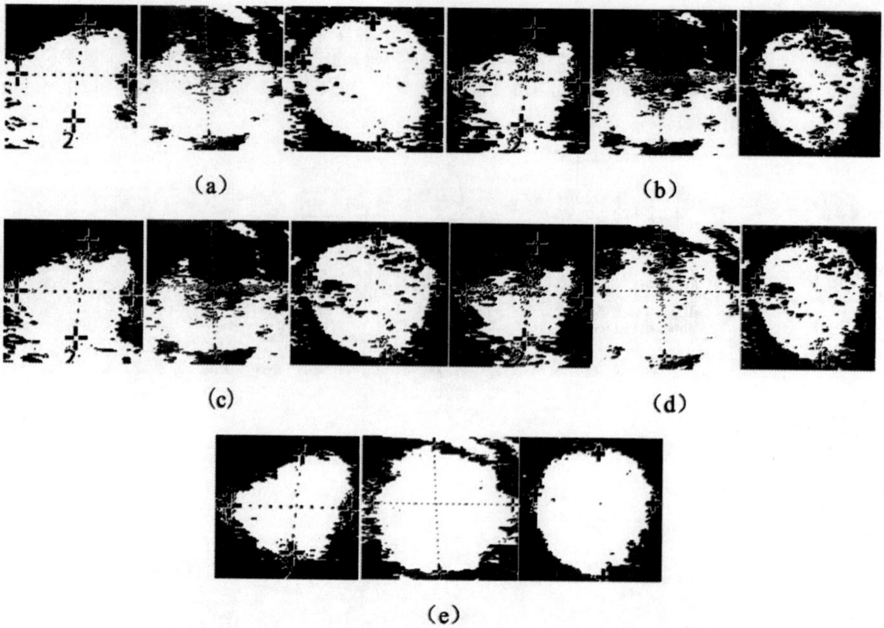

Fig. 9. Segmentation results of thyroid nodule by different algorithms. (a) OTSU algorithm; (b) histogram threshold algorithm; (c) traditional PCNN algorithm; (d) literature [19] algorithm; (e) the proposed algorithm.

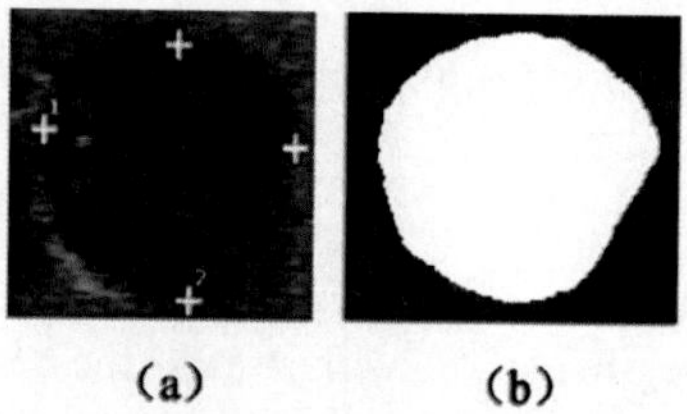

Fig. 10. The initial outline of the thyroid nodule. (a) Thyroid nodule image; (b) initial contour.

Table 2. Quantitative evaluation of segmentation results for the five models

Algorithm	MSE	PSNR	F1-Measure
OTSU	11.2416	37.6225	0.8740
Histogram threshold	50.4272	31.1042	0.7713
Traditional PCNN	31.8216	33.1036	0.8487
Ref. 20	27.7305	33.7012	0.8600
Proposed algorithm	8.4312	38.8719	0.9469

7 Concluding Remarks

In this paper, an ultrasonic image segmentation algorithm for thyroid nodule based on DPCNN is proposed, which adopts a progressive nodule target extraction method of first rough segmentation, then rough positioning, and finally fine segmentation, so as to solve the segmentation difficulties caused by low contrast of ultrasonic images and complex background region. By comparing with other segmentation algorithms, the experimental results further demonstrate the feasibility of this algorithm. This algorithm is suitable for the segmentation of ultrasound images of various thyroid nodules, especially for the edge is not clear thyroid nodule segmentation has good robustness and high efficiency, and it has a significant effect in improving the clarity and completeness of image segmentation, and the detailed information is also relatively rich. However, in the coarse segmentation of ultrasound images using DPCNN, the automatic selection of optimal segmentation cannot be achieved yet. In addition, this article does not diagnose and classify the thyroid nodules after segmentation, which will be the work that needs to be completed in the next study.

Acknowledgment. National Natural Science Foundation of China (61961037), Postgraduate Training and Curriculum Reform Project of Northwest Normal University.

References

1. Parsa, A.A., Gharib, H.: Epidemiology of thyroid nodules. In: Gharib, H. (ed.) Thyroid Nodules. Contemporary Endocrinology. Humana Press, Cham (2018)
2. Wang, P., Liu, J., Yue, W.S., et al.: The application of diagnosis guider of thyroid nodules in 2016 with ultrasound in the differentiation of benign and malignant thyroid nodules. J. Practical Med. Imaging **18**(16), 466–468 (2017)
3. Gabriel, E., Venkatesan, V., Shah, S.: Towards high performance cell segmentation in multi-spectral fine needle aspiration cytology of thyroid lesions. Comput. Methods Progr. Biomed. **98**(3), 231–240 (2010)
4. Iakovidis, D.K., Savelonas, M.A., Karkanis, S.A., et al.: A genetically optimized level set approach to segmentation of thyroid ultrasound images. Appl. Intell. **27**(3), 193–203 (2007)
5. Chang, C.Y., Huang, H.C., Chen, S.J.: Automatic thyroid nodule segmentation and component analysis in ultrasound images. Biomed. Eng. Appl. Basis Commun. **22**(2), 81–89 (2010)
6. Koundal, D., Sharma, B., Guo, Y.: Intuitionistic based segmentation of thyroid nodules in ultrasound images. Comput. Biol. Med. **121**, 8 (2020)
7. Ma, J., Wu, F., Jiang, T., Zhao, Q., Kong, D.: Ultrasound image-based thyroid nodule automatic segmentation using convolutional neural networks. Int. J. Comput. Assist. Radiol. Surg. **12**(11), 1895–1910 (2017). https://doi.org/10.1007/s11548-017-1649-7
8. Prabal, P., Christian, H., Julian, S., et al.: 3D segmentation of thyroid ultrasound images using active contours. Curr. Dir. Biomed. Eng. **2**(1), 467–470 (2016)
9. Binny, S.: Mean-shift filtering and segmentation in ultra sound thyroid images. Int. J. Res. Commer. Manag. **3**(3), 126 (2013)
10. Eckhorn, R., Reitboeck, H., Arndt, M., et al.: Feature linking via synchronization among distributed assemblies: simulations of results from cat visual cortex. Neural Comput. **2**(3), 293–307 (2014)

11. Guo, Y., Yang, Z., Ma, Y., et al.: Saliency motivated improved simplified PCNN model for object segmentation. Neurocomputing **275**(2), 2179–2190 (2018)
12. Zhou, L., Sun, Y., Zheng, J.: Automated color image edge detection using improved PCNN model. WSEAS Trans. Comput. **7**(4), 184–189 (2008)
13. Deng, X.-Y., Ma, Y.-D.: PCNN model automatic parameters determination and its modified model. Acta Electron. Sin. **5**(5), 955–964 (2012)
14. Deng, X.Y., Yang, Y.H., Qin, W.J.: An improved non-coupled PCNN model for image segmentation. IOP Conf. Ser. Mater. Sci. Eng. **790**, 884–892 (2020)

Computer-Aided Detection/Diagnosis

Information Technologies in Complex Reconstructive Maxillofacial Surgery

Svetlana Cherebylo[1], Evgeniy Ippolitov[1], Mikhail Novikov[1](✉), and Sergey Tereshchuk[2]

[1] Institute on Laser and Information Technologies RAS – Branch of the Federal Scientific Research Centre "Crystallography and Photonics" of RAS, Shatura, Russia
novikov@rambler.ru

[2] Center for Maxillofacial Surgery and Dentistry at Burdenko Main Military Clinical Hospital, Moscow, Russia

Abstract. The data presented by the Ministry of Public Health of Russia over the past 10 years show that the incidence of the malignant tumours in the population has been increasing by 1,5% annually. Unfortunately, more than 62% of oral cavity tumours were only revealed at the III and IV stages of disease. In these cases, surgical treatment is of critical importance. The operations performed at these stages result in significant defects of the maxillofacial region, their correction being an extremely complicated task. The utilization of the microvascular grafts enables the surgeon to close these defects to a great extent. The growing requirements to the patient's life quality in the postoperative period makes the surgeon search for new instruments to enhance the precision of planning and performing of the operations. The development of informational diagnostic devices and methods of high-technology cure of patients enhance the potentialities of the new approaches in processing the patient's data for planning the treatment with the use of the modern information systems: computer simulation and additive technologies. The article describes the use of information technologies for the preparation and planning of complex maxillofacial reconstructions. The use of 3D medical images (computed tomography and magnetic resonance imaging), computer-aided design and additive technologies allows you to create detailed anatomical computer models and their physical prototypes. The surgeon can use these models to plan treatment, custom design and manufacture implants, and evaluate outcomes.

Keywords: Computed tomography · Digital model · Computer modeling · Additive technologies · Reconstructive surgery

1 Introduction

The growing requirements to the patient's life quality in the postoperative period makes the surgeon search for new instruments to enhance the precision of planning and performing of the operations [1, 2]. The development of informational diagnostic devices and methods of high-technology cure of patients enhance the potentialities of the new

R. Su et al. (Eds.): MICAD 2021, LNEE 784, pp. 177–185, 2022.
https://doi.org/10.1007/978-981-16-3880-0_19

approaches in processing the patient's data for planning the treatment with the use of the modern information systems: computer simulation and additive technologies [3, 4].

The application of the computer-aided design (CAD) and additive technologies allow for production of patient's biological models and the intraoperative surgical templates in the shortest possible time [5, 6]. The creation of new materials and technologies to produce the articles for the replacement and regeneration of tissues and organs is one of the priority trends of the up-to-date biomedicine.

The clinical application of biomaterials requires that their shape, structure and biomechanical characteristics correspond to those of the organs and tissues of a living being. Thousands of restorative operations are annually performed which involves the replacement of the bone tissue with implants and endoprostheses. The main requirement imposed upon any implant is its reliability that primarily depends on a possibility of osteointegration, i.e. the firm union of the implant and the bone with no inflammatory reactions causing the implant rejection. The implant is expected to be made from a biocompatible material, possess sufficient strength and have large surface provide a maximally close between the implant and the bony defect in the damaged area. Plastic biomodels are being increasingly used in the preparation and planning of the operative intervention in the maxillofacial surgery, in the surgery of spine, thoracic surgery, orthopedics and neurosurgery, as well as in the fast fabrication of implants from biocompatible materials and their preoperative fitting. The effectiveness of the virtual surgical planning (VSP) results in the shorter time that is essential for pediatric patients for whom the time of undergoing general anesthesia is strictly limited; secondly, in the improvement of the qualitative indices, primarily, the accuracy of restoration of the contours and shapes of the lost parts of the body, which reduces the postoperative complications and the duration of the rehabilitation period; thirdly, in the reduction of the treatment cost [7, 8].

The present work illustrates the application of the 3D medical imaging in combination with the computer and telecommunication technologies in planning the reconstructive operations in maxillofacial surgery. The designed method permits to not only obtain fairly objective information on the pathology in the damaged area (even in the cases of very complex defects), but makes it possible to create the customized implants to close this defect. A unified approach to performing the operations of this kind involves obtaining and processing the computer tomography data, making a computer model, computer simulation, virtual surgical planning, fabrication of individual biomodels and templates.

2 Computer Simulation and Additive Technologies in Maxillofacial Surgery

ILIT RAS has developed and is successfully applying laser stereolithography, one of the first additive technologies based on laser polymerization of liquid photopolymer compositions [4].

In 1994, laser stereolithography was first used in ILIT RAS for the purpose of medicine within the framework of the forensic medical examination of the remains of the Russian tsar's family found near Ekaterinburg. It was the first time in Russia that a plastic copy of a human skull had been made with the accuracy feasible for performing the forensic medical examination relying on the data obtained from the computer tomograph by the method of laser stereolithography [9].

The spiral computer tomograph permits scanning of the whole skull within several minutes. High-precision reconstruction of the complex geometry of skull bone defects requires that the thickness of a section in scanning should be less than 0.5 mm. The software realized on the high-speed computer systems makes possible prompt processing of the obtained data and creating the 3D models of any defect and deformation of the skull, permits modeling of the implants closely fitted to the damaged area before performing reconstructive operations. The up-to-date methods of additive production of 3D objects, laser stereolithography, in particular, permit making the plastic copies of any fragment of the human bony skeleton. Fabrication of the medical implants presents a striking example of single-part production since each of the implants is produced for the individual patient.

Computer simulation and laser stereolithography have contributed greatly to the reconstructive maxillofacial surgery offering the improvement of both functional and cosmetic results of operative intervention [10].

The designed methods of tomography data processing enable the construction of high-precision computer 3D models to be used in restorative surgery and planning of most complex operations. In December 2007, jointly with Burdenko Main Military Clinical Hospital (Moscow, maxillofacial surgeon S.V. Tereshchuk), was carried out virtual surgical planning resection of the mandible and its primary reconstruction with fibular free flap. The main goal of this research was designing and fabricating surgical guides increasing accuracy of the operation. The primary reconstructive procedures present a priority trend in surgery since they facilitate fast enough the restoration of the vital functions during the post-operative period and favor the reduction of the patient's rehabilitation time [11].

For mandiblular reconstruction they use flaps from different donor places: rib, shoulder blade, iliac bone, radial bone, the fibular flap being the «working horse»: rib; shoulder blade; fibular bone; iliac bone; radial bone; ulnar bone; humeral bone; metatarsus.

Further will be described the algorithm of interaction between the surgeon and the technical assistant in the process of preparation, planning and performing the reconstructive operations, which is followed at the present time.

The primary inspection of the patient, diagnosing and planning of cure are carried out in the hospital. The surgeon makes a decision to perform the reconstruction of the lower jaw with the fibular free flap; then tomographic examination of the facial skeleton and both fibulas is made with the spacing no more than 1 mm. Figure 1 illustrates the patient computer tomography (CT) scans [12–14].

Based on the CT scan data of a patient a 3D composite model is build. The CT scan data in DICOM format are imported to ILIT RAS via the Internet. The downloaded tomograms are processed with the 3Dview package developed in ILIT RAS and are conversed to a 3D computer model in STL format that is used on the additive technologies. The conversion of the CT data and the construction of 3D models are illustrated by Fig. 2.

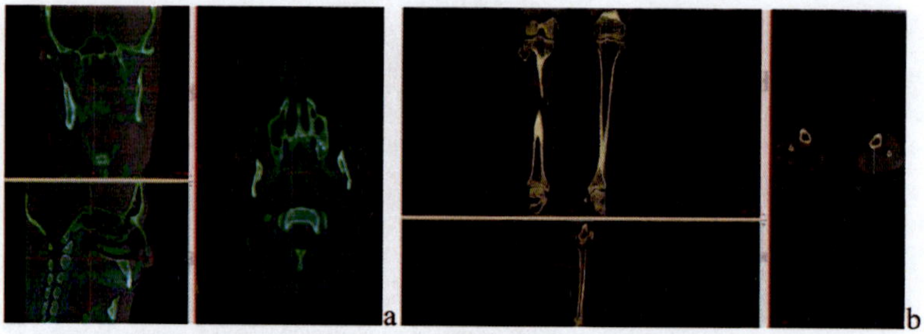

Fig. 1. CT examination of a) the patient's facial skeleton; b) the bones of lower extremities (a set of scans with the spacing of 0.4 and 0.8 mm, respectively)

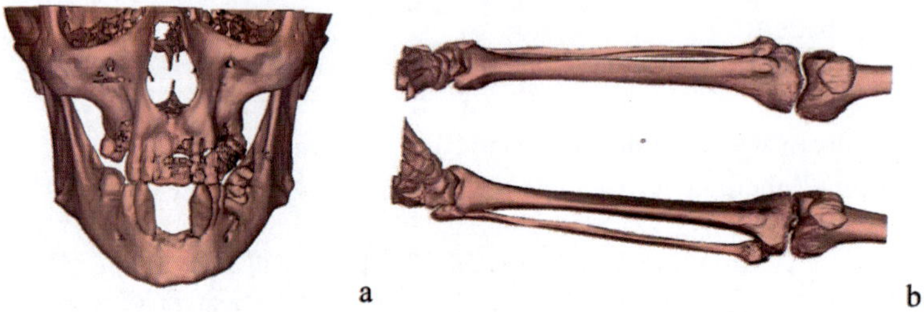

Fig. 2. Customized 3D models a) the facial skeleton, b) the lower extremities reproduced using the patient's tomography data.

The virtual resection of the patient's lower jaw was performed by a technical assistant under the direction of a surgeon during the on-line conference between ILIT RAS and Burdenko Main Military Clinical Hospital. The computer simulation was conducted by the Magics program of firm Materialise, Belgium. Materialise is a world leader in creating the software for the additive production. The main tasks at this stage are (see Fig. 3): defining the size of the bone defect; specifying the correct cutting planes.

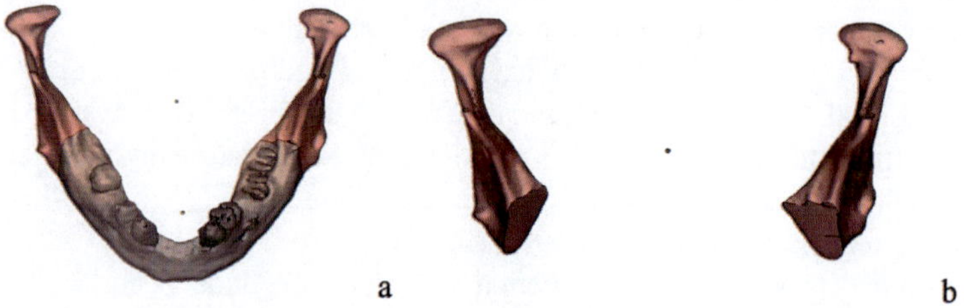

Fig. 3. Localization of the malignant region (a); the result of resection (b).

The following stage involves the formation of the fibular graft, its placement in the defect. The position of the nutrient blood vessels influences these steps (see Fig. 4).

The conditions for correct location of the graft are:

– the blood vessels of the fibula should pass along on the inner side of the graft;

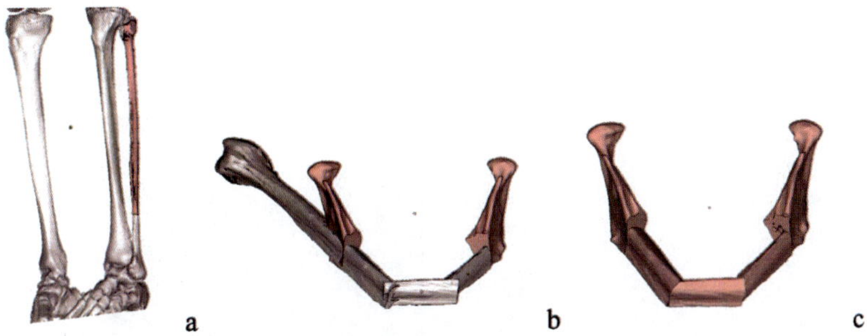

Fig. 4. Separation of a fragment of the fibular bone (a); spatial orientation and alignment of the flap graft with the lower jaw (b); formation of the autograft (c).

- when the flap is raised with a skin pad for closing skin or mucosa defects, the posterior fascial septum with skin perforator arteries should be protected from damage;
- an optimal interrelation between the graft and the upper teeth provides the conditions for the subsequent orthopedic rehabilitation of the patient;
- the anatomic position of the articular head in the temporomandibular joints is retained;
- the graft length and the position of its parts are chosen to ensure a match of the resulting occlusion with the initial one;
- the plane of the outside wall of the graft bone and the outer sides of the jaw branches coincide.

Figure 5 presents the final variant of the occlusion as compared to the resected fragment of the patient's lower jaw.

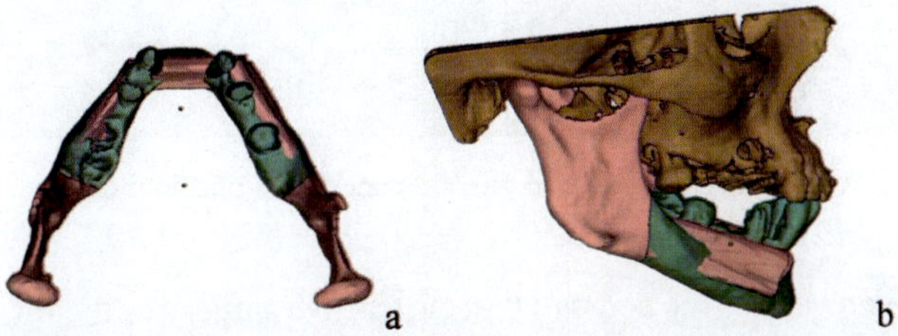

Fig. 5. A variant of the occlusion as compared to the resected fragment of the lower jaw: a) top view; b) side view.

The positive outcome of the operation depends on exact matching of the site and direction of resection of both the lower jaw and the fibular bone. To fulfill this condition, the following physical objects are designed and fabricated: 3D model of the mandible with the flap in the defect, surgical guides for resection of the mandible and osteotomy of the fibula. The computer models and plastic prototypes of the simulated objects made on the laser stereolithograph in ILIT RAS are shown in Fig. 6.

The following stage involves the fabrication of the models of lower jaw fragments and the templates from the photopolymerizing composition on the laser stereolithograph of ILIT RAS.

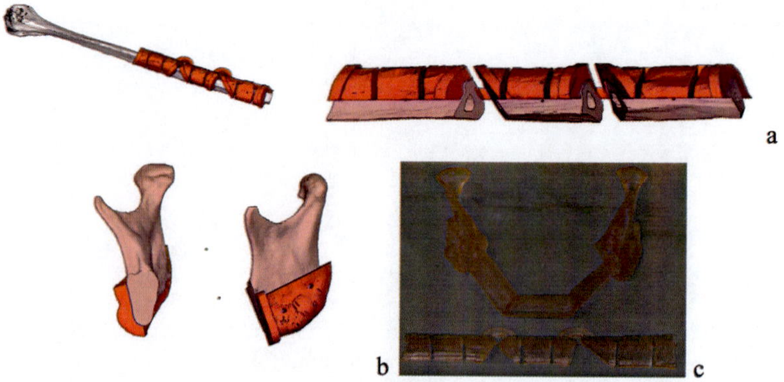

Fig. 6. Computer models of the templates for resection of a fibular bone (a), a lower jaw bone (b) and their plastic prototypes (c).

Then, the produced models and templates are delivered to the hospital for preparation and planning of the operation. For precise making and fitting of the fixation plates, a plastic stereolithography model is used, the time of the operation itself being reduced (Fig. 7). The number of the fixation plates is defined by the surgeon in accordance with the plan of operation and subsequent orthopedic rehabilitation.

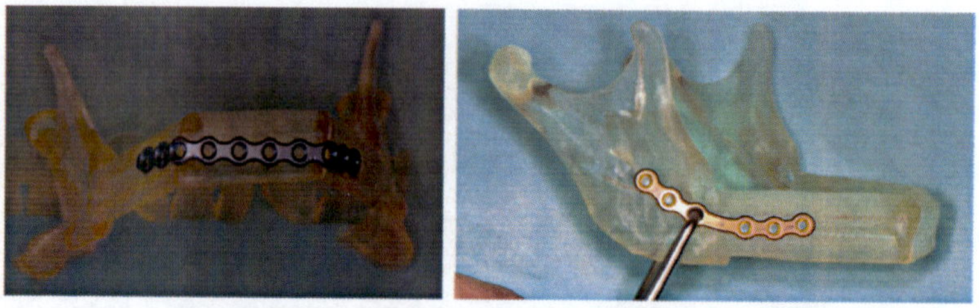

Fig. 7. Fitting of the fixture element on the plastic model.

Figure 8 demonstrates the course of reconstructive surgery of the lower jaw.

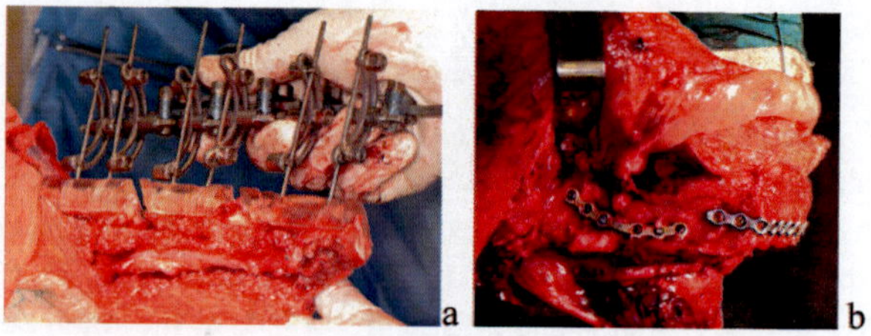

Fig. 8. The course of operation for reconstruction of the lower jaw: a) placing the template on the fibular bone; b) jointing and fastening of the graft parts on the lower jaw.

The device for fixation of the fibula during its osteotomy is optional (Fig. 8b). The application of this device is necessity for the graft gripping with the instruments, which decreases the possibility of damaging the nutrient vessels in the bone and improves the stability of the graft in osteotomy. It should be noted here that the position of the pins of the fixation device in the bone is also planned during the virtual operation, and their accurate localization is ensured by the guide placed into the holes in the template. (see Fig. 9).

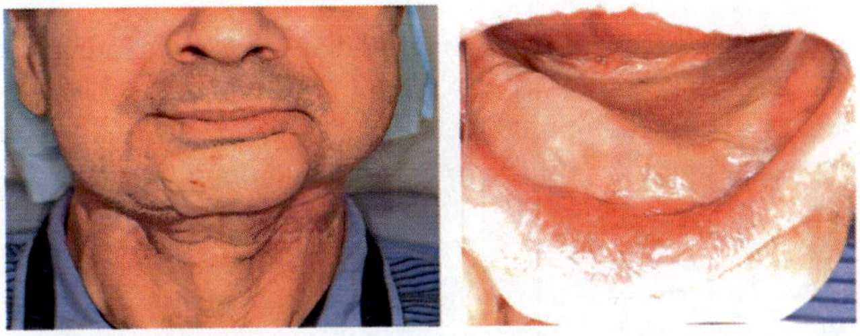

Fig. 9. The patient's appearance in 6 months after the operation.

All the stages of operation (resection of the lower jaw, sampling of the fibular bone, formation and fixation of the graft in the defect) are performed in a single process owing to the preliminary planning and template preparation, which considerably improves the operation precision, minimizes trauma and its duration, thus favoring the engraftment and fast recovery of the patient. High precision of computer simulation permits speeding up the accretion of the graft bone fragments and improving the cavity functionality. The described algorithm of planning and performing the operations of this kind has been successfully tested and is now obligatory for application in the Centre of maxillofacial surgery and stomatology of N.N. Burdenko Clinical hospital, Moscow.

The following advantages of the application of computer simulation and laser stereolithography in the reconstructive maxillofacial surgery can be pointed out [12–19]:

- a reduction of the operation performing time at the cost of its planning and fixture fitting on the plastic model and, hence, a greater chance of successful outcome of the operation;
- an increase in the accuracy of matching the jointed planes of the graft and the jaw, and, consequently, the reduction of the recovery period;
- an increase in the accuracy of the graft coincidence with the jaw initial shape and, for this reason, an improvement of functionality and a possibility of dentition restoration through implantation;
- the full recovery of the lost vital functions.

3 Conclusion

At present, the additive technologies have found their niche along with the traditional methods of producing the parts for the high-technology medicine. The additive technologies application jointly with the CAS systems increases preciseness and accuracy of the surgery owing to the science-based account of the patient's personal features, optimization of the operational process and minimization of the operative intervention, and therefore permits enhancing the quality of life of the patient in the post op period [20, 21].

The developed technique of fabrication of individual implants and templates with the use of computer simulation and laser stereolithography enables:

- the fabrication of the 3D models of biological objects relying on the tomography data of the patient;
- designing and fabrication of the individual implants and templates to close the bone defects;
- the shortening of the operating time, the improvement of the aesthetic outcomes, the shorter rehabilitation period, which is of great social importance.

Acknowledgments. This work was done with the financial support of the RFBR (Grant MK # 18-29-03238). Work on laser stereolithography is executed at financial support of the Ministry of science and higher education (State task FSRC "Crystallography and Photonics" RAS).

References

1. Sharaf, B., Levine, J., Hirsch, D., Bastidas, J., Schiff, B., Garfein, E.: Importance of computer-aided design and manufacturing technology in the multidisciplinary approach to head and neck reconstruction. J. Craniofac. Surg. **21**(4), 1277–1280 (2010)
2. Antony, A., Chen, W., Kolokythas, A., Weimer, K., Cohen, M.: Use of virtual surgery and stereolithography-guided osteotomy for mandibular reconstruction with the free fibula. J. Plast. Reconstr. Aesthet. Surg. **128**(5), 1080–1084 (2011)
3. Zhuk, D.M., Perfiliev, S.A.: CAS systems – computer-aided design systems in surgery. Electronic scientific and technical edition "Science and education", no. 3, March 2011, p. 12 (2011). http://technomag.edu.ru
4. Panchenko, V.Y.: Modern laser and information technologies, red., Interkontakt Nauka, Moscow (RUS) (2014)
5. Matthew, M., Hanasono, M.D., Roman, J.S.: Computer-assisted design and rapid prototype modeling in microvascular mandible reconstruction. Laryngoscope **123**, 597–604 (2013)
6. Modabber, A., Legros, C., Rana, M., Gerressen, M., Riediger, D.: Alireza Ghassemi Evaluation of computer-assisted jaw reconstruction with free vascularized fibular flap compared to conventional surgery: a clinical pilot study. Int. J. Med. Robot. Comput. Assist. Surg. **8**, 215–220 (2012)
7. Lethaus, B., Poort, L., Böckmann, R., Smeets, R., Tolba, R., Kessler, P.: Additive manufacturing for microvascular reconstruction of the mandible in 20 patients. J. Cranio-Maxillo-Fac. Surg. **40**, 43–46 (2012)
8. Liu, Y.F., Xu, L.W., Zhu, H.Y., Liu, S.S.Y.: Technical procedures for template-guided surgery for mandibular reconstruction based on digital design and manufacturing. BioMed. Eng. OnLine **13**, 63 (2014). http://www.biomedical-engineering-online.com/content/13/1/63
9. Evseev, A.V., Kamaev, S.V., Kotsuba, E.V., Markov, M.A., Novikov, M.M., Panchenko, V.Y., Popov, V.K.: Computer biomodeling and laser stereolithography. In: Proceedings of SPIE, Eighth International Conference on Lasers and Laser Information Technologies, vol. 5449, (21 June 2004). https://doi.org/10.1117/12.563109

10. Lethaus, B., Poort, L., Böckmann, R., Smeets, R., Tolba, R., Kessler, P.: Additive manufacturing for microvascular reconstruction of the mandible in 20 patients. J. Cra- nio-Maxillofac. Surg. **40**, 43–46 (2012)
11. Gorbulenko, V., Kozlov, S., Demenchuk, P., Tereshuk, S.V.: Primary replacement of postoperative defects of maxillofacial area after malignant tumor excision. Vestnik of N.N. Blokhin Russian oncological research centre of RAMS, vol. 20, no. 2 (Suppl. 1), p. 103 (2009)
12. Musatyan, S.A.: Sposoby segmentacii medicinskih izobrazhenij. Trudy ISP RAN **30**(4), 183–194 (2018). (RUS)
13. van Eijnatten, M., Koivisto, J., Karhu, K., Forouzanfar, T., Wolff, J.: The impact of manual threshold selection in medical additive manufacturing. Int. J. Comput. Assist. Radiol. Surg. **12**(4), 607–615 (2016). https://doi.org/10.1007/s11548-016-1490-4
14. Hou, J., Chen, M., Pan, C., et al.: Immediate reconstruction of bilateral mandible defects: management based on computer-aided design/computer-aided manufacturing rapid prototyping technology in combination with vascularized fibular osteo- myocutaneous flap. J. Oral Maxillofac. Surg. **69**, 1792–1797 (2011)
15. Modabber, A., Legros, C., Rana, M., Gerressen, M., Riediger, D., Ghassemi, A.: Evaluation of computer-assisted jaw reconstruction with free vascularized fibular flap compared to conventional surgery: a clinical pilot study. Int. J. Med. Robot. Comput. Assist. Surg. **8**, 215–220 (2012)
16. Rodby, K., Turin, S., et al.: Advances in oncologic head and neck reconstruction: systemic review and future considerations of virtual surgical planning and computer aided design/computer aided modeling. J. Plast. Reconstr. Aesthet. Surg. **67**(9), 1171–1185 (2014)
17. Crafts, T.: Three-dimensional printing and its applications in otorhinolaryngology– otolaryngol. Head Neck Surg. **156**(6), 999–1010 (2017)
18. Char, M.P., Rozen, W.M., McMenamin, P.G., Findlay, M.W., Spychal, R.T., Hunter-Smith, D.J.: Emerging applications of bedside 3D printing in plastic surgery. Front. Surg. 16 June 2015. https://doi.org/10.3389/fsurg.2015.00025
19. Zachary, G.: Applications of 3-dimensional printing in facial plastic surgery. J. Oral Maxillofac. Surg. **74**, 427–428 (2016)
20. Rodby, K.A., et al.: Antony advances in oncologic head and neck reconstruction: systematic review and future considerations of virtual surgical planning and computer aided design/computer aided modelling. J. Plast. Reconstr. Aesthet. Surg. **67**(9), 1171–1185 (2014)
21. Kim, J.H., Atala, A., Yoo, J.: Translation and applications of biofabrication. In: Ovsianikov, A., Yoo, J., Mironov, V. (eds.) 3D Printing and Biofabrication. RSBE, pp. 451–484. Springer, Cham (2018). https://doi.org/10.1007/978-3-319-45444-3_17

Machine Learning-Based Imaging in Connected Vehicles Environment

Sayon Karmakar[1,2](✉) and Seshadri Mohan[1]

[1] University of Arkansas at Little Rock, Little Rock, AR 72204, USA
{skarmakar,sxmohan}@ualr.edu

[2] National Institute of Technology Sikkim, Ravangla, Sikkim, India

Abstract. Intelligent algorithms greatly influence imaging. Machine learning techniques find applicability in correcting and highlighting medical images generated by X-rays, Computed Tomography (CT) scan, Positron Emission Tomography (PET) scan, Magnetic Resonance Imaging (MRI). Such techniques increase the reliability and quality of diagnosis to aid the doctors in devising an effective treatment. These systems have found wide applicability under clinical settings. Imaging is also an essential task in autonomous vehicle development and Connected Vehicles. Research on Connected Vehicles is evolving at a staggering rate with an objective to reduce road accidents significantly and replace drivers with fully autonomous self-driving vehicles. Driver monitoring system (DMS) is a new area of research where drivers are monitored using cameras and other medical sensor networks to detect the drivers' medical state, mental state as well as cognitive state. Objective biomarkers allow such systems to predict these states. Imaging plays an essential role in the diagnosis aided by the state of the art machine learning algorithms. This paper addresses the challenges posed by imaging under driving environments for diagnosis of medical and cognition of drivers.

Keywords: Machine learning techniques · Autonomous vehicle · Connected vehicle · Driver monitoring system · Cognitive state · Medical sensor networks · Biomarkers

1 Introduction

The medical imaging industry has derived immense benefits from fast growing field of computationally powerful machine learning algorithms. These algorithms have contributed increased reliability in imaging due to the ease of implementation of features such as image resolution correction, sharpness correction, and motion correction. Results of X-rays, MRI, CT scans must produce accurate physical structure of the target organ for proper diagnosis by the doctors. Erroneous systems produce faulty images that can lead to fatal suggestions by doctors. The new algorithms carry out filtering in a reliable manner. The entire development and functioning of such algorithms are usually carried out in a clinical setting. It means the system has lower tolerance to noise since the source of noise are generally absent or removed to produce accurate results.

R. Su et al. (Eds.): MICAD 2021, LNEE 784, pp. 186–194, 2022.
https://doi.org/10.1007/978-981-16-3880-0_20

Connected Vehicles and autonomous vehicles utilize the computer vision for varied tasks. An onboard mounted camera captures the status of traffic flow, hazardous conditions along the roads, traffic accidents, and many other essential factors that are then processed to produce appropriate steering and acceleration-braking actions. Researchers have investigated the development of a system aimed at monitoring drivers to determine their medical state, mental state and cognitive state in the form of DMS. DMS is the technology implemented in the vehicles to monitor drivers of their condition using camera as a primary sensor with a set of other medical wireless sensors network collectively working to acquire data and predict the driver's health condition. A camera that is mounted on the dashboard or in the vicinity of the driver captures the driver's facial cues. Current medical research allows early diagnosis of chronic medical conditions, mental state as well as cognition from the behavioral analysis of human emotions and ocular movements, known as objective biomarkers. Various driving models show the importance of cognition in driving and statistics of automobile accidents show the importance of proper health condition to prevent such fatalities. Imaging in clinical setting is difficult and error prone; real-time imaging for medical diagnosis is a new forte. Proper data resolution of biomarkers play a key role in the accuracy as well as the reliability of this system. Several challenges arise due to the dynamic nature of the connected vehicles' environment.

Medical imaging in open fields and real time basis is a challenge that is coming up and requires extensive research. These systems are prone to much different types of noise and hence require development of new ML algorithms to eliminate the noise. This draft addresses the key challenges of image acquisition in this environment which would predict the health condition of drivers.

The paper has been explored into following sections. Section 2 discusses the history and current advances in the medical imaging industry. Section 3 highlights the assumptions and challenges addressed physically and computationally in the environment of medical imaging. Section 4 introduces the concept of connected vehicles and its related research. Section 5 establishes the missing link between the connected vehicles' research to the medical imaging industry. Section 6 brings out the challenges in the connected vehicles environment (CVE) followed by the remedies that can be given by the intelligent ML algorithms in Sect. 7. Finally, the key findings of paper is summarized in the conclusion.

2 Current Medical Imaging Industry

The medical imaging industry heavily relies on the proper functioning of the algorithms. Reliability of the algorithm is extremely crucial for the proper diagnosis carried by the doctors. Thus, accuracy validation is a challenge in this industry for lack of availability of ground truth.

Imaging in healthcare evolved very rapidly since the discovery of X-rays 120 years ago [1]. It led the radiologists to image the human body. Currently, the imaging industry prefers the intricate methods of computed tomography, magnetic resonance imaging, positron emission tomography, ultrasound and other modalities [2]. The leap in the technology is huge that led to a very solid foundation of today's screening, diagnosis and monitoring of diseases. On the contrary, there are some risks associated to these methods. These risks include exposure to ionizing radiations, that has capacity to destroy DNA and ultimately leading to cancer [3, 4]; and plausible allergy reactions to intravenous contrast agents [5]. Moreover, the healthcare industry charges taxes on imaging which leads to the triggering of anxiety and depression in patients.

X-rays, which was accidentally discovered by Prof. Roentgen made an industrial radiograph but later was deemed suitable for evaluating the bone fracture, that become the underlying basis of today's mammography, tomography and angiography [6]. Fluoroscopy became realizable when the X-rays became powerful and with an oral injection of barium (radio-opaque in nature), diagnosed cancers, ulcers in vicinity of the stomach. Modern day image intensifiers omit the use of such contrasting agents.

Nuclear medicine utilizes positrons for imaging modality named, positron emission tomography (PET). Positron annihilates with an electron releasing photons, that is light and the emission is localized in space. It is based on positron emitting isotope of fluorine incorporated in glucose called fluorodeoxyglucose (FGD). PET measures the glucose intake, which is the mainstream diagnosis technique for cancer [7]. Therefore, a major leap is seen in this imaging industry from a feeble x-ray to an extremely sophisticated PET scan.

3 Environment of Clinical Medical Image Acquisition

The study of the environment where these imaging takes place is an essential component of this paper as it would highlight the assumptions and challenges taken care while carrying out the image acquisition. It also leads to the introduction of critical decision making steps at a computational level.

Common types of imaging modalities used in the modern medicine include x-rays, CT scans, PET scans, angiography, ultrasonography, MRI scans, mammography, etc. X-rays primarily uses electrically charged cathode tube to generate produce x-ray gamma photons which are bombarded on the area for imaging.

The rooms where these imaging is carried out must contain a proper shielding to prohibit the escape of such high energy particles to the environment. But, there must a place for the radiologist to view the patient undergoing the imaging. Thus, a glass that is extremely transparent for clear viewing but has the capacity to block the high energy particles.

4 Introduction to Connected Vehicles

Connected Vehicles is the modern complex network of automobiles communicating with each other and with other infrastructures for sharing safety critical information which has the ultimate goal to reduce traffic accidents, reduce pollution by increasing the efficiency of the transportation systems and reduce the travel time. An optimized and connected network of traffic would ensure human safety as it is of highest priority to most global organizations. Safety regulations, active and passive safety systems in vehicles, road signs even upon strict enforcement is not enough to stop the fatal accidents. 90% of the crashes are caused due to human errors [8]. The research on developing safety systems for driver led to the establishment of connected vehicles. Communication standards are being developed for supporting this disruptive and transformative technology on global level by FCC, 3GPP and ITU-T [9–11].

Safety is the primary concern and thriving force of this research. Special spectrum bands for communications are being identified and allotted only for vehicular communications. There are multiple challenges in this vehicular networks being addressed using the intelligent algorithms. Research shows multiple use cases of the immense and reliable power of these algorithms.

Advanced driver assistance systems (ADAS) is a complex system which is equipped with every automobile for providing additional information to the driver upon which the decisions are taken to guide the vehicle through safety. Some recent ADAS has the capability to avert life threating situations by controlling the vehicles' lateral and longitudinal motion. Some of these systems are Forward collision warning system, Automatic Emergency Braking, Electronic Stability Control and many more. The highest level of decision taking ADAS forms the control center of Automated Vehicles, having the capability of full automation. The pace of the research in development of fully autonomous vehicle is at its peak which utilizes these intelligent algorithms for decision taking and finding the appropriate solution.

Acquiring image from the environment which is then processed by the onboard computer to generate decisions that are responsible for directing and guiding the vehicle through the traffic, eventually reaching to the intended destination. There are some fundamental differences as well as similarities in the imaging under clinical setting and connected vehicle environment that are addressed later in the paper.

Current research on development of ADAS is shifting from a vehicle centric approach to driver centric approach where the drivers' cognitive state, mental state and medical state is being monitored by non-invasive sensors. Sensors include cameras, lidars, wireless wristbands and many such that assess the drivers' state. The majority of the role is of the camera which helps in detection and identification of objective biomarkers for assessing the driver [8].

5 Medical Imaging in Connected Vehicles

Driver monitoring system (DMS) is the new field of research which acquires data from medical sensors and utilizes the computationally powerful machine learning algorithms for assessing the condition of the driver and act accordingly. As the connected vehicles are progressing towards the onset of fully autonomous vehicles, the role of drivers are becoming less in controlling the vehicles, their staying medically fit for final decision on extremely complex driving conditions is a critical factor. Thus, image based diagnosis of drivers' health using the objective biomarkers such as ocular movements [12], saccadic changes, blinking [13] and many such, are being implemented and being deployed into the vehicles [14–16]. Since, a large portion of the detection is done by camera, the challenges pertaining to imaging needs to be identified as these images are used for preliminary diagnosis of the drivers' health. It is the essential joining link between the connected vehicles to the medical imaging research.

6 Challenges of Imaging in Connected Vehicles Environment

There are various challenges in imaging associated with the dynamically changing environment in the connected vehicle setup. The factors are 1. Luminescence 2. Vibrations 3. Field of View 4. Motion Blur 5. Resolution 6. Sharpness 7. Focusing 8. Pixelation 9. Light exposure on Camera Sensor. These factors have a very negative impact on the imaging if not tackled properly.

The real time driving environment is extremely dynamic due to change of multiple parameters in a very short period of time. The luminescence is one of the changing factors. This has direct correlation with the time of the day, month of the year, weather and road demography (tunnels, shades from trees). The facial cues of the driver is the point of interest which is exposed to varying lighting conditions. The changing lighting conditions create a possibility of false detection of cues that may be absent. Uniform lighting conditions are practically not feasible specially during night time. Thus, detection of the facial cues with varying luminescence is a challenging task.

Mechanical vibrations is another challenge that is caused due to uneven road conditions affecting the camera itself. This makes the image acquisition very challenging as the images would not be clear. Thus, it would reduce the image clarity and chances of loss of data on facial cues may occur. The loss of micro-expressions may lead to a faulty diagnosis that needs to be prevented from occurring.

Every camera has its own field of view depending upon the lens configuration. There is also a very limited availability of space for the placement of the camera in order to focus on the driver, without affecting the drivers' field of view or being a distraction. The objects (switches, gear lever, mirrors) near the vicinity of the drivers are placed scientifically such that it is easily accessible without the need to move focus from road and not being a source of visual distraction. Thus, camera's placement is extremely crucial such that it captures the drivers' faces but does not invade the visual attention zone of the drivers. There must be a computational system that searches for the driver's face and alert when the camera is obstructed.

Current on-board systems are much more computationally powerful than that were a decade ago. There is large volume of real time data processing done by these systems. Sudden jerks or unwanted movements of these computational systems can make them unreliable and they enter into phases where these systems behave in unwanted manner. Thus, image acquisition from the camera might occur but with a factor of motion blur during extraction of real time video. It generally happens when some computationally heavy processing goes on in parallel. It leads to unwanted issues that can produce faulty diagnosis or complete failure of the computational system.

Resolution of the video being captured is solely an intrinsic factor of the camera. Higher the resolution, more accurate are the details on the facial cues that leads to proper diagnosis. But, the current onboard systems have a limitation on data processing capabilities. Higher resolution leads to generation of higher volume of data whose processing takes much more time when compared to small volume. Thus, trade off on selecting appropriate resolution of camera is a challenge. Moreover, new state of the art algorithms have the capability to increase the resolution of the images.

Sharpness is the details of the images captured, which is commonly interchanged with resolution. There is a quite a possibility that higher resolution camera can capture lower sharpness image. Since, medical diagnosis based on facial cues requires good detailed image that have the capability to capture the micro-expressions and minute changes due to their medical and clinical coherence in them, sharpness is an important factor.

Focusing is another challenge that is an intrinsic property of the camera. But, there's a possibility of computationally handling this by generation of control signal for focusing. Improper focusing of the drivers face can be lead to faulty diagnosis. Constant movement of the head due to vehicle motion requires the camera to change the focal length every instant in order to keep the details of driver as sharp as possible. Such quick change of focal length in real-time is possible by intelligent algorithms.

Pixelation is another challenge in imaging which is not very frequently encountered but a probable occurrence may cause wrong diagnosis. Low light imaging, imaging in lower aperture, improper compression, size of the camera sensor are some of the major factors that causes pixelation in the images. These environmental factors can be corrected using current computational algorithms.

Light exposure on the camera sensor can be extremely difficult to handle in the dynamically changing environment. Thus, this factor can be handled computationally by altering the white balance of the videos, but there's a limitation to it. Placement of the camera also plays an important role. Placement of the camera must be such that the possibility of falling external light on its sensor is minimum.

Thus, the above factors very explicitly show the negative coherence on the quality of imaging which are a factor of the dynamically changing environment. These changes are so subtle and quick that traditional algorithms fail and is only realizable by machine learning algorithms.

7 Machine Learning for CVE

The factors discussed in the previous section allows researchers to understand the problems of real time imaging in the connected vehicle environment. Upon identification of some of the relevant challenges, the machine learning algorithms prove to be extremely useful and reliable.

The mechanical vibrations lead to a harmonic motion of the camera which leads to blurring of images captured. Removal of blurriness due to mechanical vibrations requires the estimation of the motion, followed by the compensation of the motion on the image composition [17]. These estimation of the motion is very well achieved by the machine learning algorithms and care is taken that no residual motion is added after stabilization. Research [18] has shown the video stabilization using convolutional neural network. Grundman et al. applied L1-Norm optimization for synthesizing a path consisting of simple cinematographic motions [19].

In the field of view of the camera, detection of drivers' face is a critical aspect. Numerous research has been done on face detection. The research has been extended to camera obstruction detection as well. Support vector machines were the initial machine learning algorithms that was used [20]. As the new computational power becomes powerful, new use cases of Region based convolutional neural networks (R-CNN) [21, 22], neural network based face detection [23] has been carried out with the reduction of program complexity and memory requirement. This is essential because of the limited onboard computational capabilities.

Changing luminescence is a challenge which researchers tackled with machine learning to artificially illuminate the images without the addition of noise [24]. There has been significant work done for light correction using deep learning [25]. Such correction is necessary to remove the unwanted noise of facial cues.

Image must carry proper details of the facial cues. Thus, images are needed to be focused, non-pixelated and as sharp as possible. It is then possible for the machine learning algorithms to look for the objective cues for diagnosis. Deep learning proves to be extremely useful here as well as these corrections can be very easily done by the stated [26]. Google with their TensorFlow is making their neural networks learn to correct the images [27]. There has been use cases for such focus correction of microscopic images using CNN based on U-Net architecture [28]. New adversarial neural networks based EnhancedNet has shown the true potential of machine learning algorithm for correction of low resolution input to super resolution [29]. Researchers from Duke University developed a method named PULSE on the basis of self-supervised generative models [30]. Light Exposure correction have also taken the advantage of such algorithms to enhance the image as well as capture the person of interest in best possible condition [31]. There are many more use cases of machine learning for eliminating such factors as required.

8 Conclusion

The connected vehicle paradigm is experiencing a pragmatic shift by the inclusion of drivers for critical decision making process as well as automating the driving experience to a driverless automation. Imaging under such dynamic condition is extremely challenging in itself, let alone for medical diagnosis. Thus, this paper establishes the challenges that arise in the area of imaging for the CVE and how current intelligent algorithms may tackle such challenges and resolve them. Machine learning algorithms have the potential to provide reliable solutions in comparison to the traditional algorithms.

Acknowledgement. The first author acknowledges his father, Mr. Tarakeswar Karmakar for providing key industrial insights to the research and unending support in pursuing higher research. He also acknowledges Dr. Sourav Mallick, HOD – EEE, NIT Sikkim and Dr. Kuntal Mandal, Assistant Professor, NIT Sikkim for their support.

References

1. History. https://www.nde-ed.org/EducationResources/CommunityCollege/Radiography/Introduction/history.htm
2. Scatliff, J.H., Morris, P.J.: From Roentgen to magnetic resonance imaging: the history of medical imaging. N. C. Med. J. **75**, 111–113 (2014)
3. How ionising radiation damages DNA and causes cancer – Wellcome Sanger Institute. https://www.sanger.ac.uk/news_item/how-ionising-radiation-damages-dna-and-causes-cancer/

4. Behjati, S., et al.: Mutational signatures of ionizing radiation in second malignancies. Nat. Commun. **7**, 1–8 (2016)
5. Baerlocher, M.O., Asch, M., Myers, A.: Allergic-type reactions to radiographic contrast media. CMAJ **182**, 1328 (2010)
6. Bradley, W.G.: History of medical imaging. Proc. Am. Philos. Soc. **152**(3), 349–361 (2008)
7. Berger, A.: Positron emission tomography. BMJ **326**, 1449 (2003)
8. Karmakar, S., Mohan, S.: Monitoring biomarkers of drivers with medical wireless sensor networks deployed in Connected Vehicles. Nord. Balt. J. Inf. Commun. Technol. **Vol2020**, section WWRF44, 275–296 (2021). https://doi.org/10.13052/nbjict1902-097X.2020.012
9. FCC proposes splitting 5.9GHz spectrum for vehicle comms and WiFi - Internet of Things News. https://iottechnews.com/news/2019/nov/21/fcc-spectrum-splitting-vehicle-comms-wifi/
10. 3GPP sets new timeline for next 5G specification, Release 17 | FierceWireless. https://www.fiercewireless.com/5g/3gpp-sets-new-timeline-for-next-5g-specification-release-17
11. ITU-T Recommendation database. https://www.itu.int/itu-t/recommendations/rec.aspx?id=14091
12. Sun, Q., Xia, J., Nadarajah, N., Falkmer, T., Foster, J., Lee, H.: Assessing drivers' visual-motor coordination using eye tracking, GNSS and GIS: a spatial turn in driving psychology. J. Spat. Sci. **61**(2), 299–316 (2016)
13. Karmakar, S., Gore, S., Nagesh, A., Salman, H., Milanova, M., Mohan, S.: An IoT-based machine learning system for detecting drowsiness of drivers. In: Wireless World Research Forum '41, Herning, Denmark, Oct. 30–Nov. 1 (2018)
14. Begum, S.: Intelligent driver monitoring systems based on physiological sensor signals: a review. In: IEEE Conference on Intelligent Transportation Systems, Proceedings, ITSC, pp. 282–289 (2013). https://doi.org/10.1109/ITSC.2013.6728246
15. Bylykbashi, K., Qafzezi, E., Ikeda, M., Matsuo, K., Barolli, L.: Fuzzy-based driver monitoring system (FDMS): implementation of two intelligent FDMSs and a testbed for safe driving in VANETs. Futur. Gener. Comput. Syst. **105**, 665–674 (2020)
16. Kim, W., et al.: An adaptive batch-image based driver status monitoring system on a lightweight GPU-equipped SBC. IEEE Access **8**, 206074–206087 (2020)
17. Morimoto, C., Chellappa, R.: Evaluation of image stabilization algorithms. In: Acoustics, Speech, and Signal Processing, 1988. ICASSP-88., 1988 International Conference on. 5, vol. 5, pp. 2789–2792 (1998). https://doi.org/10.1109/ICASSP.1998.678102
18. Wang, M., et al.: Deep Online Video Stabilization. https://www.youtube.com/watch?v=8vu7IDuDD64
19. Grundmann, M., Kwatra, V., Essa, I.: Auto-directed video stabilization with robust l1 optimal camera paths. In: Proceedings of the International Conference on CVPR. IEEE, 2011, pp. 225–232 (2011)
20. Osuna, E., Freund, R., Girosit, F.: Training support vector machines: an application to face detection. In: Proceedings of IEEE Computer Society Conference on Computer Vision and Pattern Recognition, San Juan, Puerto Rico, USA, 1997, pp. 130–136 (1997). https://doi.org/10.1109/CVPR.1997.609310
21. Sun, X., Wu, P., Hoi, S.C.H.: Face detection using deep learning: an improved faster RCNN approach. Neurocomputing **299**, 42–50 (2018)
22. Sawat, D.D., Hegadi, R.S.: Unconstrained face detection: a deep learning and machine learning combined approach. CSI Trans. ICT **5**(2), 195–199 (2016). https://doi.org/10.1007/s40012-016-0149-1
23. Rowley, H.A., Baluja, S., Kanade, T.: Neural network-based face detection. IEEE Trans. Pattern Anal. Mach. Intell. **20**, 23–38 (1998)

24. Researchers use AI to brighten ultra-low light images without adding noise: Digital Photography Review. https://www.dpreview.com/videos/1559702271/researchers-use-ai-to-brighten-ultra-low-light-images-without-adding-noise
25. Scene Light Correction via Deep Learning | CVisionLab. https://www.cvisionlab.com/cases/scene-light-correction-via-deep-learning/
26. Yang, S.J., Berndl, M., Michael Ando, D., et al.: Assessing microscope image focus quality with deep learning. BMC Bioinform. **19**, 77 (2018). https://doi.org/10.1186/s12859-018-2087-4
27. How Google Is Using Deep Learning To Identify Out-Of-Focus Microscope Images. https://analyticsindiamag.com/how-google-is-using-deep-learning-to-identify-out-of-focus-microscope-images/
28. ReFocus: Making Out-of-Focus Microscopy Images In-Focus Again | by Yuan Tian | Towards Data Science. https://towardsdatascience.com/refocus-making-out-of-focus-microscopy-images-in-focus-again-90e1fe98ead4
29. Sajjadi, M.S.M., Schölkopf, B., Hirsch, M.: EnhanceNet: Single Image Super-Resolution Through Automated Texture Synthesis
30. Artificial Intelligence Turns Blurry Pixelated Photos Into Hyper-Realistic Portraits – Try It Yourself. https://scitechdaily.com/artificial-intelligence-turns-blurry-pixelated-photos-into-hyper-realistic-portraits-try-it-yourself/
31. Bernacki, J.: Automatic exposure algorithms for digital photography. Multimed. Tools Appl. **79**(19–20), 12751–12776 (2020). https://doi.org/10.1007/s11042-019-08318-1

Preliminary Considerations on the Design of Multi-layered Bone Scaffold for Laser-Based Printing

Alida Mazzoli[1](✉), Marco Mandolini[2], Agnese Brunzini[2], Manila Caragiuli[2], and Michele Germani[2]

[1] Department of Materials, Environmental Sciences and Urban Planning (SIMAU), Università Politecnica delle Marche, via Brecce Bianche 12, 60131 Ancona, Italy
a.mazzoli@univpm.it

[2] Department of Industrial Engineering and Mathematical Sciences, Università Politecnica delle Marche, Ancona, Italy

Abstract. Several implant materials are used in cranial surgery. Still, each one has its drawbacks, such as the risk of infections, low mechanical strength, or low osseointegration. Implants with a porous surface are considered more effective than a smooth and rough coating. The porosity density and structure also influence the mechanical properties of the final implant. Moreover, the implant properties depend on the manufacturing method.

This study aims to present a custom-made cranial scaffold composed of two distinct layers. A compact inner one guarantees adequate structural properties to the scaffold. In contrast, a porous outer one lightens the scaffold structure and assures the correct osseointegration. The customized scaffold has been designed through a 3D free-form modeling system. It can be manufactured by 3D printing techniques such as direct metal laser sintering in titanium or via selective laser sintering using PEEK. The advantages and limitations of the multi-layered custom-made scaffold and the related design process are qualitatively described.

Keywords: Customized scaffolds · Craniofacial reconstruction · Additive manufacturing · Porous scaffolds · Multi-layered scaffolds

1 Introduction and Literature Review

The defects of the cranial vault derive mainly from tumor forms, trauma, infections, congenital and developmental deformities, and result in aesthetic and functional deficiencies that must be restored [1–6]. The autologous bone is considered the gold standard cranial implant in osseointegration and full regeneration [1, 7]. Nevertheless, synthetic materials may overcome its intrinsic drawbacks related to the harvesting site availability and complications, the size of the defect, the malleability of bone, the high resorption rate, the additional patient morbidity, and the increased surgical time [4]. Thus, other kinds of implant materials are often used in cranioplasty. Their choice

R. Su et al. (Eds.): MICAD 2021, LNEE 784, pp. 195–204, 2022.
https://doi.org/10.1007/978-981-16-3880-0_21

depends on the manufacturing technique and the implant properties (i.e., biocompatibility, osteoinductivity, toxicity, yield strength, flexural modulus, lightweightness, thermal stability, malleability, infection risk, costs) [7]. The primary implant materials used in cranial surgery are polymethylmethacrylate (PMMA), titanium, hydroxyapatite (HA), polyetheretherketone (PEEK), polyethylene (PE), and calcium phosphate [2, 3]. However, each has its drawbacks, such as the risk of infections, low mechanical strength, or low osseointegration [1, 7].

In the traditional surgical procedure, the prosthesis is carried out by the surgeon directly in the operating room. PMMA is currently the most used implant material. It comes from the polymerization of PMMA powder and liquid MMA, which are combined to form a malleable paste that can be prefabricated or intra-operatively shaped by hand or through a mold. In a few minutes, it hardens and creates the prosthesis. At the end of the hardening process, the implant often presents numerous micro-porosities (air bubbles) that cause mechanical fragility and bacterial infections that lead to rejection and, therefore, to the removal and replacement of the prosthesis [7].

Titanium (plate or mesh) is a versatile metal with high biocompatibility and a strong osseointegration potential, given a proper texture (i.e., mesh). The implant's rough surface quality promotes osseointegration with human tissues and bones [8]. However, bulk Titanium implants are responsible for developing stress shielding effects at the implant-bone interface resulting in bone resorption due to the lack of mechanical stress on the bone itself. Porous structures have been thought to compensate for large differences in the stiffness between the implant and the bone. Still, there is no clear evidence on the behavior of the porous structure, porosity, and its strength [1, 9]. Meanwhile, Zanotti et al. [10], studying porous HA implants, demonstrated that the most common complication is implant fracture (this is due to the low mechanical properties of porous HA).

A comparison of fabrication methods results that the implant infection risk decreases in materials that favor the bone growth into the implant and promote the surface interaction [7]. For this reason, implants with a porous surface are considered more effective than smooth and rough surface treatment. The pores' properties, especially the total porosity, the dimensional distribution, the morphology, the orientation, and the degree of interconnection, strongly influence the implant's penetration by the bone tissue.

The apparent density and structure also influence the mechanical properties of the final implant. The amount of porosity and the pore size depend on the manufacturing method. A high porosity with a pore size of approximately 100 μm (osteoblast cell size) is required to regenerate bone tissue [7]. Still, a pore size in the range of 500–1500 μm [11] is generally considered adequate to ensure space for cell adhesion and proliferation and to guarantee structural strength, avoiding manufacturing defects.

For example, porous PE allows obtaining semi-rigid systems that may not have good mechanical properties for specific applications (i.e., extensive defect reconstruction) [7]. For this reason, it is crucial to identify the right proportion between porosity and mechanical strength.

Conventional techniques of scaffold fabrication for tissue engineering (such as fiber bonding, solvent casting, and melt molding) generate highly porous scaffold with interconnected pores of unpredictable size and irregular shape due to their limitations in flexibility and control of porosity and distribution. Moreover, such structures are thin with low mechanical strength and structural stability [12].

Metallic porous materials can be fabricated through different techniques. In phase separation techniques (e.g., sintering-dissolution process, thermally stimulated decomposition and thermally melted elimination) and embedding cenosphere technique, the porosity, and mechanical properties can be effectively controlled by altering the concentration and size of the pore-forming agents. Recent developments on computer-aided design (CAD) and additive manufacturing (AM) techniques have allowed the possibility to fabricate reproducible customized porous structures via a layer-by-layer deposition through high-energy electron beam melting (EBM) and selected laser sintering (SLS) processes [8, 13].

Shuai et al. [14] fabricated PLGA/nano-HAP composite porous scaffolds through the SLS process, achieving a well-controlled pore structure. The authors have introduced nano-HAP as a reinforcing phase to improve mechanical properties. An approach based on fused deposition modeling (FDM) and rapid prototyping (RP) technologies was developed by Masood et al. [12] to design and fabricate a complex scaffold structure of desired porosity. Vlasea et al. [15] proposed a combined AM and microsyringe deposition approach to fabricate bio-ceramic structures with controlled micro-sized channels. Armillotta and Pelzer [16] generated an algorithm to create a porous structure of desired properties to be superimposed to a geometric model in polygon format for RP. Khaja et al. [1] designed and fabricated a patient-specific cranial implant with a controlled porous sizing and mechanical properties for aesthetic and functional restoration using electron beam melting (EBM) to ensure a patient-specific titanium implant with adequate mechanical strength. Although scientific literature highlights the benefits of porous structures on the osteointegration, insufficient evidence exists about the effects of the channels' sizes on the physical and mechanical properties of the implants. Basalah et al. [17] investigated the impact of macro-scale channels with a diameter of 1 mm on the physical and mechanical properties of 3D-printed porous titanium implants. The results demonstrated that the structure's channels' horizontal orientation might reduce its ultimate strength and induce an isotropic shrinkage after sintering. Besides, the overall porosity is affected by the number of channels in the structure [17].

The review of Zhao et al. [13] concerning the manufacturing techniques of metallic porous materials highlighted that the porosity in metallic porous materials negatively impacts the implant's mechanical properties. The papers found in the literature presented implants composed of different pore sizes and geometries and manufactured through various techniques. However, all these implants are characterized by a fully porous structure that shows low mechanical properties.

The present paper describes the design and manufacturing of a custom-made cranial scaffold composed of two distinct layers: the compact inner one and the porous outer one. The customized scaffold has been designed to be manufactured by 3D-printing techniques. The multi-layered structure guarantees the correct osseointegration (through the spongy outer part in contact with surrounding tissues) and adequate structural properties (through the compact inner part).

2 Materials and Methods

2.1 Multi-layered Porous Scaffold

The present paper aims to present a novel kind of custom-made scaffolds designed to improve the implant itself's osseointegration process, assuring adequate structural properties. We planned a patient-specific implant that contained a porous surface lattice for better osseointegration of the autogenous bone graft and a compact inner part for optimal structural support. The permeable grid has been designed to enhance bone-scaffold integration through a highly porous substrate. The custom-made scaffold can be subsequently printed using direct metal laser sintering in titanium or selective laser sintering using PEEK. We treated a patient affected by an osteoma on the right parietal bone of the skull.

2.2 Design and Manufacture Procedure for Multi-layered Scaffold

The custom-made implant has been designed and manufactured following the workflow in Fig. 1. The Computed tomography (CT) images of a patient affected by an osteoma were imported into the commercial software for image processing MIMICS (Materialise NV, Belgium) and segmented through a proper threshold to extract the bony components. By stacking the segmented slices, it was possible to reconstruct the 3D anatomical model through the marching cubes algorithm, a well-known algorithm in 3D reconstruction. The 3D visual model was then converted in STL (Standard Triangulation Language) format, the de facto standard interface from CAD to rapid manufacturing. The custom-made scaffold was virtually designed in a haptic environment, given that a traditional CAD modeling software would not ensure accurate reconstruction of such a complex and irregular defect. The STL file of the segmented cranial defect resulting from the previous phase was imported into the free-form modeling system (3D Systems Haptic Device) equipped with the PHANToM Omni. Haptic free-form modeling provides the practitioner with tools for direct interaction with the virtual model. It gives force feedback to the operator to render the sense of touch when sculpting the virtual clay representing the model.

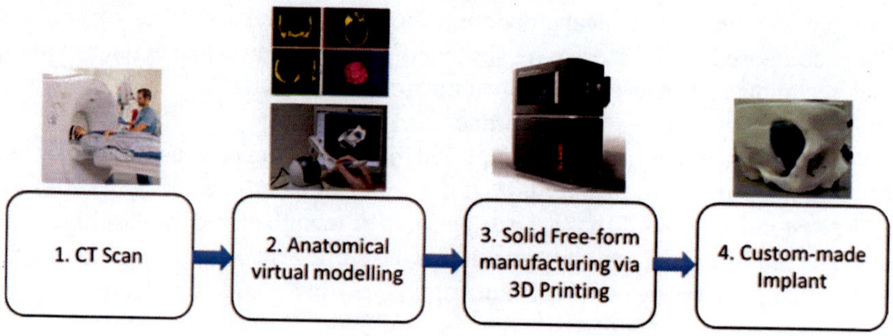

Fig. 1. Modeling and manufacturing chain

The operator can thus orient the anatomical model to obtain the best view of the defect and draw the defect site's contour even for irregularly shaped defect geometry. The osteoma has been resected freehand using the command 'construct clay' combined with the plane drawings of the part that should have been resected (command 'sketch') as showed in Fig. 2.

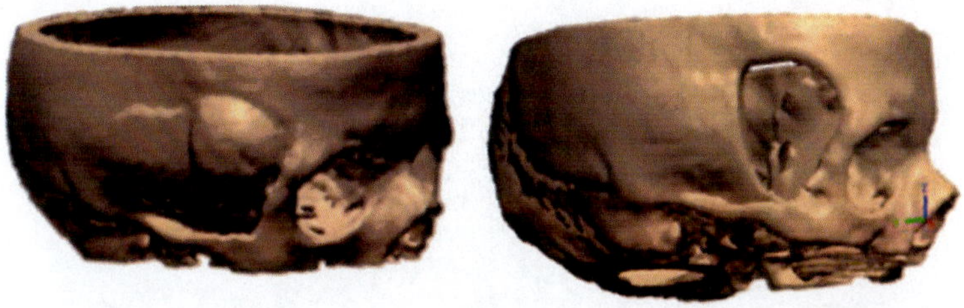

Fig. 2. 3D model of the osteoma (left) and after the resection (right)

Using this modeling approach, the osteoma has been extruded from the skull. Hereafter the implant has been designed using the symmetric portion of the patient's skull. The plate has been smoothed and adapted to the resection in the head. At this point, the implant's external surface has been manipulated to apply a porous texture that can stimulate the growth of the surrounding bone tissue once implanted. In this way, the implant can be directly 3D-printed, showing a roughened multi-layered structure without recurring to any chemical or physical post-processing and augmenting the osseointegration possibilities of the implant itself. Using the MIMICS software's editing and boolean commands, the implant has been split into two areas, an inner core and an external shell 3 mm thick, as can be seen in Fig. 3.

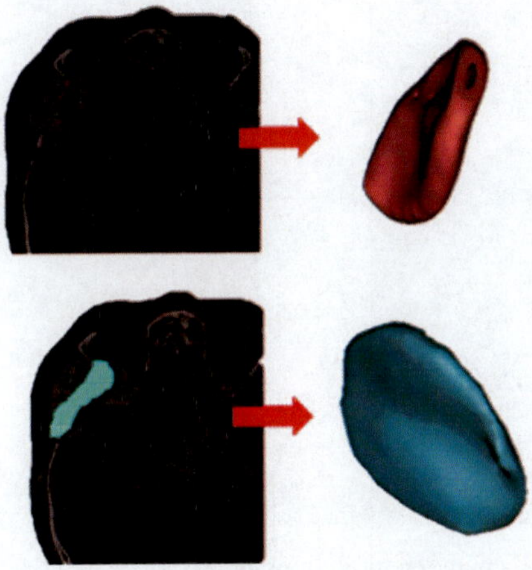

Fig. 3. 3D model of the external shell (upper) and inner core (lower)

The obtained STL files have been imported in FreeForm to use the haptic device to apply the surface porosity. The porous surface has been designed as a texture. A cubic cell, 0.5 mm x/y/z, chosen in the FreeForm library, has been repeated all over the implant's external surface shell to obtain the porous structure. Once the outer shell has been finished, it has been merged with the inner part to get the cranial plate, showed in Fig. 4 (left). It can be saved in STL format and 3D-printed using a biocompatible material such as PEEK.

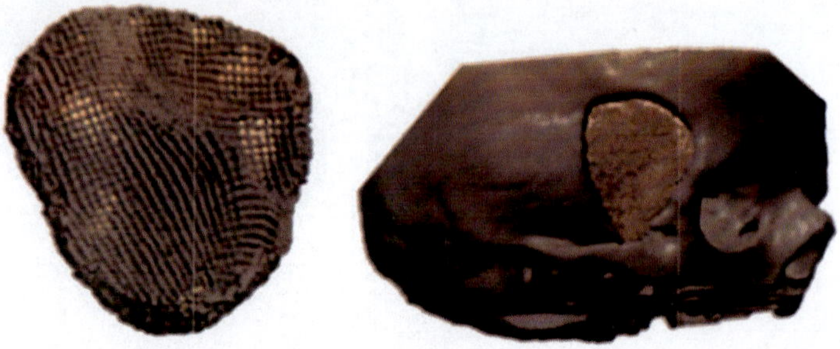

Fig. 4. Multi-layered designed cranial implant (left) and positioning in the cranial slot (right)

Before the 3D-printing process, the entire implant has been resized to perfectly fit the implant in the cranial place, as shown in Fig. 4 (right). It was necessary because the free-form modeling process induced some changes to the whole scaffold. The implant has been manufactured by Selective Laser Sintering using PEEK. SEM images of the manufactured implant, external shell (right), and inner core (left) are reported in Fig. 5.

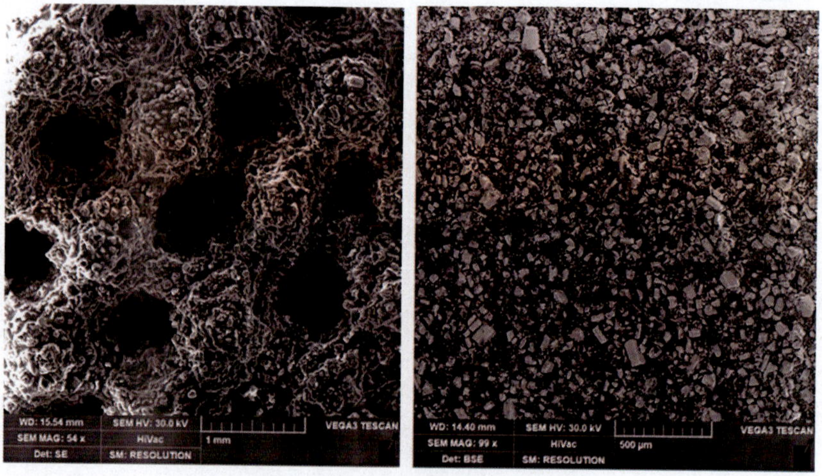

Fig. 5. SEM images of the manufactured implant, external shell (right), and inner core (left).

3 Results and Discussion

The multi-layered custom-made implant and the related design process described in the previous section present several advantages and limitations compared with the respective ones commented in the proposed literature review.

The main advantages are:

- The freeform modeling software tool allows controlling the implant porosity in terms of global porosity and local distribution, orientation, and porosity interconnection. All these factors influence the growth of bone and cartilaginous tissues (pore size more significant than 100 μm). The pores interconnection, showed in Fig. 5, allows circulation and exchange of body fluid, ion diffusion, nutritional content, penetration of osteoblasts, and vasculature (pore size smaller than 50 μm). According to a study into porous implants [18], pores sized 75–100 μm result in significant bone growth, but the optimal range is 100–135 μm. Many studies recommended pores exceeding 300 μm for bone formation and enhanced vascularisation and oxygenation, promoting direct osteogenesis. Conversely, pores smaller than 300 μm can encourage osteochondral ossification. However, it is crucial to identify the upper limits in pore size without compromising the scaffolds' mechanical properties by increasing void volume [18].

  - By adopting different textures, it is possible to create a multi-density surface designed according to medical requirements. High porosity, where the implant is connected to the bone to speed up the osseointegration. Low porosity, in the middle, for fostering the growth of cartilaginous tissues;
  - The implant porosity can be created through standard (e.g., cylinder, tetrahedron, parallelepiped, etc.) or customized shapes. The porosity is realized through a texturing process, where a texture is applied to the surface to treat. Such a solution is an extremely flexible design process. The textured shape will depend on the bone conditions where the prosthesis will be implanted;
  - The porosity is completely controlled during the design stage. It does not depend on any parameters of the chemical or physical post-processing typically used for creating the porosity of the implant surface;
  - The external porosity contributes to reducing the weight of the implant.

The main limitation met during the design process is the following:

- The texturing process and the software tool used for this test case lead to a uniform porosity in the case of simple surfaces (i.e., developable surfaces). For freeform shapes, typical of custom-made implants, the dimension of the pores varies through the surface. Figure 6 shows the porosity deviation in terms of hole dimensions, where as Fig. 7 shows the variation in hole depth. In conclusion, in the release used for this case study, such a software tool does not permit to realize a uniform texturized surface.

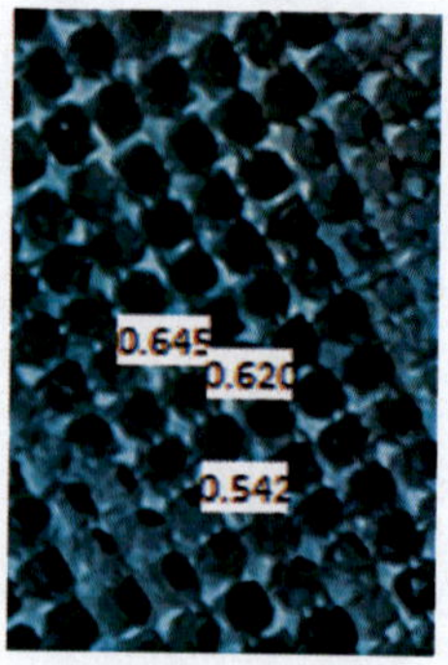

Fig. 6. External implant surface obtained with the texturing process. Values express the dimensions of the pores (mm)

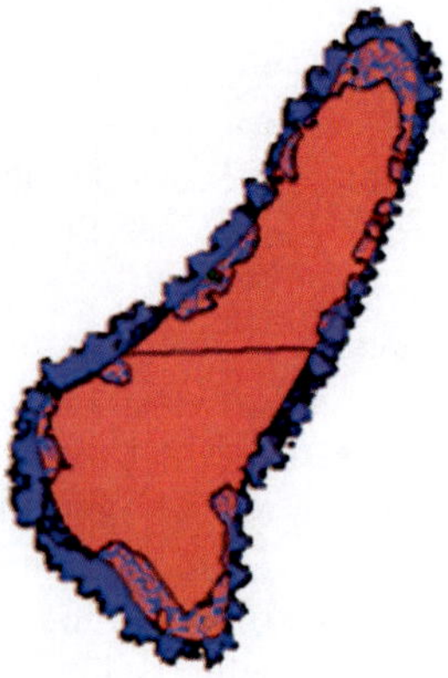

Fig. 7. Cross-section of the multi-layered custom-made implant is visible in the implant's inner core (smooth) and the external shell (speckled).

4 Conclusions

This paper aims to approach the qualitative advantages and limitations of a multi-layered designed custom-made cranial scaffold concerning the one-layered ones. In literature, authors have designed and developed one-layered customized implants with traditional manufacturing techniques. Those allow realizing completely porous and completely compact implants in a 'one-step' production or multi-layered implants with a 'more-steps' production. In this paper, we proposed a preliminary procedure for designing multi-layered scaffolds via a unique manufacturing step. By combining a free-form modeling system and 3D-printing, it is possible to overcome the literature by speeding up the implant development process and assuring the perfect fitting and integration of the implant to the bone.

References

1. Khaja, M., Saied, D., Abdulrahman, A.A., Sherif, E., Ashfaq, M., Wadea, A.: Structural and mechanical characterization of custom design cranial implant created using additive manufacturing. Electron. J. Biotechnol. **29**, 22–31 (2017). https://doi.org/10.1016/j.ejbt.2017.06.005
2. Parthasarathy, J.: 3D modeling, custom implants and its future perspectives in craniofacial surgery. Ann. Maxillofac. Surg. **4**(1), 9–18 (2014). https://doi.org/10.4103/2231-0746.133065
3. Mandolini, M., Brunzini, A., Germani, M., Manieri, S., Mazzoli, A., Pagnoni, M.: Selective laser sintered mould for orbital cavity reconstruction. Rapid Prototyping J. **25**(1), 95–103 (2019). https://doi.org/10.1108/RPJ-05-2017-0098
4. Cho, H.R., Roh, T.S., Shim, K.W., Kim, Y.O., Lew, D.H., Yun, I.S.: Skull reconstruction with custom made three-dimensional titanium implant. Arch. Craniofac. Surg. **16**(1), 11–16 (2015). https://doi.org/10.7181/acfs.2015.16.1.11
5. Mandolini, M., Brunzini, A., Serrani, E.B., Pagnoni, M., Mazzoli, A., Germani, M.: Design of a custom-made cranial implant in patients suffering from Apert syndrome. In: Proceedings of the 22nd International Conference on Engineering Design (ICED19), Delft, The Netherlands, 5–8 August 2019. https://doi.org/10.1017/dsi.2019.75
6. Brunzini, A., et al.: Orbital wall reconstruction by selective laser sintered mould. In: Proceedings of the IASTED International Conference Biomedical Engineering (BioMed 2017), 20–21 February 2017. Innsbruck, Austria (2017). https://doi.org/10.2316/P.2017.852-045
7. Kwarcinski, J., Boughton, P., Ruys, A., Doolan, A., van Gelder, J.: Cranioplasty and craniofacial reconstruction: a review of implant material, manufacturing method and infection risk. Appl. Sci. **7**, 1–17 (2017). https://doi.org/10.3390/app7030276
8. Mandolini, M., Caragiuli, M., Brunzini, A., Mazzoli, A., Pagnoni, M.: A procedure for designing custom-made implants for forehead augmentation in people suffering from apert syndrome. J. Med. Syst. **44**(9), 1 (2020). https://doi.org/10.1007/s10916-020-01611-9
9. Zanotti, B., et al.: Surgical pitfalls with custom made porous hydroxyapatite cranial implants. Plast. Aesthetic Res. **2**(1), 7–11 (2015). https://doi.org/10.4103/2347-9264.149364
10. Saptaji, K., Gebremariam, M.A., Azhari, M.A.B.M.: Machining of biocompatible materials: a review. Int. J. Adv. Manufact. Technol. **97**(5–8), 2255–2292 (2018). https://doi.org/10.1007/s00170-018-1973-2
11. Otsuki, B., Takemoto, M., Fujibayashi, S., Neo, M., Kokubo, T., Nakamura, T.: Pore throat size and connectivity determine bone and tissue ingrowth into porous implants: three dimensional micro-CT based structural analyses of porous bioactive titanium implants. Biomaterials **27**, 5892–5900 (2006). https://doi.org/10.1016/j.biomaterials.2006.08.013
12. Masood, S.H., Singh, J.P., Morsi, Y.: The design and manufacturing of porous scaffolds for tissue engineering using rapid prototyping. Int. J. Adv. Manufact. Technol. **27**, 415–420 (2005). https://doi.org/10.1007/s00170-004-2187-3
13. Zhao, B., Gain, A.K., Ding, W., Zhang, L., Li, X., Fu, Y.: A review on metallic porous materials: pore formation, mechanical properties, and their applications. Int. J. Adv. Manufact. Technol. **95**(5–8), 2641–2659 (2017). https://doi.org/10.1007/s00170-017-1415-6
14. Shuai, C., Yang, B., Peng, S., Li, Z.: Development of composite porous scaffolds based on poly(lactide-co-glycolide)/nano-hydroxyapatite via selective laser sintering. Int. J. Adv. Manufact. Technol. **69**(1–4), 51–57 (2013). https://doi.org/10.1007/s00170-013-5001-2
15. Vlasea, M., Shanjani, Y., Bothe, A., Kandel, R., Toyserkani, E.: A combined additive manufacturing and micro-syringe deposition technique for realization of bio-ceramic structures with micro-scale channels. Int. J. Adv. Manufact. Technol. **68**(9–12), 2261–2269 (2013). https://doi.org/10.1007/s00170-013-4839-7

16. Armillotta, A., Pelzer, R.: Modeling of porous structures for rapid prototyping of tissue engineering scaffolds. Int. J. Adv. Manufact. Technol. **39**, 501–511 (2008). https://doi.org/10.1007/s00170-007-1247-x
17. Basalah, A., Esmaeili, S., Toyserkani, E.: Mechanical properties of additive-manufactured porous titanium bio-structures with oriented macro-scale channels. Int. J. Adv. Manufact. Technol. **84**(9–12), 2239–2246 (2015). https://doi.org/10.1007/s00170-015-7849-9
18. Murphy, C.M., Haugh, M.G., O'Brien, F.J.: The effect of mean pore size on cell attachment, proliferation and migrationin collagen–glycosaminoglycan scaffolds for bone tissue engineering. Biomaterials **31**, 461–466 (2010). https://doi.org/10.1016/j.biomaterials.2009.09.063

Two-Stage Convolutional Neural Network for Knee Osteoarthritis Diagnosis in X-Rays

Kang Wang[1](✉), Xin Niu[1], Yong Dou[1], Di Yang[1], Dongxing Xie[2], and Tuo Yang[3]

[1] National Laboratory for Parallel and Distributed Processing, School of Computer, National University of Defense Technology, Changsha 410073, China
wangkang@nudt.edu.cn

[2] Department of Orthopaedics, Xiangya Hospital, Central South University, Changsha 410008, China

[3] Department of Health Management Center, Xiangya Hospital, Central South University, Changsha 410008, China

Abstract. Knee osteoarthritis (OA) is a common musculoskeletal illness. To solve the problem that inaccurate knee joint localization and inadequate knee OA features extracted from plain radiographs affect the accuracy of knee OA diagnosis in X-rays, we propose a novel Two-Stage Convolutional Neural Network (TS-CNN) method, consisting of the KneeDetnet and the KLnet. The KneeDetnet with two small multi-task convolutional neural networks is proposed to locate knee joints, improving the accuracy of knee joint localization. Then KLnet is designed to assess knee OA, where a shared Siamese network via ResNet is used to extract more discriminative deep learning features that are fused with gender information for obtaining richer features. Our method is evaluated on public OAI and MOST datasets. The highest detection accuracy of knee joints can reach 99.93% and 99.02% on two datasets, respectively. The KLnet algorithm achieves 78.85% and 68.20% prediction accuracy on the OAI and MOST datasets, respectively. Experimental results show that our method outperforms the existing workhorse. The proposed approach may become a potentially useful tool for assisting physicians.

Keywords: Knee osteoarthritis · Two-stage convolutional neural network · Feature fusion · Gender information · X-rays

1 Introduction

Knee osteoarthritis (OA) [18,31] causes frequent physical, psychological damages to human health; worse yet, such a common disease may even lead to disability [3, 6]. Nowadays, it is still challenging to cure an OA patient. *An ounce of prevention is worth a pound of cure.* The studies on the early prevention of OA are very necessary and thus have achieved great improvements in past decade. People

R. Su et al. (Eds.): MICAD 2021, LNEE 784, pp. 205–217, 2022.
https://doi.org/10.1007/978-981-16-3880-0_22

mainly use the radiography (X-ray)[1] [4] to assess knee OA by checking the major pathological features, aka, knee joint space narrowing, osteophytes formation and sclerosis [15,20,21]. However, the visual diagnosis of doctors is highly dependent on personal medical experience and thus very subjective. What worse is that such a diagnosis is very time-consuming and labor-intensive. A natural idea is *why not use the computer?* It can effectively solve the problems just mentioned that may exhaust a doctor. Existing researches about computer-aided knee OA diagnosis [20] specifically grade knee OA, which can be regarded as a fine classification problem [30]. Traditionally, Kellgren-Lawrence (KL)[2] [9] is the gold standard for initial assessment of knee OA.

Previous work about knee OA diagnosis usually consists of two main stages [1]: the first one is the location and extraction of knee joint areas, and the second one is the prediction of knee OA grades. The first stage of current routines focuses on extracting traditional features with classifiers to locate knee joints. However, the high missed and false detection rates hurt subsequent identification. What follows is that people need to exploit manual intervention to extract knee joint areas, which are nonautomatic and time-consuming. Although in the second stage, the current knee OA prediction have used deep learning methods, extracted knee OA features are still inadequate and the prediction accuracy needs to be further improved.

1.1 Our Approaches

Thus, we propose a novel Two-Stage Convolutional Neural Network (TS-CNN) method to assess the severity of knee OA:

- **Stage 1** Replacing the traditional machinery with neural networks to detect knee joints, we then propose a KneeDetnet that consists of two multi-task convolutional neural networks, and the detection accuracy of knee joints is improved.
- **Stage 2** At first, the knee joint areas are further cropped and repositioned via key points. The repositioned knee joints as critical knee joints are divided into two parts with symmetry: the left part and the right part. Then the right part is flipped horizontally. The two patches are sent to a shared Siamese network via ResNet [7] to extract local features. And then, the prediction uses local features from two parts and gender information of patients that concatenated with fully connected layers. The network of assessing knee OA is called KLnet.

1.2 Contributions

Complementary to previous efforts of two-stage knee OA diagnosis, the main contributions in this paper can be summarized in threefold.

[1] In fact various medical imaging categories [14,17], such as magnetic resonance imaging (MRI) and ultrasound imaging, are used in medicine. However, X-ray is a favourite one due to its economic aspect.

[2] The details of KL are described in the Sect. 3.

(1) We propose the KneeDetnet method to locate knee joints and key points simultaneously, which leverages the advantages of deep learning compared to traditional classifier.
(2) In order reduce redundancy, the detected knee joint regions are further relocated according to key points.
(3) The ResNet-based Siamese network with shared weights is proposed for KL prediction by fusing knee joint features and gender information.

1.3 More Related Works

Shamir et al. proposed the WND-CHARM [16,22,23] to manually extract features from original and transformed images with computer-aided analysis. Recently, convolutional neural networks have achieved successful results in many computer vision tasks, such as image recognition [10], automatic detection [13] and segmentation [11], image retrieval [29], video classification [28]. Compared to manually extracted features, convolutional neural networks can learn more efficient features to represent images and videos. Convolutional neural networks have also been applied to the knee OA diagnosis. Antony et al. [2] migrated pre-trained convolutional neural networks via the ImageNet dataset [19], such as VGG16 [24], VGG-M-128 [5] and CaffeNet [8], and performed the fine-tuning on the knee OA classification task. However, their knee joints located method is based on Sobel horizontal image gradient features and SVM, which has a low detection accuracy. They need to manually label knee joint regions for subsequent recognition tasks. Antony et al. [1] later proposed FCN-based method [12] for knee joint localization, and a six-layer convolutional neural network was cascaded to assess knee OA with mean square error loss function and the cross-entropy loss function. However, FCN-based localization method needs to generate binary images and splits knee joints at the pixel level, which is time-consuming. And a shadower network is used during knee OA recognition, the recognition rate can be improved. A 7-layer Siamese convolutional neural network with shared parameters was introduced by Tiulpin et al. [26] to diagnose knee OA, where symmetrically relative features are learned. Due to shared network parameters in Siamese network, the number of learnable parameters are reduced. However, they use HOG and SVM method proposed by them [27] to detect knee joint areas. The mislocalised knee joint areas are manually re-annotated and used for subsequent identification task. The detection accuracy of knee joint areas still has potential for improvement. In addition, during knee OA diagnosis stage, image patches are extracted with fixed pixels, which has certain errors. Also, the deeper shared Siamese convolutional neural network and feature fusion strategy are unused, and the prediction accuracy can be further improved.

2 Methods

The details of our algorithms are shown as Fig. 1. Firstly, the KneeDetnet is presented for accurate location of the knee joints and six key points from original knee images. Then six key points are used to further crop detected knee joints for generating critical knee joints. Finally, critical knee joints are equally divided into two patches via their symmetry. The two separated parts and gender information of patients are drained into the KLnet to prediction KL.

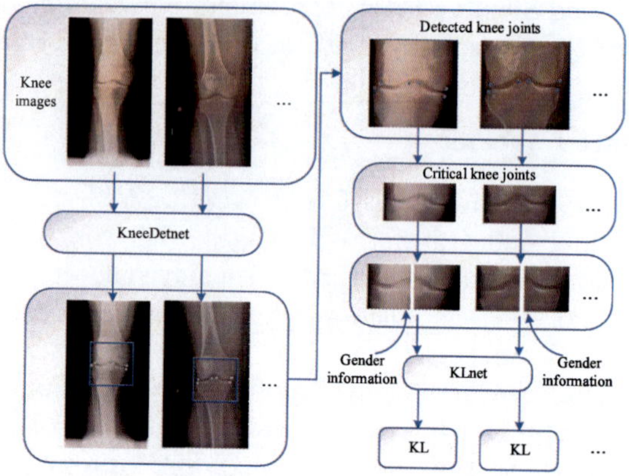

Fig. 1. The pipeline for the proposed TS-CNN method.

2.1 Data Preprocessing

Figure 2 illustrates the specific procedure of data preprocessing. The original data are X-ray medical images including the left and right knees with non-uniform bright-dark phenomenon. At first, we use a pixel inversion to unify the bright-dark property of the images. And then, all original X-ray images are transformed into images with dark background and bright legs. On the other hand, double-knee images are converted into single-knee images, which are turned into 8-bit uint images and processed by histogram equalization.

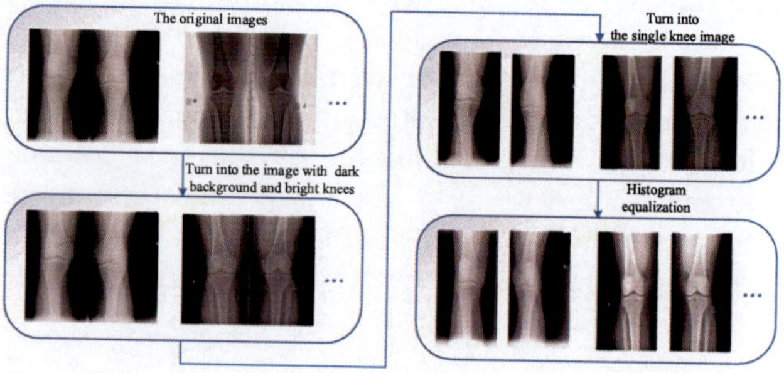

Fig. 2. The pipeline for data preprocessing.

2.2 KneeDetnet for Knee Joint Localization

This paper improves the algorithm proposed by Zhang et al. [32] and proposes two small multi-task convolutional neural networks to complete the localization of knee joints and six key points, which is called KneeDetnet. In our algorithm, we need to train two cascaded neural networks. The whole learning target can be described as

$$
\begin{aligned}
&\min \left\{ \sum_{i=1}^{N} \left[\sum_{j \in \mathcal{A}} \alpha_j \cdot \text{Loss}_i^j \right] \right\}, \mathcal{A} := \{\text{det}, \text{box}, \text{key points}\} \\
\text{Loss}_i^{\text{det}} &= -\left[y_i^{\text{det}} \log(p_i) + (1 - y_i^{\text{det}})(1 - \log(p_i)) \right], \\
\text{Loss}_i^{\text{box}} &= \left\| \hat{y}_i^{\text{box}} - y_i^{\text{box}} \right\|_2^2, \\
\text{Loss}_i^{\text{key points}} &= \left\| \hat{y}_i^{\text{key points}} - y_i^{\text{key points}} \right\|_2^2,
\end{aligned} \tag{1}
$$

where N is the number of training samples and α_j represents the task importance. $\text{Loss}_i^{\text{det}}$ stands for the cross-entropy loss of knee/non-knee classification task. $y_i^{\text{det}} \in \{0, 1\}$ represents the true label of the sample x_i, p_i is the probability generated by the network that regards x_i as the knee. $\text{Loss}_i^{\text{box}}$ denotes the Euclidean loss of knee joint detection task. y_i^{box} is true coordinate for the i-th sample and $y_i^{\text{box}} \in \mathbb{R}^4$. $\hat{y}_i^{\text{box}}$ is the bounding box regression vector predicted by the network. $\text{Loss}_i^{\text{key points}}$ is the Euclidean loss for key point localization. $y_i^{\text{key points}}$ is true coordinate for the i-th sample and $y_i^{\text{key points}} \in \mathbb{R}^{12}$. $\hat{y}_i^{\text{key points}}$ is the located coordinate of six key points. In the first network, we set $\alpha_{\text{det}} = 1$, $\alpha_{\text{box}} = 0.5$ and $\alpha_{\text{key points}} = 0$. In the second network, we set $\alpha_{\text{det}} = 0.8$, $\alpha_{\text{box}} = 0.6$ and $\alpha_{\text{key points}} = 1.5$.

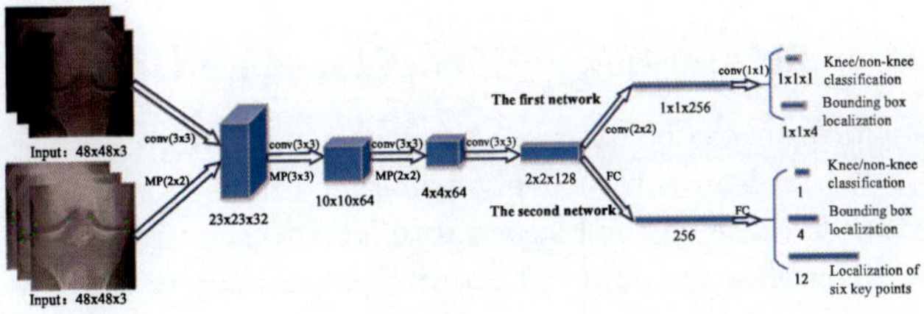

Fig. 3. Training neural network for KneeDetnet.

In the following, we introduce the network proposed by us for training and test. It is worth mentioning that the training networks are similar to test ones except for the different inputs[3]. The specific structure of the training networks

[3] The training data needs to be normally sized as $48 \times 48 \times 3$ while test ones need to generate the pyramid.

is presented in Fig. 3, in which the shared part stands for that the two networks has the same structure in the hidden layers. The first network includes six layers and performs two tasks: knee/non-knee classification and knee joint detection. The second network also contains six layers and builds three tasks: knee/non-knee classification, knee joint detection and key point localization. The practical training highly depends on the generated data, whose details will be reported in the numerical part. As for the test network in Fig. 4, at first, each knee image is resized into different scales to generate image pyramid. Then image pyramid of each knee image is sent to the first network, which is a fully convolutional neural network, to obtain available candidate knee joints. The sequence procedure is the use of the non-maximum suppression (NMS) to merge highly overlapped candidate regions. In addition, a second network is designed to reject false candidates and output the desired objects, as a result.

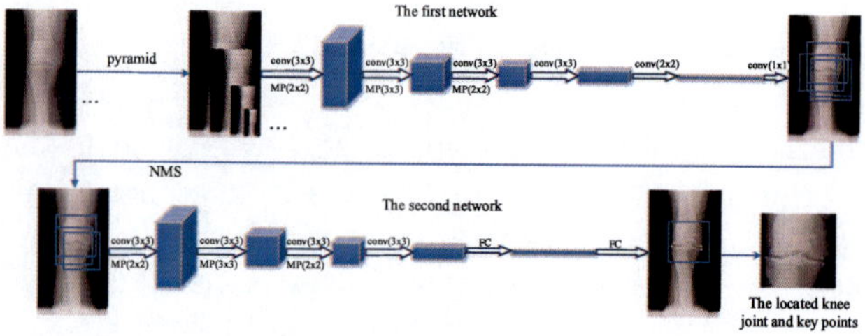

Fig. 4. The KneeDetnet for knee joints localization.

Different from previous work [32], in the first network, we add extra layers to extract more details about the feature. In the experiments, a very interesting finding is that two networks can beat the three-network results. Thus, in our algorithm, two networks rather than three are used.

2.3 User-Friendly Assessment: KLnet for Knee OA

This part provides an easily used assessment method for the doctors' clinical diagnosis as shown in Fig. 5. Intuitively, the knee image from the KneeDetnet is a little bit redundant due to the disease is reflected around the knee joint space. Thus, the KneeDetnet's outputs are cropped according to six key points with critical knee joints obtained adaptively. Existing methods employ fixed scales to resize. However, such a fixation way may not be appropriate due to the diversity of knee joint width. Therefore, we carry out a flexible scheme: The first question is how to describe the knee joint width mathematically. Here, we denote largest distance of the x-coordinates of the six key points as the width. We observe that the heights of the knee joint spaces are much smaller than the width. The desired area is contained in a rectangle, which is chosen as: The maximum ordinate of six points increases by 0.2 times of knee joint width as the top of relocated knee joints; The minimum ordinate of six points is reduced by 0.2 times of knee joint width as the bottom of relocated knee joints[4]. The relocated regions keep the previous widths but with cropped heights.

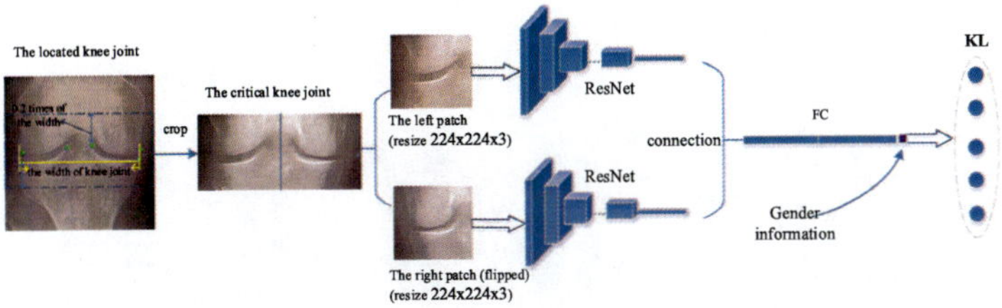

Fig. 5. The KLnet for knee OA assessment.

After relocating key areas, we equally divide them into left and right parts, and the right image patches are horizontally flipped. Both two parts are input into the shared ResNet-based Siamese convolutional neural network to extract local deep learning features. Considering the difference features caused by the gender, thus, multi-information features fusion strategy is applied for obtaining richer features. Here, the extracted local features of two image patches and the gender information with one dimensional vector of patients are connected in series to form fused features with better representations, which are fed to FC layers to evaluate the knee OA severity. Here, we use the deeper ResNet-based Siamese network architecture to learn features of each image side with shared weights, which not only reduces the number of learnable parameters, but also can learn more discriminative relative features between two image sides in one knee image. This method can extract more detailed features to describe knee joint images.

3 Results

3.1 Datasets

Experiments are conducted on two widely used public datasets: the OAI dataset (https://oai.epi-ucsf.org/datarelease/) and the MOST dataset (http://most.ucsf.edu). The OAI dataset contains the data from 4796 subjects. The MOST database is similar to the OAI database but excluded in the OAI dataset. The MOST dataset contains the data from 3026 participants. Both datasets include follow-up data with different months from men and women aged between 50–79 and 45–79 years old.

KL grades range five different labels: KL0, KL1, KL2, KL3 and KL4. As the Fig. 6 shown, KL0 means no knee OA symptoms, i.e., the normal knee joint. KL1 indicates doubtful diseases about knee OA. KL2 represents early knee OA

[4] The coefficient 0.2 can be chosen as others.

troubles. KL3 means moderate accident. The worst is KL4, which has "broke" your leg.

Here, we select data with KL labels from the part of OAI and MOST databases. And the experimental platform we used is Ubuntu 16.04, Python 3.6, PyTorch 0.4 and 2080Ti GPU.

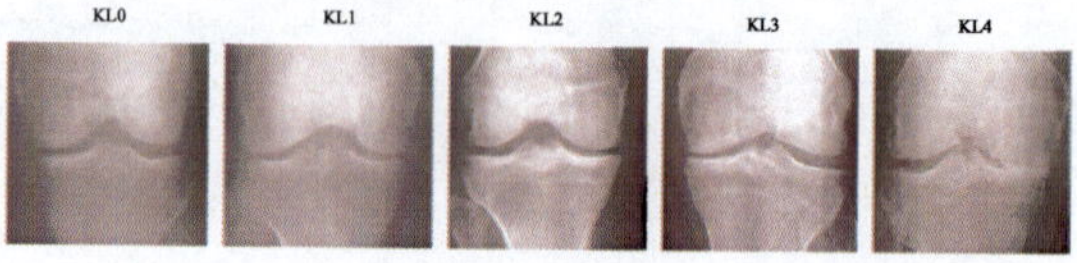

Fig. 6. Knee images with different grades.

3.2 Experimental Results and Analysis of the Knee Joint Localization

5448 single-knee images from the OAI 00m dataset are manually marked with six key points to generate the ground-truth of the knee joint region as shown in Fig. 7. We calculate the mean of six key points as the center point. The ordinate of the center point adds 0.65 times of the knee joint width and subtracts 0.65 times of the knee joint width, which is as the height of the ground-truth of the bounding box. Just like the method ahead, the abscissa of the center point adds 0.65 times of the knee joint width and subtracts 0.65 times of the knee joint width, which is regarded as the width of the ground-truth of the bounding box. In the Fig. 7, red marked bounding box is the ground-truth of the knee joint area. Then 4086 images are selected from 5448 images to generate the training data of the KneeDetnet. We randomly select bounding boxes from each single-knee image, which are compared with its ground-truth via Intersection Over Union (IOU). Generated training samples include positive samples with IOU ≥ 0.65, partial samples with $0.4 \leq$ IOU < 0.65 and negative samples with IOU < 0.3, all of which are resized into 48×48. Training samples are augmented by mirror operations. In the end, the training data for the first network contains 40131 positive samples, 220166 negative samples and 39363 partial samples. The training data of the second network are based on results obtained from the first network and re-generated according to the IOU. The training data for the second network includes 18450 positive samples, 7151 negative samples, 4993 partial samples and 20132 samples for key points localization.

After several explorations, we found that the first network can achieve quite good performance when the training parameters are set as follows: the *epoch* is set as 10, the *learning rate (lr)* is set as 0.001, and the *batch_size* is set as 500. The training parameters of the second network are set as follows: the *epoch* is set as 10, the *learning rate (lr)* is set as 0.0001, and the *batch_size* is set as 500.

The remaining 1362 images are used for verifying KneeDetnet method, where knee joint areas of 1360 images are detected. Thus, the detection accuracy of

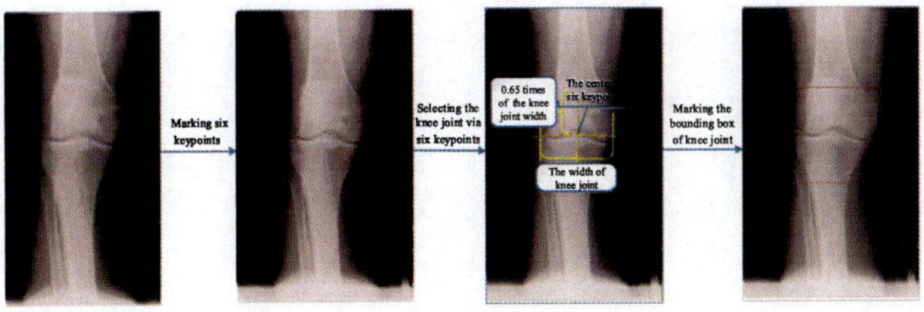

Fig. 7. The process of generating the ground-truth of the bounding box for KneeDetnet.

the knee joint areas on the validation set is 99.85%. Then we test KneeDetnet method on two datasets. Table 1 show that the OAI dataset has 45110 single knee images, where only 32 images fail to be identified with our method. The average detection accuracy is 99.93%, which is 0.48% higher than the MTCNN method, and 8.2% higher than the HOG+SVM method. As shown in Table 2, although HOG+SVM shows the better performance on the MOST V0, V1, V2 datasets, the HOG+SVM method detects the 19034 knee joints among 19383 single knee images. The KneeDetnet method detects 19194 sheets, and the average detection accuracy of which is 99.02%. That is 0.82% higher than the detection accuracy (98.20%) of the HOG+SVM method and 1.4% higher than the MTCNN method. Therefore, the proposed KneeDetnet algorithm in this paper shows superior performance in knee joint localization and can be directly used for subsequent knee OA identification.

Table 1. The number and detection accuracy comparisons of detected knee joints on the OAI dataset with different months.

Dataset								
Method	The number (accuracy)							
	00 m	12 m	24 m	36 m	48 m	72 m	96 m	Total (average)
The original number	8626 (–)	8362 (–)	7372 (–)	7050 (–)	6918 (–)	3349 (–)	3433 (–)	45110 (–)
HOG+SVM [27]	7077 (82.04%)	7073 (84.59%)	6895 (93.53%)	6897 (97.83%)	6774 (97.92%)	3294 (98.36%)	3369 (98.14%)	41379 (91.73%)
MTCNN [32]	8570 (99.35%)	8317 (99.46%)	7326 (99.38%)	7010 (99.43%)	6875 (99.38%)	3343 (99.82%)	3421 (99.65%)	44862 (99.45%)
Ours (KneeDetnet)	**8621 (99.94%)**	**8355 (99.91%)**	**7367 (99.93%)**	**7045 (99.93%)**	**6908 (99.86%)**	**3349 (100.00%)**	3433 (100.00%)	**45078 (99.93%)**

Table 2. The number and detection accuracy comparisons of detected knee joints on the MOST dataset with different months.

Dataset						
Method	The number (accuracy)					
	V0	V1	V2	V3	V5	Total (average)
The original number	6019 (–)	574 (–)	5125 (–)	4039 (–)	3626 (–)	19383 (–)
HOG+SVM [27]	**5969 (99.17%)**	**572 (99.65%)**	**5059 (98.71%)**	3919 (97.03%)	3515 (96.94%)	19034 (98.20%)
MTCNN [32]	5845 (97.11%)	556 (96.86%)	4960 (96.78%)	3982 (98.59%)	3578 (98.68%)	18921 (97.62%)
Ours (KneeDetnet)	5933 (98.57%)	565 (98.43%)	5051 (98.56%)	**4027 (99.70%)**	**3618 (99.78%)**	**19194 (99.02%)**

3.3 Experimental Results and Analysis of the Knee OA Diagnosis

We divide detected 45078 images from the OAI dataset into 25040 training sets, 5006 validation sets, and 15032 test sets. The detected 19194 knee joints of the MOST dataset are also the test set. They are input into the shared ResNet-based Siamese network, such as ResNet18, ResNet34, ResNet50, and ResNet101. To deal with the illumination and angle changes and over-fitting problems [25], we use the data augmentation [7,24]: illumination contrast enhancement, gamma correction, rotation and translation, etc.

In order to verify effectiveness of the knee joint relocation after KneeDetnet's detection, the comparison experiments are carried out with repositioning and non-repositioning methods on the OAI and MOST datasets when the gender information from patients is absent in ResNet models. As shown in Table 3, the highest accuracy of 78.59% is obtained on the OAI dataset under knee relocation method via ResNet 101. The highest accuracy of 67.86% on the MOST dataset is based on the knee relocation method via ResNet34. We can find that relocated methods are better than non-relocated methods. Experimental results illustrate that knee relocation method we proposed is beneficial to KL grades prediction, reducing redundancy information and highlighting key position information.

Table 3. Performance comparison with and without knee repositioning on the OAI and MOST datasets.

Method		OAI dataset				MOST dataset			
		Learning rate	Accuracy	Kappa	MSE	Learning rate	Accuracy	Kappa	MSE
Without knee repositioning	via ResNet18	10-6	72.24%	0.8559	0.4317	10-6	67.36%	0.8599	0.5414
	via ResNet34	10-6	73.69%	0.8652	0.4057	10-6	67.36%	0.8627	0.5328
	via ResNet50	10-6	73.51%	0.8727	0.3808	10-6	66.00%	0.8604	0.5374
	via ResNet101	10-6	73.96%	0.8722	0.3867	10-6	67.55%	0.8654	0.5275
With knee repositioning	via ResNet18	10-5	74.55%	0.8746	0.3796	10-5	67.40%	0.8737	0.4947
	via ResNet34	10-5	76.92%	0.8826	0.3525	10-5	**67.86%**	**0.8744**	**0.4907**
	via ResNet50	10-5	77.23%	0.8903	0.3313	10-5	67.31%	0.8717	0.5014
	via ResNet101	10-5	**78.59%**	**0.8945**	**0.3177**	10-5	67.14%	0.8693	0.5129

As for KL prediction results shown in Table 4, our method achieves the highest accuracy (78.85%), the highest kappa coefficient (0.8970) and the lowest mean square error (MSE) of 0.3074 on the OAI dataset. The accuracy of our method is 8.19% higher than that of Tiulpin et al. On the MOST dataset, the proposed TS-CNN (ResNet34+gender) method achieves 68.20% accuracy, which is 0.27% lower than the method of Tiulpin et al. But its kappa coefficient is the highest (0.8756) and the MSE is the lowest (0.4855). Table 4 presents that it is more effective to integrate the gender information of patients than gender information free cases. The results demonstrate our method has promising performance in KL prediction of knee OA.

Table 4. Performance comparison with state-of-the-art methods on the OAI and MOST datasets.

Method	OAI dataset				MOST dataset			
	Learning rate	Accuracy	Kappa	MSE	Learning rate	Accuracy	Kappa	MSE
Antony et al., 2017 [1]	10-4	62.65%	0.7612	0.7648	10-4	67.05%	0.8505	0.6126
Tiulpin et al., 2018 [26]	10-3	70.66%	0.8498	0.4579	10-3	**68.47%**	0.8638	0.5354
TS-CNN (ResNet18+nogender)	10-5	74.55%	0.8746	0.3796	10-5	67.40%	0.8737	0.4947
TS-CNN (ResNet34+nogender)	10-5	76.92%	0.8826	0.3525	10-5	67.86%	0.8744	0.4907
TS-CNN (ResNet50+nogender)	10-5	77.23%	0.8903	0.3313	10-5	67.31%	0.8717	0.5014
TS-CNN (ResNet101+nogender)	10-5	78.59%	0.8945	0.3177	10-5	67.14%	0.8693	0.5129
TS-CNN (ResNet18+gender)	10-5	74.89%	0.8749	0.3741	10-5	68.08%	0.8701	0.5005
TS-CNN (ResNet34+gender)	10-5	77.27%	0.8852	0.3454	10-5	68.20%	**0.8756**	**0.4855**
TS-CNN (ResNet50+gender)	10-5	77.34%	0.8910	0.3267	10-5	66.74%	0.8722	0.4962
TS-CNN (ResNet101+gender)	10-5	**78.85%**	**0.8970**	**0.3074**	10-5	66.82%	0.8681	0.5088

4 Conclusions

To improve the accuracy of assessing knee OA, a novel Two-Stage Convolutional Neural Network (TS-CNN) method is proposed in this paper. Our methods are based on a two-stage neural network technique together with gender information fusion, whose efficiency is strongly demonstrated by the numerical results. Although the proposed method has achieved non-trivial outperformance in the knee OA diagnosis, it may be improved in the perspective of the accuracy (the current accuracy ranges about 66%–79%). We list three possible future works. The first one is the integration of the knee joint spaces and osteophytes information for decision-level fusion. While the second one might use multi-task and even the multi-network in the diagnosis. The last one may investigate an end-to-end deep learning system by combining these steps.

Acknowledgments. This work is supported by the National Key Research and Development Program of China under No. 2018YFB0204301.

References

1. Antony, J., McGuinness, K., Moran, K., O'Connor, N.E.: Automatic detection of knee joints and quantification of knee osteoarthritis severity using convolutional neural networks. In: International Conference on Machine Learning and Data Mining in Pattern Recognition, pp. 376–390. Springer (2017). https://doi.org/10.1007/978-3-319-62416-7_27
2. Antony, J., McGuinness, K., O'Connor, N.E., Moran, K.: Quantifying radiographic knee osteoarthritis severity using deep convolutional neural networks. In: 2016 23rd International Conference on Pattern Recognition (ICPR), pp. 1195–1200. IEEE (2016). https://doi.org/10.1109/ICPR.2016.7899799
3. Arden, N., Nevitt, M.C.: Osteoarthritis: epidemiology. Best Pract. Res. Clin. Rheumatol. **20**(1), 3–25 (2006). https://doi.org/10.1016/j.berh.2005.09.007
4. Braun, H.J., Gold, G.E.: Diagnosis of osteoarthritis: imaging. Bone **51**(2), 278–288 (2012). https://doi.org/10.1016/j.bone.2011.11.019

5. Chatfield, K., Simonyan, K., Vedaldi, A., Zisserman, A.: Return of the devil in the details: delving deep into convolutional nets. arXiv preprint arXiv:1405.3531 (2014). https://doi.org/10.5244/C.28.6
6. Cross, M., et al.: The global burden of hip and knee osteoarthritis: estimates from the global burden of disease 2010 study. Ann. Rheumat. Dis. **73**(7), 1323–1330 (2014). https://doi.org/10.1136/annrheumdis-2013-204763
7. He, K., Zhang, X., Ren, S., Sun, J.: Deep residual learning for image recognition. In: Proceedings of the IEEE Conference on Computer Vision and Pattern Recognition, pp. 770–778 (2016). https://doi.org/10.1109/CVPR.2016.90
8. Jia, Y., et al.: Caffe: convolutional architecture for fast feature embedding. In: Proceedings of the 22nd ACM International Conference on Multimedia, pp. 675–678. ACM (2014). https://doi.org/10.1145/2647868.2654889
9. Kellgren, J., Lawrence, J.: Radiological assessment of osteo-arthrosis. Ann. Rheumat. Dis. **16**(4), 494 (1957). https://doi.org/10.1136/ard.16.4.494
10. Kong, F.: Facial expression recognition method based on deep convolutional neural network combined with improved LBP features. Pers. Ubiquit. Comput. 1–9 (2019). https://doi.org/10.1007/s00779-019-01238-9
11. Liu, C., et al.: Automatic segmentation of the prostate on CT images using deep neural networks (DNN). Int. J. Radiat. Oncol.* Biol.* Phys. **104**(4), 924–932 (2019). https://doi.org/10.1016/j.ijrobp.2019.03.017
12. Long, J., Shelhamer, E., Darrell, T.: Fully convolutional networks for semantic segmentation. In: Proceedings of the IEEE Conference on Computer Vision and Pattern Recognition, pp. 3431–3440 (2015). https://doi.org/10.1109/CVPR.2015.7298965
13. Nguyen, C.C., Tran, G.S., Nghiem, T.P., Burie, J.C., Luong, C.M.: Real-time smile detection using deep learning. J. Comput. Sci. Cybern. **35**(2), 135–145 (2019). https://doi.org/10.15625/1813-9663/35/2/13315
14. Norman, B., Pedoia, V., Majumdar, S.: Use of 2D U-net convolutional neural networks for automated cartilage and meniscus segmentation of knee MR imaging data to determine relaxometry and morphometry. Radiology **288**(1), 177–185 (2018). https://doi.org/10.1148/radiol.2018172322
15. Oka, H., et al.: Fully automatic quantification of knee osteoarthritis severity on plain radiographs. Osteoarthritis Cartilage **16**(11), 1300–1306 (2008). https://doi.org/10.1016/j.joca.2008.03.011
16. Orlov, N., Shamir, L., Macura, T., Johnston, J., Eckley, D.M., Goldberg, I.G.: WND-CHARM: multi-purpose image classification using compound image transforms. Pattern Recogn. Lett. **29**(11), 1684–1693 (2008). https://doi.org/10.1016/j.patrec.2008.04.013
17. Pedoia, V., Norman, B., Mehany, S.N., Bucknor, M.D., Link, T.M., Majumdar, S.: 3D convolutional neural networks for detection and severity staging of meniscus and PFJ cartilage morphological degenerative changes in osteoarthritis and anterior cruciate ligament subjects. J. Magn. Reson. Imaging **49**(2), 400–410 (2019). https://doi.org/10.1002/jmri.26246
18. Puig-Junoy, J., Zamora, A.R.: Socio-economic costs of osteoarthritis: a systematic review of cost-of-illness studies. In: Seminars in Arthritis and Rheumatism, vol. 44, pp. 531–541. Elsevier (2015). https://doi.org/10.1016/j.semarthrit.2014.10.012
19. Russakovsky, O., et al.: ImageNet large scale visual recognition challenge. Int. J. Comput. Vis. **115**(3), 211–252 (2015). https://doi.org/10.1007/s11263-015-0816-y

20. Shamir, L., Ling, S.M., Scott, W., Hochberg, M., Ferrucci, L., Goldberg, I.G.: Early detection of radiographic knee osteoarthritis using computer-aided analysis. Osteoarthritis Cartilage **17**(10), 1307–1312 (2009). https://doi.org/10.1016/j.joca.2009.04.010
21. Shamir, L., et al.: Knee x-ray image analysis method for automated detection of osteoarthritis. IEEE Trans. Biomed. Eng. **56**(2), 407–415 (2008). https://doi.org/10.1109/TBME.2008.2006025
22. Shamir, L., Orlov, N., Eckley, D.M., Macura, T., Johnston, J., Goldberg, I.: WND-CHARM: multi-purpose image classifier. Astrophysics Source Code Library (2013)
23. Shamir, L., Orlov, N., Eckley, D.M., Macura, T., Johnston, J., Goldberg, I.G.: Wndchrm-an open source utility for biological image analysis. Sour. Code Biol. Med. **3**(1), 13 (2008). https://doi.org/10.1186/1751-0473-3-13
24. Simonyan, K., Zisserman, A.: Very deep convolutional networks for large-scale image recognition. arXiv preprint arXiv:1409.1556 (2014)
25. Srivastava, N., Hinton, G., Krizhevsky, A., Sutskever, I., Salakhutdinov, R.: Dropout: a simple way to prevent neural networks from overfitting. J. Mach. Learn. Res. **15**(1), 1929–1958 (2014)
26. Tiulpin, A., Thevenot, J., Rahtu, E., Lehenkari, P., Saarakkala, S.: Automatic knee osteoarthritis diagnosis from plain radiographs: a deep learning-based approach. Sci. Rep. **8**(1), 1727 (2018). https://doi.org/10.1038/s41598-018-20132-7
27. Tiulpin, A., Thevenot, J., Rahtu, E., Saarakkala, S.: A novel method for automatic localization of joint area on knee plain radiographs. In: Scandinavian Conference on Image Analysis, pp. 290–301. Springer (2017). https://doi.org/10.1007/978-3-319-59129-2_25
28. Tran, D., Wang, H., Torresani, L., Feiszli, M.: Video classification with channel-separated convolutional networks. arXiv preprint arXiv:1904.02811 (2019)
29. Wiggers, K.L., Britto Jr., A.S., Heutte, L., Koerich, A.L., Oliveira, L.S.: Image retrieval and pattern spotting using siamese neural network. arXiv preprint arXiv:1906.09513 (2019). https://doi.org/10.1109/IJCNN.2019.8852197
30. Yang, S.: Feature engineering in fine-grained image classification. Ph.D. thesis (2013). http://hdl.handle.net/1773/23376
31. Yoo, T.K., Kim, D.W., Choi, S.B., Park, J.S.: Simple scoring system and artificial neural network for knee osteoarthritis risk prediction: a cross-sectional study. PLoS ONE **11**(2), e0148,724 (2016). https://doi.org/10.1371/journal.pone.0148724
32. Zhang, K., Zhang, Z., Li, Z., Qiao, Y.: Joint face detection and alignment using multitask cascaded convolutional networks. IEEE Signal Process. Lett. **23**(10), 1499–1503 (2016). https://doi.org/10.1109/LSP.2016.2603342

The Art-of-Hyper-Parameter Optimization with Desirable Feature Selection

Optimizing for Multiple Objectives: Ransomware Anomaly Detection

Priynka Sharma(✉), Kaylash Chaudhary, and M. G. M. Khan

School of Computing, Information and Mathematical Sciences, University of the South Pacific, Suva, Fiji
{priynka.sharma,kaylash.chaudhary,mgm.khan}@usp.ac.fj

Abstract. The development of cyber-attacks carried out with ransomware has become increasingly refined in practically all systems. Attacks with pioneering ransomware have the best complexities, which makes them considerably harder to identify. The radical ransomware can obfuscate much of these traces through mechanisms, such as metamorphic engines. Therefore, predictions and detection of malware have become a substantial test for ransomware analysis. Numerous Machine Learning (ML) algorithm exists; considering each algorithm's Hyper-parameter (HP) just as feature selection strategies, there exist a huge number of potential options. This way, we deliberate more about the issue of simultaneously choosing a learning algorithm and setting its HPs, going past work that tends to address the issues in isolation. We show this issue determined by a completely automated approach, utilizing ongoing developments in ML optimizations. We also show that modifying the information preprocessing brings about more significant progress towards better classification recalls.

Keywords: HP · Feature Selection · Optimization · Ransomware · ML classification algorithms · Data imbalance

1 Introduction

The earlier decade has seen a detonation of ML exploration besides applications; particularly, deep learning strategies have empowered key advances in numerous application areas, for example, computer vision, speech processing, and game-playing [1]. In any case, the performance of numerous ML strategies is exceptionally delicate to a plethora of design decisions, which establishes an extensive obstruction for new users. This is especially valid in the booming field of deep learning, where designers' requisite to choose the right models, formulating approaches in addition to tuning HPs of these segments with sufficient executions [1, 3]. Although, this procedure only needs to rehash for individual applications. Even experts are frequently left with monotonous acts of experimentation until they recognize a decent arrangement of decisions for a specific dataset. The field of automated ML (AutoML) plans to settle on choices that are based

R. Su et al. (Eds.): MICAD 2021, LNEE 784, pp. 218–227, 2022.
https://doi.org/10.1007/978-981-16-3880-0_23

on information-driven and objectives in an automated way [3]. AutoML makes state-of-the-art ML approaches available to domain researchers who are keen on applying ML yet do not have enough assets to realize the advancements in detail. However, the best-performing models for some modern applications of ML are getting bigger and in this way more computationally costly to organize. Therefore, authorities want to set as many HPs automatically as expected under any circumstances. A vast assortment of learning strategies exists, extending from artificially invigorated neural systems [1, 3] over kernel techniques to ensemble models [1, 11]. A typical attribute in these techniques is parameterization by a lot of HPs λ, which is set appropriately by the user to intensify the usefulness of the learning approaches. HPs are to design different parts of the ML learning algorithms and can have uncontrollably fluctuating consequences for the subsequent model and the situation demo levels [4, 5].

HP combs are usually performed manually, through dependable guidelines, or by testing sets of HPs on a predefined lattice [6]. Automating HP search is accepting total measures of consideration in machine learning, for example using benchmarking suites in addition to different activities. Automated methodologies previously appeared to outflank manual searches through authorities on a few subjects [5]. The limitations call for practical answers for the HPOs enhancement that satisfies numerous desiderata. Consequently, choosing the best arrangement of HP values for an ML model yielding directly with performance level. Although there exist several automatic optimization methods, yet these usually take significant resources, increasing the dynamic complexity to obtain a vast level of accuracy rate. HPO finds a tuple of HPs that yields an optimal model that minimizes a predefined loss function on given independent data [5]. The objective function takes a tuple of HPs and returns the associated loss. Cross-validation is often used to estimate this generalization for performances [5].

Our research displays a review of the quick-moving field of AutoML and precision optimization in the ML algorithm through HP tuning. This curiosity will, in the long run, lead to an ideal isolating hyper-plane realistic in both linear and non-linear classification problems towards ransomware anomaly detection.

1.1 Hyper-parameter Optimization (HPO)

In machine learning, model parameters are the properties of training information that will learn without a person during training by the classifiers. Model HPs are valued in ML models that can require various imperatives, loads, or learning rates to produce various information patterns, for example, the number of neighbors in K-Nearest Neighbors (KNN). HPs are significant by the fact that they legitimately control the practices of the training algorithms and influence the presentation of the models prepared. Selecting appropriate HPs undertakes a basic effort in the performance levels of ML models. HPs improvement is the way forward for a perfect model recognition [7, 8]. Reasonably, HPs tuning is only to streamline over model learning to locate the procedure in prompting the least error on the approval set. Therefore, HPs are the only knobs that can tune when as-assembling the appropriate ML algorithm model for anomaly detection or to any application as in Fig. 1.

Figure 1 Highlights the model logic in any ML tuned environment. It shows the logical scheme and confirms on the calculation that Model design added with HP of individual parameters results in enhanced model parameters.

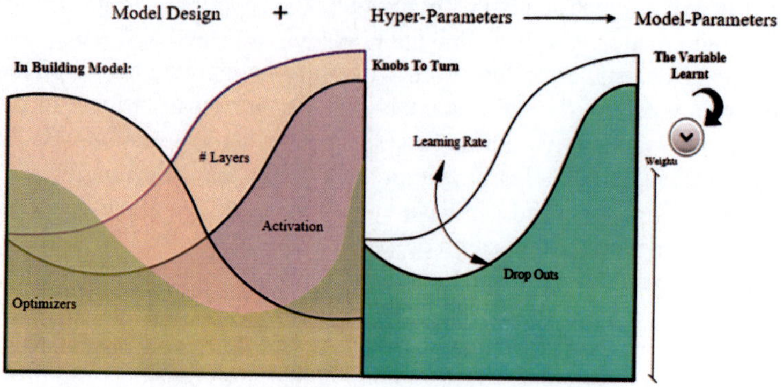

Fig. 1. Momentary portrayal of the HP scheme.

Following [8], HP λ_p is restrictive on another HP λ_i, if λ_p it is dynamic and HP λ_j takes in approvals from a given set VP (I) $\subseteq \wedge_i$, then we call λ_i the parent of λ_p. However, the restrictive HPs on the other hand can only be guardians of other dependent HPs, contributing to rising to a tree-organized space otherwise, sometimes, referred to as a directed acyclic graph (DAG) [2, 9]. The objective of HP improvement is to decide the HPs λ*optimizing hypothetical execution of $A_{\lambda *}$ depends on a restricted measure of training information does = $\{(x_1, y_1)\ldots(Xn, y_n)\}$. Hypothetical execution is approximated by parting into split training, and approval sets (Ds $_{(p)\ \text{train}}$ and $_{(p)\ \text{valid}}$). The learning volumes can be applied by $A_{\lambda *}$ to Ds $_{(p)\ \text{train}}$ and assessing the presentation of these volumes on Ds $_{(p)\ \text{valid}}$. This permits the HPs improvement into subject composed as:

$$C(\lambda) = \frac{1}{k}\sum\nolimits_{P=1}^{k} l\left(A_{\lambda},\ Ds_{(p)\,\text{train}},\ Ds_{(p)\,\text{valid}}\right) \tag{1}$$

$$\lambda * \epsilon \frac{argmin}{\lambda\epsilon\bigwedge} c(\lambda) \tag{2}$$

1.2 Model Selection

In model selection accountabilities, we attempt to locate the correct coherence among prediction and estimation of errors. If our learning algorithm ignores to discover an indicator with a little threat, it is imperative to understand over-fitting or under-fitting.

Under-fitting: The classifier learned on the training set is not sensitive enough to account for the data provided. In this case, both the training error and the test error will be high, as the classifier does not account for relevant information present in the training set.

Over-fitting: The classifier learned on the training set is too specific, and cannot be used to infer anything about unseen data accurately. Although training error continues to decrease over time, test error will begin to increase again as the classifier begins to make decisions based on patterns that exist only in the training set and not in the broader distribution.
The over-fitting and under-fitting will result in poor performance in any given model. Therefore, to refrain from these problems during an analysis phase of an ML model it is vital to follow a technique out from the given four techniques as depicted in Fig. 2.

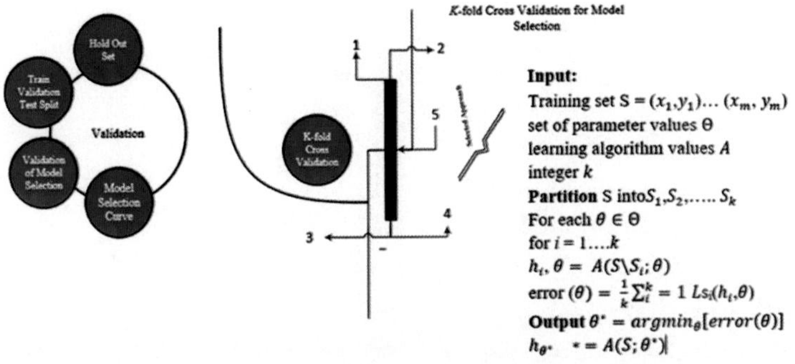

Fig. 2. Model selection approaches.

K-fold Cross-Validation (Selected Method)
In specific applications, information is rare, and we would prefer not to "misuse" information on validation. The k-overlap, cross-validation methods intended to give a precise gauge of the genuine error without squandering an excessive amount of information. In k-overlap cross-validation, the first training set is parceled into k subsets (folds) of size m/k (for straightforwardness, expect that m/k is a number). For each fold, the algorithm prepares for a connection with different overlays thus the error is achieved through overlays. However, K-overlap, cross-validation is often applied for model selection (or parameter tuning).

1.3 The Common Optimization Strategy

A typical optimization procedure defines the possible set of hyper-parameters and the metric to be maximized or minimized for a given problem. Hence, in practice, any optimization procedure follows these classical steps as depicted in Fig. 3.

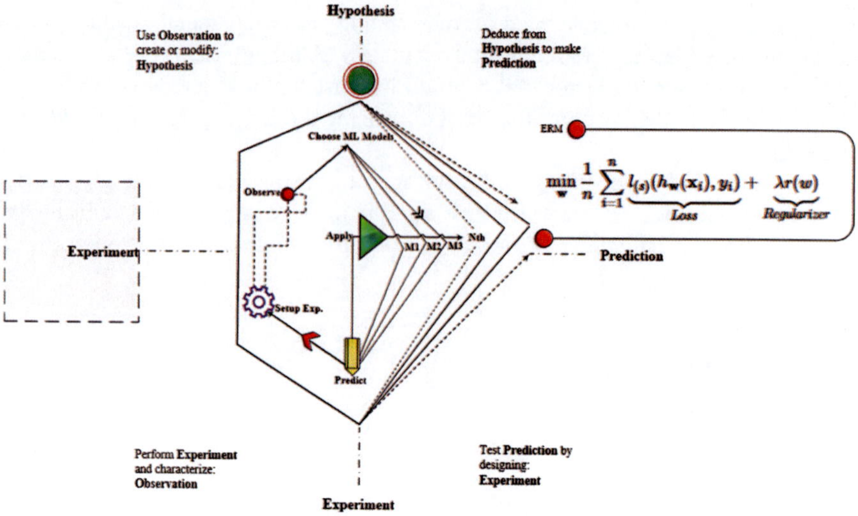

Fig. 3. Illustrates an optimization strategy.

2 Result and Discussion

The experiment dataset was downloaded from VirusShare4, a website that keeps up a continuously updated database of malware for a few [10]. Table 1. Below reports the full list of ransomware families utilized in our research. To analyze the samples, the initial researches used Cuckoo Sandbox to automate the analysis.

To achieve the objective of this research, the classification methods on ransomware detection datasets were applied, through the WEKA environment. WEKA is an information mining structure made by the University of Waikato in New Zealand that executes information mining algorithms working on the JAVA language [12]. WEKA is the best state-of-the-art facility for making, ML systems, and their application to genuine information mining anomalies. It comprises ML algorithms for information mining assignments [12]. WEKA executes algorithms for information preprocessing, classification, regression, clustering, and association rules. The new plans can similarly be made with this pack. In particular, WEKA is an open-source application given under General Public License [12]. The information record usually used by Weka is in the ARFF file-group, which involves labeling to reveal different attributes in the information file. It has many areas, all of which can be used to play out a particular work. At the point when a dataset has been stacked, one of the various panes in the Explorer can be applied to perform further examination.

Table 1. Data description for experiment test set.

Data set	Selected attributes		
Name: Ransomware	Missing: 0%	Distinct: 12	Unique: 0%
Type: Nominal			
Data set	Ransomware Anomaly Detection		
	Features	*Instances*	*Class*
Selected attribute	16382	1524	12
After feature selection	14631	992	Samples used
0	942.0 wt.		Goodware
1	50.0 wt.		Critroni
2	107.0 wt.		CryptLocker
3	46.0 wt.		CryptoWall
4	25.0 wt.		Kollah
5	64.0 wt.		Kovter
6	97.0 wt.		Locker
7	59.0 wt.		Matsnu
8	4.0 wt.		PGPCoder
9	90.0 wt.		Reveton
10	6.0 wt.		TeslaCrypt
11	34.0 wt.		Trojan-Ransom

Most Relevant Features of Each Class Used

We determined the most relevant features through the knowledge based on dataset observation in comparison with feature evaluator and feature model as below:

Dataset Observations: Percentage of the Most Relevant Features for Each Class.

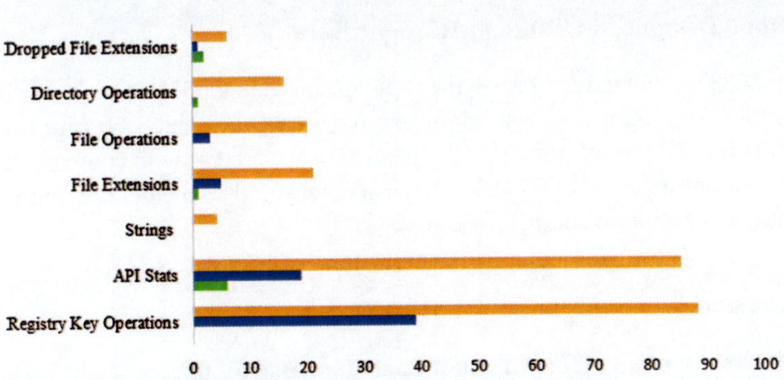

Fig. 4. Most relevant features of each class

Feature Evaluator (supervised, Class (nominal): 16382 Class): WEKA Information Gain Ranking Filter.
Evaluation Mode: Evaluate all training data.
We determined from Fig. 4. Above that Registry Keys and API Stats are the two most pertinent sets, yet different sets are also useful depending on the areas in need. Among every one of these features, several features are for ransomware comportment, together with different features of malware behavior, prompted with an impressive detection rate.

2.1 Finest Features in Descending Approach - Top Twenty

We then again managed to determine our finest features as depicted in Table 2. Table 2 highlights, top five features ranked in descending order based on the average weights. The finest features turn out to be considered essential when the quantity of features is enormous. From this research, it is evident that the finest feature, giving preferable outcomes over a complete set of features for a similar algorithm. The finest features empower the machine learning algorithm to prepare quicker as well as lessens the complex nature of a model and makes it simpler to interpret.

Search Method: WEKA Feature Ranking.
Extracted Features: 14631.

Table 2. Top five ranked attributes (feature selection)

Ranked attribute	Abbreviation	Set Id	Avg. weight
API Stat	API	119	0.431262
Directory operation	DIR	14265	0.407925
Dropped file extensions	DROP	330	0.330449
File extension	FILES_EXT	11684	0.327463
API stats	API	167	0.275793

2.2 Method Obtained in Tuning ML Algorithms

There are 14631 extracted features with 1524 instances loaded. Hence, in total for each ML algorithm, six algorithm configurations were each evaluated 50 times, or 5-fold cross-validation (CD) multiplied by 10 repeats (R). We are going to compare each algorithm configuration based on the percentage accuracy. All of the default configurations are adjusted as per below control measures.

2.3 Discussion

The results are impressive. Ten ML algorithms were used for this research. Feature ranking and file transformations in `ARFF` file were furthermore performed, with the WEKA tool. In each model analysis, we set K= 10, whereK encapsulates the number of base classifiers. Additionally, we took N= 5 for the cross-validation and weight assignments independently. However, ML algorithms can be intended to motivate particular behavior. This is important since it allows the behavior of the model to be acclimated to the main points of our machine learning problem. In this way, one must tune the setup of each ML algorithm to a given problem. This is as often called algorithm tuning or algorithm HPO. For this research, we have chosen the ransomware dataset used to assess the distinctive algorithm configurations. We have additionally included frequent events of all ten algorithms (carried out in Weka) and each with an alternate algorithm arrangement as portrayed in Table 3. To achieve the best outcome. The feature selection method, along with the tuning methodology, has shown an impact on the performance level of the learned model as portrayed in Table 3.

Table 3. Tuning test control

ML algorithms	Common parameter tuning controls
An Iteration Control Set of 10 Repeats; 5-Fold Cross-Validation	
1. IBK 2. J48 3. JRip 4. Naïve Bayes 5. Part 6. Random Tree 7. Random Forest 8. SMO 9. Rep Tree 10. OneR	• Analysis for distance measure: Euclidean or Manhattan • K-values tested for {1,3,7} for both distance measures • Iteration control set to 10 repeats • MinNumObj tested for {2,3,5} • MinNumObj: 2 • NumFolds tested for {3,5,7} • Confidence Factor: 0.25 • Optimization 2 and 5 • MinBucketSize = 6 • NumDecimalPlaces = 2

Table 4 Provides a list of WEKA algorithms with the Receiver Operating Characteristic (ROC) area. Each value on ROC highlights the sensitivity in correspondence with a particular decision threshold. The ROC curve additionally reveals the correctly classified instances as positive values and incorrectly classified instances as a negative value. Whereas, Kappa stats provides the correlation coefficient in our performed experiment. Though the value of Kappa squared is responsible for the accurate amount of data, due to the similarity with our data correctors. Moreover, the False Positive (FP) in our case is in charge of depicting the number of detected ransomware anomaly values and the True Positive (TP) reveals the instances that are effectively anticipated as normal. Finally, after several trials and tuning, we managed to achieve the improved percentage model accuracy performance as in Table 4.

Table 4. Final results (with and without HPO).

Algorithms		ROC Area	FPR	Recall	Precision	Model (%) Performance	Rank
IBK	*With HPO*	0.977	0.974	0.95	0.967	97.83	2
	Without HPO	0.916	0.047	0.811	0.821	81.1	
PART	*With HPO*	0.89	0.754	0.977	0.821	85.01	
	Without HPO	0.899	0.618	0.804	0.803	80.38	
SMO	*With HPO*	0.989	0.034	0.867	0.961	86.67	3
	Without FS	0.923	0.057	0.841	0.835	84.1	
J48	*With HPO*	0.805	0.457	0.087	0.804	80.72	
	Without FS	0.907	0.076	0.805	0.796	80.51	
Jrip	*With HPO*	0.871	0.071	0.782	0.777	78.37	
	Without FS	0.735	0.317	0.745	0.756	74.54	
OneR	*With HPO*	0.51	0.41	0.512	0.574	65.32	
	Without FS	0.57	0.506	0.646	0.664	64.56	
RF	*With HPO*	0.978	0.981	0.97	0.961	98.01	1
	Without FS	0.959	0.08	0.846	0.812	97.89	
RT	*With HPO*	0.61	0.51	0.57	0.589	79.1	
	Without FS	0.863	0.068	0.775	0.785	77.5	
RepT	*With HPO*	0.615	0.541	0.63	0.714	78.01	
	Without FS	0.919	0.773	0.773	0.751	77.3	

3 Conclusion

The outcomes just indicated that Auto-WEKA is powerful at advancing it's given objective. Though, the amount of HPs of an ML algorithm develops and so does its potential for overfitting. The use of cross-validation significantly increments Auto-WEKA's robustness against overfitting. In this work, we have presented the irresistible issue of simultaneously choosing an algorithm selection in addition to HPOs that can be settled by a completely automated tool. This is made promising by recent optimization techniques that iteratively assemble models of the algorithm HP landscape and influences these models to distinguish new focuses on the space that requires investigation. Auto-WEKA, which draws on the full scope of learning algorithms in WEKA and makes it simple for non-specialists to assemble great classifiers for giving application situations.

A broad observational examination of ransomware detection datasets showed that Auto-WEKA regularly beat standard algorithm selection and HPO techniques, particularly on substantial data sets.

References

1. Bergstra, J., Bardenet, R., Bengio, Y., Kégl, B.: Algorithms for hyper-parameter optimization. Adv. Neural. Inf. Process. Syst. **24**, 2546–2554 (2011)
2. Shahhosseini, M., Hu, G., Pham, H.: Optimizing ensemble weights and hyperparameters of machine learning models for regression problems, *arXiv preprint* arXiv:1908.05287 (2019)
3. Falkner, S., Klein, A., Hutter, F.: BOHB: Robust and efficient hyperparameter optimization at scale, *arXiv preprint* arXiv:1807.01774 (2018)
4. Claesen, M., De Smet, F., Suykens, J., De Moor, B.: EnsembleSVM: a library for ensemble learning using support vector machines, *arXiv preprint* arXiv:1403.0745 (2014)
5. Claesen, M., De Moor, B.: Hyperparameter search in machine learning, *arXiv preprint* arXiv:1502.02127 (2015)
6. Pedregosa, F., et al.: Scikit-learn: machine learning in python. J. Mach. Learn. Res. **12**, 2825–2830 (2011)
7. Mantovani, R.G., Horváth, T., Cerri, R., Vanschoren, J., de Carvalho, A.C.: Hyper-parameter tuning of a decision tree induction algorithm. In: 2016 5th Brazilian Conference on Intelligent Systems (BRACIS). IEEE, pp. 37–42 (2016)
8. Bae, K.: Bayesian model-based approaches with MCMC computation to some bioinformatics problems. Texas A and M University (2005)
9. Escalante, H.J., Montes, M., Sucar, L.E.: Particle swarm model selection. J. Mach. Learn. Res. **10**(2) (2009)
10. Sgandurra, D., Muñoz-González, L., Mohsen, R., Lupu, E.C.: Automated dynamic analysis of ransomware: benefits, limitations and use for detection. *arXiv preprint* arXiv:1609.03020 (2016)
11. Breiman, L., Friedman, J., Olshen, R.: Classification and regression trees Routledge (2017)
12. Garner, S.R.: Weka: The waikato environment for knowledge analysis. Proc. New Zealand Comput. Sci. Res. Stud. Conf. **1995**, 57–64 (1995)
13. Alsoghyer, S., Almomani, I.: Ransomware detection system for android applications. Electronics **8**(8), 868 (2019)

Data Augmentation for Breast Cancer Mass Segmentation

Luc Caselles, Clément Jailin(✉), and Serge Muller

GE Healthcare, 78530 Buc, France
clement.jailin@ge.com

Abstract. In medical imaging, a major limitation of supervised Deep Neural Network is the need of large annotated datasets. Current data augmentation methods, though quite efficient to enhance the performance of deep learning networks, do not include complex transformations. This paper presents a realistic image transformation model mimicking multiple acquisitions obtained from the analysis of a mammography database composed of screening acquisitions with priors. Our transformation model results from the combination of a registration algorithm, an invariant meshing strategy and a reduced model describing motion and local intensity variation in paired images. The extracted data variability was then transferred trough data augmentation to a small database for the training of a deep learning-based segmentation algorithm. Significant improvements are observed compared to usual data augmentation techniques.

Keywords: Breast cancer mass detection · Deep learning · Data augmentation · Statistical models · Image registration

1 Introduction

Worldwide, breast cancer is the most common type of cancer for women. Detected at an early stage, the chances of survival are important as it can be effectively treated [1]. Being able to diagnose breast cancers at the earliest stage is thus of upmost importance. The recent development of Computer Aided Detection (CAD) based on Deep Learning (DL) has been a breakthrough in medical image classification [2] and in breast cancer detection on screening mammography [3,4]. However, in order to obtain robust models, the training through supervised approaches require large datasets including labels assessed by radiologists [4,5]. The difficult access to annotated data is one of the main limitations of such approaches in medical image analysis.

Data augmentation is a method commonly used to enrich the dataset and partially compensate the lack of data. It consists in applying predefined transformations with random amplitudes on the training dataset. Applying transformations on the training set allows creating invariance or equivariance in the

R. Su et al. (Eds.): MICAD 2021, LNEE 784, pp. 228–237, 2022.
https://doi.org/10.1007/978-981-16-3880-0_24

model. Usual augmentation techniques [6,7] are composed of geometrical transformations (rotation, translation, shear, etc..) and/or intensity transformations (brightness/contrast, noise, etc..). Though it may not add considerable variability it was proven to be efficient in many cases [8] including breast cancer mass segmentation (*e.g.,* with rigid motions [4] or random deformation fields [9]). However, such augmentations do not capture the variety of transformations that could be derived from the analysis of a given dataset.

In those works, the chosen type of transforms and their amplitudes are not well characterized and rely on manual specification, making data augmentation an implicit form of feature engineering. In addition, non realistic augmentations - sometimes called aggressive transformations - may train the model to learn improbable representations and even wrongly influence the model (*e.g.,* rotational invariance in 6–9 classifications in MNIST [10]). A data augmentation method based on the analysis of motion has been recently proposed for the heart segmentation from MRI images [11]. Unlike previous approaches, this augmentation is designed to create realistic images which prevents the neural network to learn unrealistic patterns. From a small dataset (5 to 100 training subjects) of beating heart sequences, the measured displacement of the heart was used to design a motion model allowing the generation of new instances. The gain in performance using this augmentation was significant when compared to classical augmentation methods (especially with small training dataset). In [12], the authors developed a similar method aiming at reproducing the anatomical variability of brains and knees in MRI sequences (less than 60 training patients). It consisted in interpolations in a geodesic registration space to generate new geometrical transformations. None of the previous studies leveraged both geometrical and intensity variations and allowed a transfer of the learnt transformation model in other databases. In addition, the large variability in size and shape of the breasts imaged in mammography constitutes an additional challenge we had to face in our study, as it impacts the support where the transformations are applied.

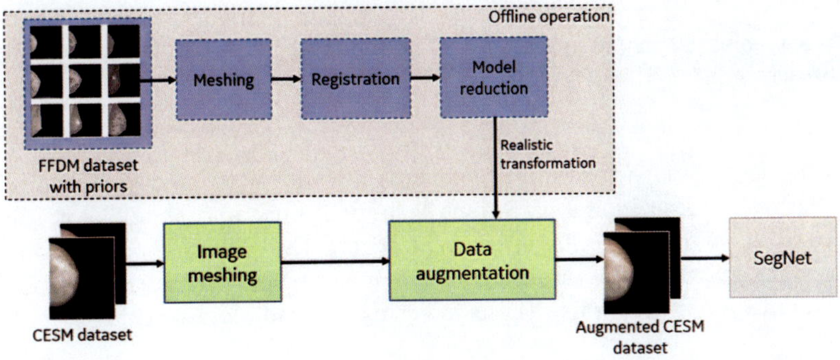

Fig. 1. Data augmentation procedure.

This paper investigates the space of realistic transformations in mammography imaging aiming at designing a data augmentation method mimicking multiple image acquisitions of the same breast. The data augmentation, obtained from a screening dataset with patient history analysis, will be used to increase a segmentation model trained on another smaller breast imaging dataset (Fig. 1). The novelty of this work lies in the introduction of geometrical and intensity transformations extracted from the inherent variability in images of the same breast imaged under different compressions and at different dates, leveraging a geometric and intensity registration process.

The paper is organized as follow: in Sect. 2 we describe the proposed procedure for generating realistic image transformations and how they can be used for data augmentation. Then, Sect. 3 presents the performance in breast cancer mass segmentation obtained with our data augmentation procedure compared to usual data augmentation methods.

2 New Data Augmentation Based on Multiple Acquisition Modeling

In a screening program, the patient undergoes multiple exams at different dates (spaced by few years). The image variations between acquisitions (Fig. 2) are hence composed of 1. physical breast texture evolution in time, 2. changes in breast positioning on the detector and 3. intensity variations due to a change in acquisition parameters.

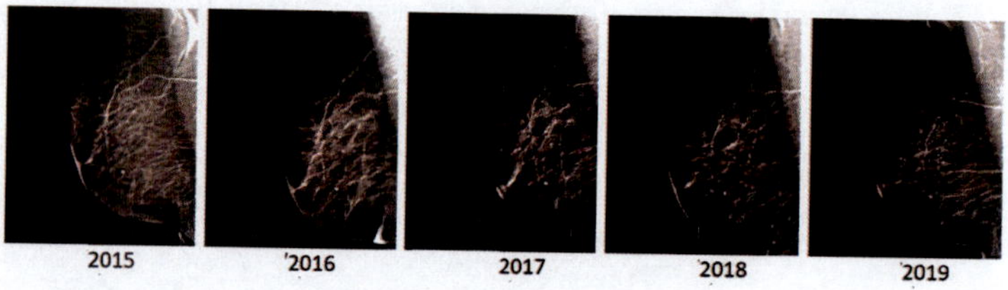

Fig. 2. Screening history with geometrical and intensity variations (MLO views of the right breast).

If a patient were to take multiple exams during the same day, the variations would correspond to image variations 2. and 3. only and should not lead the radiologist to a different diagnostic concerning the presence of a lesion. It is proposed to leverage this transformation invariance to perform anatomically realistic data augmentation without affecting the radiologist decision.

2.1 Realistic Transformation Model Based on Image Meshing and Registration

The transformation fields mapping different acquisitions of the same patient are modeled and identified with a registration algorithm based on an optical flow conservation.

Among many registration techniques proposed in the literature, the one used in this paper is an intensity-based registration method called Digital Image Correlation [13]. The goal of the procedure is the registration of a given pair of mammography images, $I_1 \in \mathbb{R}^{N\times M}$ acquired at a time t_1 and $I_2 \in \mathbb{R}^{N\times M}$ acquired at a time t_2. The Lagrangian displacement field mapping I_2 from I_1 is denoted $v \in \mathbb{R}^{2\times N\times M}$. The acquisition system and parameters evolve between two different exams and highly affect the measured intensity. As the goal is to register the two images based on the optical flow conservation, identifying a brightness correction field, written $a(x)$, is essential. The approach aims to minimize, over the region of interest (ROI) Ω, the residual ρ defined by $\rho(v, a, x) = I_1(x) - a(x)I_2(x + v(x)),\ \forall x \in \Omega$.

$$U, b = \underset{v\in\mathbb{E}, a\in\mathbb{E}}{\text{Argmin}} \int_{\Omega} (I_1(x) - a(x)I_2(x + v(x)))^2 dx \tag{1}$$

As the problem is severely ill-posed, it is required to regularize the solution field in the sense that we assume there is a link between neighboring pixels. For this reason, we propose to use a finite element framework. The displacement is written as a mesh kinematics composed of N_u nodes and a basis of shape functions $\phi(x)$ defining the vector space $\mathbb{E}$. The motion can thus be written in its regularized form $u(x) = \sum_{l=1}^{N_u} u_l\phi_l(x)$, with u_l the nodal displacements. This regularized approach is called global approach [14]. In the exact same spirit, the brightness correction field is also regularized on the same subspace $\mathbb{E}$.

The non-linear problem is solved using an alternating multi-scales iterative Gauss-Newton method, starting with the displacement identification at step k, with $U^{(k+1)} = U^{(k)} + \delta U^{(k)}$ and $b^{(k+1)} = b^{(k)} + \delta b^{(k)}$:

$$\begin{cases} \delta U_j^{(k)} & = \langle S_i, S_j\rangle^{-1}\langle S_i, \rho(U^{(k)}, b^{(k)}, x)\rangle \\ \delta b_m^{(k)} & = \langle \tilde{S}_m, \tilde{S}_n\rangle^{-1}\langle \tilde{S}_n, \rho(U^{(k+1)}, b^{(k)}, x)\rangle \end{cases}$$

The notation $\langle\cdot,\cdot\rangle$ denotes the inner product (*i.e.*, contraction over $x \in \Omega$) and the sensitivity fields (image variation with respect to each nodal parameter): $S_i = \phi_i(x)\nabla I_1(x)$ and $\tilde{S}_n = \phi_n(x)I_1(x)$. The analysis of the entire patient database requires to study all transformations on a common support. To express the transformation fields at the same relative breast position, we used an invariant meshing procedure based on breast tissues nodes. In order to satisfy this constraint, we propose a simple method based on a solution introduced by Feng *et al.* [15] based on a contour discretization of the breast. Few nodes are placed inside the breast to capture texture motion. This approach was validated by comparing the mesh of multiple mammography pairs acquired at different times.

The displacements between the pairs of meshes match the one computed by the registration method with only small errors (average of 1 pix).

The registration is applied on a full field digital mammography (FFDM) dataset with priors acquired on a Senographe Pristina system (GE Healthcare, Chicago, IL, USA). Our dataset contains $P = 583$ CC and MLO views with priors. No radiological findings were found by radiologists in this database. Images are 2294×1914 pixels with a detector pitch of 100 μm.

For each image pair, the mesh composed of 24 nodes was positioned on breast tissues (it was verified that the results were mesh-invariant). The procedure efficiency can be quantified by comparing the ratio of the standard deviation in the image over the standard deviation of the residual measured in the ROI defined by the mesh. Indeed, we observed an increase from 4.4 before to 83.2 after registration. Some errors remain and are due to 3D transformations of the breast that cannot be registered from 2D images.

The P solution fields are then $\{\mathbf{U}^j,\ j \in [1, P]\}$ for the motion fields and $\{\mathbf{b}^j,\ j \in [1, P]\}$ the brightness changes.

2.2 Reduced Model of Realistic Transformations

The generation of a reduced model from all measured fields allows (i) constructing an interpretable model with a controlled complexity, (ii) designing a generative process to create new realistic transformation fields.

Each $\mathbf{U}^j$ is being reshaped as columns in a matrix $\mathcal{M} \in \mathbb{R}^{2n \times P}$, each column being the concatenation of horizontal and vertical displacements. A similar data preparation is applied for the brightness fields. Principal component analysis (PCA) is then applied to decompose the matrix $\mathcal{M}$

$$\mathcal{M}_{ij} = \hat{\mathcal{M}} + \sum_{m=1}^{n_c} \Gamma_{mi} \beta_{mj} \lambda_m \tag{2}$$

with $\hat{\mathcal{M}}$ being the average field. One can see that each of the n_c modes is composed of a spatial nodal component Γ_{mi}, a patient amplitude component β_{mj} and an eigenvalue λ_m. The first spatial components of displacements are shown in Fig. 3 (ordered by λ_m). It is interesting to note that components 2 and 4 correspond to an evolved version of respectively a scaling factor and a rotation. Those two fields are often chosen heuristically in standard data augmentation methods and are here found as indeed contributive.

The variance analysis of the principal components indicates that 6 components (on a 24-dimension space) account for 90% of the variability of the displacement fields in our dataset. Same results are observed for intensity fields.

While PCA leads to linearly uncorrelated components, non-linear couplings (that would complicate the design of new realistic instances) where not found visually from the inspection of the pairwise projections: (β_{mi}, β_{nj}).

Finally, we model the β_i distributions by centered normal laws $\mathcal{N}(0, \sigma_i)$ with standard deviations σ_i computed by maximizing the likelihood with normal distributions (Fig. 3).

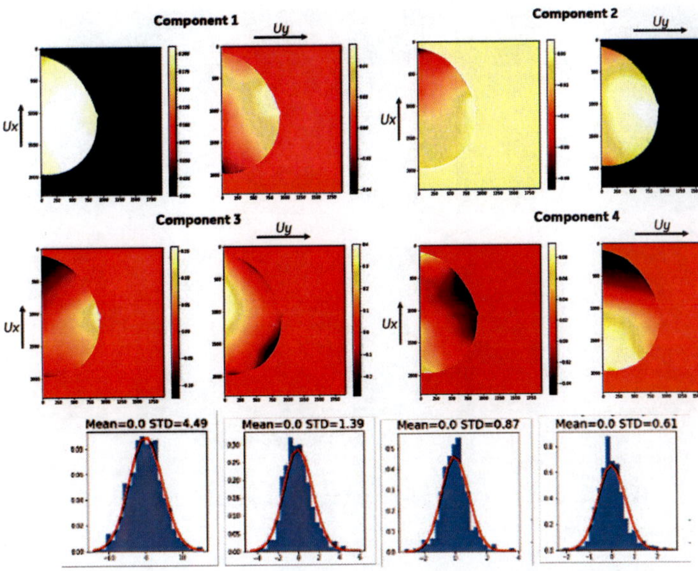

Fig. 3. (Top) The four first principal spatial components in displacement field Γ_{mi} for the CC views. (Bottom) Distributions of the corresponding β_i patient components modeled with a normal distribution.

2.3 Realistic Data Augmentation Model

Synthetic real transformation fields on the nodes can be generated based on a combination of the eigenvectors modeled by independent random variables $X_i \sim \mathcal{N}(0, \sigma_i)$, $i \in [1, N]$, with N the truncation order. As $\hat{\mathcal{M}}$ is negligible (on average, 1.6% of the norm of the transformation fields in our application), the generated centered transformation fields α^t can be written as:

$$\alpha^t(x) = \sum_{m=1}^{N^t} X^t_m \Gamma^t_m(x) \lambda^t_m \tag{3}$$

where $t = [U, b]$ denotes intensity and displacement indexes. Realistic transformation fields are generated using this method and applied over FFDM images (Fig. 4).

In the next section, we leverage our proposed data augmentation model to transfer the variability of an initial FFDM database to a smaller Contrast Enhanced Mammography [16–18] (CESM) database with the objective to improve the performance of a deep learning based segmentation algorithm. We used a dataset composed of 204 pathological CESM exams (108 MLO, 96 CC views) including lesion contours drawn by radiologists. CESM exams lead to two channel images: a low energy (*i.e.*, standard FFDM) and a recombined image (contrast uptakes) that will be the input of the deep learning model.

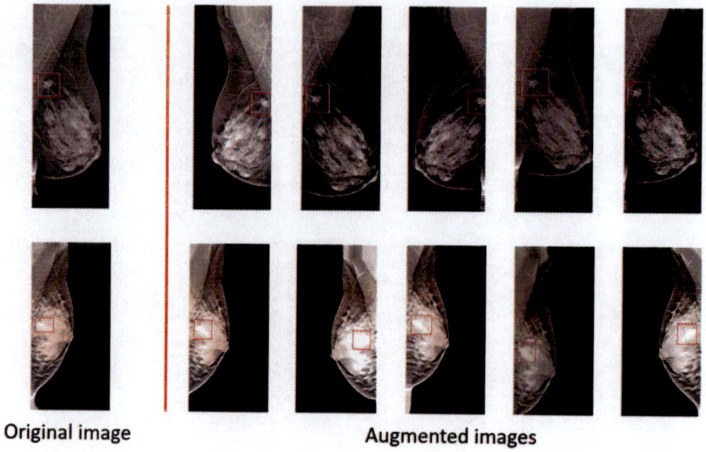

Fig. 4. Multiple transformations of FFDM images: original images (left), transformed images (right).

3 Contribution of Data Augmentation in Deep Learning Based Segmentation

In previous sections, a method to build from a FFDM dataset a model of realistic displacement/intensity variation fields occurring between mammography screening exams has been described. We now want to leverage this model to train a deep neural network that performs lesion segmentation on a small CESM dataset and compare the gain in performance of our method compared to usual data augmentation.

Among various architectures used in the medical imaging literature for the segmentation of breast cancer findings, U-Net is one of the most used algorithms [19]. Therefore, we used U-Net architecture with ResNet blocks to segment the lesions on CESM images [20–22]. Because of the small available dataset, we chose a small network (only 8 features on first convolution layers then doubling at each of the four scales) to avoid overfitting. The training was performed using *TensorFlow 2* with a combination of Dice and binary cross-entropy as loss function and Adam as optimizer. Validation and test sets, fixed for all experiments, were made up of respectively 40/50 {images,labels}. Early stopping based on validation loss was used to prevent overfitting of the training dataset. As the network will be used with different augmentation strategies, the results must be considered in terms of relative performance. We do not state that U-Net is optimal for the segmentation of lesions in CESM images.

The performance of our segmentation model was evaluated using the proposed data augmentation approach based on realistic transformations compared to usual data augmentation methods. Classic data augmentation transformations and manually optimized parameters consisted in centered rotation in the range $[-15°, 15°]$, translation in the range of $[-20 \text{ pixels}, 20 \text{ pixels}]$, shear (30 pixels of maximal displacement), horizontal flip (50 % probability). The performance of the trained deep learning models were evaluated using Dice.

Figure 5 illustrates the performance of our segmentation model applied to CESM images when trained with no data augmentation, with usual data augmentation and with our proposed data augmentation approach. The performance was quantified for different dataset sizes (32, 45, 60 and 100 images). Figure 5(a) shows significant gain in performance using realistic data augmentation over no augmentation or classic data augmentation approaches. This gain over the latter is especially important when very few data data are available (see Table 1). The trends in Dice as function of the training dataset size (also observed in [9,12]) is expected as when the dataset becomes very large (compared to the model size) the relative effect of data-augmentation becomes smaller. In other contexts, a data augmentation could still be relevant when confronted to unbalanced or biased classes. Moreover, the transformation model (build in previous section) is data-dependent as it "learns" the input distribution (FFDM dataset). Applying these transformations to the CESM dataset having different properties is a mean to transfer variability to this dataset.

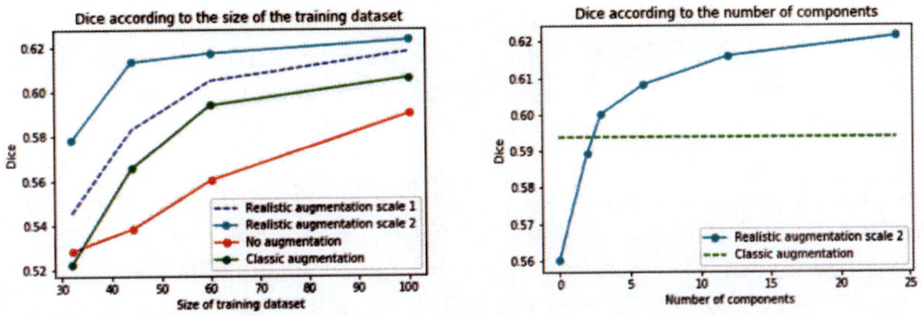

(a) (b)

Fig. 5. (a) Model performance for different data augmentation strategies. (b) Dice according to the number of modes used for data augmentation

Table 1. Gain in performance with respect to no augmentation in Dice

Augmentation/dataset size	32	44	60	100
Realistic	+9.4%	+13.9%	+10.2%	+5.6%
Classical	−1.1%	+5.1%	+6.0%	+2.7%

Each generated realistic transformation field is constructed with a chosen number of modes. The data augmentation performance with different number of modes is illustrated in Fig. 5(b) for 0 (no augmentation), 2, 3, 6 and 12 components. The evolution of the Dice curve as function of the number of components matches the cumulative variance evolution of the PCA. This result seems fundamental as it confirms the link between the performance gain and the variance brought to the dataset by the reduced model.

4 Conclusions

A data augmentation method based on realistic transformations has been proposed. One of our contributions on the design of a data augmentation method is the introduction of a framework enabling the evaluation of real transformations from pairs of images acquired at different dates. It leverages a reliable registration algorithm and an invariant meshing strategy. Another contribution is the introduction of a reduced model of these realistic transformations in screening images, enabling a generative process to create new realistic transformation fields from a limited number of observed transformations. Finally, the assessment of the relative performance of contrast uptake segmentation in CESM images showed a significant improvement over Dice metrics when using the proposed realistic data augmentation. This is a consequence of applying a wide range of realistic transformations whereas classic data augmentation strategies only slightly increase the variability of the dataset used to train a DL-based segmentation model. Moreover, as the transformations are realistic, the neural network does not have to learn unrealistic patterns which may improve the convergence and enhance the overall segmentation performance.

Acknowledgements. The authors would like to acknowledge Pablo Milioni de Carvalho, Zhijin Li, Andrei Petrovskii and Ann-Katherine Carton (all working at GE Healthcare, Buc, France) for their help in data collection and insights in mammography. We wish to point out the absence of conflicts of interest related to our study.

Compliance with Ethical Standards. This research study was conducted retrospectively using anonymized human subject data made available by research partners (Dr Philippe Benillouche, CSE-Paris, France; Dr Weijun Peng, Shanghai Cancer Center, Fudan University, China; Dr Guixiang Zhang, Shanghai First People's Hospital, Medical College, Shanghai Jiaotong University, China). Applicable law and standards of ethic have been respected.

References

1. Torre, L.A., Bray, F., Siegel, R.L., Ferlay, J., Lortet-Tieulent, J., Jemal, A.: Global cancer statistics, 2012. CA: Cancer J. Clin. **65**(2), 87–108 (2015)
2. Zhou, S.K., Greenspan, H., Shen, D.: Deep Learning for Medical Image Analysis. Academic Press, Cambridge (2017)
3. Sahiner, B., et al.: Deep learning in medical imaging and radiation therapy. Med. Phys. **46**(1), e1–e36 (2019)
4. Shen, L., Margolies, L.R., Rothstein, J.H., Fluder, E., McBride, R., Sieh, W.: Deep learning to improve breast cancer detection on screening mammography. Sci. Rep. **9**(1), 1–12 (2019)
5. Benzebouchi, N.E., Azizi, N., Ayadi, K.: A computer-aided diagnosis system for breast cancer using deep convolutional neural networks. In: Computational Intelligence in Data Mining, pp. 583–593. Springer (2019)

6. Taylor, L., Nitschke, G.: Improving deep learning using generic data augmentation. IEEE (2017)
7. Shorten, C., Khoshgoftaar, T.M.: A survey on image data augmentation for deep learning. J. Big Data **6**(1), 60 (2019)
8. Hussain, Z., Gimenez, F., Yi, D., Rubin, D.: Differential data augmentation techniques for medical imaging classification tasks. In: 2017 AMIA Annual Symposium Proceedings, vol. 2017, p. 979. American Medical Informatics Association (2017)
9. Castro, E., Cardoso, J.S., Pereira, J.: Elastic deformations for data augmentation in breast cancer mass detection. In: IEEE EMBS International Conference on Biomedical & Health Informatics (BHI) (2018)
10. Hauberg, S., Freifeld, O., Larsen, A.B.L., Fisher, J., Hansen, L.: Dreaming more data: class-dependent distributions over diffeomorphisms for learned data augmentation. In: Artificial Intelligence and Statistics, pp. 342–350 (2016)
11. Acero, J., et al.: SMOD - data augmentation based on statistical models of deformation to enhance segmentation in 2D cine cardiac MRI, pp. 361–369, May 2019
12. Shen, Z., Xu, Z., Olut, S., Niethammer, M.: Anatomical data augmentation via fluid-based image registration. In: International Conference on Medical Image Computing and Computer-Assisted Intervention, pp. 318–328. Springer (2020)
13. Sutton, M.A., Orteu, J.J., Schreier, H.: Image Correlation for Shape, Motion and Deformation Measurements: Basic Concepts. Theory and Applications. Springer, Heidelberg (2009)
14. Besnard, G., Hild, F., Roux, S.: "Finite-element" displacement fields analysis from digital images: application to portevin-le châtelier bands. Exp. Mech. **46**(6), 789–803 (2006)
15. Feng, S.S.J., Patel, B., Sechopoulos, I.: Objective models of compressed breast shapes undergoing mammography. Medical Physics **40**(3), 031902 (2013)
16. Skarpathiotakis, M., et al.: Development of contrast digital mammography. Med. Phys. **29**(10), 2419–2426 (2002)
17. Dromain, C., et al.: Dual-energy contrast-enhanced digital mammography: initial clinical results. Eur. Radiol. **21**(3), 565–574 (2011)
18. James, J.J., Tennant, S.L.: Contrast-enhanced spectral mammography (CESM). Clin. Radiol. **73**(8), 715–723 (2018)
19. Ronneberger, O., Fischer, P., Brox, T.: U-net: convolutional networks for biomedical image segmentation. In: International Conference on Medical image computing and computer-assisted intervention, pp. 234–241. Springer (2015)
20. Gurummunirathnam, V., Yarlapati, N., Little, S., O'Connor, N.E.: A deep residual architecture for skin lesion segmentation. In: OR 2.0 Context-Aware Operating Theaters, Computer Assisted Robotic Endoscopy, Clinical Image-Based Procedures, and Skin Image Analysis, pp. 277–284. Springer (2018)
21. Zhuang, Z., Li, N., Joseph Raj, A.N., Mahesh, V.G.V., Qiu, S.: An RDAU-NET model for lesion segmentation in breast ultrasound images. PloS One **14**(8), e0221535 (2019)
22. Weng, C.-H., et al.: Artificial intelligence for automatic measurement of sagittal vertical axis using ResUnet framework. J. Clin. Med. **8**(11), 1826 (2019)

Check for updates

Dual-Attention Network for Acute Pancreatitis Lesion Detection with CT Images

Jinyi Zhang and Daoqiang Zhang(✉)

Nanjing University of Aeronautics and Astronautics, Nanjing 211106, China
dqzhang@nuaa.edu.cn

Abstract. Deep learning technique has been widely applied in medical image analysis, whereas no work has been done for recognition or detection for acute pancreatitis, which is one of the most common digestive disorders. Most of current detection architectures are not sufficiently robust to deal with scale variation of all kinds of acute pancreatitis lesions, resulting in inaccurate detection and sometimes false positive small lesions near large lesions. To address this, we proposed a method that modifies classic detection network by employing the idea of attention mechanism in backbone and detector neck. Specifically, channel-wise attention is used to capture the relationship between channels of feature maps to pale the uninformative and meaningless channels unrelated to AP lesions, and spatial attention is applied to prompting the network focus on the area more relevant to AP lesions. The experiment conducted on a real acute pancreatitis dataset verifies the performance improvement the proposed method brings to the original detection model.

Keywords: Lesion detection · Attention mechanism · Acute pancreatitis · CT

1 Introduction

As one of the most common digestive disorders, acute pancreatitis is the main reason for hospital admissions due to gastrointestinal diseases in many countries, with an annual incidence density rate varying from 0.13‰ to 0.45‰. Acute pancreatitis is the second highest cause of hospitalization and the fifth leading cause of hospital death [1]. In a systematic review, the mortality rate of all acute pancreatitis, interstitial pancreatitis and necrotizing pancreatitis cases is about 5%, 3%, and 17% [2]. Severe acute pancreatitis causes persistent (more than 48 h) organ failure and complications, most of which may progress to pancreatic necrosis, and the mortality rate could even reach 30% [3]. Acute pancreatitis endangers the lives of patients with high incidence, fast onset, many complications, and high mortality. The key to improving the prognosis of acute pancreatitis lies in timely detection and intervention. Therefore, it is critical to accurately diagnose acute pancreatitis and determine its severity.

Most common clinical scoring systems for acute pancreatitis includes the Ranson score, the BISAP, APACHE [4] series, SOFA, etc. CT scanning is one of the best imaging methods for detecting pancreatic necrosis and edema, and CECT has been regarded as

R. Su et al. (Eds.): MICAD 2021, LNEE 784, pp. 238–250, 2022.
https://doi.org/10.1007/978-981-16-3880-0_25

the best standard for diagnosis of acute pancreatitis. CTSI [5] is the most common imaging scoring system, which combines Balthazar CT grading with grading of the degree of pancreatic necrosis, and the modified CTSI [6] assigns weights for extra-pancreatic complications and the presence of pleural effusion or ascites. Clinical data analysis of acute pancreatitis has been applying machine learning techniques, such as XGBoost and random forest, on physiological indicators to facilitate diagnosis. In terms of medical image analysis of acute pancreatitis, the mainstream remains designing or discovering features manually depending on prior medical knowledge, without going further to extract higher-level and more discriminant information from images. Doctors diagnose acute pancreatitis with CT scans by figuring out lesions manually, with low diagnosis speed and low accuracy. It is of great significance to apply deep learning technology to processing and analyzing AP's medical images for doctor's diagnosis, whereas nothing related has been done.

Due to the complex pathology, the course, imaging and prognosis of patients with acute pancreatitis vary greatly from patient to patient. On the one hand, as a small, soft and flexible organ, pancreas has a high degree of anatomical variability compared to other organs (like kidney, liver, heart, etc.) and the location, shape, and size of the pancreas vary from person to person as in Fig. 1. Local complications include pancreatic pseudocyst, acute peripancreatic fluid collection, and wall-off necrosis as in Fig. 2. And the lesions of acute pancreatitis are not only limited to the pancreas itself, peripancreatic tissues may also show fluid accumulation, edema, and hemorrhage due to complications and the area of lesion varies greatly as in Fig. 3. Thus, the recognition and lesion detection of acute pancreatitis is not just about identifying or locating pancreas.

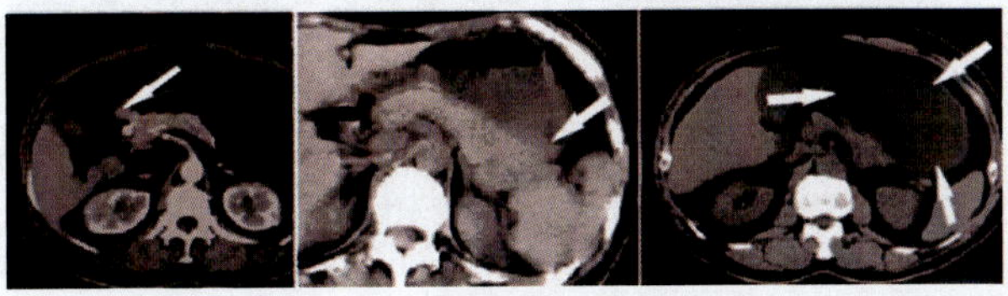

Fig. 1. Anatomical variability of pancreas. Left: pancreas head; middle: pancreas tail; right: pancreas body.

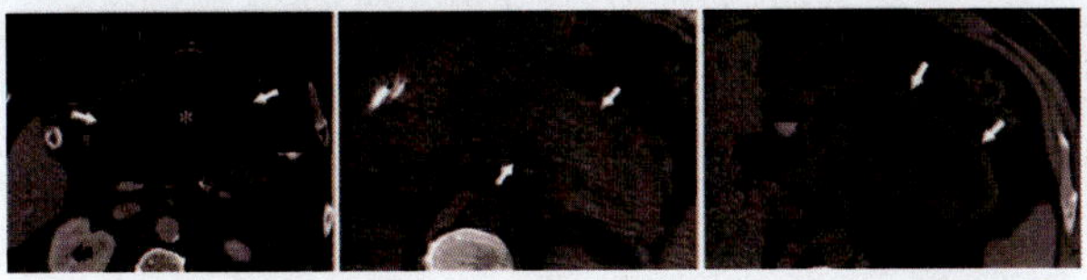

Fig. 2. Local complications of acute pancreatitis. Left: pancreatic pseudocyst, middle: acute necrotic collection, right: wall-off necrosis.

Nowadays, as an effective tool for data analysis, deep learning has been widely used in computer-aided diagnosis or detection, but it has not been applied in acute pancreatitis. Previous studies have achieved organ segmentation of the pancreas with CNNs on CT images or MR images [7–10]. Hitherto, no work based on deep learning has been done for acute pancreatitis lesion detection on CT images. And most of current detection architectures are not sufficiently robust to deal with scale variation of all kinds of acute pancreatitis lesions. We proposed an attentional detection network for acute pancreatitis lesion detection, which modifies classic detection model by applying attention mechanism in detector backbone and neck. The main contributions of this paper are listed as below:

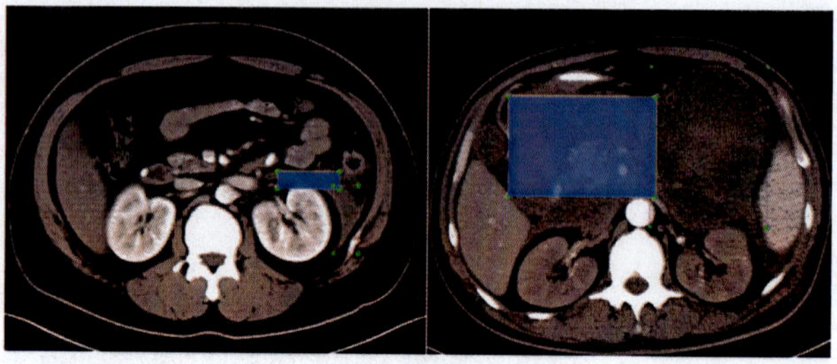

Fig. 3. Variation of lesion area of acute pancreatitis.

- We proposed a detection network for lesion detection of acute pancreatitis, which fills the blank of deep learning methods of medical image analysis for acute pancreatitis.
- We use a dual-attention network as the detector backbone to educe more informative and more discriminant features of acute pancreatitis.
- We utilize channel-wise attention and spatial attention in the detector neck to help filter out the less informative channel-wise features and spatial features.

The rest of this paper is organized as follows. The related work including detection architecture and attention mechanism is reviewed in Sect. 2. The proposed method is presented in Sect. 3. The experiment is conducted and results are shown in Sect. 4. Finally, this paper is concluded in Sect. 5.

2 Related Work

2.1 Detection Architecture

Object detection is one of the most significant tasks in imaging analysis. Before deep learning arose in the field of computer vision, traditional hand-crafted features are utilized in image recognition or object detection, for example, the CTSI for acute pancreatitis diagnosis, which is inefficient and laborious.

The mainstream detectors include one-stage detectors like YOLO [11], SSD [12], and two-stage detectors like Faster R-CNN [13]. The former directly predict the location of the lesion resulting in higher speed, the latter has additional optimization of the lesion location resulting in higher accuracy. FPN [14] combines deep features with semantic information and shallow features with sufficient resolution, therefore facilitates recognition and locating. FPN has become one of the most popular detection modules.

Following the framework in YOLOv4 [15], as shown in Fig. 4, a detection model, one-stage or two-stage, is generally composed of a backbone network and a detection head. The backbone realizes feature extraction of input, and detector neck processes feature obtained by backbone for enhancement, for instance, features fusion of different scales or different abstract levels. Detection head learns target's category and location with features processed and supervised information.

R-CNN [16] is the pioneering work of the two-stage detection model, as the name suggests, abstracting the whole process as two stages. The first is to select a number of regions in the image that may contain the detection target, i.e., region proposals. The second uses classification branch to obtain the categories of objects in each area, and regression branch to obtain coordinate positions. On the basis of R-CNN, SPPNet [17] proposed spatial pyramid pooling to obtain a fixed-length output, thereby avoiding deformation or cropping of fixed-size input required by R-CNN, which leads to performance reducing. Fast RCNN [18] replace the original subsequent SVM classification and regression stages with a network, and uses ROI polling to convert feature maps of different size to a same size. Faster RCNN [13] proposed RPN (Region Proposal Network) to replace the selective search algorithm, and the whole process of generating region proposal, feature extraction, coordinate regression and classification are jointly trained, finally the entire detection task become completely end-to-end.

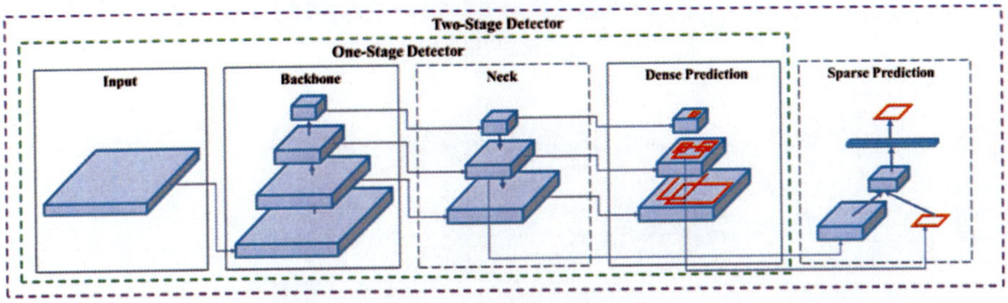

Fig. 4. Detector structure

2.2 Attention Mechanism

At present, there is no unified systematic mathematical definition of attention mechanism. The essence of attention mechanism is utilizing the relevance of data to highlight significant information and suppress the unimportant. Considering the influence of Transformer [19], here we continue to use its expression of attention mechanism. Attention can be considered as a mapping between a series of key-value pairs, and each query has a corresponding value under this mapping, as shown in Fig. 5. The specific calculation process of attention is shown in Fig. 6. Firstly, calculate the similarity between the query and each key as

$$c_i = Similarity(Query, Key_i) \tag{1}$$

The method of measuring similarity varies according to the specific problem. Most common methods include cosine similarity, inner product similarity, splicing similarity, etc. Secondly, introduce the Softmax function to normalize the scores in order to highlight the important ones, as

$$Weight_i = Softmax(c_i) = e^{c_i} / \sum_{j \in \Omega} e^{c_j} \tag{2}$$

Thirdly, perform a weighted summation of the corresponding values to obtain the attention, calculated as

$$Attention\left(Query, \{Key\}_{i \in \Omega}, \{Value\}_{i \in \Omega}\right) = \sum_{i \in \Omega} Weigth_i \cdot Value_i \tag{3}$$

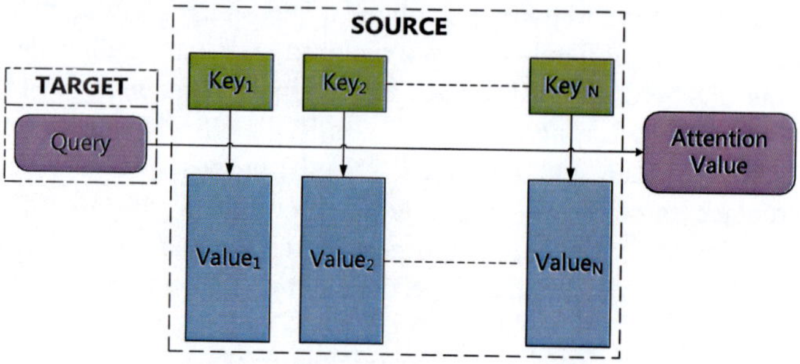

Fig. 5. Attention mechanism.

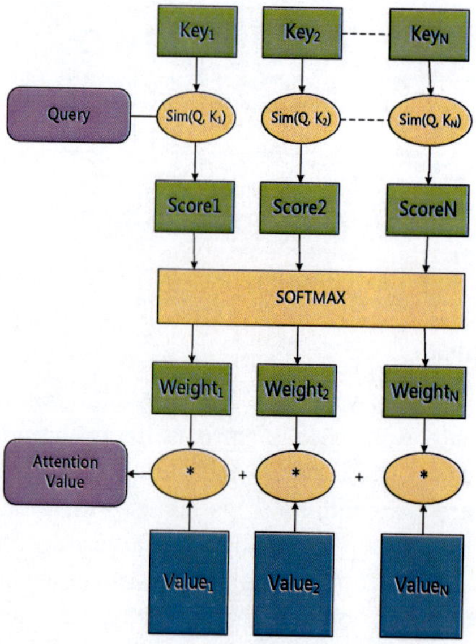

Fig. 6. Calculation of attention

Attention has been widely employed in tasks in the field of computer vision, for instance, image recognition [20–26], object location [27, 28], image generation [29,

30], image segmentation [31, 32]. The semantic information and context information extracted by network have a strong connection to the network performance of tasks including object detection, semantic segmentation and instance segmentation. In CNN, limited by the receptive field, convolutional layers capture local features. In order to enrich context information, stack of convolutional layers of small kernel size are often used to increase the receptive field, but this is adequately efficient. However, attention mechanism is a simple and efficient way to enrich global context information.

3 Proposed Method

We use a two-stage detection model, DA_Det, for lesion detection of acute pancreatitis. With DA_ResNet we previously proposed for acute pancreatitis diagnosis the backbone to educe features to construct a feature pyramid network, we utilize two attention modules in detector neck after FPN. Both channel-wise and spatial attention are used in sequence for each level of features to facilitate focusing on the more informative features. Finally, we use a sparse prediction detector head as in Faster-RCNN. The whole model is shown in Fig. 7.

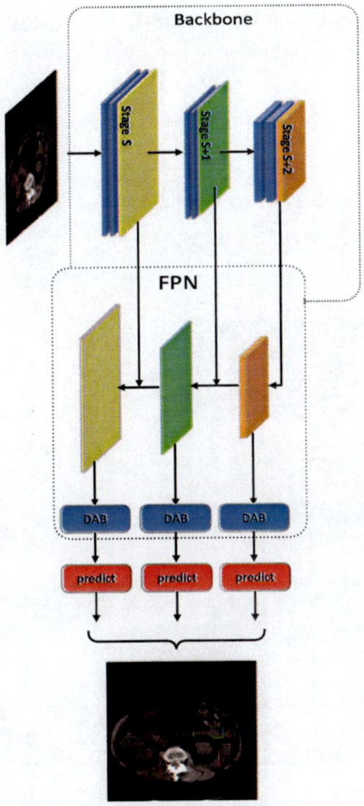

Fig. 7. Structure of DA_Det. (DAB for dual attention block)

We highlight all parts of the proposed model in details in following subsections.

3.1 Backbone

The DA_ResNet based on ResNet [33] utilizes spatial attention to focus on the more informative features and exploits global information of the features to produce weight for feature of each convolution stage to obtain local attention feature. Channel-wise attention is used to model channel interdependencies to improve performance. And finally, the prediction is made with fusion of all local attention features.

Multi-scale Spatial Attention. As seen in Fig. 8, L^s denotes the response after the sth convolution stage, and L_i^s denotes the response of L^s at spatial position *i*. $\boldsymbol{g}$ denotes the global feature which is the output before the final layer for classification. Then with a function $\mathcal{F}$ that evaluates the similarity of two tensors of the same channel, the similarity of L^s and $\boldsymbol{g}$ is defined as

$$\mathcal{F}\left(\widehat{\mathcal{L}}^s, \boldsymbol{g}\right) = \left\{\mathcal{F}\left(\widehat{\mathcal{L}}_i^s, \boldsymbol{g}\right)\right\}^i = \left\{c_i^s\right\}^i \tag{4}$$

where $\widehat{\mathcal{L}}^s$ is a tensor obtained by a mapping from l_i^s to $\boldsymbol{g}$. This mapping converts the number of tensor's channels and can be learned. And then the normalized similarity can be formulated as

$$a_i^s = \exp\left(c_i^s\right) / \sum\nolimits_j exp\left(c_j^s\right) \tag{5}$$

Then the local attention feature can be described as $\boldsymbol{g}_a^s = \mathcal{A}_i^s \otimes \mathcal{L}^s$. And the fusion of all local attention features is written as $\boldsymbol{g}_a = [g_a^{S1}, g_a^{S2}, \cdots, g_a^{Sm}]$.

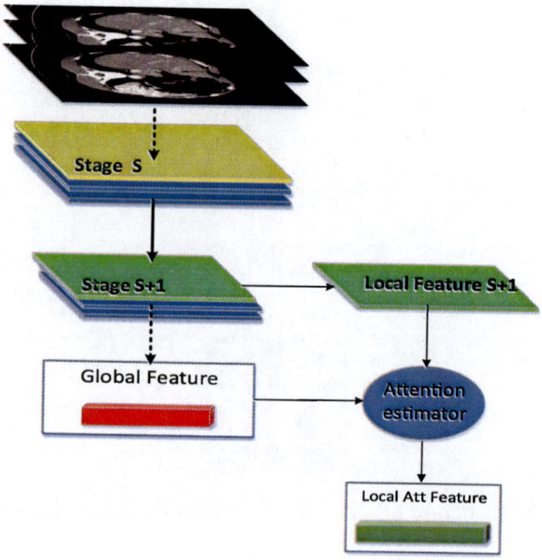

Fig. 8. Multi-scale spatial attention module

Here, without loss of generality, the similarity function we choose is, adding the two tensors element by element, the similarity is obtained through a learned linear mapping, calculated as $c_i^s = \langle u, \hat{l}_i^s + g \rangle$ where u is the learned mapping.

Channel-wise Attention. As shown in Fig. 9, inspired by SENet [34], it empathizes informative features and suppress useless ones by capturing explicit relationship between channels of convolution layers. Global average pooling is performed for each channel to ignore spatial information as

$$comp_c^s = \frac{1}{W \times H} \sum\nolimits_1^{\mathrm{H}} \sum\nolimits_1^{W} L_c^s(i, j) \tag{6}$$

Where L_c^s is the cth channel. Then we learn nonlinear interaction between channels through two fully connected layers as

$$sc = \sigma(\mathbf{W}_2 \delta(\mathbf{W}_1 comp^s)) \tag{7}$$

where $\mathbf{W}_1$ and $\mathbf{W}_2$ are the weights of the fully connected layers, respectively. The final output of each layer of the attention convolution is $\tilde{L}^s = sc \odot L^s$ where $\odot$ is a channel-wise multiplication.

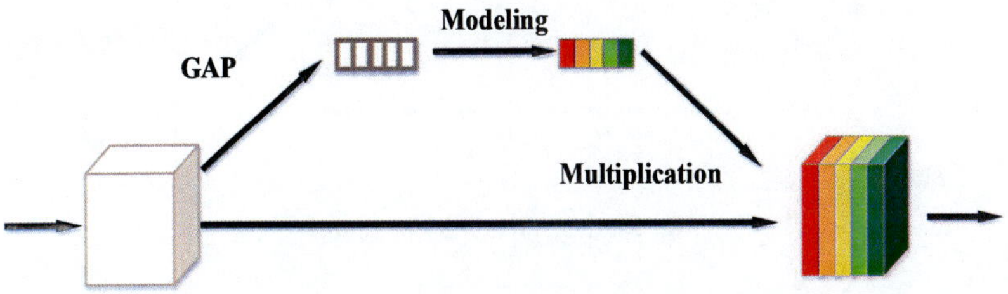

Fig. 9. Channel-wise attention module

3.2 Channel-Wise Attention

For a certain type of acute pancreatitis lesion, the corresponding response may only reside in some certain channels. An intuitive thought is to utilize channel-wise attention to adjust the weight of the channels. The module utilizes context information of the features to produce weight for each feature channel. The compression process is also by global average pooling, written as

$$\mathrm{F}_{ch}(L^s) = \mathcal{F}_{avg}(L_C^s) \tag{8}$$

Then feature map is excited by a 1×1 convolution layer as

$$scaler = \mathrm{F}_{ch}(L_C^s) * \mathbf{W}_{1\times 1} \tag{9}$$

where $\mathbf{W}_{1\times 1}$ is the parameters of convolution layer. Finally, the reweighted feature map can be described as $\tilde{L}^s = scaler \odot L^s$, where $\odot$ is a channel-wise multiplication.

3.3 Spatial Attention

The spatial attention module, as shown in Fig. 10, is after the channel-wise attention module It increases acute pancreatitis lesion response within features, which prompts the network to focus on the ROIs related to certain kind of acute pancreatitis lesion and reduce distraction. The compression process is also by global max pooling as

$$F_{sp}\left(L^{s}\right) = \mathcal{F}_{max}\left(L_{C}^{s}\right) \tag{10}$$

Then the activation process by a 3 × 3 convolution layer can be described as

$$scaler = \mathrm{F}_{sp}\left(L_{C}^{s}\right) * \mathbf{W}_{3\times 3} \tag{11}$$

where $\mathbf{W}_{3\times 3}$ denotes the parameters of convolution layer. Finally, the re-weighted feature map can be described as $\overline{L}^{s} = scaler \otimes L^{s}$ where ⊗ is a position-wise multiplication.

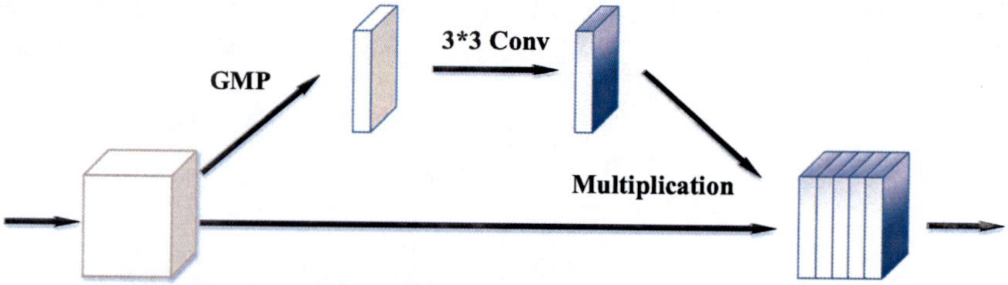

Fig. 10. Spatial attention module

4 Experiment

4.1 Dataset

The proposed method is evaluated on dataset collected by Affiliated Jinling Hospital, Medical School of Nanjing University. The dataset consists of 5045 CT slices collected from 45 patients admitted to the hospital who underwent CT imaging, of which 20 had infected pancreatic necrosis, 11 had acute necrotic collection (ANC), 10 had wall-off necrosis (WON) and the rest had pancreatic pseudocysts or hemorrhage. All images were reviewed by experienced specialists. Each patient was scanned from the top of the diaphragm to the anterior superior iliac spine. For each patient 25–50 consecutive axial CT images were selected, with slice thicknesses ranging from 6mm to 10mm and slice size of 512 pixel * 512 pixel. Number of lesions ranges from 1 to 4 in each slice. We finetune the network from a pre-trained model which is learnt on COCO dataset with extra data that is not used in later experiment.

Table 1. Performance comparison of the proposed network and the original one

Methods	AP (%)	$AP_{0.5}$(%)	$AP_{0.75}$(%)	AP_l (%)	AP_m (%)
ResNet + Faster RCNN	62.36	87.46	58.08	64.13	71.28
ResNet + Faster RCNN + DAB	65.31	**89.27**	61.95	68.08	71.64
DA_ResNet + Faster RCNN	64.03	88.08	64.78	65.23	72.49
DA_ResNet + Faster RCNN + DAB	**67.97**	88.66	**69.16**	**69.98**	**73.22**

4.2 Experiment Result

Mean average precision have been employed for the experimental comparative. As shown in Table 1, the backbone with dual attention improves performance, and so do the attentions utilized in detector neck.

4.3 Ablation Study

The dual attention module (denoted as DAB) utilized in detector neck includes spatial attention (denoted as SP) and channel-wise attention (denoted as CH). We test the performance improvement of different modules, with DA_ResNet as the backbone. The result is shown in Table 2. The spatial attention can bring about 0.9% improvement in mAP, and the channel-wise attention can bring about 2% performance improvement. The spatial attention is relatively insignificant compared with the channel-wise attention. We speculated that the FPN integrates features of different scales so that the spatial attention improvement is less apparent. The predictions of models with different configurations on the same image are shown in Fig. 11. The ground truth is shown in the first line, and below is the prediction results of 4 models under different configurations. It can be seen that the model without attention mechanism is misjudged near the large lesion.

Table 2. Performance comparison of different configurations with backbone DA_ResNet

Methods	mAP (%)	AP0.5(%)	$AP_{0.75}$(%)	AP_l (%)	AP_m (%)
origin	64.03	88.08	64.78	65.23	72.49
SP	64.96	88.96	62.43	65.07	70.73
CH	66.06	88.73	63.27	68.10	72.14
DAB	**67.97**	88.66	**69.16**	**69.98**	**73.22**

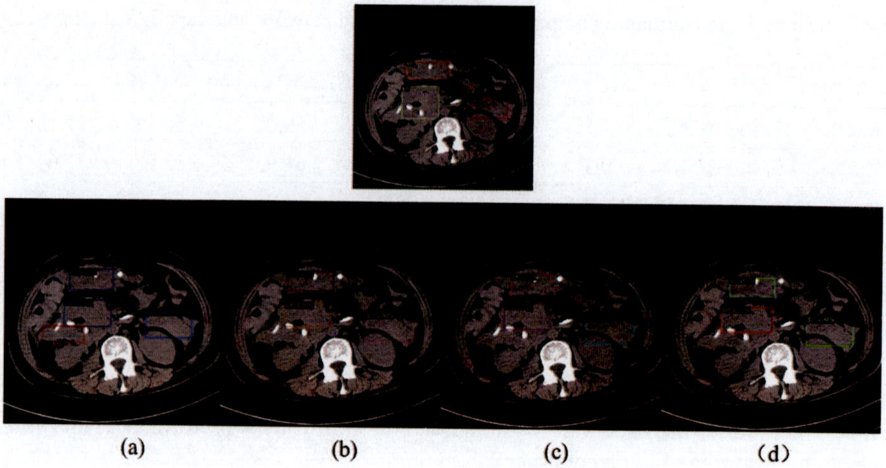

Fig. 11. Visual effect of attention mechanism in the proposed network. a: origin; b: SP; c: CH; d: DAB

5 Conclusion

Lesion detection for acute pancreatitis is never done before, and most of current detection architectures are not sufficiently robust to deal with scale variation of all kinds of acute pancreatitis lesions, resulting inaccurate results. We proposed DA_Det for acute pancreatitis lesion detection. It has been shown that attention mechanism in both backbone and neck facilitates learning more discriminative information. Compared to the original Faster RCNN, the proposed network obtains more accurate detection results and has less false positive result.

References

1. Tuennemann, J., Mössner, J., Beer, S.: Der Internist **55**(9), 1045–1056 (2014). https://doi.org/10.1007/s00108-014-3580-0
2. Banks, P.A., Freeman, M.L.: Practice guidelines in acute pancreatitis. Am J Gastroenterol **101**(10), 2379–2400 (2006)
3. Besselink, M., Santvoort, H., Freeman, M.: IAP/APA evidence-based guidelines for the management of acute pancreatitis. Pancreatology 13(4, suppl 2), E1-E15 (2013)
4. Knaus, W.A., et al.: APACHE II: a severity of disease classification system. Crit. Care Med. **13**(10), 818–829 (1985)
5. Balthazar, E.J., Robinson, D.L., et al.: Acute pancreatitis: value of CT in establishing prognosis. Radiology **174**(2), 331–336 (1990)
6. Mortele, K.J., Wiesner, W., Intriere, L.: A modified CT severity index for evaluating acute pancreatitis: improved correlation with patient outcome. AJR Am J Roentgenol **183**(5), 1261–1265 (2004)
7. Farag, A., et al.: A bottom-up approach for pancreas segmentation using cascaded superpixels and (deep) image patch labeling. IEEE Trans. Image Process. **26**(1), 386–399 (2017)

8. Roth, H.R., et al.: DeepOrgan: Multi-level Deep Convolutional Networks for Automated Pancreas Segmentation. In: Navab, N., Hornegger, J., Wells, W.M., Frangi, A.F. (eds.) MICCAI 2015. LNCS, vol. 9349, pp. 556–564. Springer, Cham (2015). https://doi.org/10.1007/978-3-319-24553-9_68
9. Cai, J., Lu, L., Zhang, Z., Xing, F., Yang, L., Yin, Q.: Pancreas Segmentation in MRI Using Graph-Based Decision Fusion on Convolutional Neural Networks. In: Ourselin, S., Joskowicz, L., Sabuncu, M.R., Unal, G., Wells, W. (eds.) MICCAI 2016. LNCS, vol. 9901, pp. 442–450. Springer, Cham (2016). https://doi.org/10.1007/978-3-319-46723-8_51
10. Roth, H.R., Lu, L., Farag, A., Sohn, A., Summers, R.M.: Spatial Aggregation of Holistically-Nested Networks for Automated Pancreas Segmentation. In: Ourselin, S., Joskowicz, L., Sabuncu, M.R., Unal, G., Wells, W. (eds.) MICCAI 2016. LNCS, vol. 9901, pp. 451–459. Springer, Cham (2016). https://doi.org/10.1007/978-3-319-46723-8_52
11. Redmon, J., Divvala, S., Girshick, R., et al.: You only look once: unified, real-time object detection. In: Proceedings of 2016 IEEE Conference on Computer Vision and Pattern Recognition (CVPR), pp. 779–788. IEEE, Las Vegas (2016)
12. Liu, W., et al.: SSD: Single Shot MultiBox Detector. In: Leibe, B., Matas, J., Sebe, N., Welling, M. (eds.) ECCV 2016. LNCS, vol. 9905, pp. 21–37. Springer, Cham (2016). https://doi.org/10.1007/978-3-319-46448-0_2
13. Ren, S., He, K., Girshick, R., et al.: Faster r-cnn: Towards real-time object detection with region proposal networks. IEEE Trans. Pattern Anal. Mach. Intell. **39**(6), 1137–1149 (2016)
14. Lin, T.Y., Dollár, P., Girshick, R., et al.: Feature pyramid networks for object detection. In: Proceedings of the 2017 IEEE Conference on Computer Vision and Pattern Recognition (CVPR), pp. 936–944. IEEE, Honolulu (2017)
15. Bochkovskiy, A., Wang, C.Y., Liao, H.Y.M.: YOLOv4: optimal Speed and Accuracy of Object Detection. arXiv preprint arXiv:2004.10934 (2020)
16. Girshick, R., Donahue, J., Darrell, T., et al.: Rich feature hierarchies for accurate object detection and semantic segmentation. In: Proceedings of the 2014 IEEE conference on Computer Vision and Pattern Recognition (CVPR), pp. 580–587. IEEE, Columbus (2014)
17. He, K., Zhang, X., Ren, S., et al.: Spatial pyramid pooling in deep convolutional networks for visual recognition. IEEE Trans. Pattern Anal. Mach. Intell. **37**(9), 1904–1916 (2015)
18. Girshick, R. Fast r-cnn. In: Proceedings of the IEEE International Conference on Computer Vision (ICCV), pp. 1440–1448. IEEE, Santiago (2015)
19. Vaswani, A., Shazeer, N., Parmar, N., et al.: Attention is all you need. Adv. Neural. Inf. Process. Syst. **30**, 5998–6008 (2017)
20. Hu, H., Gu, J., Zhang, Z., et al.: Relation networks for object detection. In: Proceedings of the 2018 IEEE Conference on Computer Vision and Pattern Recognition (CVPR), pp. 3588–3597. IEEE, Salt Lake City (2018)
21. Wang, X., Girshick, R., Gupta, A., et al.: Non-local neural networks. In: Proceedings of the 2018 IEEE Conference on Computer Vision and Pattern Recognition (CVPR), pp. 7794–7803. IEEE, Salt Lake City (2018)
22. Gu, J., Hu, H., Wang, L., Wei, Y., Dai, J.: Learning Region Features for Object Detection. In: Ferrari, V., Hebert, M., Sminchisescu, C., Weiss, Y. (eds.) ECCV 2018. LNCS, vol. 11216, pp. 392–406. Springer, Cham (2018). https://doi.org/10.1007/978-3-030-01258-8_24
23. Huang, Z., Wang, X., Huang, L., et al.: Ccnet: criss-cross attention for semantic segmentation. In: Proceedings of the 2019 IEEE International Conference on Computer Vision (ICCV), pp. 603–612. IEEE, Seoul (2019)
24. Zhao, H., et al.: PSANet: Point-wise Spatial Attention Network for Scene Parsing. In: Ferrari, V., Hebert, M., Sminchisescu, C., Weiss, Y. (eds.) ECCV 2018. LNCS, vol. 11213, pp. 270–286. Springer, Cham (2018). https://doi.org/10.1007/978-3-030-01240-3_17

25. Fu, J., Liu, J., Tian, H., et al.: Dual attention network for scene segmentation. In: Proceedings of the 2019 IEEE Conference on Computer Vision and Pattern Recognition (CVPR), pp. 3146–3154. IEEE, Long Beach (2019)
26. Guo, H., Zheng, K., Fan, X., et al.: Visual attention consistency under image transforms for multi-label image classification. In: Proceedings of the 2019 IEEE Conference on Computer Vision and Pattern Recognition (CVPR), pp. 729–739. IEEE, Long Beach (2019)
27. Choe, J., Shim, H.: Attention-based dropout layer for weakly supervised object localization. In: Proceedings of the 2019 IEEE Conference on Computer Vision and Pattern Recognition (CVPR), pp. 2219–2228. IEEE, Long Beach (2019)
28. Zheng, H., Fu, J., Zha, Z.J., et al.: Looking for the devil in the details: Learning trilinear attention sampling network for fine-grained image recognition. In: Proceedings of the 2019 IEEE Conference on Computer Vision and Pattern Recognition (CVPR), pp. 5012–5021. IEEE, Long Beach (2019)
29. Zhang, H., Goodfellow, I., Metaxas, D., et al.: Self-attention generative adversarial networks. In: International Conference on Machine Learning, pp. 7354–7363. PMLR (2019)
30. Xu, T., Zhang, P., Huang, Q., et al.: Attngan: Fine-grained text to image generation with attentional generative adversarial networks. In: Proceedings of the 2018 IEEE Conference on Computer Vision and Pattern Recognition (CVPR), pp. 1316–1324. IEEE, Salt Lake City (2018)
31. Lu, X., Wang, W., Ma, C., et al.: See more, know more: Unsupervised video object segmentation with co-attention Siamese networks. In: Proceedings of the 2019 IEEE Conference on Computer Vision and Pattern Recognition (CVPR), pp. 3623–3632. IEEE, Long Beach (2019)
32. Ye, L., Rochan, M., Liu, Z., et al.: Cross-modal self-attention network for referring image segmentation. In: Proceedings of the 2018 IEEE International Conference on Computer Vision (CVPR), pp. 10502–10511. Salt Lake City (2018)
33. He, K., Zhang, X., Ren, S., et al.: Deep residual learning for image recognition. In: Proceedings of the 2016 IEEE Conference on Computer Vision and Pattern Recognition (CVPR), pp. 770–778. IEEE, Las Vegas (2016)
34. Hu, J., Shen, L., Sun, G.: Squeeze-and-excitation networks. In: Proceedings of the 2018 IEEE Conference on Computer Vision and Pattern Recognition (CVPR), pp. 7132–7141. IEEE, Salt Lake City (2018)

Measurement of Q Factor from Two Dimensional Images of Osteoarthritic Knee Braces

Chetana Krishnan, Sasya Subramanyam Vishnuvazzla, and S. Pravin Kumar(✉)

Sri Sivasubramaniya Nadar College of Engineering, Kalavakkam, Chennai, India
chetana1808@bme.ssn.edu.in, pravinkumars@ssn.edu.in

Abstract. Osteoarthritis is one of the common joint arthritis that occurs due to the inflammation of cushion endings of the bone and cartilage wearing. The condition affects millions of people each year in India especially among the age groups above 55. Compared to other curatives, knee braces are mostly preferred as they have many advantages. Knee braces come with a lot of different designs and functionality which are discussed in this paper. 2D images of the brace will not be sufficient for the quantitative analysis. In order to analyze the image in rotational motion, there is a need for the conversion to 3D models and finite element mesh (FEM) generation. FEM analysis is one of the most widely used methods for calculating the load and energy distributions of a knee brace. The proposed paper compares different braces in terms of Q factor using ordinary differential equations and Gaussian curves. The curve gives the details about the suspension levels of the brace when integrated with the joint and concludes the objective analysis of the knee brace. The Q Factor jointly determines the loading and unloading distribution of knee brace without the need for individual analysis which makes the process simpler and easier.

Keywords: Q factor · Triangulated mesh · Osteoarthritis

1 Introduction

Osteoarthritis (OA) is assessed into four stages depending on the amount of cartilage wear and the amount of pain caused due to inflammation. Though radiographic images do not help in visualizing cartilage wear, it helps in determining the joint space width between the thigh and the shin bone (Fig. 1).

1.1 Types of Braces [3, 4]

Prophylactic braces protect the joint from injury, usually when sports are played. They are used to reduce the valgus and varus stress in the case of OA. Upon wearing the brace, they provide moderate subjective movement that flexes up to 35°. Cork screw knee braces are one of the best examples of prophylactic braces where they provide soft cushion-based protection when athlete crash happens.

R. Su et al. (Eds.): MICAD 2021, LNEE 784, pp. 251–259, 2022.
https://doi.org/10.1007/978-981-16-3880-0_26

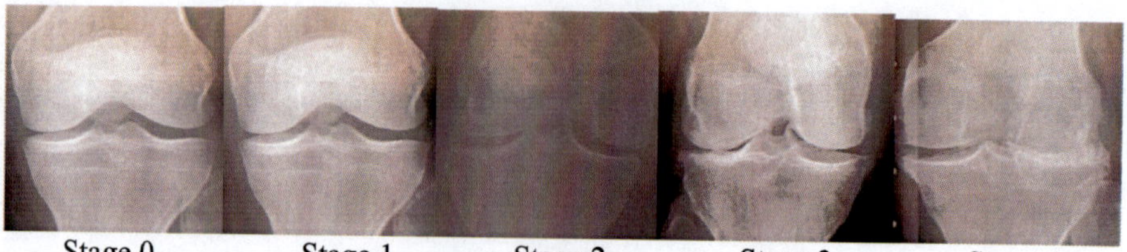

Fig. 1. Radiographic images indicating different stages of OA

Functional or supportive braces support the joint when there is an injured joint. They stabilize the knee through rotational and anteroposterior forces. The force distribution across the joint is balanced by a linkage mechanism at the specific clamping point located a few inches away from the joint. Functional knee braces resemble cast made of fibers to avoid joint cracks.

Rehabilitative braces help in limiting the extensor and flexor movements of a joint, giving significant time for the joint to heal. There are mainly used to keep up the join to a position post-surgery to avoid external disturbances and stress. Their main function is to compensate for the original functionality of the knee before the injury. These braces provide only limited extension movement to avoid frequent knee instabilities. Rehabilitative braces resemble external splints with linear angle to promote stiffness of the knee.

Unloader or off loader braces are the recommended knee braces for patients with osteoarthritis. They help in transferring the stress from the affected area to the healthier area to reduce pain and inflammation. However, since these braces are custom-designed, it is important to consider the skin properties and walking habits of the user. Some of the examples of unloader braces are quantum style (provides friction in four rotational dimensions), free style (provides friction in positions where maximum stress is applied by the user), linear style (provides friction in the strap or clamped region) and linkage style (offloaded the pressure by linkage mechanism).

1.2 Finite Element Method

The Finite element method is the procedure of analyzing the 3D models in the form of their surface mesh for loading and energy distribution calculation by applying certain boundary conditions. However, they provide only subjective and Qualitative analysis. FEM is only possible to calculate:

- Calculate points in the stress-strain curve
- Find out the force constants to know the design's maximum volatility (Table 1).

Table 1. FEM vs proposed method [3]

FEM limits	Proposed solution
A large amount of data is required as input for the mesh used in terms of nodal connectivity and other parameters depending on the problem	A single mesh as a whole is enough to analyze the whole design instead of large surface points
It requires a digital computer and fairly extensive	A free MATLAB version can be used
It requires a longer execution time compared with FEM	A single code run can produce results for up to 3000 trials
The output results will vary considerably	The result comes with RMSE oriented constants and hence provides reliable output
Only loading properties are determined, unloading properties are not considered	Loading and unloading characteristics are plotted as a hysteresis plot
Subjective factors are only considered	Objective factors like suspension and reserve capacity are considered

2 Proposed Solution

2.1 System Architecture

The proposed solution follows a sequence of operations to be followed to achieve the given output which are divided into two architectural points as shown in Fig. 2. The detailed steps that are followed in the prerequisite region starting from Hill's constants determination to mesh generation are described in analysis 1 and the steps followed for conducting the analysis and comparison are described in analysis 2 of system architecture.

2.2 Equations Involved in Analysis

Hill and Limerick were the firsts to model the design mesh using ordinary differential equations [2]. By solving these equations, we can calculate the FEM parameters for a given surface mesh. Limerick's equations were used for low-level models with few surface points and Hill's equations is an advanced version equation whose compatibility can be extended to all types of braces ranging from about 1900 to 5000 surface points. The equations supporting this theory are

$$F = kx + \eta \text{v}$$

$$RMSE = \left(\sum |Fi, model - Fi, average|\right)^{1/2}$$

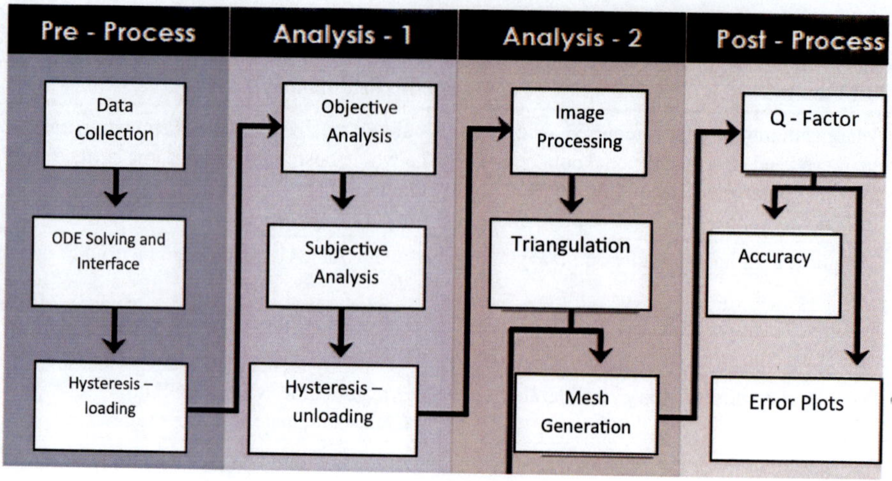

Fig. 2. System architecture 1

By solving the above equations, we get Hill's constants. In the below equation, the RE and WE are complements of A and B (Hill's constants). The density of the surface mesh is pre imported using a range of values and MATLAB chooses the right one during run time [5, 6]

$$RE = \rho.\ \mu.d/\mu$$

$$WE = \rho.\ \mu.\mu.d/\sigma$$

To determine the accuracy of interfaced Hill's parameters with the brace meshes, a regression plot was made using the standard brace load values (Fig. 3). The corresponding ANOVA table was plotted to find out the number of points not following the fixed-line [7].

Real-time data can be fed the MATLAB GUI and compile-time comparison between various 3D meshes can be done using this algorithm. The proposed idea uses a one-way ANOVA mechanism (compares measure with standard). Two-way ANOVA mechanisms are used when unsupervised learning algorithms are used (Compare and Calibrate).

2.3 Generating Models from 2D Mesh

Android offers mobile version AUTOCAD and other 3d Modeling software where 2D images can be imported or drawn using sketches and converted into 3D models. The principle behind the conversion is the use of triangulation which considers each matrix point in the 2D image and plots them in 3D coordinates [1]. The same can be achieved through MATLAB. The triangulated model can also be converted into a four-dimensional model using tetrahedron features. This feature is mainly used when the model is analyzed for any internal cracks or defects. The empty lattices in the 3D plot are zero-padded to achieve conversion accuracy. These 3D models are later converted into meshes using

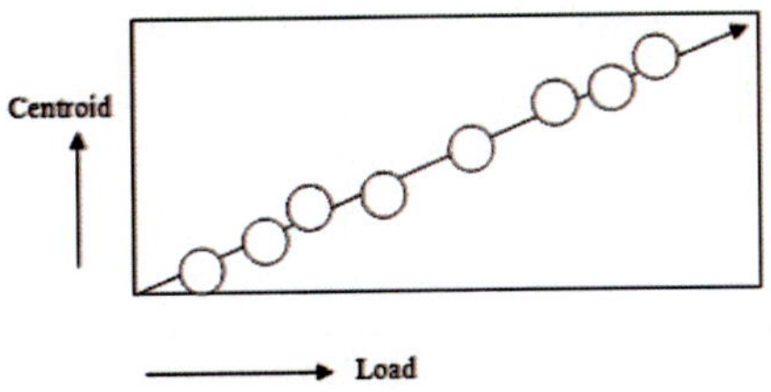

Fig. 3. Regression plot. All the points (indicated by crosses) lie on the fixed-line. This proves that Hill's models can be as accurate as FEM analysis. X axis indicates load distribution and Y axis indicates Centroid

online SimScale Software. This method allows easy modeling of 3D designs and their conversions. Given below is a sample example. Figure 4 shows the Triangulated 3D plot where the coordinates of the plot represent the 2D matrix points. The surface lattice of the figure (surface plane) is contained with lower and upper triangles of the diagonal elements in the 2D image matrix. The 2D discrete image matrix points and its corresponding 3D triangulation matrix is displayed in Fig. 4 (Tables 2 and 3).

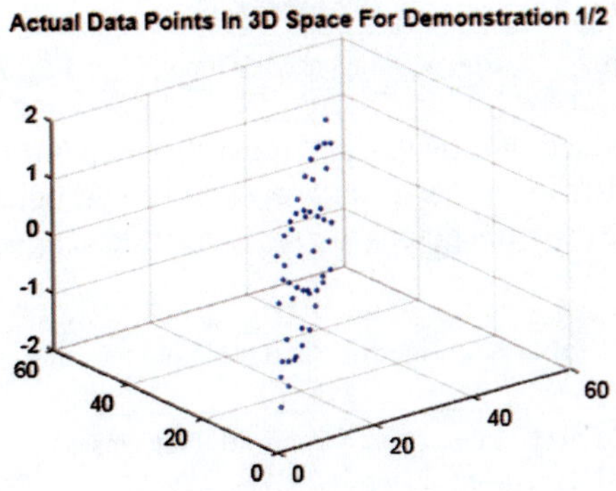

Fig. 4. Triangulation 3D plot

Table 2. 2D input matrix.

2.5	8
6.5	8
2.5	5
6.5	5
1.0	6.5
8.0	6.6

$$O = \left[1\ 2.5\ 5.0\ 2.5\ 8\right]$$

Table 3. Connectivity matrix

5	3	1
3	2	1
3	4	2
4	6	2

This matrix is the output matrix called the triangulated matrix. Figures 5, 6 and 7 show the 2D sketch, 3D model and converted 3D mesh, respectively.

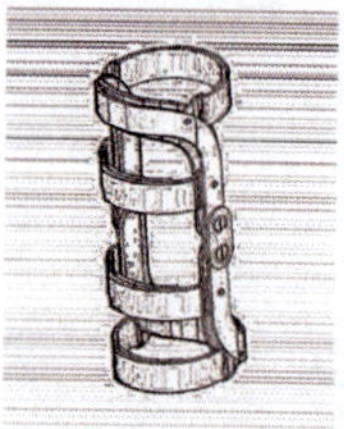

Fig. 5. 2D sketch

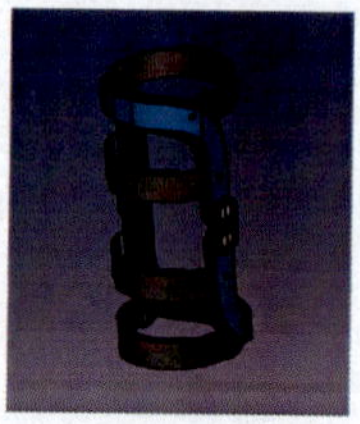

Fig. 6. Converted 3D model

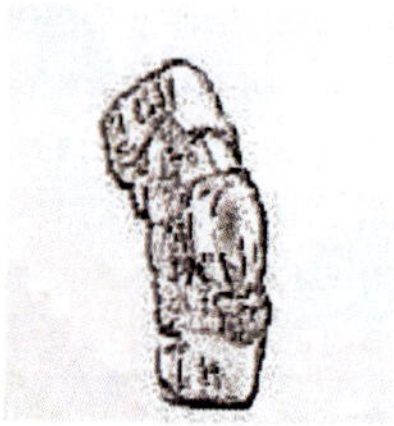

Fig. 7. Converted 3D mesh

The analysis is divided into two steps. In the first step, 10 Different meshes from different brace types [10] are chosen and are operated on the equations to determine the parameters and plot the gaussian graphs to determine its loading and unloading features.

Table 4. Suspension and force points value

Blob	Fmax N	Fflex Deg	Fext Deg	Centroid	Suspension %	Eff/Aff No unit
1	2693	18.6	32.5	0.1	73	235
2	1899	17.4	56.6	0.3	74	243
3	2725	19..2	34.7	0.7	71	90
4	1840	12.8	25.8	0.1	75	105
5	2796	19.1	45.7	0.1	65.8	263
6	2564	18.9	34.6	0.2	69	241
7	2648	17.6	43.5	0.67	74	114

It is clear from Table 4 that sample 4 has lower Fmax values compared to other samples. The threshold values for a good brace depend on the person's muscle and joint properties [8, 9]. For analysis purposes, we have considered the mannequin datasets. The top 6 samples that show similarity with the threshold values are taken for the next step analysis where around 3000 trials are conducted on a single run and the error of the model is determined. The loading and unloading parameters of the braces are plotted using Gaussian curves (Fig. 8). The peak value of each curve determines the maximum load point beyond which any mobility events in the brace will lead to unloading (Table 5).

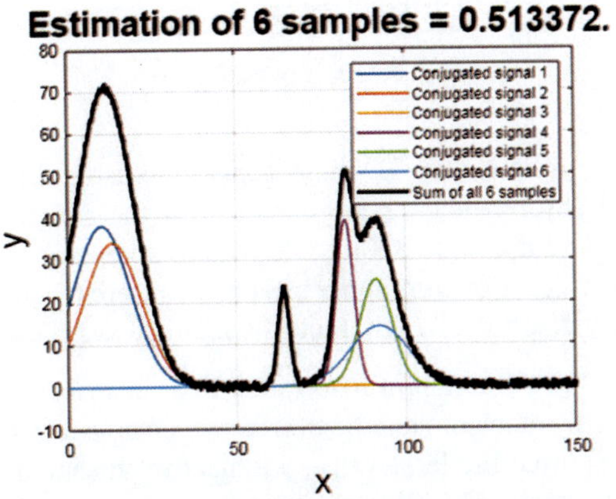

Fig. 8. Gaussian - loading and unloading parameters [X axis indicates pixel strength; Y axis indicates peak parameters. The estimated value indicates the combined RMSE value of the entire sample considered]

Table 5. Command window output

Beginning to run lipo3.m			
Sample	Suspension	Reserve capacity	Q factor
1	17.0	3.0	13.0
2	24.0	63.0	8.0
3	10.0	75.0	6.0
4	40.0	11.00	81.0
5	26.0	82.0	5.0
6	34.0	92.0	12.0

**Q factor: Q factor is a combined term used for the properties of brace which includes objective and subjective properties. Involving the Q factor reduces execution and analysis time [12]. **

3 Discussion

The FEM method and the proposed idea was compared in terms of execution time and boundary conditions. 3D models were generated from 2D images using triangulation and

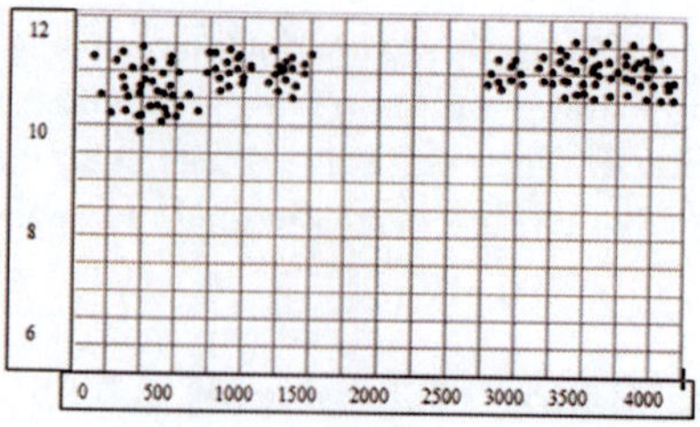

Fig. 9. Error plot of model

tetrahedron principles followed by 3D mesh generation using Simscale. The proposed method did not use any boundary conditions to test the samples and the execution time was around 0.24 s for around 3000 trials. The triangulation method provides easy generation of meshes. Types of commonly used braces were taken as samples and were compared objectively in terms of 2 Parameters which are as follows.

Subjective: This includes maximum load/force (Load distribution that the brace provides around the joint), extension, and flexion angles (Angle improvement in users). In this case, sample 4 showed the least values. Subjective threshold values depend from brace to brace. For example, rehabilitation braces require low values as they need low mobility whereas an unloader brace needs higher extension and flexion values.

Objective: This includes Suspension level (Extend up to which the brace interfaces with the human body), reserve capacity (Minimum customized load barrier parameter of brace), Q factor (Combined parameter combination), and centroid (Hysteresis peak value). In this case, linkage-based braces show poor to medial objective accuracy which is mainly unloader braces.

An accuracy model was plotted for 3000 trials and the number of errors was negligible compared to the number of trials conducted. The error plot in Fig. 9 shows sparse error distributions. This is because the proposed idea considers a different Hill's constant every time the code runs. The time taken for the compiler to shift from one constant to another is plotted as an error. This process is called Multi Phasing [13]. However, the regression plot adds up additional accuracy data making the proposed idea efficient and reliable. Since the whole methodology uses online versions of software, they are cost-effective [11].

References

1. Dessery, Y., Belzile, E.L., Turmel, S., Corbeil, P.: Comparison of three knee braces in the treatment of medial knee osteoarthritis. Knee **21**, 1107–1114 (2014)
2. Duivenvoorden, T., Brouwer, R.W., van Raaij, T.M., Verhagen, A.P., Verhaar, J.A.N., Bierma-Zeinstra, S.M.A.: Braces and orthoses for treating osteoarthritis of the knee. Cochrane Database Syst. Rev. **2015**(3). Accessed 02 Aug 2021. https://doi.org/10.1002/14651858
3. Khosravi, M., Arazpour, M., Vaziri, A.S.: An evaluation of the use of a lateral wedged insole and a valgus knee brace in combination in subjects with medial compartment knee osteoarthritis (OA). Assist Technol. **33**(2), 87–94 (2021). https://doi.org/10.1080/10400435.2019.1595788

4. Richards, J.D., Sanchez-Ballester, J., Jones, R.K., Darke, N., Livingstone, B.N.: A comparison of knee braces during walking for the treatment of osteoarthritis of the medial compartment of the knee. J. Bone Jt. Surg. **87-B**(7)
5. Miller, R.H.: Hill-based muscle modeling. In: Müller, B., et al. (eds.) Handbook of Human Motion, pp. 1–22. Springer, Cham (2018). https://doi.org/10.1007/978-3-319-30808-1_203-2
6. Romero, F., Alonso, F.J.: A comparison among different Hill-type contraction dynamics formulations for muscle force estimation. Mech. Sci. **7**, 19–29 (2016)
7. Lichtwark, G.A., Wilson, A.M.: Is Achilles tendon compliance optimised for maximum muscle efficiency in locomotion? J. Biomech. **40**, 1768–1775 (2007)
8. Johnson, F., Leitl, S., Waugh, W.: The distribution of load across the knee. A comparison of static and dynamic measurements. J. Bone Joint Surg. Br. **62**, 346–349 (1980)
9. Schipplein, O., Andriacchi, T.P.: Interaction between active and passive knee stabilizers during level walking. J. Orthop. Res. **9**, 113–119 (1991)
10. Pollo, F.E., Otis, J.C., Backus, S.I., Warren, R.F., Wickiewicz, T.L.: Reduction of medial compartment loads with valgus bracing of the osteoarthritic knee. Am. J. Sports Med. **30**(3), 414–421 (2002)
11. Kutzner, I., Küther, S., Heinlein, B., Dymke, J., Bender, A., Halder, A.M., et al.: The effect of valgus braces on medial compartment load of the knee joint—in vivo load measurements in three subjects. J. Biomech. **44**(7), 1354–1360 (2011)
12. Palladino, J.L.: Functional requirements of a mathematical model of muscle contraction. In: 2019 41st Annual International Conference of the IEEE Engineering in Medicine and Biology Society (EMBC) (2019)
13. Kim, Y., Hori, Y.: Muscle group activation estimation in the human leg during gait using recursive least squares embodying Hill's muscle model. In: 5th IEEE RAS/EMBS International Conference on Biomedical Robotics and Biomechatronics (2014)

Machine Learning and Deep Learning

2Be3-Net: Combining 2D and 3D Convolutional Neural Networks for 3D PET Scans Predictions

Ronan Thomas[1](✉), Elsa Schalck[1], Damien Fourure[2], Antoine Bonnefoy[1], and Inaki Cervera-Marzal[1]

[1] Eura Nova, Marseille, France
{ronan.thomas,inaki.cerveramarzal}@euranova.eu
[2] Eura Nova, Mont-Saint-Guibert, Belgium

Abstract. Radiomics - high-dimensional features extracted from clinical images - is the main approach used to develop predictive models based on 3D Positron Emission Tomography (PET) scans of patients suffering from cancer. Radiomics extraction relies on an accurate segmentation of the tumoral region, which is a time consuming task subject to inter-observer variability. On the other hand, data driven approaches such as deep convolutional neural networks (CNN) struggle to achieve great performances on PET images due to the absence of available large PET datasets combined to the size of 3D networks. In this paper, we assemble several public datasets to create a PET dataset large of 2800 scans and propose a deep learning architecture named "2Be3-Net" associating a 2D feature extractor to a 3D CNN predictor. First, we take advantage of a 2D pre-trained model to extract feature maps out of 2D PET slices. Then we apply a 3D CNN on top of the concatenation of the previously extracted feature maps to compute patient-wise predictions. Experiments suggest that 2Be3-Net has an improved ability to exploit spatial information compared to 2D or 3D-only CNN solutions. We also evaluate our network on the prediction of clinical outcomes of head-and-neck cancer. The proposed pipeline outperforms PET radiomics approaches on the prediction of loco-regional recurrences and overall survival. Innovative deep learning architectures combining a pre-trained network with a 3D CNN could therefore be a great alternative to traditional CNN and radiomics approaches while empowering small and medium sized datasets.

Keywords: Deep learning architecture · 2D and 3D convolutional neural network · PET

1 Introduction

18 F-fluorodeoxyglucose (FDG) in positron emission tomography (PET) enables to highlight areas with high glucose metabolism, which is characteristic of tumor cells. PET is often associated with computerized tomography (CT) in a PET-CT exam, a hybrid imaging modality that allows to correlate metabolic and anatomic information to improve lesion localisation and characterisation. PET-CT is a useful tool for diagnosis,

R. Su et al. (Eds.): MICAD 2021, LNEE 784, pp. 263–271, 2022.
https://doi.org/10.1007/978-981-16-3880-0_27

prognosis, staging or re-staging of patients affected by cancer, and has been widely used in many studies [1–3].

Two main approaches are generally considered to exploit these 3D images. A first approach consists in the extraction of radiomics [4], defined as high-dimensional imaging features extracted from a segmented region of interest (ROI): the tumor. Radiomics features allow to quantitatively describe a tumor and can be divided into 4 groups: tumor shape, intensity, texture, and statistical features extracted after applying filters or mathematical transformations to the image. Radiomics can lead to the discovery of new quantitative bio-markers. Standardized Uptake Value (SUV) is a common metric describing tumor uptake normalized to the injected dose of FDG and patient's body weight. SUV is used in clinical routine and is a precious indicator to differentiate benign from malignant tumors and provides important prognostic and diagnostic information [5–8]. Several studies [9–11] illustrate the interest of using radiomics for applications such as prognosis, non-invasive disease tracking, treatment response or clinical outcome prediction tasks. Despite their good performances, radiomics robustness and replicability is questioned [12]. One of the most limiting points is linked to the difficulty of producing standardised images prior to radiomic extraction. In addition, tumor segmentation, a requirement for radiomics extraction, remains a complicated task. This step, either done manually or by a semi-automatic algorithm, introduces biases and raises several issues related to the experience reproducibility, its consistency and therefore hinders their deployment in clinical routine.

The second main approach consists in the use of convolutional neural networks that recently demonstrated great performances on vision tasks such as image classification, semantic segmentation or object detection. A major contribution to this success relies on the massive amount of training data with detailed and accurate annotations. Natural images models often rely on a transfer from large datasets such as the ImageNet dataset [13]. However, due to data sensitivity, it remains extremely challenging to build large datasets in the medical imaging domain. As a consequence, no large PET dataset has been made available so far.

Different CNN methods were applied on PET images. Because of the 3D nature of PET images, 3D CNN are logic architectures fitting PET scans dimensionality. However, the use of 3D convolutions implies an increased number of parameters and therefore requires large sets to be trained, where a training example corresponds to a scan. The limited size of PET datasets increases 3D CNN tendency to overfitting and degrades their performances. Studies applying 3D CNN on PET images therefore rely on consequent data augmentation to improve their model robustness [14, 15]. Other solutions reformulated the problem in 2D enabling the exploitation of pre-trained models or the use of lighter 2D CNN [16–18]. However, using 2D models also implies losing rich 3D spatial information, which results in sub-optimal performances. Some publications [19–21] illustrated that pre-training some of the network layers can help to accelerate training, convergence speed and increase the accuracy of the target model. Zhou [22] trained a shared 3D encoder associated with 8 decoding branches to segment different organs. Then they used the encoder as a backbone architecture to the classification of pulmonary nodules. Clark [23] trained several auto encoders (AE), each specific to an image modality (MRI, CT, X-ray). Training was done through image restoration which allowed the AEs to learn on unlabeled data specific information in the image such as appearance, texture or context. They transferred the learned AE on several tasks as brain tumor segmentation or nodule classification and illustrated an improvement in performances. They also demonstrated that their 3D models outperform their 2D versions, confirming the importance of 3D spatial information.

As illustrated by these recent works, traditional CNN approaches either 2D or 3D have both advantages and inconveniences. We decided to take advantage of their assets by combining a 2D pre-trained feature extractor with a predictive model such as a 3D CNN. Such a combination hasn't been studied much yet and could result in a more stable network than a complete 3D CNN. Moreover, we justify the use of a 2D pre-trained network by the information learned on millions of images, where an equivalent training from scratch on a PET dataset would not have been possible. The contributions of this work are summarized as follows:

- We introduce an innovative deep neural network entitled "2Be3-Net" combining a 2D pre-trained model to a 3D CNN
- We illustrated through predicting patient gender that the proposed pipeline integrates an increased ability to exploit spatial information compared to traditional CNN
- We evaluated the proposed architecture on the prediction of several clinical outcomes of the head-neck cancer and illustrated that it achieves superior performances on two out of the three tasks compared to PET radiomics.

2 Method

We propose an architecture entitled "2Be3-Net", described in Fig. 1, that enables exploitation of raw 3D PET scans by associating a 2D feature extractor to a 3D CNN predictor. K randomly (but ordered) slices are sampled out of the 3D PET image to form a batch of k 2D input images. A 2D feature extractor is applied on each slice independently, resulting in k groups of 2D features maps. A concatenation layer is used to create one group of 3D features maps that are fed to a 3D classifier to get the final prediction.

The feature extractor is a pre-trained 2D model that extracts feature maps out of 2D PET slices. We choose to use a ResNet-50 [24] pre-trained on the ImageNet dataset [13]. As the network is trained with 3 channels RGB images, we transform each PET slice into a gray scale image with 3 channels. Deep neural networks are known to learn hierarchical features, going from textural features in the network first layers to semantic features in the last layers. We believe that the textural features learned by an ImageNet pretrained network are useful for PET scan images but that the gap between PET scans and natural images is too high for the semantic features to be useful. Knowing that, we decided to keep only the 5 first layers of the pretrained network and, because of our small amount of data, decided to freeze these layers instead of finetuning them.

We concatenate the feature maps extracted from each slice and apply a predictive model, whose objective is to correlate the spatial and metabolic available information to compute patient-wise predictions. The predictive model is a typical framework of a CNN that applies three 3D convolutional blocks to reduce feature map size, followed by fully connected (FC) layers to realize the prediction.

PET scans have variable resolutions and numbers of slices. We considered these constraints as opportunities to do data augmentation. We randomly select a fixed number of slices and crop them. Random slice selection ensures that the network can't rely on specific slices in the scan, which further increases its robustness, while cropping decreases the size of the feature maps outputted by the feature extractor.

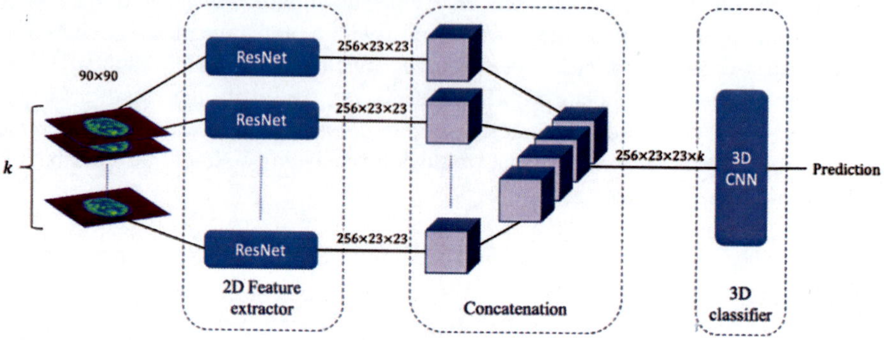

Fig. 1. 2Be3-Net global pipeline

3 Experiments

3.1 Experimental Setup

Studies applying CNN models on medical images often train and evaluate their models on small datasets. In this work, we collected and assembled 10 public datasets available in The Cancer Imaging Archive [25–35]. These datasets contain images from different modalities, pathologies and centers, which implies a large variety of data characteristics, spatial resolution, range of pixel intensities and acquisition protocols. We selected PET with attenuated correction (AC) scans and normalized raw pixel values to SUV scale using the definition[1] provided by the Quantitative Imaging Biomarkers Alliance (QIBA). Scans containing SUV outliers were dropped before conversion to NIFTI format, resulting in a PET dataset containing 2834 scans. We split this dataset in two to create two sub-datasets for specific tasks: gender and clinical outcomes prediction (loco-regional recurrences (LR), distant metastases (DM) and overall survival (OS)). The clinical outcomes dataset is included in the gender dataset, but no overlapping exists between the validation set of the clinical outcomes dataset and the gender training set.

The number of input slices is set to k = 66 as it corresponds to the number of slices of the smallest scan. We also chose a resolution of 90 × 90 pixels per slice. To match this resolution, we crop the slices at their center. Finally, we apply random flip and rotation (−10°, +10°) as data augmentation. Models were implemented in Python 3.7 and Pytorch 1.6 [36]. Experiments were conducted on a Ubuntu 18.04 system equipped with a Nvidia GeForce GTX 1070 with 8 Gb GPU memory and CUDA 11.0.

[1] https://qibawiki.rsna.org/index.php/Standardized_Uptake_Value_(SUV).

3.2 Experiment 1: Ability to Exploit Spatial Information

We compare 2Be3-Net capacity to exploit spatial information with a 2D and a 3D CNN. The 2D model is the 2D version of 2Be3-Net, where we replace the 3D blocks by their 2D alternative. The feature maps outputted by the ResNet-50 are provided as input to the 2D blocks and are flattened before applying FC layers. The full 3D CNN is composed of four 3D convolutional blocks similar to the ones of 2Be3-Net, followed by 2 FC layers. Batch size is set to 6, due to limited GPU memory.

In order to evaluate their capacity to exploit spatial information, we predict patient gender based on transverse slices. As transverse slices don't provide a whole body visualization, models should exploit the spatial information contained in the feature maps to compute predictions. The gender dataset used in this experiment contains 2459 scans in the training set and 377 in the validation set. The dataset is also imbalanced, as 77.2% of patients are men. We address this issue by using a weighted binary cross-entropy loss associated with Adam optimizer with an initial learning rate of 1e−5 and a weight decay of 1e−2. We evaluate models' performances with the area under the curve (AUC) of receiver characteristic operator (ROC) associated with sensitivity (SENS), specificity (SPEC) and accuracy (ACC). Experimental results are displayed in Table 1. The experiment shows that 2Be3-Net achieved a better result than the 2D version, showing the importance of taking into account the 3D spatial information while the full 3D CNN struggles in this task.

Table 1. Results of experiment 1

Metric	AUC	ACC	Sensitivity	Specificity
2Be3-Net	0.94	0.92	0.91	0.97
ResNet + Conv 2d	0.92	0.91	0.90	0.93
3D CNN	0.7	0.75	0.79	0.61

3.3 Experiment 2: Prediction of Clinical Outcomes

We compare the CNN models previously described to the radiomics approach developed by Vallières [37] on the prediction of clinical outcomes of head-and-neck cancer. To ease comparisons, we compare our results with 2 of their models. The PET radiomics model applies a logistic regression on different variables specific to each outcome. The best radiomics model uses random forests to combine PET and/or CT radiomics to clinical data. On the other side, we decline the 2Be3-Net in two versions. The first version entitled 2Be3-Net-[WS] takes as input 66 slices randomly selected in the whole scan. The second version, named 2Be3-Net-[H&N], takes as input 66 slices extracted from the head-neck region, following the intuition that this area is more inclined to contain relevant information for these tasks. As a pre-training, we use the weights of the models trained on gender prediction to initialize CNN models weights.

The clinical outcomes dataset used follows the dataset [37], at the difference of 9 patients (5 in the training set and 4 in the validation set), excluded due to image errors, initial data curation error (detected by TCIA) or missing information to calculate SUV. The resulting dataset contains 187 scans in the training set and 102 in the validation set. This dataset presents a pronounced class imbalance (LR: 14.6%, DM: 13.6% and OS: 18.4%). We apply the same strategy as experiment 1 to address this issue. Same data augmentation as before is applied to improve network robustness. Experiment results displayed in Table 2 show that both versions of 2Be3-Net outperforms the PET radiomics for LR and OS predictions, but achieves inferior performances in DM prediction.

Table 2. Clinical outcomes prediction results

	Metric	ResNet + Conv2D	3D CNN	2Be3-Net [WS]	2Be3-Net [H&N]	PET radiomics [41]	Best radiomics model [41]
LR	ACC	0.58	0.83	0.6	0.73	0.67	0.67
	AUC	0.64	0.69	0.68	0.72	0.53	0.69
	SENS	0.71	0.5	0.79	0.71	0.38	0.63
	SPEC	0.56	0.89	0.57	0.73	0.7	0.68
DM	ACC	0.70	0.71	0.68	0.76	0.68	0.77
	AUC	0.67	0.71	0.78	0.71	0.8	0.86
	SENS	0.64	0.71	0.93	0.64	0.85	0.86
	SPEC	0.71	0.71	0.64	0.77	0.66	0.76
OS	ACC	0.75	0.68	0.71	0.71	0.64	0.62
	AUC	0.72	0.65	0.76	0.74	0.62	0.74
	SENS	0.68	0.59	0.86	0.79	0.58	0.79
	SPEC	0.76	0.7	0.66	0.69	0.66	0.57

4 Discussion

We first evaluated 2Be3-Net capacity to exploit spatial information through predicting patient gender based on transverse PET slices. The proposed pipeline achieves a 0.94 AUC, achieving the best score on this task. We attribute this performance to the 3D convolutional blocks that exploited the spatial information contained in the concatenated feature maps. In the ResNet + Conv 2D model, the 3D convolutional blocks were replaced by 2D convolutional blocks, which prevented the exploitation of feature maps spatial information. By contrast, we attribute the full 3D CNN poor results to it's deep architecture and it's training from scratch, where more training samples would have been required to improve its results.

We studied the gender predictions made by our CNN and found that 70% of mis-predicted scans in the validation set have less than 180 slices. These scans only cover the body upper region and represent 25.2% of the total dataset size. As the whole body cannot be visualised on these scans, it is difficult for models to identify the gender and therefore are more prone to mispredictions.

We predicted different clinical outcomes of head-neck cancer (LR, DM, OS), and compared the deep learning models to a radiomics approach. CNN models took advantage of a pre-training on gender prediction, which improved their performances compared to training from scratch. In this experiment, all deep learning models achieved better results than PET radiomics on LR and OS predictions. We also note that both versions of 2Be3-Net achieved at least equivalent AUC and improved sensitivity compared to the best radiomics model. These results seem promising as the best radiomics model combined information from PET-CT scans associated with clinical data while our models only had access to the PET scan. The improved sensitivity implies that the proposed 2Be3-Net correctly identified more examples of the minority class than the radiomics models. It is also important to note that specificity wasn't compromised while sensitivity increased. We also note that 2Be3-Net-[H&N] presents results more stable compared to 2Be3-Net-[WS] as the gap between sensitivity and specificity decreased. This difference can be attributed to the slice selection area, where 2Be3-Net-[H&N] used slices selected in the head-neck region, and was therefore able to focus on tumor related information. However, CNN models achieved inferior results on DM prediction compared to the radiomics models. The radiomics models were specific to each outcome, and reached their best score on DM prediction. Thus, we attribute radiomics superior results on DM prediction to the specific design of the radiomics DM model. On the other hand, both 2Be3-Net versions were designed to predict all clinical outcomes and achieved stable results on those.

In the light of these experimental results, alternative deep learning architectures seem promising alternatives to radiomics and CNN approaches. The proposed 2Be3-Net accepts as input 3D PET scans with SUV conversion as the only preprocessing step, and is able to predict clinical outcomes of head-neck cancer from a training done on a small size dataset.

5 Conclusion

This paper introduces 2Be3-Net, a new architecture allowing direct exploitation of 3D PET scans through the association of a 2D pre-trained network with a 3D CNN, which enables exploitation of spatial information between the feature maps extracted. We compared 2Be3-Net to a traditional 2D CNN, a 3D CNN and a radiomics approach on the prediction of clinical outcomes of head-neck cancer. Experiments illustrated that the proposed architecture is a good alternative to classic CNN models and radiomics approaches. Moreover, it accepts as input entire PET scans requiring few preprocessing steps.

We used a ResNet-50 pre-trained on natural images as a feature extractor. Future works could focus on using a model pre-trained on PET images. In this matter, autoencoder architectures seem promising as they can be trained in an unsupervised manner, which solves the requirement of large annotated datasets and could further improve the relevance and quality of the feature maps extracted.

References

1. Krause, B.J., et al.: FDG PET and PET/CT. Recent Results Cancer Res. **187**, 351–369 (2013). https://doi.org/10.1007/978-3-642-10853-2_12
2. Gallamini, A., et al.: FDG-PET scan: a new paradigm for follicular lymphoma management. Mediterr. J. Hematol. Infect. Dis. **9**(1), e2017029 (2017). https://doi.org/10.4084/MJHID.2017.029
3. Fletcher, J.W., et al.: Recommendations on the use of 18F-FDG PET in oncology. J. Nucl. Med.: Off. Publ. Soc. Nucl. Med. **49**(3), 480–508 (2008). https://doi.org/10.2967/jnumed.107.047787
4. Mayerhoefer, M.E., et al.: Introduction to radiomics. J. Nuc. Med.: Off. Publ. Soc. Nucl. Med. **61**(4), 488–495 (2020). https://doi.org/10.2967/jnumed.118.222893
5. Bastiaannet, E., et al.: The value of FDG-PET in the detection, grading and response to therapy of soft tissue and bone sarcomas; a systematic review and meta-analysis. Cancer Treat. Rev. **30**(1), 83–101 (2004). https://doi.org/10.1016/j.ctrv.2003.07.004
6. Slot, K.M., et al.: Prediction of meningioma WHO grade using PET findings: a systematic review and meta-analysis. J. Neuroimaging (2020). https://doi.org/10.1111/jon.12795
7. Bailly, C., et al.: Interest of FDG-PET in the management of mantle cell lymphoma. Front. Med. **6**, 70 (2019). https://doi.org/10.3389/fmed.2019.00070
8. Xie, P., et al.: 18F-FDG PET or PET-CT to evaluate prognosis for head and neck cancer: a meta-analysis. J. Cancer Res. Clin. Oncol. **137**, 1085–1093 (2011). https://doi.org/10.1007/s00432-010-0972-y
9. Ha, S., et al.: Radiomics in oncological PET/CT: a methodological overview. Nucl. Med. Mol. Imaging **53**, 14–29 (2019). https://doi.org/10.1007/s13139-019-00571-4
10. Aerts, H.J., et al.: Decoding tumour phenotype by noninvasive imaging using a quantitative radiomics approach. Nat. Commun. **5**, 4006 (2014). https://doi.org/10.1038/ncomms5006
11. Lucia, F., et al.: Prediction of outcome using pretreatment 18F-FDG PET/CT and MRI radiomics in locally advanced cervical cancer treated with chemoradiotherapy. Eur. J. Nucl. Med. Mol. Imaging **45**(5), 768–786 (2017). https://doi.org/10.1007/s00259-017-3898-7
12. Bogowicz, M., et al.: CT radiomics and PET radiomics: ready for clinical implementation? Q. J. Nucl. Med. Mol. Imaging: Off. Publ. Ital. Assoc. Nucl. Med. (AIMN) Int. Assoc. Radiopharmacol. (IAR) Sect. Soc. **63**(4), 355–370 (2019). https://doi.org/10.23736/S1824-4785.19.03192-3
13. Russakovsky, O., et al.: ImageNet large scale visual recognition challenge. Int. J. Comput. Vis. **115**(3), 211–252 (2015). https://doi.org/10.1007/s11263-015-0816-y
14. Islam, J., et al.: Understanding 3D CNN behavior for Alzheimer's disease diagnosis from brain PET scan (2019). arXiv:1912.04563
15. Khvostikov, A., et al.: 3D CNN-based classification using sMRI and MD-DTI images for Alzheimer disease studies (2018)
16. Han, X., et al.: MR-based synthetic CT generation using a deep convolutional neural network method. Med. Phys. **44**, 1408–1419 (2017). https://doi.org/10.1002/mp.12155
17. Kawauchi, K., et al.: A convolutional neural network-based system to prevent patient misidentification in FDG-PET examinations. Sci. Rep. **9**(1), 7192 (2019). https://doi.org/10.1038/s41598-019-43656-y
18. Ding, Y., et al.: A deep learning model to predict a diagnosis of alzheimer disease by using 18F-FDG PET of the brain. Radiology **290**(2), 456–464 (2019). https://doi.org/10.1148/radiol.2018180958
19. Ravishankar, H., et al.: Understanding the mechanisms of deep transfer learning for medical images. In: Carneiro, G., et al. (eds.) LABELS/DLMIA -2016. LNCS, vol. 10008, pp. 188–196. Springer, Cham (2016). https://doi.org/10.1007/978-3-319-46976-8_20

20. Tajbakhsh, N., et al.: Convolutional neural networks for medical image analysis: full training or fine tuning? IEEE Trans. Med. Imaging **35**(5), 1299–1312 (2016). https://doi.org/10.1109/TMI.2016.2535302
21. Erhan, D., et al.: The difficulty of training deep architectures and the effect of unsupervised pre-training. In: Proceedings of the Twelfth International Conference on Artificial Intelligence and Statistics, in PMLR, vol. 5, pp. 153–160 (2009)
22. Zhou, Z., et al.: Models genesis: generic autodidactic models for 3D medical image analysis. In: Shen, D., et al. (eds.) MICCAI 2019. LNCS, vol. 11767, pp. 384–393. Springer, Cham (2019). https://doi.org/10.1007/978-3-030-32251-9_42
23. Chen, S., et al.: Med3D: transfer learning for 3D medical image analysis (2019)
24. Kaiming, H., et al.: Deep residual learning for image recognition. In: Proceedings of the IEEE Conference on Computer Vision and Pattern Recognition (2016)
25. Clark, K., et al.: The cancer imaging archive (TCIA): maintaining and operating a public information repository. J. Digit. Imaging **26**(6), 1045–1057 (2013). https://doi.org/10.1007/s10278-013-9622-7
26. Vallières, M., et al.: Data from head-neck-PET-CT. The Cancer Imaging Archive (2017). https://doi.org/10.7937/K9/TCIA.2017.8oje5q00
27. Walter, R.B., et al.: Data from Head-Neck_Cetuximab. The Cancer Imaging Archive (2015). https://doi.org/10.7937/K9/TCIA.2015.7AKGJUPZ
28. Zuley, M.L., et al.: Radiology data from the cancer genome atlas head-neck squamous cell carcinoma [TCGA-HNSC] collection. The Cancer Imaging Archive (2016). https://doi.org/10.7937/K9/TCIA.2016.LXKQ47MS
29. Grossberg, A., et al.: M.D. Anderson Cancer center head and neck quantitative imaging working group. HNSCC. The Cancer Imaging Archive (2020). https://doi.org/10.7937/k9/tcia.2020.a8sh-7363
30. Beichel, R.R., et al.: Data from QIN-HEADNECK. The Cancer Imaging Archive (2015). https://doi.org/10.7937/K9/TCIA.2015.K0F5CGLI
31. Kinahan, P., et al.: Data from the ACRIN 6668 Trial NSCLC-FDG-PET [Dataset]. The Cancer Imaging Archive (2019). https://doi.org/10.7937/tcia.2019.30ilqfcl
32. Bakr, S., et al.: Data for NSCLC radiogenomics collection. The Cancer Imaging Archive (2017). https://doi.org/10.7937/K9/TCIA.2017.7hs46erv
33. Albertina, B., et al.: Radiology data from the cancer genome atlas lung adenocarcinoma [TCGA-LUAD] collection. The Cancer Imaging Archive (2016). https://doi.org/10.7937/K9/TCIA.2016.JGNIHEP5
34. Kirk, S., et al.: Radiology data from the cancer genome atlas lung squamous cell carcinoma [TCGA-LUSC] collection. The Cancer Imaging Archive (2016). https://doi.org/10.7937/K9/TCIA.2016.TYGKKFMQ
35. Muzi, P., et al.: Data from RIDER Lung PET-CT. The Cancer Imaging Archive (2015). https://doi.org/10.7937/K9/TCIA.2015.OFIP7TVM
36. Paszke, A., et al.: PyTorch: an imperative style, high-performance deep learning library. In: Advances in Neural Information Processing Systems, vol. 32, pp. 8026–8037. Curran Associates, Inc. (2019). 1912.01703
37. Vallières, M., et al.: Radiomics strategies for risk assessment of tumour failure in head-and-neck cancer. Sci. Rep. **7**(1), 10117 (2017). https://doi.org/10.1038/s41598-017-10371-5

Check for updates

Covid-19 Chest CT Scan Image Classification Using LCKSVD and Frozen Sparse Coding

Kaveen Liyanage, Fereshteh Ramezani, and Bradley M. Whitaker(✉)

Montana State University, Bozeman, MT 59717, USA
bradley.whitaker1@montana.edu

Abstract. The coronavirus disease 2019 (COVID-19) is a fast transmitting virus spreading throughout the world and causing a pandemic. Early detection of the disease is crucial in preventing the rapid propagation of the virus. Although Computed Tomography (CT) technology is not considered to be a reliable first-line diagnostic tool, it does have the potential to detect the disease. While several high performing deep learning networks have been proposed for the automated detection of the virus using CT images, deep networks lack the explainability, clearness, and simplicity of other machine learning methods. Sparse representation is an effective tool in image processing tasks with an efficient algorithm for implementation. In addition, the output sparse domain can be easily mapped to the original input signal domain, thus the features provide information about the signal in the original domain. This work utilizes two sparse coding algorithms, frozen dictionary learning, and label-consistent k-means singular value decomposition (LC-KSVD), to help classify Covid-19 CT lung images. A framework for image sparse coding, dictionary learning, and classifier learning is proposed and an accuracy of 89% is achieved on the cleaned CC-CCII CT lung image dataset.

Keywords: COVID-19 · CT image · Sparse coding · KSVD · Frozen dictionary · LC-KSVD

1 Introduction

[1]The coronavirus disease 2019 (COVID-19) is a fast transmitting virus spreading throughout the world and causing a pandemic [1]. Early detection of the disease is crucial in preventing the rapid propagation of the virus. As of now, authorized assays for viral testing include those that detect SARS-CoV-2 nucleic acid or antigen [2]. However, due to the high demand and lack of onsite testing, the turnout time for the test results have increased [3].

[1] **CAUTION:** This work should not be used as a diagnostic method for any disease without the proper approval of a licensed medical practitioner.

R. Su et al. (Eds.): MICAD 2021, LNEE 784, pp. 272–281, 2022.
https://doi.org/10.1007/978-981-16-3880-0_28

Computed Tomography (CT) technology is not considered to be a reliable first-line diagnostic or screening tool for COVID-19 due to lack of specificity, risk of spreading, and resource management [4–6]. However, CT images of the chest are useful in symptomatic, suspected, or high-risk cases where real-time reverse transcription-polymerase chain reaction (RT-PCR) testing is unavailable, delayed, or negative. As such, CT technology has the potential to be used as a diagnostic tool for the detection of the disease [7–9].

Several deep learning networks have been proposed for the automated detection of the virus using CT images [10–12]. While deep learning may be successful in classification, deep networks lack the transparency and simplicity of other machine learning (ML) methods [13]. Recent developments in sparse representations algorithms in the field of image processing provides the user with efficient algorithms that easily relate the sparse output to the original input feature space [14]. Sparse coding has been proposed for the use of CT image de-noising in [15] where the authors have implemented a patch-based parallel algorithm for fast execution.

In this article, we are proposing a patch-based sparse coding framework that uses the statistics of the dictionary atom utilization for classifier learning. The framework is applied to the cleaned CC-CCII dataset [16,17] for the classification of lung CT scan images. We employ two sparse coding algorithms—frozen dictionary learning [18] and label-consistent k-means singular value decomposition (LC-KSVD) [19]—in a complementary manner to learn a more descriptive dictionary. The final dictionary is composed by augmenting two separate dictionaries learned using the frozen dictionary and LC-KSVD algorithms. Frozen dictionary learns the expertly identified [16] lung CT image features in a hierarchical order. These features are ground-glass opacity (GGO) and consolidations (CO) [20]. LC-KSVD learns a discriminative dictionary according to class labels and classification error. By combining these properties we hope to achieve an effective representation for classification tasks between the classes common pneumonia (CP), novel coronavirus pneumonia (NCP), and Normal CT scans.

2 Data Set

The lack of publicly available CT scan data sets and standards are some of the main obstacles in developing a robust framework [21]. However, CT image relating to COVID-19 reporting standards are published by [22] and categorical CT assessment guidelines are published by [23]. Some of the popular publicly available datasets are Covid-CT dataset [24], China Consortium of Chest CT Image Investigation (CC-CCII) dataset [16], and COVID-19 Image Data Collection [25,26]. Full comparisons of the datasets can be found in [11,12,27]. Since datasets like Covid-CT dataset and COVID-19 Image Data Collection have curated the images by collecting data from previously published works, websites, and papers, the image quality has deteriorated and lacks full metadata supporting the images [6]. Hence, they hinder the ability of ML algorithms to be more standardized. However, authors of the COVID-CT dataset argue that even with low-resolution images, radiologists can distinguish features proficiently [24].

For this paper we will be using a subset of (CC-CCII) dataset[2] [16] as it contains a large collection of high-quality images with the sources. The dataset consists of three class labeled CT images belonging to novel coronavirus pneumonia (NCP) due to SARS-CoV-2 virus infection, common pneumonia (CP), and normal (NORMAL) controls. Additionally, 750 CT image slices were manually segmented by experts into the background, lung field (LF), ground-glass opacity (GGO), and consolidations (CO). This manual segmentation information can be utilized to learn specific features.

We will be utilizing the dataset pre-processing done by [17] with the CC-CCII dataset. He *et al.* have manually filtered/cleaned out the dataset to remove the corrupted, duplicated, out-of-order, and mismatched formats of the images. They have finally selected a subset of the images according to Table 1.

Table 1. Cleaned CC-CCII dataset [17]

Classes	#Patients		#Scans	
	Train	Test	Train	Test
NCP	726	190	1,213	302
CP	778	186	1,210	303
Normal	660	158	772	193
Total	2,164	534	3,195	798

Since the CC-CCII dataset consists of lung segmented and non-segmented scan images, He *et al.* have used a K-means-based, openly available[3] method to segment the lung area from the background for all the images to achieve consistency. In this paper, we will be using this segmented and cleaned CC-CCII image dataset[4]. At the moment the He *et al.* work has not yet been peer-reviewed, and therefore there are no other independent works on this dataset. However, we observed that a well formatted publicly available dataset is beneficial in developing and testing of new frameworks for diagnosis.

He *et al.* have applied transfer learning with some popular pre-trained networks (ResNet, DenseNet, etc.) and also proposed a CNN based mixup data augmented deep learning model called, MNas3DNet41 which was able to gain an accuracy of 87.14% [17]. They have carried out slice sampling and slice processing to conform to the input standards of pre-trained networks. In the slice sampling stage, the number of slices per scan was kept consistent. In the slice sampling stage, the image resolutions were decreased and then cropped to a size of 128×128. Both $2d$ and $3d$ pre-trained models were evaluated on the dataset.

Our method does not resize the image as we are considering small size image patches. Since we are discarding the empty patches from the lung segmented

[2] http://ncov-ai.big.ac.cn/download?lang=en.
[3] https://github.com/booz-allen-hamilton/DSB3Tutorial.
[4] https://github.com/arthursdays/HKBU_HPML_COVID-19.

images, the increase in computational requirements is minimal. Also, we are evaluating the presence of disease slice-by-slice as a $2d$ greyscale image. Even though this might not be able to identify $3d$ lesion features, we are hoping that $2d$ features will be sufficient for satisfactory results. However, we can expand the proposed method to cater to $3d$ image processing also without any major modifications.

3 Sparse Representation

There has been a growing interest in the search for sparse representations of signals in recent years. In the field of computer vision it can be reasonably assumed that image patches do not populate or sample the whole input domain [28]. Sparse coding is a representation learning method which aims to find a sparse representation of an n dimensional input signal $y_i \in \mathbb{R}^n$ in the form of a sparse linear combination, such that the reconstructed data is $\tilde{y}_i = \alpha_{i,1}d_1 + \alpha_{i,2}d_2 + ... + \alpha_{i,K}d_K$. Where $\alpha_i \in \mathbb{R}^K$ is the the sparse vector and $d_i \in \mathbb{R}^n$ are the dictionary elements (atoms) of a Dictionary $\mathbf{D}$. Sparse representation algorithms optimize (1) with a l_0 regularization term:

$$\underset{D,\alpha}{\text{argmin}}\, ||\mathbf{Y} - \mathbf{D}\alpha||_2^2 \;\; s.t. \;\; \forall i, ||\alpha_i||_0 \leq S, \tag{1}$$

where $\mathbf{Y} = [y_1, y_2, .., y_N] \in \mathbb{R}^{n \times N}$ denotes the N number of input signals, $\mathbf{D} = [d_1, d_2, ..., d_K] \in \mathbb{R}^{n \times K}$ is the learned dictionary of size K, $\alpha = [\alpha_1, \alpha_2, ..., \alpha_N] \in \mathbb{R}^{K \times N}$ is the sparse representation of the input signal, and S is the sparsity constraint of α_i (maximum number of non-zero elements). Usually $K > n$, in which case the dictionary is called over-complete. If $K = n$ the dictionary is called complete and if $K < n$ it is called under-complete.

Equation (1) can be solved by alternating between the following two stages. First, sparse coding is to calculate α with a fixed over-complete dictionary D. Second, dictionary learning is performed to update D with a fixed α. K-means Singular Value Decomposition (K-SVD) [14,29] has emerged as an effective and popular algorithm for sparse representation tasks. K-SVD first initializes a random dictionary. It then alternates between the two stages by utilizing Orthogonal Matching Pursuit (OMP) [30,31] for the sparse coding and generalized k-means with Singular Value Decomposition (SVD) for the dictionary update. K-SVD efficiently learns an over-complete dictionary and has been effectively utilized for tasks including de-noising, restoration, and classification.

For classification tasks, in order to improve the performance a more discriminatory representation is required. Jiang *et al.* [19,32] have presented a Label Consistent K-SVD (LC-KSVD) algorithm as an extension of the K-SVD framework, which is a supervised learning algorithm to learn a compact and discriminative dictionary. In LC-KSVD, class-specific dictionary elements are trained separately as an initialization and then combined to learn a discriminative dictionary. A label consistent constraint called "discriminative sparse-code error", reconstruction error and classification error terms are combined to structure a unified objective function to optimize the discriminated dictionary. Due to the class constraints in the sparse coding and dictionary update stages, the input data will forced to be mapped to the dedicated dictionary atoms according to the label information. Consequently in the sparse dictionary domain, a majority of the input signals will be projected to a subspace belonging to a certain class. Hence, a lower order classifier can be trained for the classification.

Traditional dictionary learning models do not take into account the class imbalances of the training data. Hence the dictionary atoms can be biased towards the larger class. The segmented lung CT scan training images have consisted mainly of lung field (LF) class patches and the rare occurrences abnormalities (GGO and CO) image patches. Therefore to address the class imbalances and the structure, a separate dictionary learning algorithm is also employed. Frozen dictionary learning modifies the dictionary learning process as a hierarchical structure to learn a dictionary that can effectively model imbalanced datasets [18]. In this algorithm, first, the dictionary learning step is carried out using the K-SVD algorithm on "normal" (LF) training data. Then the learned dictionary elements are frozen (held constant) and the dictionary is augmented with additional elements by dictionary elements is trained again on image patches containing abnormalities (GGO and CO). This process is repeated for all the remaining classes, by keeping the previously learned dictionaries frozen. The frozen elements of the dictionary represent the "normal" aspects of the data, hence the new elements (non-frozen) learn to represent the anomalous aspects of the data that are not present in the "normal" data. The frozen dictionary approach could be generally used and applied to the problems including data with or without abnormalities.

4 Methodology

Figure 1 gives a visual overview of the full framework presented in this paper. First, 750 images from 150 patients (manually segmented by experts) were divided into patches of size $p \times p$ with an overlap of $0.3p$. Then the patches containing lung field (LF), ground-glass opacity (GGO), and consolidations (CO) are extracted if the patch contains at least 25% of the region of interest. The patch sizes ($p = 24$) were chosen such that sufficient spatial features of the GGO and CO are captured within a patch. Extracting overlapping patches will ensure that the feature locations are distributed across the patches for more generality. Next, these patches were used to train the frozen dictionary atoms of the dictionary. In the dictionary training, sparsity shall be kept to a minimum with low reconstruction error. The dictionary composition for each section is chosen to roughly represent the distribution of each segment (LF: 250, GGO: 150, CO: 100). The frozen dictionary is trained in the order of LF, GGO and CO while keeping the previously learned dictionary frozen and then augmenting.

After learning the frozen dictionary, all the lung segmented images are redivided into the same sized patches as above. The patches which overwhelmingly contain only the background are discarded. This drastically reduces the computational cost. Since GGO and CO are not specific enough for detecting COVID-19,

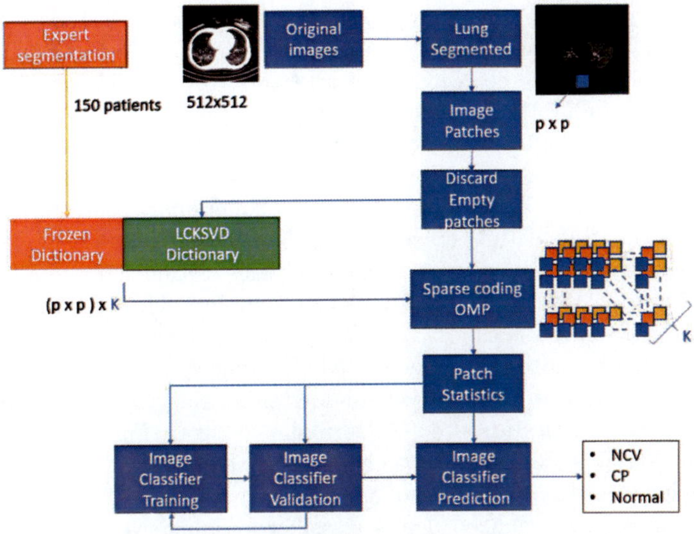

Fig. 1. Framework

LC-KSVD is used to automatically learn any underlying features which could differentiate the class labels. A random portion (~10%) of the lung-segmented cleaned CC-CCII train dataset is divided into the same sized ($p = 24$) patches as above. These patches are used to learn the LC-KSVD dictionary as the same size(~500) as a frozen dictionary. Parameters for the LC-KSVD training are chosen such that it would have a higher discriminating power even with a high reconstruction error.

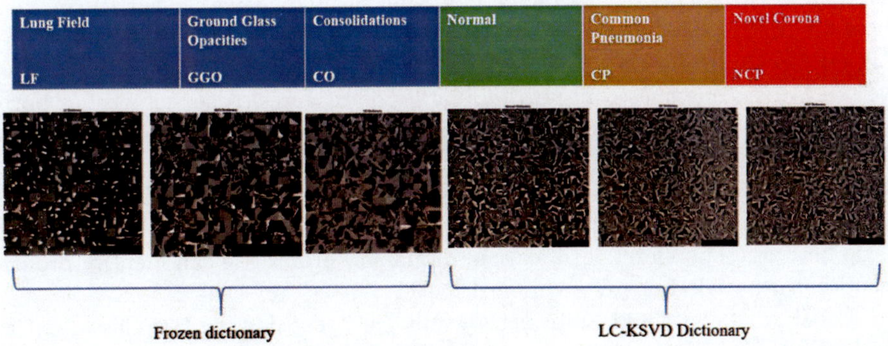

Fig. 2. Dictionary composition. The top row describes the dictionary composition. The second row shows dictionary elements learned from frozen dictionary learning and LC-KSVD.

Then the two sets of dictionary atoms, frozen and LC-KSVD are appended to construct one discriminative dictionary. In the sparse coding stage, the parameters are set such that the reconstruction error will be minimal with sparsity $S = 20$. Hence the OMP algorithm will likely find a solution from both sets of dictionary atoms. The learned dictionary atom samples and the composition is shown in Fig. 2. The dictionary elements associated with each type of lung tissue or disease are visually distinct, indicating that dictionary learning produced a highly discriminative feature space.

The remainder of the training, validation, and testing sets are all subjected to patch-based sparse coding via the OMP algorithm. Then the dictionary utilization statistics of patches for each slice image is calculated. Statistics calculated are mean, variance, and non-zero count of the sparse coefficients per each patient scan. Since our dictionary is divided according to the class labels and features, these statistics are used to learn the classifier. Furthermore, since we have an over-representation based sparse coding the resulting statistics will also be sparse, hence justifying the use of a lower order classifier. The statistics of the coefficients will be normalized before classifier learning. Normalization is done by dividing each statistic of each dictionary segment by the segment's absolute maximum parameter value to preserve the sparsity of the coefficients. Finally, a Support Vector Machine (SVM) optimized classifier is trained using MATLAB classifier learner.

5 Results and Conclusion

When the learned dictionaries are examined, it can be observed that the frozen dictionary learning has learned distinct dictionaries for each lung feature as seen in Fig. 2. The LF features are composed of more lung structural elements and more detailed lesion structures are leaned for GGO and CO respectively. However, in LC-KSVD, the dictionary does not seem to have a clear distinction between the CP and NCP classes. This could be explained because, in the training process, whole image slices were used with labeled as CP or NCP, whereas very few image patches contain the lung lesion features. Also, sometimes both CP and NCP exhibit the same features in the CT scans, hence the lack of specificity. Since the two dictionaries are complimentary, this is somewhat mitigated. Furthermore, in both cases the dictionary atoms are in the same domain as the input image patches, so the model performance is much more intuitive than a deep network. Therefore, with learned dictionary atoms, we can identify prominent features underlying the system.

For the classification results as shown in Fig. 3, considering two classes, NCP and Non-NCP (CP and Normal), our method yields an accuracy of 89% with an F_1 measure of 0.859, precision of 0.8413, recall of 0.8775 with a cubic SVM classifier. This compares favorably to Table VII of He et al. [17], where the highest accuracy is 87.83% with an F_1 score of 0.8604 when using ResNet3D34 out of a variety pre-trained Neural networks. In our method, by introducing a misclassification cost matrix, the F_1 score can be slightly improved with the expense of accuracy. For three-class classification, we achieved an accuracy of 82.6%. Our model produces results that are on par with deep networks [17] while also providing an intuitive relationship between classifier and features.

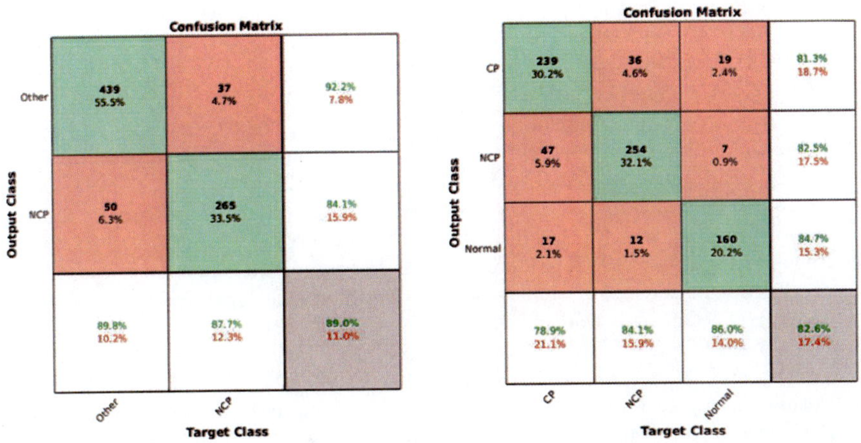

Fig. 3. Confusion matrix for classification results. (a) Two class: NCP and other (CP and normal) (b) Three class: CP, NCP and normal.

This work does not take into account the patient metadata provided with the dataset. These data could provide additional information regarding disease progression and severity. One of the assumptions in our work is that image acquisition is performed uniformly with compatible intensity and resolution. However this may not be the practical case and further tests should be carried out to determine the robustness of the learned dictionary elements and the classifiers during the presence of variations in resolution, noise, and intensities. Further, it would be beneficial to improve the system to output the results according to the CO-RADS guidelines [23].

Here we have presented a patch-based end-to-end framework for the utilization of sparse representation for the detection of COVID-19 through lung CT scans. Although the CT scan should not be used as a diagnostic model at present, the development of robust frameworks will be beneficial in understanding the disease diagnostics and fast deployment in future pandemics. As per future work, we plan to develop a $3d$ sparse representation model to learn $3d$ spatial features following the industry standards. Also, a parallel computational pipeline would improve the computational time. Further, this framework can be applied to other Covid-19 CT lung image data sets and the effects of other hyper-parameters should be further investigated.

References

1. WHO: Coronavirus disease (COVID-19) pandemic (2020). https://www.who.int/emergencies/diseases/novel-coronavirus-2019. Accessed 4 Dec 2020
2. CDC: Overview of testing for SARS-CoV-2 (COVID-19) (2020). https://www.cdc.gov/coronavirus/2019-ncov/hcp/testing-overview.html. Accessed 21 Oct 2020
3. Beeching, N.J., Fletcher, T.E., Beadsworth, M.B.J.: Covid-19: testing times. **369**(8241), BMJ m1403 (2020)
4. ACR: ACR recommendations for the use of chest radiography and computed tomography (CT) for suspected COVID-19 infection (2020). Accessed 22 Mar 2020
5. CAR: Canadian society of thoracic radiology and the Canadian association of radiologists' statement on COVID-19 (2020). Accessed 26 Mar 2020
6. Tizhoosh, H.R., Fratesi, J.: COVID-19, AI enthusiasts, and toy datasets: radiology without radiologists. Eur. Radiol. **31**, 3553–3554 (2020)
7. Revel, M.P., et al.: COVID-19 patients and the radiology department - advice from the European society of radiology (ESR) and the European society of thoracic imaging (ESTI). Eur. Radiol. **30**(9), 4903–4909 (2020)
8. Francone, M., et al.: Chest CT score in COVID-19 patients: correlation with disease severity and short-term prognosis. Eur. Radiol. **30**(12), 6808–6817 (2020)
9. Bernheim, A., et al.: Chest CT findings in coronavirus disease-19 (COVID-19): relationship to duration of infection. Radiology **295**(3), 200463 (2020)
10. Ozsahin, I., Sekeroglu, B., Musa, M.S., Mustapha, M.T., Ozsahin, D.U.: Review on diagnosis of COVID-19 from chest CT images using artificial intelligence. Comput. Math. Methods Med. **2020**, 1–10 (2020)
11. Pham, T.D.: A comprehensive study on classification of COVID-19 on computed tomography with pretrained convolutional neural networks. Sci. Rep. **10**(1), 1–8 (2020)
12. Bizopoulos, P., Vretos, N., Daras, P.: Comprehensive comparison of deep learning models for lung and COVID-19 lesion segmentation in CT scans (2020)
13. Berenguer, A.D., et al.: Explainable-by-design semi-supervised representation learning for COVID-19 diagnosis from CT imaging, November 2020
14. Aharon, M., Elad, M., Bruckstein, A.: K-SVD: an algorithm for designing overcomplete dictionaries for sparse representation. IEEE Trans. Signal Process. **54**(11), 4311–4322 (2006)
15. Bartuschat, D., Borsdorf, A., Köstler, H., Rubinstein, R., Stürmer, M.: A parallel K-SVD implementation for CT image denoising. Dept. Comput. Sci. **10**, 1–26 (2009)
16. Zhang, K., et al.: Clinically applicable AI system for accurate diagnosis, quantitative measurements, and prognosis of COVID-19 pneumonia using computed tomography. Cell **181**(6), 1423–1433.e11 (2020)
17. He, X., et al.: Benchmarking deep learning models and automated model design for COVID-19 detection with chest CT scans (2020)
18. Carroll, B.T., Whitaker, B.M., Dayley, W., Anderson, D.V.: Outlier learning via augmented frozen dictionaries. IEEE/ACM Trans. Audio Speech Lang. Process. **25**(6), 1207–1215 (2017)
19. Jiang, Z., Lin, Z., Davis, L.S.: Label consistent K-SVD: learning a discriminative dictionary for recognition. IEEE Trans. Pattern Anal. Mach. Intell. **35**(11), 2651–2664 (2013)
20. Byrne, D., et al.: RSNA expert consensus statement on reporting chest CT findings related to COVID-19: interobserver agreement between chest radiologists. Can. Assoc. Radiol. J. 084653712093832 (2020)

21. Shuja, J., Alanazi, E., Alasmary, W., Alashaikh, A.: COVID-19 open source data sets: a comprehensive survey. Appl. Intell. **51**, 1296–1325 (2020)
22. Simpson, S., et al.: Radiological society of north America expert consensus document on reporting chest CT findings related to COVID-19: endorsed by the society of thoracic radiology, the American college of radiology, and RSNA. Radiol.: Cardiothorac. Imaging **2**(2), e200152 (2020)
23. Prokop, M., et al.: CO-RADS: a categorical CT assessment scheme for patients suspected of having COVID-19–definition and evaluation. Radiology **296**(2), E97–E104 (2020)
24. Yang, W., Yan, F.: Patients with RT-PCR-confirmed COVID-19 and normal chest CT. Radiology **295**(2), E3 (2020)
25. Cohen, J.P., Morrison, P., Dao, L.: COVID-19 image data collection, March 2020
26. Cohen, J.P., Morrison, P., Dao, L., Roth, K., Duong, T.Q., Ghassemi, M.: Covid-19 image data collection: prospective predictions are the future, June 2020
27. Sarosh, P., Parah, S.A., Mansur, R.F., Bhat, G.M.: Artificial intelligence for COVID-19 detection - a state-of-the-art review, November 2020
28. Elad, M.: Sparse and Redundant Representations: From Theory to Applications in Signal and Image Processing. Springer, Heidelberg (2010)
29. Rubinstein, R., Peleg, T., Elad, M.: Analysis k-SVD: a dictionary-learning algorithm for the analysis sparse model. IEEE Trans. Signal Process. **61**(3), 661–677 (2013)
30. Pati, Y., Rezaiifar, R., Krishnaprasad, P.: Orthogonal matching pursuit: recursive function approximation with applications to wavelet decomposition. In: Proceedings of 27th Asilomar Conference on Signals, Systems and Computers, pp. 40–44. IEEE, IEEE Computer Society Press (1993)
31. Davis, G., Mallat, S., Avellaneda, M.: Adaptive greedy approximations. Constr. Approx. **13**(1), 57–98 (1997)
32. Jiang, Z., Lin, Z., Davis, L.S.: Learning a discriminative dictionary for sparse coding via label consistent K-SVD. In: CVPR 2011. IEEE (2011)

A Hybrid Deep Model for Brain Tumor Classification

Hamail Ayaz[1](✉), Muhammad Ahmad[2], David Tormey[1], Ian McLoughlin[3], and Saritha Unnikrishnan[1]

[1] Faculty of Engineering and Design and Centre for Precision Engineering, Materials and Manufacturing Research, Institute of Technology Sligo, Sligo 91 YW50, Ireland
hamail.ayaz@mail.itsligo.ie, unnikrishnan.saritha@itsligo.ie
[2] Department of Computer Science, National University of Computer and Emerging Sciences, Islamabad, Chiniot-Faisalabad Campus, Chiniot 35400, Pakistan
[3] Department of Computer Science and Applied Physics, Galway-Mayo Institute of Technology, Galway, Ireland

Abstract. Classification of brain tumors from Magnetic Resonance Images (MRIs) using Computer-Aided Diagnosis (CAD) has faced some major challenges. Diagnosis of brain tumors such as glioma, meningioma, and pituitary mostly rely on manual evaluation by neuro-radiologists and is prone to human error and subjectivity. In recent years, Machine Learning (ML) techniques have been used to improve the accuracy of tumor diagnosis with the expense of intensive pre-processing and computational cost. Therefore, this work proposed a hybrid Convolutional Neural Network (CNN) (i.e., AlexNet followed by SqueezeNet) to extract quality tumor biomarkers for better performance of the CAD system using brain tumor MRI's. The features extracted using AlexNet and SqueezeNet are fused to preserve the most important biomarkers in a computationally efficient manner. A total of 3064 brain tumors (708 Meningioma, 1426 Glioma, and 930 Pituitaries) MRIs have been experimented. The proposed model is evaluated using several well-known metrics, i.e., Overall accuracy (94%), Precision (92%), Recall (95%), and F1 score (93%) and outperformed many state of the art hybrid methods.

Keywords: Hybrid model · Ensemble learning · Brain tumor · Classification

1 Introduction

Brain tumors are the second most fatal medical emergency after Alzheimer's and they are found in every age group [19]. The mass of abnormal cells formed inside the brain is considered as tumor and generally, there are many types of brain tumors, in which, Glioma (also known as "Intra-axial") is the most aggressive one [20]. Glioma is found in brain cells such as ependymal, glial, and astrocytes and is likely to be spread inside the brain. Pituitary tumors are adenomas, which usually appear between the hypothalamus and the pineal gland. Meningioma are benign intracranial tumors that cover the brain and spinal cord [2].

R. Su et al. (Eds.): MICAD 2021, LNEE 784, pp. 282–291, 2022.
https://doi.org/10.1007/978-981-16-3880-0_29

Brain tumor patients suffer serious headaches, fits, eye-sight loss, stress, depression, and death in extreme cases [9]. Classification of the above mentioned tumors mostly relies on advanced medical imaging such as Computed Tomography (CT) and Magnetic Resonance (MR) imaging. CT is predominant in dealing with the medical emergency of bones, and chest based assessments whereas, MR Imaging (MRIs) is to asses' brain tumors. Manual identification of tumor through MRIs is highly dependent on the experience of radiologists and neurologists, which are subject due to manual operation and limited capacity to use the previous knowledge based on thousands of MRIs [19].

Automated image recognition through computer vision and machine learning techniques have proven the potential in the identification and classification of brain tumors using T1/MRIs [5]. MR images have also been used by segmentation methods such as histogram of gradient (HoG), scale-invariant feature (SIFT) and Local binary patterns (LBP) followed by supervised learning algorithms such as Support Vector Machine (SVM), K-Nearest Neighbour (KNN), Linear Regression (LR), and clustering techniques [3].

For instance, Cheng et al. [6] proposed a study on brain tumor classification of glioma, meningioma, and pituitary abnormal cells. In Cheng's work, a total of 3064 T1-weighted Contrast-Enhanced MRI (CE-MRI) were used for classification using gray level co-occurrence matrix (GLCM), histogram intensities, and bag-of-words (BoW) to extract Region of Interest (RoI) as feature vectors and later fed to SVM, KNN, and, sparse representation-based classification (SRC). This method achieved an overall accuracy of 82.31% (histogram intensities), 84.75% (GLCM), and 88.19% (BoW). In another work, Cheng et al. [7] used fisher vector method to achieve higher precision of 94.62% on the similar data. Amin et al. [1], discussed automatic detection of high grade and low grade glioma and ischemic stroke lesions through an unsupervised clustering approach for tumor segmentation. Several conventional feature extraction methods (such as Gabor wavelet features (GWF), Histograms of Oriented Gradient (HOG), Local Binary Pattern (LBP), and Segmentation-based Fractal Texture Analysis (SFTA) features) were fused to perform the classification through RF classifier.

However, traditional machine learning algorithms with T1 images require more processing (i.e., data augmentation, image segmentation, Region of interest selection), which decreases the effectiveness of classification and increases the computational cost [21]. Irrespective of these techniques, deep learning provides more accurate results for classification of tumor biomarkers [10]. For instance, Paul et al. [17], used Convolution Neural Network (CNN) to classify Glioma, Meningioma, and Pituitary brain tumors and achieved an overall accuracy of 91.43%. Pashaei et al. [16] proposed a study of CNN with Extreme Learning Machines (ELM) by using the same tumor data and achieved an overall accuracy of 93.68%.

Later in 2019, Deepak et. al., [8] proposed a study to use transfer learning with the GoogleNet model to classify Glioma, Meningioma, and Pituitary brain tumor with an overall accuracy of 92.3%. Similarly, Rehman et al. [18] proposed a transfer learning approach by studying AlexNet, GoogLeNet, and VGGNet architecture that achieved an overall accuracy of 98.69% through VGGNet-16. Ghosal et al. [11] proposed an ensemble learning approach by ResNet-101 and SqueezeNet architectures that achieved an overall accuracy of 89.93% for real tumors data and increased by 3.9% by using the augmentation techniques i.e., flipping, rotate and degree transformation.

However, the above-mentioned studies consume a large number of convolution operations and have high time consumption for an efficient CAD tool. Therefore, this work proposes a hybrid deep learning model, which automates the classification system for three types of brain tumors (i.e., Glioma, Meningioma, and Pituitary) with minimum convolutional operations in a computationally efficient manner. In a nutshell, the following contributions are made in this study:

1. Constructing two different networks with minimal operations.
2. Merging and extraction of features to make an efficient hybrid deep network. 3. evaluating the model through statistical evaluation metrics

The rest of the paper is structured as follows: Sect. 2 explain the proposed methodology. Section 3 present the results of our proposed model with discussion on the existing models. Finally, Sect. 4 concludes the paper with possible future research directions.

2 Methodology

2.1 Deep Networks

In computer vision, deep convolutional neural networks (DCNN) is widely used in classification related applications of medical imaging (brain tumor) [11]. DCNN has overcome the limitations of traditional machine learning such as image segmentation and Region of Interest (RoI's) extraction by implementing deep learning models such as AlexNet, ResNet, DesNet, VggNet, and Inception net [18]. Additionally, they have also been used in hybrid approaches to consume less time, complexity, and normally, 2D-DCNN are learned by using the following (1) [14];

$$X_{ab}^{lm} = f\left(\sum_{n=0} \sum_{h=o}^{H_l-1} \sum_{w=0}^{W_m-1} K_{lmn}^{hw} O_{(l-1)n}^{(a+h)(b+w)} + B_{lm}\right) \tag{1}$$

where, B_{lm} represents the bias, $O_{(l-1)n}^{(a+h)(b+w)}$ gives the feature output learned by the previous layer through a kernel function K_{lmn}^{hw} through n^{th} feature map at the given value at h and w, with height H and width W of the entire Kernel. Finally, X_{ab}^{lm} is the final output learned at the position [a, b], with l layers and m feature maps.

The tumor biomarkers learned by the deep models are usually smaller than the entire MRIs. The number of convolution operations on each MRIs extract quality features however, due to numerous layers the existing model are prone to consume greater epochs and high computational complexity. The proposed model uses minimal number of convolutional operations followed by a kernel moderate function, which help's in extracting standard quality features.

AlexNet. AlexNet (AX) was designed in 2012 and is the most common and widely used deep model [13]. AX is a fully connected network with five convolution layers and three dense layers. The model uses numerous training parameters to predict the outcome. Whereas, in this work, three convolution layers (3 × 3) with 4 kernel filters at each layer is implemented to extract the minimum features, which followed three max-pooling layers after every convolution to down sample the feature size. Finally, one flatten layer to vectorized the feature map. The activation function used in the model for each layer is the rectified linear unit (*Relu*).

SqueezeNet. SqueexeNet (SQ) [12] is an optimized version of AX model, with a smaller fire block of 9 architectures. SQ uses lesser parameters than the AX model to achieve high precision and test accuracy. Therefore, in this work, a single fire block of SQ architecture is formulated, which is organized as the traditional 5 convolutional layer network with the rectified linear unit (*Relu*) as an activation function. Initially, the 3 × 3 convolutional layer is implemented with 8 kernel filters as the input layer (256 × 256 × 1). The learned features are fed to the fire block of SQ model by using 3 convolution layers (1 × 1) and 8, 4, and 4 kernel filters respectively. Finally, the merged fire block is stride down by using a max-pool layer and flattened to form a feature vector.

2.2 Proposed Classification Framework

The proposed classification framework used in this study consists of two stateof-the-art deep learning models (AlexNet and SqueezeNet) as shown in Fig. 1, which have been explored widely in brain tumors classification [18]. The two networks are formulated by passing an input image separately with the size of (256 × 256 × 1) and vectorized through flattening feature layer by using the (2) [11];

$$A : I \rightarrow O, I \xi P^{(h,w)}, O \xi P^{(h,w)} \tag{2}$$

where I is the input feature with the h, w is the height and width of an image. Whereas O represents the output feature map learned by performing convolutions. Initially, the input feature (I) is passed to the SQ architecture, and then the same feature map is fed to the AX model to acquire the final feature vector.

2.3 Train and Validation Model

The flatten vector features learned from the AX and SQ are merged through concatenation operation to form a fully connected vector and examined on 3064 labeled samples, which was further divided into 80: 20 ratio for train and test data. The actual acquire data was 512 × 512 in dimensions, which was reduced to the size of 256 × 256 for computational purposes. To compile the proposed model, several optimizers were experimented one after the other. To reduce the effect of the over-fitting early stopping was implemented to eliminate the training session if validation loss did not improve after 5 epochs. Finally, to validate the claims K = 10 fold cross-validation (CV) process is adopted for higher precision and improved accuracy.

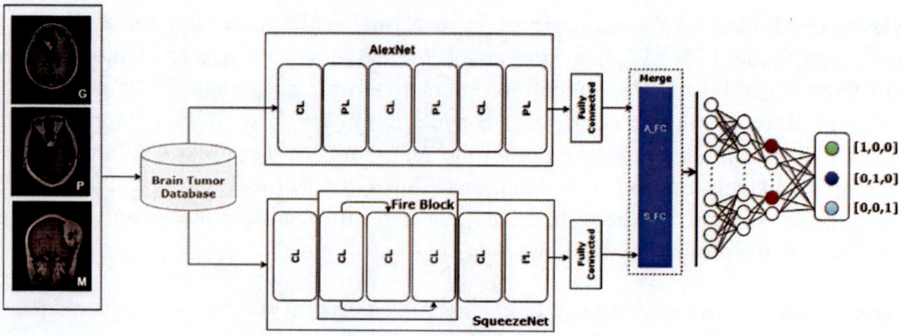

Fig. 1. The proposed Hybrid model using AlexNet and SqueezeNet architecture. G represents glioma as green; P represents pituitary as blue; and M represents meningioma as sky blue; whereas, CL is convolution layer; and PL is pooling layer.

3 Result and Discussion

3.1 Dataset Description and Its Pre-processing

The employed dataset for this study is from figshare; openly available storage space and is commonly used for brain tumor classification. The collected data of brain tumor covers the duration of 2005 to 2010 from two different hospitals (Nanfang, Tianjin General) in China [5]. The whole dataset contains 3064 MRIs of 233 brain tumor patients having glioma, meningioma, and pituitary tumors. The MRIs belonged to the T1-modality and contrast-enhanced axial, sagittal, and coronal views. A total of 89 patients were used to gather 1426 MRI of glioma tumor, 82 to capture 708 cases of meningioma and 62 belong to 930 cases of pituitary tumor. MRI of each case covers the dimensions of 512 $\times$ 512 for 3049 slices and 15 images were left with the lesser resolution of 256 $\times$ 256.

To evaluate the experimental analysis the data is first converted from mat extension to *png* for lesser computation. Initially, the given data is normalized to the range of -0.5 to 1.5 to construct a validated model, which is then resized to a static size of 256 $\times$ 256 to eliminate the difference of size in the entire dataset and also to limit the computations. The experimental evaluation is then carried out through several statistical tests such as recall and F1-score for the classification of brain tumors. In general, the experiment was carried out on an online platform Google Colab [4]. A total of 12.72 GB RAM with 68.4 GB of storage (cloud) is used with graphical processing unit (GPU) as run-time processing for data computation.

3.2 Learning Parameters and Model Structure

Deep models subjugate the use of traditional machine learning by preserving non-linear features such as shape, edges, corners, and intensities. Therefore, several experiments were conducted on 2415 train set MRIs and tested on 613 MRIs using seven optimizers. The detailed analysis and their achieved overall accuracy (OA) can be observed in Table 1, which gives the highest accuracy of 94% with RMSprop optimizer through standard learning rate (0.001) and lowest with adadelta (0.1) due to its higher step size. Other parameters for RMSprop includes rho (ρ) = 0.8, momentum = 0.00, and epsilon = $1e^{-07}$ and is evaluated with 10 epochs using 10 fold CV as shown in Fig. 2.

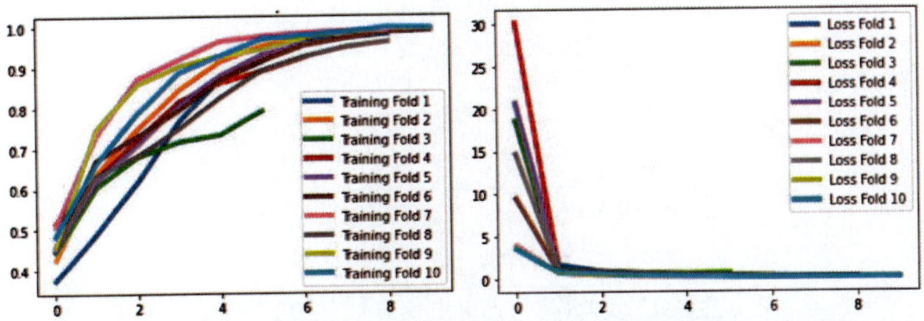

(a) Training Accuracy vs Epochs (b) Training loss vs Epochs

Fig. 2. Represents the learning curves with ten number of epochs

Table 1. Achieved accuracy of the proposed model for several different optimizer.

Class	Adam	Adamax	Nadam	Adadelta	SGD	Adagard	RMSprop
Glioma	0.93	0.90	0.89	0.77	0.88	0.91	0.91
Meningioma	0.75	0.70	0.71	0.27	0.70	0.68	0.97
Pitutary	0.94	0.98	0.98	0.83	0.96	0.98	0.97
OA	90	88	88	67	86	88	**94**

Further, during the construction of the merge deep model, fitting (under and over) issues may occur. To avoid this process a dropout technique along with early stopping is implemented. The detailed analysis of the model can be seen in Table 2 in which merge networks are dense with 64, 32, and 24 units at the neuron level with the drop out of 0.1 after each layer.

Table 2. The summary of the SQ-DCNN and AX-DCNN model.

SQ-DCNN			AX-DCNN		
Layers	**Output**	**# of Param**	**Layers**	**Output**	**# of Param**
Input Layer	(256, 256, 1)	—	Input Layer	(256, 256, 1)	—
Conv Layer	(254, 254, 8))	72	Conv Layer	(254, 254, 4)	40
Conv Layer	(254, 254, 8))	72	Pool Layer	(127, 127, 4))	0
Conv Layer	(254, 254, 4))	36	Conv Layer	(25, 125, 4))	148
Conv Layer	(254, 254, 4))	36	Pool Layer	(62, 62, 4))	0
Concat Layer	(254, 254, 8))	0	Conv Layer	(60, 60, 4))	148
Conv Layer	(252, 252, 4))	292	Pool Layer	(30, 30, 4))	0
Pool Layer	(126, 126, 4))	0	—	—	—
Flatten Layer	(63504)	0	Flatten Layer	(3600)	0

Layer	Output	# of Param
Concatenation Layer	(67104)	0
Dense	(64)	4294720
Dropout	(64)	—
Dense	(32)	2080
Dropout	(32)	—
Dense	(24)	792
Dropout	(24)	—
Dense	(# of Classes)	75
Total Trainable Parameters = 4 ,298 519		

3.3 Experimental Matrices

The proposed hybrid networks are thoroughly examined using several experimental evaluations. Therefore, overall accuracy (OA), precision, recall, and $F1 - score$ of the test set is evaluated by using the following mathematical equations [15];

$$OA = \frac{1}{P}\sum_{K=1}^{P} TP_K \tag{3}$$

$$Precision = \frac{1}{P}\sum_{K=1}^{P} \frac{TP_K}{TP_K + FP_K} \tag{4}$$

$$Recall = \frac{1}{P}\sum_{K=1}^{P} \frac{TP_K}{TP_K + FN_K} \tag{5}$$

$$F1 - Score = 2 \times \frac{(Recall \times Precision)}{(Recall + Precision)} \tag{6}$$

where p is the number of test samples, TP and TN is true positives and true negatives. FP and FN are false positives and false negatives respectively. The entire evaluations are computed with confusion matrices, which yield 94% OA with 97% accuracy for pitutary and meningioma classes and reduce to 91% for the glioma class as shown in Fig. 3. The statistical test is also presented in Table 3, which gives the validation of the proposed model through the F1-score of 0.94 and 0.98 for glioma and pitutary MRIs and 0.88 for meningiomas through poor balance between precision and recall.

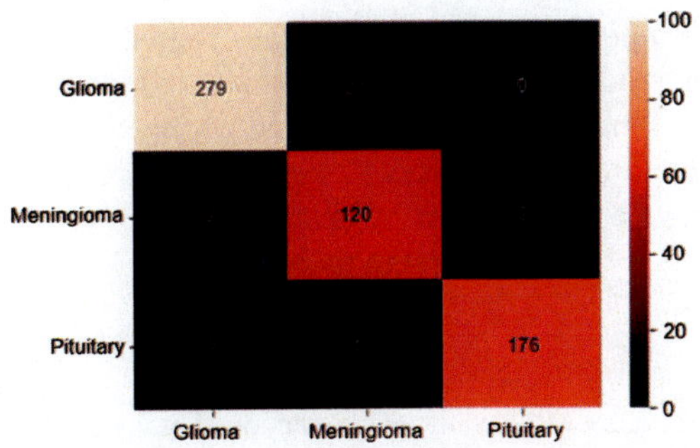

Fig. 3. Confusion matrix of the blind test set using RMSprop optimizer

Table 3. Statistical test of the proposed hybrid deep model.

Class	Glioma	Meningioma	Pitutary
Precision	0.98	0.81	0.98
Recall	0.91	0.97	0.97
F1-score	0.94	0.88	0.98
OA = 0.94			

3.4 Comparison With State-of-the-Art Deep Models

In comparison to the proposed hybrid model, the standard classical model such as mini-VGGNet, AlexNet, SqueezeNet and ResNet-50 consumed more processing time with 0.001 learning rate. The accuracy of mini-VGGNet was 88%, which has unstable validation loss. The overall accuracy achieved by AlexNet was 85%, squeezeNet was 88% and ResNet was 91%. The batch size of 32 is implemented for each model with 10 epochs to converge, whereas, the proposed model outperformed the existing models by achieving an overall accuracy of 94%. Additionally, the work of Ghosal *et al.* [11] achieved an overall accuracy of 89.93% with similar dataset through 29 epochs and needed intense convolutions to achieve higher precision. Furthermore, the transfer learning techniques [8] with similar dataset have achieved 92% accuracy but are limited to data pre-processing steps such as data augmentation and ROI selection, which make the processing time even more expensive with 100 epochs. The proposed work outperformed the previous work by achieving an OA of 94% using only 10 epochs and twelve layers of feature operation.

4 Conclusion

This work investigates the hybrid deep model for the classification of three brain tumors glioma, meningioma, and pitutary. The proposed method uses two different set of deep models squeezeNet and AlexNet to extract features from brain MRI's. The overall accuracy achieved by the hybrid model is 94% with only 10 epochs and minimal pre-processing of an accurate CAD tool. However, multiple improvements remain: Firstly, the model needs fusion to reduce the redundancies caused by the merging of two networks. Secondly, the model need some improvement to reduce the miss-classification of meningioma class. Finally, the data needs to be enriched with more tumor types. In coming future, the research will address the issues to overcome the above mentioned limitations by feeding the hybrid model to autoencoders.

References

1. Amin, J., Sharif, M., Raza, M., Yasmin, M.: Detection of brain tumor based on features fusion and machine learning. J. Ambient Intell. Hum. Comput. 1–17 (2018)
2. Arnold, D.L., Emrich, J.F., Shoubridge, E.A., Villemure, J.G., Feindel, W.: Characterization of astrocytomas, meningiomas, and pituitary adenomas by phosphorus magnetic resonance spectroscopy. J. Neurosurg. **74**(3), 447–453 (1991)
3. Bakas, S., et al.: Identifying the best machine learning algorithms for brain tumor segmentation, progression assessment, and overall survival prediction in the brats challenge. arXiv preprint arXiv:1811.02629 (2018)
4. Bisong, E.: Google colaboratory. In: Building Machine Learning and Deep Learning Models on Google Cloud Platform, pp. 59–64. Springer, Heidelberg (2019)
5. Cheng, J.: Brain tumor dataset. figshare. dataset (2018)
6. Cheng, J., et al.: Enhanced performance of brain tumor classification via tumor region augmentation and partition. PloS One **10**(10), e0140381 (2015)
7. Cheng, J., et al.: Retrieval of brain tumors by adaptive spatial pooling and fisher vector representation. PloS One **11**(6), e0157112 (2016)
8. Deepak, S., Ameer, P.: Brain tumor classification using deep CNN features via transfer learning. Comput. Biol. Med. **111**, 103345 (2019)
9. Forsyth, P.A., Posner, J.B.: Headaches in patients with brain tumors: a study of 111 patients. Neurology **43**(9), 1678 (1993)
10. Ghassemi, N., Shoeibi, A., Rouhani, M.: Deep neural network with generative adversarial networks pre-training for brain tumor classification based on MR images. Biomed. Signal Process. Control **57**, 101678 (2020)
11. Ghosal, P., Nandanwar, L., Kanchan, S., Bhadra, A., Chakraborty, J., Nandi, D.: Brain tumor classification using resnet-101 based squeeze and excitation deep neural network. In: 2019 Second International Conference on Advanced Computational and Communication Paradigms (ICACCP), pp. 1–6. IEEE (2019)
12. Iandola, F.N., Han, S., Moskewicz, M.W., Ashraf, K., Dally, W.J., Keutzer, K.: SqueezeNet: AlexNet-level accuracy with 50x fewer parameters and <0.5 mb model size. arXiv preprint arXiv:1602.07360 (2016)
13. Krizhevsky, A., Sutskever, I., Hinton, G.E.: Imagenet classification with deep convolutional neural networks. Commun. ACM **60**(6), 84–90 (2017)
14. Li, Y., Zhang, H., Shen, Q.: Spectral–spatial classification of hyperspectral imagery with 3D convolutional neural network. Remote Sens. **9**(1), 67 (2017)
15. Narmatha, C., Eljack, S.M., Tuka, A.A.R.M., Manimurugan, S., Mustafa, M.: A hybrid fuzzy brain-storm optimization algorithm for the classification of brain tumor MRI images. J. Ambient Intell. Hum. Comput. 1–9 (2020)
16. Pashaei, A., Sajedi, H., Jazayeri, N.: Brain tumor classification via convolutional neural network and extreme learning machines. In: 2018 8th International Conference on Computer and Knowledge Engineering (ICCKE), pp. 314–319. IEEE (2018)

17. Paul, J.S., Plassard, A.J., Landman, B.A., Fabbri, D.: Deep learning for brain tumor classification. In: Medical Imaging 2017: Biomedical Applications in Molecular, Structural, and Functional Imaging, vol. 10137, p. 1013710. International Society for Optics and Photonics (2017)
18. Rehman, A., Naz, S., Razzak, M.I., Akram, F., Imran, M.: A deep learning-based framework for automatic brain tumors classification using transfer learning. Circ. Syst. Signal Process. **39**(2), 757–775 (2020)
19. Ucuzal, H., Yaşar, Ş., Çolak, C.: Classification of brain tumor types by deep learning with convolutional neural network on magnetic resonance images using a developed web-based interface. In: 2019 3rd International Symposium on Multidisciplinary Studies and Innovative Technologies (ISMSIT), pp. 1–5. IEEE (2019)
20. Wong, D., Yip, S.: Pathology of primary brain tumors—gliomas. In: Comprehensive Overview of Modern Surgical Approaches to Intrinsic Brain Tumors, pp. 121–137. Elsevier (2019)
21. Zhou, M., et al.: Radiomics in brain tumor: image assessment, quantitative feature descriptors, and machine-learning approaches. Am. J. Neuroradiol. **39**(2), 208–216 (2018)

A Systematic Literature Review of Machine Learning Applications for Community-Acquired Pneumonia

Daniel Lozano-Rojas[1](✉), Robert C. Free[1](✉), Alistair A. McEwan[2](✉), and Gerrit Woltmann[3](✉)

[1] University of Leicester, Leicester LE1 7HR, UK
{dlr10,rob.free}@leicester.ac.uk
[2] University of Derby, Derby DE22 1GB, UK
A.McEwan@derby.ac.uk
[3] Department of Respiratory Medicine, University Hospitals of Leicester NHS Trust, Leicester, UK

Abstract. Community acquired pneumonia (CAP) is an acute respiratory disease with a high mortality rate. CAP management follows clinical and radiological diagnosis, severity evaluation and standardised treatment protocols. Although established in practice, protocols are labour intensive, time-critical and can be error prone, as their effectiveness depends on clinical expertise. Thus, an approach for capturing clinical expertise in a more analytical way is desirable both in terms of cost, expediency, and patient outcome. This paper presents a systematic literature review of Machine Learning (ML) applied to CAP. A search of three scholarly international databases revealed 23 relevant peer reviewed studies, that were categorised and evaluated relative to clinical output. Results show interest in the application of ML to CAP, particularly in image processing for diagnosis, and an opportunity for further investigation in the application of ML; both for patient outcome prediction and treatment allocation. We conclude our review by identifying potential areas for future research in applying ML to improve CAP management. This research was co-funded by the NIHR Leicester Biomedical Research Centre and the University of Leicester.

Keywords: Community acquired pneumonia · Machine Learning · CAP prediction · CAP outcome prediction · CAP treatment

1 Introduction

Pneumonia is a respiratory condition that represents a worldwide public health concern, since it involves high mortality, affects Intensive Care Unit (ICU) capacity, and results in high costs for health systems [1]; with annual costs for care and management of €2.5 billion in Europe and $9.5 billion in the United States [2,3].

R. Su et al. (Eds.): MICAD 2021, LNEE 784, pp. 292–301, 2022.
https://doi.org/10.1007/978-981-16-3880-0_30

Community acquired pneumonia (CAP) occurs when infection is transmitted outside hospitals and in people over the age of 16. CAP management comprises diagnosis, severity prediction, and treatment with or without hospital and/or ICU admission. Individuals are diagnosed using X-rays to identify "shadowing clusters" in the lungs. If admitted, Hospital-based severity assessment generally employs standardized scoring systems evaluating severity based on patient's symptoms and signs - for instance CURB65, PSI, ADROP. Assessments include baseline physiological observations as well as biochemical and haematological tests. CAP treatment may be delivered on general respiratory wards or involve ICU care, and most importantly involves pathogen directed antibiotic therapies and also other measures [1].

Machine Learning (ML) and Artificial Intelligence (AI) have been successfully applied to respiratory medicine conditions. For instance, Angelini et al. discussed the detection of pulmonary tuberculosis from radiographs, and identification of pathologically enlarged intrathoracic nodes from computed tomographies (CTs) [4]. Complementary, Chumbita et al. briefly discussed whether ML can be employed to improve CAP management [5].

This paper presents a structured review of peer-reviewed literature of ML applied to CAP management, classifying studies and results with the aim of identifying areas that may benefit from further research. The paper is structured as follows: in Sect. 2, we set out the approach used to carry out our review; Sect. 3 presents the papers that meet the review criteria and their clinical classifications; and in Sect. 4, findings of our review are discussed along with our conclusions and potential further study.

2 Methodology

The review was carried out using the methodology of Petersen et al. [6], and following the PRISMA statement checklist for systematic reviews in healthcare science [7]. The steps taken included: i) define the research questions (RQ) (Sect. 2.1); ii) define search terms and screen results (Sect. 2.2); and iii) classification and extraction of information (Sect. 2.3).

2.1 Research Questions

A total of five research questions were proposed:

1. What ML and data-based approaches have been employed to support CAP management? Identifies main clinical outputs where ML has contributed to CAP management.
2. What kind of data and features have been used and which sources studied? Evaluates relevance of data used in studies and consequently the generalisation and validation of those studies.
3. What statistical and AI approaches have been tested? Maps the extent, and complexity of ML techniques applied to CAP.

4. How have the AI models been assessed and compared? Enables performance assessment of algorithms and models used in literature, thus enabling definition of state-of-the-art in the domain.
5. What is the level of interpretability that models have reached? Lack of interpretability is regarded as a limitation for use of models in clinical settings.

2.2 Searching and Screening

A comprehensive search was performed using three major scholarly international libraries—PubMed, ScienceDirect, and Web of Science. The search term is given in Fig. 1, and only articles published in peer reviewed conferences or journals between January 1990 and June 2020 were considered. This period gathers the main articles in the field.

("artificial intelligence" OR "data science" OR "machine learning" OR "adaptive models") AND ("severity" OR "outcome" OR "mortality" OR "prediction" OR "diagnosis") AND ("pneumonia")

Fig. 1. Searched terms in scholarly international libraries

Articles were screened for inclusion or exclusion in two stages. In the first stage they were considered based on title, keywords, and abstract. Then, Articles were screened based on full content. Those that addressed any phase of CAP management using ML or adaptive models (not necessarily AI) were included. Those where content is not novel research (reviews, case reports, opinions etc.), or relate to respiratory disease that is not pneumonia, or do not present adaptive/AI models were excluded. Articles primarily relating to COVID-19 were also excluded.

2.3 Classification and Data Extraction

Included articles were subjected to classification considering both clinical utility and ML output. Four categories were considered: *diagnosis* (presence of the disease in patients), *outcome prediction* (severity, course of disease, and mortality), *ICU admission prediction* (ICU outcomes), and *treatment* (predicted treatment for specific patients). For each study we extracted the following information:

Data: Our study considered the analysis of types of data (such as images, text, time series, tabular); the size of data sets (number of records); and the data source. These considerations are necessary as ML models use data to calculate hyper parameters that determine patterns between features and target values that are then used to classify new data.

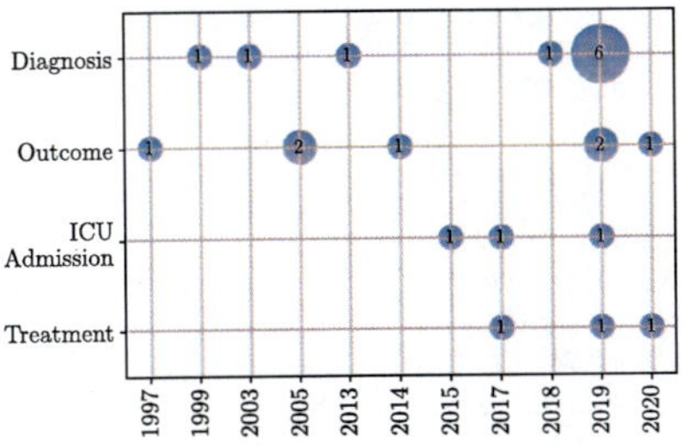

Fig. 2. Year and clinical contribution

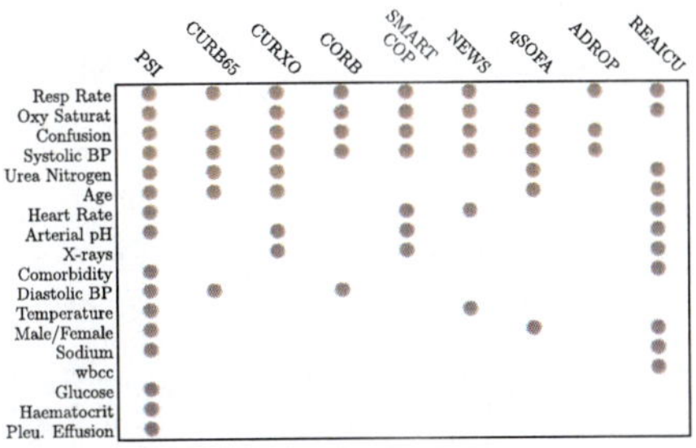

Fig. 3. CAP scoring and features

Algorithms: The study considered different classifications of algorithms including relational models: Causal Probabilistic Networks, Markov Chains, Bayesian networks, logistic regression (LR), Decision Trees, Random Forest (RF), Support Vector Machines (SVM), rule based heuristics. And non relational models: Boosting methods, Neural Networks (NN), Convolutional NN (CNN), Generalised Additive Models (GAM).

Performance: The study considered different performance measurements including precision, sensitivity, specificity, F1 and mainly AUROC curves that present variation of trade-off between sensitivity and specificity depending on decision threshold.

3 Results

Initial searching found 578 articles—201 in PubMed, 239 in Science Direct, and 138 in Web of Science. First stage screening reduced this to 94, and second stage, to 23 articles that were deemed relevant. Classification is shown in Fig. 2: 10 on diagnosis, 7 on outcome prediction, 3 on ICU admission prediction, and 3 on treatment. CAP specific data was used in 15, the other 8 were not specific about the type of data although their approach suggested it may be CAP specific.

The majority of studies were published from 2017 onwards with the earliest in 1997 (Fig. 2)—indicating significant previous and recent interest in the area. In terms of the types of data (Fig. 4), hospital admissions data was the most frequent (12), followed by chest X-ray images (6), time series of electronic health records (EHR) (2), text medical reports (2), and statistical meta-data (1). In terms of size, four studies used data sets with fewer than 1000 samples, four greater than 20000, and the rest an intermediate size. Moreover, features employed were mostly associated to data relevant to CAP severity scores such as oxygen saturation, respiratory rate and those presented in Fig. 3.

In terms of techniques, the most common were relational algorithms. CNN and DL algorithms were mainly used for classification of image diagnosis. Studies involving NN presented before 2012 (5) were simpler than those after (2)—fewer hidden layers and without regularisation methods. Most of the studies (13) use AUROC for performance and accuracy measurement.

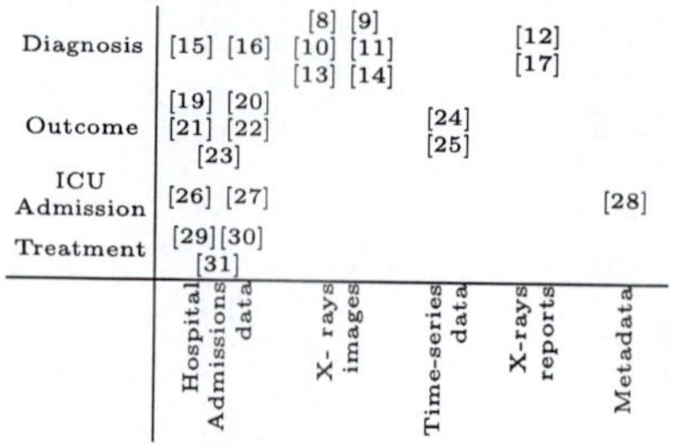

Fig. 4. Distribution of articles

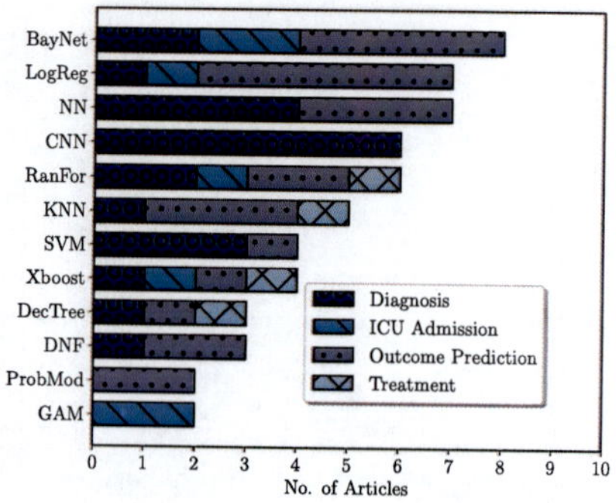

Fig. 5. Frequency of algorithms

3.1 Diagnosis

Diagnosis is the primary topic of ten articles, seven of which focus on image classification [8–14], and three apply the model to clinical data [15–17].

Two established datasets were identified as primary sources for these studies. These consist of ChestX-Ray14 from Kaggle (112,120 frontal chest X-ray images from 30,085 patients [10]) and CheXpert (a set of chest X-rays for automated interpretation of different chest conditions, labelled by radiologists [18]).

Models were mainly directed to identify shadowing clusters in lungs, with results defined as a diagnosis classification. These image processing studies are the most recent corresponding to those published between 2018 and 2020 in Fig. 2.

Knok et al. implemented a VGG16 CNN with 94% accuracy using ChestX-Ray14, also fine-tuned the network using a drop-outs technique in the final three dense layers [9], although this model would benefit from further evaluation as the validation set was small and unbalanced (532 images and 73% as health lungs). Varshni et al. used different CNN architectures (XCeption, VGG16-19, ResNet50, DenseNet121-169) as feature extractors, with classification performed using relation methods (SVM, Naïve Bayes, KNN and RF) resulting in a total of 24 models tested [10]. In this work, the best AUROC reported was 0.8 using a DenseNet169 ensemble with a SVM classifier. Vijendran et al. reported a NN employing online sequential learning with an accuracy of 92% for the same dataset [13].

CheXpert was used to interpret real-time chest images for different lung conditions reporting an AUROC of 0.9 for pneumonia diagnosis, 0.88 for pleural effusion and 0.79 for multilobar anomaly [12].

Alternative models have exhibited less accuracy. O'Quinn et al. pre-process data to balance the number of positive and negative samples, resulting in an accuracy of 72% [11]. A comparison of CNN and classic classifiers reports CNN with the best performance at 84% [14]. While an accuracy of 83% was obtained by identifying affected regions of the lungs on the image [8].

DeLisle et al. describe studies that evaluate text data and assess their models with recall, precision, and specificity using a heuristic incorporating EHR reports to diagnose acute respiratory disease [15]. Additionally, Chapman et al. present statistical frameworks that analyse X-ray reports to predict CAP, the best of which is a Bayesian Network [17].

3.2 Outcome Prediction

CAP scoring systems and features are depicted in Fig. 3 and are used as a benchmark for ML models to predict mortality or severity. Studies of clinical outcome prediction have utilised relational algorithms [19–21]. LR and single layer networks have been used to greater effect, showing the promise that ML, and more complex models, may deliver [21].

In more recent articles, rules-based models were proposed to predict 90-day mortality, with a highest AUROC reported of 0.78 [24]. In another study, the SepsisFinder model was developed in and predicted 30-day mortality and bacteraemia [22]. At 0.811, the AUROC reported for this model is higher than that reported for PSI (0.799) and CURB65 (0.75), although a comparison with other ML models is not presented. Shimzizu et al. developed three models to assess the risk of in-hospital mortality: XGBoost, LR, and RF with AUROCs of 0.88, 0.84 and 0.83, respectively [23].

Use of Markov Chains based on qSOFA scores for time series analysis produces an outcome prediction matrix [25]. Although the authors note that it is limited as it does not consider systematic implications of the disease. Nevertheless, this study is the most advanced in terms of predicting evolution of the disease over time.

3.3 ICU Admission Prediction

Hospital admissions have been studied based on the likelihood of readmission to ICU. In one study, decision trees based on Bayesian models complementing CURB65 were used to determine whether a patient should be treated as an outpatient or ICU patient [28]. Unfortunately the use of metadata from another study meant that direct comparisons could not be drawn, since results were the variance analysis of the model (ANOVA) rather than the validation of it. Possible re-admissions to hospitals have been considered using LR, RF, Boosting, and GAM reporting an AUROC of 0.78 [26, 27]. The benefit of the GAM model is that it can also evaluate interactions between features.

3.4 CAP Treatment

Treatment is a relevant area with few reported studies. Konig et al. created decision trees determining best use of antibiotic combination therapy involving macrolides. It is important to note that although macrolides therapy can be beneficial for CAP management, it is also associated with cardiovascular toxicity.

However, results of this study suggest significantly reduced mortality (27%) when utilised based on their model [29].

Khajehali et al. considered clinical factors affecting admission state and prediction of length of stay. Their model involved imputation of missing values. Bayesian boosting produced the best result in this study with an accuracy of 95.17%—they also reported use of Meropenem as antibiotic to reduce length of stay in patients admitted with CAP [30].

Aetiology (whether the disease is viral or bacterial) was studied using 43 clinical and 17 biological features [31]. Relevance of the features was assessed using LR and predictions were made using an RF classifier on a dataset of 93 samples. This work did not include validation using larger datasets, or evaluation relative to other models.

4 Discussion and Conclusion

This section considers the results of our review relative to the questions presented in Sect. 2.

RQ 1: The main classification or prediction approaches of ML for CAP are: diagnosis, mortality prediction, hospital admission status, and treatment. Diagnosis is the area that has received most attention from an ML perspective particularly analysis of X-ray imaging. There has been limited focus on treatment prediction, lack of studies offering support for intervention and antibiotic selection represents a gap in the field and could prove to be a rewarding area for the application of deep ML models to stratified treatment.

RQ 2: A number of the studies used relatively small datasets (12 with fewer than 3000 samples), mostly from hospital admissions. Non-image based studies included from 7 to 160 data features, with the most relevant presented in (Fig. 3). There is a lack of time-series data, and few studies reported management of missing values or dirty data. Another common issue uncovered in our study concerns the size, reproducibility and scalability of data sets used for evaluation including distribution and characteristics of data, which vary widely. A clear state-of-the-art approach appears not to have emerged yet.

RQ 3: Most studies employed relational algorithms—LR, RF, Bayesian Networks—as shown in Fig. 5. Bayesian networks were mostly naive, implying independence of features, which is unlikely to have clinical utility. Poor LR performance has shown many non-linear dependencies, and unbalanced data in CAP data.

For outcome prediction and ICU admission prediction, NNs have been used, although architectures do not go over three hidden layers. There is certainly scope for further study in this area as Deep Learning and ensemble models have previously been shown to offer benefits in other clinical applications [1,4,5]. There may also be opportunities to exploit transfer learning in this area, or other emerging models such as recurrent NN. At this stage the most promising technique would depend on the research question and data available.

Only one study suggested a fine-tuning process [9]. This group presented the evolution of training and validation sets to identify when the model identified general patterns of data, rather than specifics of training set (overfitting).

RQ 4: AUROC curves are the generally accepted method of reporting and comparing performance of binary classification models, although in some cases accuracy, sensitivity, and specificity are used. This can create issues when drawing comparisons.

RQ 5: Interpretability is as important as performance in clinical settings. Most studies reported typically consider performance without considering this or clinical availability. Typically, due to their nature relational and statistical models exhibit more interpretability than non-relational and DL models.

In summary, this is the first systematic review studying ML applied to CAP. It followed guidelines in both the engineering and clinical domains enabling it to take an interdisciplinary view. There is also an overlap between CAP and other acute respiratory and non-respiratory diseases that may provide further insights. Although the article search was wide and structured, it is possible that other studies—such as those published in libraries that were not included—have been missed.

There are still a lack of key criteria to enable proper assessment, suggesting the field is still in an exploratory stage and further research is required. Classification employed in our study have enabled us to identify some areas that will benefit from further research in terms of clinical processes. Firstly, validation of models for interpretation of diagnostic images. Secondly, the use of time-series and the application of DL to hospital admissions data for mortality and disease progression prediction. Thirdly, research into the application of DL on the predicted effectiveness of interventions and treatment—an area in which there is still paucity of published work, but evidence of clinical demand.

Finally, an increasingly helpful trend in the literature is the reporting of results that follow the TRIPOD checklist [32]—a method of reporting multi variable prediction models that is commonly adopted in medical sciences but less so in DL/ML communities. Although this checklist still presents gaps—for instance standardised metrics, greater adoption of this checklist would facilitate a like-for-like comparison and evaluation of models from different studies.

Acknowledgments. This research was co-funded by the NIHR Leicester Biomedical Research Centre and the University of Leicester.

References

1. Cillóniz, C., Dominedò, C., Pericàs, J.M., Rodriguez-Hurtado, D., Torres, A.: Community-acquired pneumonia in critically ill very old patients: a growing problem. Eur. Respir. Rev. (2020). https://doi.org/10.1183/16000617.0126-2019
2. Gibson, G., Gibson, C., Loddenkemper, R., Sibille, Y., Society, E.R., Lundbäck, B.: The European lung white book: respiratory health and disease in Europe. European Respiratory Society (2013)

3. America-Thoracic-Society (ATS): Top 20 pneumonia facts - 2019 (2019). https://www.thoracic.org/patients/patient-resources/resources/top-pneumonia-facts.pdf
4. Angelini, E., Dahan, S., Shah, A.: Unravelling machine learning: insights in respiratory medicine. Eur. Respir. J. **54**(6), 3–6 (2019). https://doi.org/10.1183/13993003.01216-2019
5. Chumbita, M., et al.: Can artificial intelligence improve the management of pneumonia. J. Clin. Med. **9**(1), 248 (2020). https://doi.org/10.3390/jcm9010248
6. Petersen, K., Vakkalanka, S., Kuzniarz, L.: Guidelines for conducting systematic mapping studies in software engineering: an update. Inf. Softw. Technol. **64**, 1–18 (2015). https://doi.org/10.1016/j.infsof.2015.03.007
7. Moher, D., Liberati, A., Tetzlaff, J., Altman, D.: PRISMA 2009 flow diagram (2009). https://doi.org/10.1371/journal.pmed1000097
8. Sirazitdinov, I., Kholiavchenko, M., Mustafaev, T., Yixuan, Y., Kuleev, R., Ibragimov, B.: Deep neural network ensemble for pneumonia localization from a large-scale chest x-ray database. Comput. Electr. Eng. **78**, 388–399 (2019). https://doi.org/10.1016/j.compeleceng.2019.08.004
9. Knok, Ž, Pap, K., Hrnčić, M.: Implementation of intelligent model for pneumonia detection. Tehn. Glasnik **13**(4), 315–322 (2019). https://doi.org/10.31803/tg-20191023102807
10. Varshni, D., Thakral, K., Agarwal, L., Nijhawan, R., Mittal, A.: Pneumonia detection using CNN based feature extraction. In: Proceedings of 2019 3rd IEEE International Conference on Electrical, Computer and Communication Technologies, ICECCT 2019, pp. 1–7 (2019). https://doi.org/10.1109/ICECCT.2019.8869364
11. O'Quinn, W., Haddad, R.J., Moore, D.L.: Pneumonia radiograph diagnosis utilizing deep learning network. In: Proceedings of 2019 IEEE 2nd International Conference on Electronic Information and Communication Technology, ICEICT 2019, pp. 763–767 (2019). https://doi.org/10.1109/ICEICT.2019.8846438
12. Dean, N., Irvin, J.A., Samir, P.S., Jephson, A., Conner, K., Lungren, M.P.: Real-time electronic interpretation of digital chest images using artificial intelligence in emergency department patients suspected of pneumonia. In: Respiratory Infections, p. OA3309. European Respiratory Society (2019). https://doi.org/10.1183/13993003.congress-2019.OA3309
13. Vijendran, S., Models, A.S.: Deep online sequential extreme learning machines and its application in pneumonia detection. In: 2019 8th International Conference on Industrial Technology and Management Deep, vol. 3, pp. 311–316. IEEE (2019)
14. Jakhar, K., Hooda, N.: Big data deep learning framework using keras: a case study of pneumonia prediction. In: 2018 4th International Conference on Computing Communication and Automation, ICCCA 2018, August 2019 (2018). https://doi.org/10.1109/CCAA.2018.8777571
15. DeLisle, S., et al.: Using the electronic medical record to identify community-acquired pneumonia: toward a replicable automated strategy. PLoS One **8**(8), 2–9 (2013). https://doi.org/10.1371/journal.pone.0070944
16. Heckerling, P.S., Gerber, B.S., Tape, T.G., Wigton, R.S.: Prediction of community-acquired pneumonia using artificial neural networks. Med. Decis. Making **23**(2), 112–121 (2003). https://doi.org/10.1177/0272989X03251247
17. Chapman, W.W., Haug, P.J.: Comparing expert systems for identifying chest x-ray reports that support pneumonia. In: Proceedings/AMIA ... Annual Symposium. AMIA Symposium, pp. 216–220 (1999)
18. Irvin, J., et al.: CheXpert: a large chest radiograph dataset with uncertainty labels and expert comparison. In: Proceedings of the AAAI Conference on Artificial Intelligence, vol. 33, pp. 590–597 (2019). https://doi.org/10.1609/aaai.v33i01.3301590

19. Cooper, G.F., et al.: Predicting dire outcomes of patients with community acquired pneumonia. J. Biomed. Inform. **38**(5), 347–366 (2005). https://doi.org/10.1016/j.jbi.2005.02.005
20. Visweswaran, S., Cooper, G.F.: Patient-specific models for predicting the outcomes of patients with community acquired pneumonia. In: AMIA Annual Symposium Proceedings, pp. 759–763 (2005)
21. Cooper, G.F., et al.: An evaluation of machine-learning methods for predicting pneumonia mortality. Artif. Intell. Med. **9**(2), 107–138 (1997). https://doi.org/10.1016/S0933-3657(96)00367-3
22. Ward, L., et al.: A machine-learning model for prediction of mortality among patients with community-acquired pneumonia. In: European Congress for Clinical Micrbiology and Infectious Diseases (ECCMID), vol. 779 (2019)
23. Shimizu, S., Hara, S., Fushimi, K.: PRS55 predicting the risk of in-hospital mortality in adult community-aquired pneumonia patients with machine learning: a retrospective analysis of routinely collected health data. Value Health **22**, S882 (2019). https://doi.org/10.1016/j.jval.2019.09.2544
24. Wu, C., Rosenfeld, R., Clermont, G.: Using data-driven rules to predict mortality in severe community acquired pneumonia. PLoS One **9**(4) (2014). https://doi.org/10.1371/journal.pone.0089053
25. Przybilla, J., et al.: Markov state modelling of disease courses and mortality risks of patients with community-acquired pneumonia. J. Clin. Med. **9**(2), 393 (2020). https://doi.org/10.3390/jcm9020393
26. Makam, A.N., et al.: Predicting 30-day pneumonia readmissions using electronic health record data. J. Hosp. Med. **12**(4), 209–216 (2017). https://doi.org/10.12788/jhm.2711
27. Caruana, R., Lou, Y., Gehrke, J., Koch, P., Sturm, M., Elhadad, N.: Intelligible models for healthcare: predicting pneumonia risk and hospital 30-day readmission. In: Proceedings of the 21th ACM SIGKDD International Conference on Knowledge Discovery and Data Mining, KDD 2015, pp. 1721–1730. Association for Computing Machinery, New York (2015). https://doi.org/10.1145/2783258.2788613
28. Baez, A.A., Cochon, L., Nicolas, J.M.: A Bayesian decision support sequential model for severity of illness predictors and intensive care admissions in pneumonia. BMC Med. Inform. Decis. Mak. **19**(1), 1–9 (2019). https://doi.org/10.1186/s12911-019-1015-5
29. König, R., et al.: Macrolide combination therapy for hospitalised CAP patients. An individualised approach supported by machine learning. Eur. Respir. J. (2019)
30. Khajehali, N., Alizadeh, S.: Extract critical factors affecting the length of hospital stay of pneumonia patient by data mining (case study: an Iranian hospital). Artif. Intell. Med. **83**, 2–13 (2017). https://doi.org/10.1016/j.artmed.2017.06.010
31. Lhommet, C., et al.: Predicting the microbial cause of community-acquired pneumonia: can physicians or a data-driven method differentiate viral from bacterial pneumonia at patient presentation? BMC Pulm. Med. **20**, 1–9 (2020)
32. Collins, G.S., et al.: Transparent reporting of a multivariable prediction model for individual prognosis or diagnosis (TRIPOD): explanation and elaboration. Ann. Intern. Med. (2015). https://doi.org/10.7326/M14-0698

Photograph to X-ray Image Translation for Anatomical Mouse Mapping in Preclinical Nuclear Molecular Imaging

Eleftherios Fysikopoulos[1,2](✉), Maritina Rouchota[1,2], Vasilis Eleftheriadis[2], Christina-Anna Gatsiou[2], Irinaios Pilatis[2], Sophia Sarpaki[2], George Loudos[1,2], Spiros Kostopoulos[1], and Dimitrios Glotsos[1]

[1] Biomedical Engineering Department, University of West Attica, Athens, Greece
[2] Bioemission Technology Solutions (BIOEMTECH), Lefkippos Attica Technology Park, N.C.S.R Demokritos, Athens, Greece

Abstract. We present preliminary results of an off-the-shelf approach for the translation of a photographic mouse image to an X-ray scan for anatomical mouse mapping, but not for diagnosis, in functional 2D molecular imaging techniques, such radionuclide and optical imaging. It is well known that preclinical molecular imaging accelerates the drug development process. However, commercial imaging systems have high purchase cost, require high service contracts, special facilities and trained staff. As an alternative, planar molecular imaging systems provide several advantages including lower complexity and decreased cost among others, making them affordable to small and medium sized groups which work in the field, bridging the gap between biodistributions studies and 3D imaging systems. A pix2pix network was trained to predict a realistic X-ray mouse image from a photographic one (simplifying the hardware and cost requirement compared to standard X-rays), giving the potential to have an anatomical map of the mouse, along with the functional information of a molecular planar imaging modality.

Keywords: Image-to-image translation · Molecular nuclear imaging · Artificial X-ray · PET · SPECT · Deep learning · pix2pix

1 Introduction

Molecular imaging techniques play an important role in the drug development process by allowing the non-invasive study of several biological and biochemical phenomena during preclinical and clinical studies. It is well known that the time from synthesis to market of a new pharmaceutical compound is between 12 and 15 years. [1]. This is the daily mission of thousands research teams worldwide. It is well proven that small animal imaging speeds up this work, increases accuracy and decreases cost [2–4]. Radionuclide molecular imaging techniques, such as Positron emission tomography (PET) and single photon emission computed tomography (SPECT) have their merit throughout the drug discovery process and can be used as decision-makings tools at the early stages of testing a new compound [1–4].

R. Su et al. (Eds.): MICAD 2021, LNEE 784, pp. 302–311, 2022.
https://doi.org/10.1007/978-981-16-3880-0_31

The last decade, the combined use of conventional anatomic imaging (i.e. X-ray computed tomography (CT) or magnetic resonance imaging (MRI)) with functional imaging (i.e. PET or SPECT) has led to the development of multimodality systems (PET/CT, SPECT/CT, PET/MRI etc.) increasing the reliability of the diagnostic data by using both imaging techniques simultaneously [5, 6]. On the other hand, several limitations arise due to increased complexity and purchase and maintenance costs [7, 8]. Thus, the majority of research groups, that work in the field, rely on biodistribution studies and do not use imaging in their research [9–11].

Bridging the gap between biodistributions and 3D imaging systems, planar imaging may prove to be a good alternative, since it can be effectively be used to track a new tracer from zero point in time post-injection and over a long period. Optical imaging is a well-established method for this purpose [12], offering high sensitivity, simplicity and decreased cost, while not quantitative with low depth penetration and limited clinical translation [2]. On the other hand, radioisotope planar imaging provides semi-quantitative images of high spatial resolution and clinical translation retaining also simplicity, low cost and high throughput properties at the expense of access to radioactivity [13, 14]. Both techniques have been used, either in commercial systems (In-Vivo MS FX PRO, Bruker) or prototypes [15], along with X-ray imaging, which provide useful anatomic information, at the expense of increased complexity and cost.

In this work, we present preliminary results of an off-the-shelf approach for the translation of a photographic mouse image to an X-ray scan for anatomical mouse mapping in functional 2D molecular imaging techniques. A wide variety of problems have been previously be expressed as translation of an input image to an output image including enhancement tasks (i.e. in terms of sharpening, color balance, contrast etc.) or mapping to a different scene (i.e. aerial photo to map, sketch to photo etc.) [16]. During the last five years, image-to-image translation techniques have also been used in medical imaging for several tasks, including segmentation, denoising, super-resolution, modality conversion, and reconstruction [17]. The motivation, of the current study, is to produce artificially X-ray images for animal mapping and not for diagnosis, using simple hardware, such as a conventional image sensor and deep learning techniques. Thus, enhancing 2D functional imaging signals from radionuclide or optical imaging systems, with useful localization information without adding complexity and increase the cost of manufacture.

2 Methodology

We chose to treat the problem of X-ray prediction from a photographic image, as an image-to-image translation task, using a well-known pix2pix network [18]. In that work, instead of tackling the task of translating an input image to an output image with separate, special-purpose machinery related to specific datasets, authors propose a common framework, based on conditional Generative Adversarial Networks (cGANs), in order to predict pixels from pixels in any dataset, in which the aligned image pairs vary in the visual representation, but the renderings, for e.g. edges stay the same. The methodology of current work consists of 2 stages: (a) Data collection and preprocessing; (b) Modelling and performance evaluation.

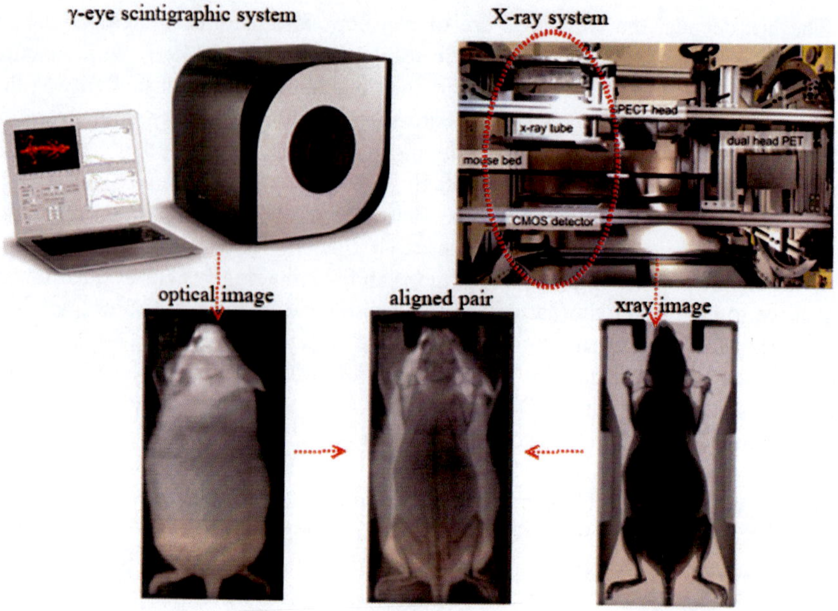

Fig. 1. γ-eye scintigraphic system used to acquire optical images (left); X-ray system used to acquire the corresponding X-ray images (right).

2.1 Data Collection and Preprocessing

We have acquired, up to now, a set of 380 input/output images, in order to train and test the pix2pix network [18]. Input image refer to a photographic mouse image, while output image to the corresponding X-ray image of the same animal. In order to acquire the input images, we use a commercial planar scintigraphic imager, which contains a simple photographic sensor to provide a static optical image of the animal, giving the outline of the mouse as an anatomical mapping solution ("γ-eye", BIOEMTECH, Greece) (Fig. 1 - left). The corresponding X-ray images were acquired using an X-ray tube (Source-Ray Inc., US) and a CMOS detector (C10900D, Hamamatsu, Japan), both mounted on a rotating Gantry (Fig. 1 - right). Both systems are optimized for small mice imaging providing a field of view of 50 mm × 100 mm.

All animal procedures were approved by the General Directorate of Veterinary Services (Athens, Attica Prefecture, Greece) and the Bioethical Committee of the Institution (Permit number: EL 25 BIO 022). In order to reduce the number of animals used in the current study, we acquire 5 paired images for each animal by placing it in 5 different poses upon the hosting bed. We assumed that this procedure will not affect the results as the small mice used in molecular imaging studies have similar dimensions and weight. Animals were anesthetized with isoflurane in all cases and kept warmed during the scans. The study involved, up to now, 62 white and 14 black swiss albino mice, leading to a total number of 380 input/output images. The dataset is currently unbalanced as far as concern the mouse color, due to the limited access to black mice. On the other hand, the number of black mice is enough in order to give us a feedback regarding the balance

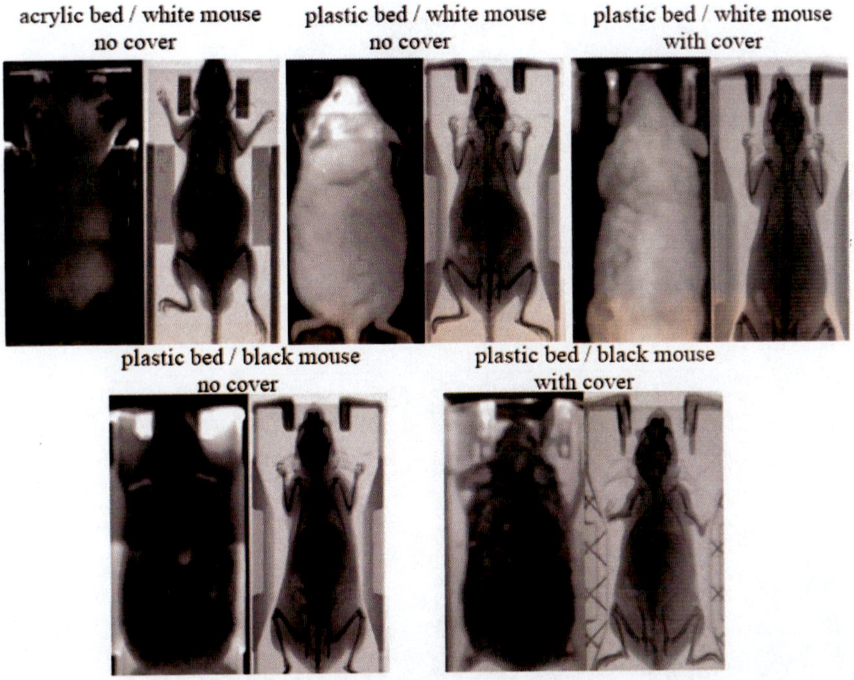

Fig. 2. Aligned image pairs used for training and testing. The pix2pix network was evaluated against the following parameters: mouse color; different background due to different material and color of the animal hosting bed and the presence or absence of acrylic cover.

that the training dataset should have, highlighting potential limitations of the method in the current problem. Except mouse color the method was evaluated against different animal hosting beds (plastic bed with white color and black mice; plastic bed with black color and white mice; acrylic transparent bed and white mice) with or without acrylic cover, usually used in small animal imaging applications to avoid potential escape of the animal due to anesthesia malfunctioning during the experiment.

These parameters lead to different background in both input and output images. The potential pairs used for training and testing are illustrated in Fig. 2. Finally, the pair images have been processed in terms of alignment (Fig. 1-down middle). The size of each input/output image, used to train and test the pix2pix network, was 512 × 1024 pixels corresponding to the 50 mm × 100 mm field of view. Table 1 summarizes the different categories along with the number of paired images used for training and testing from each category. We tried to keep a ratio higher than 10% between the test images and the total dataset in each occasion. The unbalanced nature of the dataset leads to different ratios in each category, however as the dataset grow, we aim to achieve a 10% ratio between test images and total dataset in each category.

Table 1. Train and test dataset detailed characteristics.

Mouse color	Bed color	Cover	Train	Test
White	Black plastic	No	175	20
White	Black plastic	Yes	8	2
White	Acrylic transparent	No	90	15
Black	White plastic	No	44	5
Black	White plastic	Yes	17	4
Total			**334**	**46**

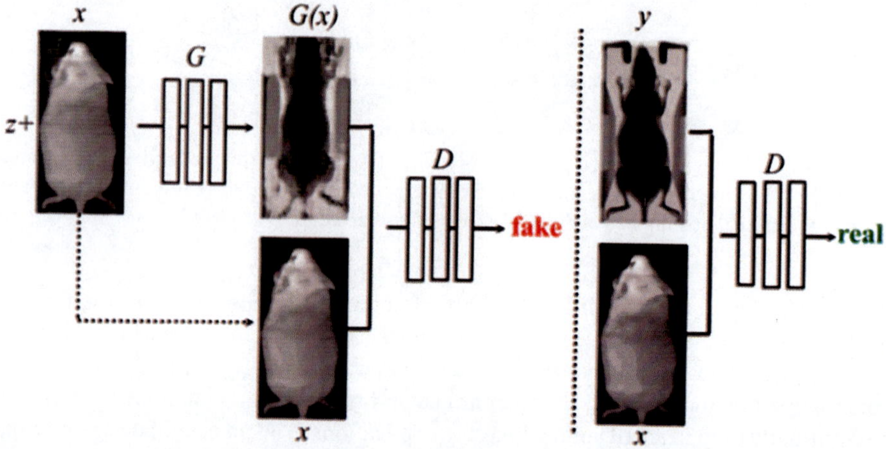

Fig. 3. Training procedure of the conditional GAN used in the present study. The discriminator, *D*, learns to classify between fake (synthesized by the generator X-ray images) and real {optical, X-ray} tuples. The generator, *G*, learns to fool the discriminator.

2.2 Modelling and Performance Evaluation

A cGAN learns a mapping from an input image x and random noise vector z to output image y, $G : \{x, z\} \rightarrow y$. The random noise vector z is required to prevent the generator from producing deterministic outputs and hence fail to match new distributions. The generator G was trained to produce realistic X-ray images that cannot be distinguished from real X-ray images (used as ground truth), by an adversarially trained discriminator, D, which is trained to do as well as possible at detecting the generator's "fakes". The procedure is illustrated in Fig. 3. For generator the model uses a "U-Net"-based architecture [18, 19] and for the discriminator a convolutional "PatchGAN" classifier is used [18]. The pix2pix network was trained with 200 epochs.

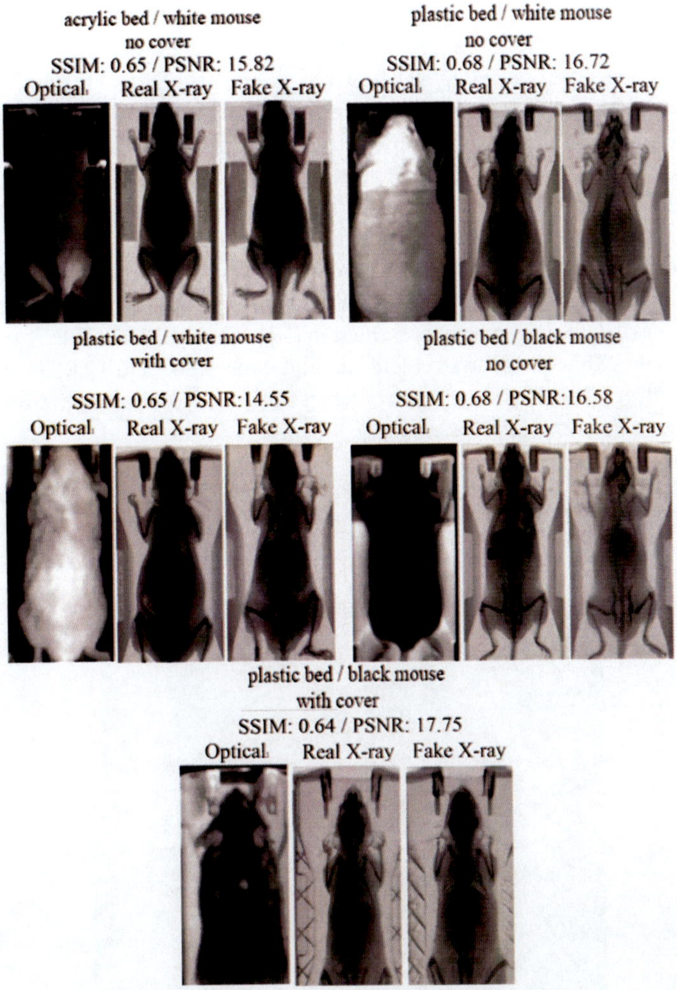

Fig. 4. Test results for trained pix2pix network. Indicative "fake" produced X-ray, along with the input optical image and ground truth for all five different occasions studied.

After the training process, the generator, G, was used to produced realistic X-ray images from given input optical images in the test dataset (refer to Table 1). Finally, we evaluated the performance of the pix2pix network, to the above described dataset using two metrics: (a) peak signal-to-noise ratio (PSNR) and (b) structural similarity index measure (SSIM). These metrics have been used previously to assess the quality of cGAN results quantitatively in comparison to other metrics such as mean absolute error (MAE) and mean square error (MSE), which in some cases are not appropriate for evaluating the results of the GAN approach [20–22].

3 Results

Figure 4 presents indicative test results of the five different occasions studied in the current work. "Fake" produced images from the trained generator of the pix2pix network are presented along with the corresponding input/optical image and the ground truth. These preliminary results show the ability of the pix2pix network to solve the problem of the translation of a photographic mouse image to a pseudo-Xray one that can be used for anatomical mapping, but not for diagnosis, along with molecular functional imaging techniques. The SSIM and PSNR mean values on the test dataset were calculated equal to 0.69 and 16.95. Values are comparable with those presented in [22], in which 4 approaches (including pix2pix network, which was used as a baseline) were evaluated on a well-known dataset primarily presented in [23]. The SSIM and PSNR values of the pix2pix model on that dataset was calculated equal to 0.2863 and 12.8684 respectively. Although a different problem is presented in that study the close correlation of the metrics shows the success of our approach.

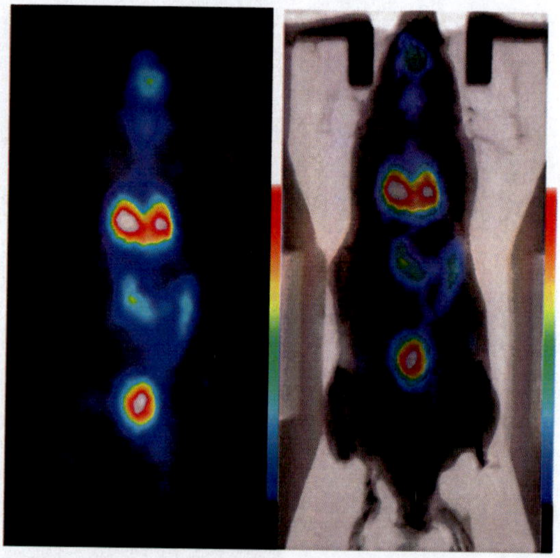

Fig. 5. 99mTc-MDP nuclear image of a healthy mouse fused with the optical image provided in the γ-eye scintigraphic system (left) and the X-ray produced from the pix2pix trained network. The color bar indicates the difference in accumulated activity.

In order to further evaluate the proposed method, a healthy mouse was administered through lung installation with 50 uCi/50 uL of 99mTc-MDP, to study the kinetics of the tracer through this administration route and imaged in the γ-eye scintigraphic system. Figure 5 shows the nuclear image fused with the optical one provided in the γ-eye system and with the predicted X-ray image produced from the pix2pix network. The nuclear image shows the clear targeting of the compound and the biodistribution in kidneys and tumor, as main organs of accumulation. The produced X-ray provides the anatomical map of the small animal enhancing the overall image information.

4 Conclusion and Future Work

Preliminary results of an off-the-shelf approach for the translation of a photographic mouse image to an X-ray scan for anatomical mouse mapping have been presented. We trained a well-established image to image translation network with aligned pairs of optical/X-ray images. The results show that the network predicts an X-ray image with sufficient accuracy for mouse anatomical mapping but not for diagnosis. The calculated metrics are comparable with those achieved in the evaluation of other networks, including also pix2pix, on several datasets [22]. The proposed method can be used in order to enhance planar radionuclide or optical preclinical systems by providing anatomic information along with the functional one, without increasing the manufacture cost and the complexity of the design.

Future work contains the balancing of the dataset in terms of mouse color and different background, in order to optimize the prediction in many potential realistic inputs. Train and test in paired images of lower resolution (128×256, 256×512 pixels) will be performed and metrics will be compared with the presented results. The output image is intended to be used for animal mapping and thus lower resolution may be acceptable if provide better estimation. Finally, a preprocessing step will be developed, in order to extract the background in the X-ray images that are used as the ground truth, as is useless. Image segmentation approaches will be considered as a preprocess step before pix2pix network training.

Acknowledgements. We thank Giorgos Tolias, assistant professor at the Czech Technical University in Prague, for helpful discussions.

This research is co-financed by Greece and the European Union (European Social Fund-ESF) through the Operational Program "Human Resources Development, Education and Life-long Learning 2014–2020" in the context of the project "Deep learning algorithms for molecular imaging applications" (MIS-5050329).

The publication of this research is funded by the University of West Attica, Greece.

References

1. Gomes, C., Abrunhosa, A., Ramos, P., Pauwels, K.: Molecular imaging with SPECT as a tool for drug development. Adv. Drug Deliv. Rev. **63**(7), 547–554 (2010). https://doi.org/10.1016/j.addr.2010.09.015
2. Willmann, J., van Bruggen, N., Dinkelborg, L., Gambhir, S.: Molecular imaging in drug development. Nat. Rev. Drug Disc. **7**, 591–607 (2008). https://doi.org/10.1038/nrd2290
3. Waaijer, S., et al.: Molecular imaging in cancer drug development. J. Nucl. Med. **59**, 726–732 (2018). https://doi.org/10.2967/junmed.116.188045

4. Cherry, S.: In vivo molecular and genomic imaging: new challenges for imaging physics. Phys. Med. Biol. **3**(7), R13 (2004). https://doi.org/10.1088/0031-9155/49/3/r01
5. Cherry, S.: Multimodality imaging: beyond PET/CT and SPECT/CT. Semin. Nucl. Med. **39**(5), 348–353 (2009). https://doi.org/10.1053/j.semnuclmed.2009.03.001
6. Vandenberghe, S., Marsden, P.: PET-MRI: a review of challenges and solutions in the development of integrated multimodality imaging. Med. Biol. **60**, R115 (2015). https://doi.org/10.1088/0031-9155/60/4/r115
7. Zanzonico, P.: Principles of nuclear medicine imaging: planar, SPECT, PET, multimodality, and autoradiography systems. Radiat. Res. **177**, 349–364 (2012). https://doi.org/10.1667/rr2577.1
8. Zaidi, H. (ed.): Molecular Imaging of Small Animals: Instrumentation and Applications. Springer, New York (2014). https://doi.org/10.1007/978-1-4939-0894-3
9. Kumar, D., et al.: Development of technetium-99m labeled ultrafine gold nanobioconjugates for targeted imaging of folate receptor positive cancers. Nucl. Med. Biol. **93**, 1–10 (2020). https://doi.org/10.1016/j.nucmedbio.2020.11.001
10. Vorobyeva, A., et al.: Optimal composition and position of histidine-containing tags improves biodistribution of ^{99m}Tc-labeled DARPin G3. Scient. Rep. **9**, 1–11 (2019). https://doi.org/10.1038/s41598-019-45795-8
11. De Kruijff, R., et al.: Elucidating the influence of tumor presence on the polymersor time in mice. Pharmaceutics **11**, 241 (2019). https://doi.org/10.3390/pharmaceutics11050241
12. Ntziachristos, V., et al.: Planar fluorescence imaging using normalized data. J. Biomed. Opt. **10** (2005). https://doi.org/10.1117/1.2136148
13. Georgiou, M., Fysikopoulos, E., Mikropoulos, K., Fragogeorgi, E., Loudos, G.: Characterization of "γ-eye": a low-cost benchtop mouse-sized gamma camera for dynamic and static imaging studies. Mol. Imag. Biol. **19**(3), 398–407 (2016). https://doi.org/10.1007/s11307-016-1011-4
14. Zhang, H., et al.: Performance evaluation of PETbox: a low cost bench top preclinical PET scanner. Mol. Imag. Biol. **13**(5), 949–961 (2011). https://doi.org/10.1007/s11307-010-0413-y
15. Rouchota, M., et al.: A prototype PET/SPET/X-rays scanner dedicated for whole body small animal studies. Hell. J. Nucl. Med. **20**, 146–153 (2017). https://doi.org/10.1967/s0022449910556
16. Eslami, M., Tabarestani, S., Albarqouni, S., Adell, E., Navab, N., Adjouadi, M.: Image to images translation for multi-task organ segmentation and bone suppression in chest X-ray radiography. IEEE Trans. Med. Imag. **39**, 2553–2565 (2020). https://doi.org/10.1109/TMI.2020.2974159
17. Kaji, S., Kida, S.: Overview of image-to-image translation by use of deep neural networks: denoising, super-resolution, modality conversion, and reconstruction in medical imaging. Radiol. Phys. Technol. **12**(3), 235–248 (2019). https://doi.org/10.1007/s12194-019-00520-y
18. Isola, P., Zhu, J.-Y., Zhou, T., Efros, A.: Image-to-image translation with conditional adversarial networks. In: IEEE Conference on Computer Vision and Pattern Recognition Proceedings (2017). arXiv:1611.07004
19. Ronneberger, O., Fischer, P., Brox, T.: U-Net: convolutional networks for biomedical image segmentation. In: Navab, N., Hornegger, J., Wells, W.M., Frangi, A.F. (eds.) MICCAI 2015. LNCS, vol. 9351, pp. 234–241. Springer, Cham (2015). https://doi.org/10.1007/978-3-319-24574-4_28
20. Salimans, T., Goodfellow, I., Zaremba, W., Cheung, V., Radford, A., Chen, X.: Improved techniques for training GANs. In: NIPS (2016)
21. Kupyn, O., Budzan, V., Mykhailych, M., Mishkin, D., Matas, J.: DeblurGAN: blind motion deblurring using conditional adversarial networks. In: Proceedings of the IEEE Conference on Computer Vision and Pattern Recognition, Salt Lake City, USA, 18–22 June (2018)

22. Yoo, J., Eom, H., Choi, Y.: Image-to-image translation using a cross-domain auto-encoder and decoder. Appl. Sci. **9**(22), 4780 (2019)
23. Cordts, M., et al.: The cityscapes dataset for semantic urban scene understanding. In: Proceedings of the IEEE Conference on Computer Vision and Pattern Recognition (2016)

Active Strain-Statistical Models for Reconstructing Multidimensional Images of Lung Tissue Lesions

Vladimir Kulagin, Dmitry Akimov, Ekaterina O. Guryanova(✉), and Sergey Pavelyev

Russian Technological University (MIREA), Moscow, Russia
guryanova@mirea.ru

Abstract. Coupling augmented reality data with data from previous medical studies is most useful for surgeries on organs with little movement and deformation (e.g., skull, brain, and pancreas), as there is an opportunity to more clearly define the edges of the organ. The proposed coupling methods can be used in other operations. Besides, organ imaging techniques can compensate for the lack of tactile feedback during laparoscopic surgery by providing the surgeon with visual cues, improving hand-eye coordination, including robotic surgery. Using the combined image of MRI, CT-angiography, and ultrasound, individual adjustment of incisions and cutting planes, optimal positioning of paracentesis needles, and position display of the organ's main components are realized.

Keywords: Knowledge bases · Surgeon assistance · Hybrid reality · Augmented reality · Pattern recognition · Active strain-statistical models

1 Introduction

Blood vessel structure data can be superimposed on the surgical cavity using vessel contour recognition. For this purpose, a model for identifying vessel contours in the video stream was developed using active strain-statistical models for recreating multidimensional images.

The training procedure for active appearance models begins with normalizing all shapes' position to compensate for differences in scale, tilt, and offset. For this purpose, the so-called generalized Procrustean analysis is used.

The learning process here consists of the following steps: extraction from the training images of the textures that best match the basic shape; region mapping is carried out using piecewise interpolation of the training image resulting from triangulation to the corresponding regions of the texture to be formed; a matrix is formed from the textures, each column containing the pixel values of the corresponding texture (similar to the S matrix). The textures used for training were single-channel (grayscale) and multi-channel (RGB color space).

R. Su et al. (Eds.): MICAD 2021, LNEE 784, pp. 312–315, 2022.
https://doi.org/10.1007/978-981-16-3880-0_32

2 Computer Model of Contour Selection

To date, empirical methods are fast, reasonably easy to implement and configure but usually show a high percentage of false contour detection in large image sets. Methods based on constructing a model of the lungs' affected area and deformable models give relatively high recognition rates on extensive collections of images with a potentially large number of lung images [1–3].

The mathematical apparatus of active appearance models has been actively developed. At the moment, two approaches to the construction of such models can be distinguished: the classical one (initially proposed by Coutes) and inverse composition based (proposed by Matthews and Baker in 2003 [4]).

First, consider the common parts of the two approaches. Two parameters are modeled in active appearance models: shape-related parameters (shape parameters) and parameters related to a statistical image model or texture (appearance parameters). Before use, the model must be trained on a set of pre-marked images. Markup of images is done manually or in semi-automatic mode when using an algorithm to find approximate mark locations, and then they are clarified by an expert. Each mark has its number and defines a characteristic point that the model will have to find during adaptation to the new image. Example of a markup (lung base) (see Fig. 1).

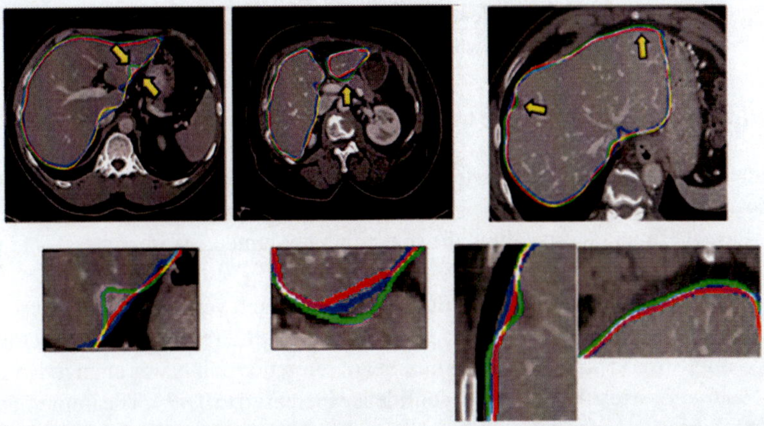

Fig. 1. Active strain-statistical models superimposed on the texture.

The training procedure for active appearance models begins with normalizing all shapes' position to compensate for differences in scale, tilt, and offset. For this purpose, the so-called generalized Procrustean analysis is used [8].

In a model of this type, the authors also need to calculate the vector of combined parameters, which is given by the following formula:

$$b = \begin{bmatrix} W_s b_s \\ b_t \end{bmatrix} = \begin{bmatrix} W_s \Phi_s^T (s - s_0) \\ \Phi_t^T (t - t_0) \end{bmatrix}, \tag{1}$$

where W_s is a diagonal matrix of weight values that allows balancing the contribution of pixel distances and pixel intensities. For each element of the training sample (the texture-shape pair), its vector b is calculated. Then the resulting set of vectors is combined into a matrix, and its main components are found. In this case, the synthesized vector of combined shape and texture parameters is defined by the following expression: $b = \Phi_c c$.

Here Φ_c is the matrix of principal components of the combined parameters, and C is the vector of combined appearance parameters [6]. From here, obtained new expressions for the synthesized shape and texture:

$$s = s_0 + \Phi_s W_s^{-1} \Phi_{c,s} c, \; t = t_0 + \Phi_t \Phi_{c,t} c, \; \Phi_c = \begin{bmatrix} \Phi_{c,s} \\ \Phi_{c,s} \end{bmatrix} \tag{2}$$

In practice, the matrix Φ_c is also subjected to removing noise components to reduce the effect of overfitting and reduce the number of calculations performed.

After calculating the shape, appearance, and combined parameters, the so-called prediction matrix R is required, which in the sense of the minimum root-mean-square error would satisfy the following linear equation:

$$\delta p = R \delta t \tag{3}$$

where $\delta t = t_{image} - t_{model}$, and δp is the perturbation of the position vector and the combined appearance parameters.

Various methods have been developed to solve the above equation. Their detailed consideration is carried out in the works [4–6].

3 Analysis of the Active Form Model

Experimental procedures were carried out on computed tomography images of the lungs with the affected part.

For the experimental procedure, the selection of volunteers (researchers) – 15 people was carried out [9–11].

The model of active deformable forms was trained and verified to identify contours. Preliminary training gave a confidence score of 0.75 – the result is unsatisfactory. The training sample was expanded, and the number of reference points was changed to 128 per closed contour. As a result of training, confidence increased to 0.937. The implementation of contour detection was performed with a confidence of at least 0.88, in contrast to the level of 0.73 for the gradient method [12, 14, 15]. The level of confidence enhancement achieved in the model for detecting closed loops exceeded the directive level. The model training accuracy is 0.1 mm.

4 Conclusion

A method for constructing a model of the contours of lung segments to identify affected tissues is shown. Strain-statistical models are used to reconstruct multidimensional images to build contours. The model showed an accuracy of detecting contours equal to 0.1 mm, which meets the requirements for detecting affected lung tissue and can be used in medical systems for early diagnosis.

Acknowledgment. The project is supported by the Foundation for Assistance to Small Innovative Enterprises in Science and Technology. (Russian Federation). Project No. 63437, application NTI-84099 within the framework of the implementation of the innovative project "Development of an intelligent software package for the preventive diagnosis of human respiratory diseases based on active deformation and statistical models for recreating multidimensional images using an immersive environment" to implement "HealthNet" action plans ("road maps").

References

1. Axelrod, R.: The Structure of Decision: Cognitive Maps of Political Elites, p. 342. Princeton University Press, Princeton (1976)
2. Baker, S., Gross, R., Matthews, I.: Lucas-Kanade 20 years on: a unifying framework: Part 3. Technical report CMU-RI-TR-03-35, Carnegie Mellon University Robotics Institute (2003)
3. Baker, S., Gross, R., Matthews, I.: Lucas-Kanade 20 years on: a unifying framework: Part 1. Technical report CMU-RI-TR-02-16, Carnegie Mellon University Robotics Institute (2002)
4. Baker, S., Gross, R., Matthews, I.: Lucas-Kanade 20 years on: a unifying framework: Part 2. Technical report CMU-RI-TR-03-01, Carnegie Mellon University Robotics Institute (2003)
5. Cootes, T.F., Edwards, G.J., Taylor, C.J.: Active appearance models. In: Burkhardt, H., Neumann, B. (eds.) ECCV 1998. LNCS, vol. 1407, pp. 484–498. Springer, Heidelberg (1998). https://doi.org/10.1007/BFb0054760
6. Cootes, T.F., Edwards, G.J., Taylor, C.J.: Active appearance models. IEEE Trans. Pattern Recognit. Mach. Intell. **23**(6), 681–685 (2001)
7. Cootes, T.F., Taylor, C.J.: Statistical models of appearance for medical image analysis and computer vision. In: Proceedings of the SPIE Medical Imaging, vol. 1, pp. 236–248. SPIE (2001)
8. Cootes, T.F., Taylor, C.J.: Constrained active appearance models. In: Proceedings of the Eighth IEEE International Conference on Computer Vision, ICCV 2001, vol. 1, pp. 748–754 (2001)
9. OpenCV Library User Guide. Intel Research Lab, p. 420 (2000)
10. Gorban, A.N.: Training of Neural Networks. SP ParaGraph, Moscow (1990)
11. Van Dijk, T.A.: Critical discourse analysis. In: Tannen, D., Schiffrin, D., Hamilton, H. (eds.) Handbook of Discourse Analysis. Blackwell, Oxford (2001)
12. Akimov, D.A., Potapov, D.A.: Identification of speech constructions that increase the accuracy of the information retrieval system. In: Modern Science: Actual Problems of Theory and Practice, no. 1, pp. 41–43 (2017)
13. Landauer, T., Foltz, P.W., Laham, D.: Introduction to latent semantic analysis. Discourse Process. **25**(2–3), 259–284 (1998). https://doi.org/10.1080/01638539809545028
14. Levy, O., Golberg, Y., Dagan, I.: Improving distributional similarity with lessons learned from word embeddings. http://www.aclweb.org/anthology/Q15-1016. Accessed 01 June 2018
15. Mansoor, A., et al.: Segmentation and image analysis of abnormal lungs at CT: current approaches, challenges, and future trends. Radiograph. Rev. Publ. Radiol. Soc. North Am. Inc. **35**(4), 1056–1076 (2015). https://doi.org/10.1148/rg.2015140232

A New Content-Based Image Retrieval System for SARS-CoV-2 Computer-Aided Diagnosis

Gabriel Molina[1], Marcelo Mendoza[1](✉), Ignacio Loayza[1], Camilo Núñez[1], Mauricio Araya[2], Víctor Castañeda[3], and Mauricio Solar[1]

[1] Department of Informatics, Universidad Técnica Federico Santa María, Valparaíso, Chile
marcelo.mendoza@usm.cl

[2] Department of Electronics, Universidad Técnica Federico Santa María, Valparaíso, Chile

[3] Centro de Informática Médica y Telemedicina-CIMT, Universidad de Chile, Santiago, Chile

Abstract. Medical images are an essential input for the timely diagnosis of pathologies. Despite its wide use in the area, searching for images that can reveal valuable information to support decision-making is difficult and expensive. However, the possibilities that open when making large repositories of images available for search by content are unsuspected. We designed a content-based image retrieval system for medical imaging, which reduces the gap between access to information and the availability of useful repositories to meet these needs. The system operates on the principle of query-by-example, in which users provide medical images, and the system displays a set of related images. Unlike metadata match-driven searches, our system drives content-based search. This allows the system to conduct searches on repositories of medical images that do not necessarily have complete and curated metadata. We explore our system's feasibility in computational tomography (CT) slices for SARS-CoV-2 infection (COVID-19), showing that our proposal obtains promising results, advantageously comparing it with other search methods.

Keywords: Deep learning · Content-based image search · SARS-CoV-2

1 Introduction

The use of automatic data processing techniques based on deep learning has gained attention from the medical imaging community in the last years [18]. Inductive learning's relevance to support decision-making and computer aided diagnosis has pushed the community to have more and better methods that can help in these initiatives. In addition, the rapid advance of deep learning techniques, which introduce representation learning within artificial neural network architectures, has allowed advances in the area [1]. Their results address various problems related to image processing, improving these techniques' skills in many tasks.

Medical imaging and computer-aided diagnosis have a long history of development. Many of the assisted support strategies for medical imaging-based diagnoses use classical image processing techniques to construct representations of images based on visual

R. Su et al. (Eds.): MICAD 2021, LNEE 784, pp. 316–324, 2022.
https://doi.org/10.1007/978-981-16-3880-0_33

descriptors, such as SIFT descriptors [16]. Classic automatic classification techniques are often used on these representations to train diagnostic classifiers. These techniques have been predominant in computer-aided diagnosis [11].

A complementary approach to image classification is to search for related images [13]. In a search system, the user provides an example image, often without meta-data, from which the system must identify related images based on their content. In content-based search systems, the image's characteristics, such as color, morphology, and intensity, are essential. However, image search is difficult. Searching for an image in a repository based on its content often returns false positives. One of the problem's difficulties is that the images can be similar according to their content but correspond to different diagnoses. The challenge is to encode the image's content so that the system can distinguish non-evident differences. Search systems can be much more informative than classifiers. They provide many related results, helping users and patterns between results, facilitating identifying relevant cases, or suggesting alternative diagnoses. The interest in developing effective systems of this type is important, but it runs into the difficulty that their development has important technical challenges.

We propose a new content-based medical image search system. Our system uses deep learning architectures to generate representations of the images indexed by a nearest neighbor query engine. Deep learning is used for two purposes. First, it allows us to build representations of the images in a low dimensional space. Low-dimensional representations are useful since they favor the use of functions such as the Euclidean distance, which deteriorates its performance in high-dimensional spaces due to the curse of dimensionality. The second purpose is to incorporate latent information that deep learning uses to build high-performance classifiers. In this way, the representations of the images encode their content and encode latent features used by these architectures to solve diagnostic classification tasks.

We combine two deep learning architectures to facilitate searches over an image repository. First, we use an image segmentation architecture called Ce-Net (Context Encoder Network) [6], allowing 2D medical images to be processed. This architecture allows obtaining image embeddings by training the Ce-Net to solve a segmentation problem. Then, the embeddings are used as the encoding of the images to train a diagnostic-based classifier. For this purpose, we use an Xception architecture [5], which builds a new representation of the images to solve a classification task. Both embeddings are concatenated and indexed in a nearest neighbor query engine. When the user provides an example image, the system uses the Ce-Net and Xception models to obtain the example image encoding, projecting it into the same space in which the repository images were encoded. Next, the example image's encoding is processed in the query engine, which returns its nearest neighbors.

The main contributions of this paper are:

- We combine two deep learning architectures supporting medical imaging nearest neighbor searches, providing valuable information to computer-aided diagnosis systems.
- We systematically validate our system's precision, comparing our system's performance favorably with its most direct competitors.

– We use open datasets to conduct our experiments for SARS-CoV-2 diagnosis, favoring reproducible research in this relevant topic.

The rest of the paper is organized in the following way. In Sect. 2, we review related work. Our proposal is introduced in Sect. 3. In Sect. 4, we report experimental results. Finally, we conclude in Sect. 5, providing concluding remarks and commenting on future work.

2 Related Work

Content-based retrieval of image search is a difficult task because there is a semantic gap between the low-level visual information captured by algorithms and the high-level information perceived by the human evaluators. Deep learning reduces this gap without using handcrafted features by encoding/combining low-level and high-level features [11]. This is the reason why current content-based medical image search techniques use deep learning architectures to extract image descriptors [1].

Anavi *et al.* [2] uses trained convolution networks (CNNs) to classify X-ray images, extracting the network's weights to represent the images in a low dimensional space. A similar approach was examined by Liu *et al.* [12], who uses the weights of a fully connected layer connected to a CNNs output to construct a representation of the images. Prostate MR image searching was studied by Shah *et al.* [15], who also used CNNs to extract characteristics from images, combining them with hashing forests. Hashing allowed them to work with low dimensional representations, which is a key aspect to process this type of images. Deep convolutional neural networks as the VGG-19 have been used to extract representations from contrast-enhanced magnetic resonance images (CE-MRI) to support brain tumor imaging [16]. Deep learning has shown great advantages in this task compared to classical methods of extraction of characteristics, motivating the exploration of these techniques in other tasks. For example, Hamidinekoo *et al.* [7] used CNNs to retrieve hematoxylin and eosin breast histology images in mammograms, with promising results. Camalan *et al.* [4] explored the use of image retrieval for the early detection of eardrum. Recently, Haq *et al.* [8] have applied deep learning to develop a search system for X-ray images, with promising results in a large-scale repository.

Although most medical image retrieval systems use CNNs, deep learning shows that other novel architectures are more efficient in image processing. Baur *et al.* [3] explored the use of Fully Convolutional Networks (FCNs) for MRI segmentation for multiple sclerosis lesions detection. The proposal based on the U-Net architecture [14], outperforms CNNs and also can be trained with partially labeled data. As the proposal combines diagnostic data with a segmentation task, can be very competitive, which is the reason why we will use it to compare the performance of our method in image search. Currently, FCNs are widely used in medical imaging, becoming the new state of the art for complex segmentation tasks such as head and neck cancer radiotherapy [17].

Despite the growing interest in the development of medical image retrieval systems, these efforts are expected to increase exponentially in the coming years [18]. It is expected that the greater availability of medical image datasets could push this area with a specific focus on multi-modal image retrieval tasks [13].

3 Proposal

3.1 Motivation

We combine two image processing architectures based on deep learning to facilitate searches over an image repository. First, we use an image segmentation architecture called Ce-Net (Context Encoder Network) [6], allowing 2D medical images to be processed (see Fig. 1). The Ce-Net architecture is an extension of the U-Net architecture [14], which is based on the encoder-decoder architecture. Encoder-decoder architectures work with a tandem of layers, building a representation of the input in a lower-dimensional space known as latent space. Another sequence of layers transforms the encoding from the latent space to the original space, retrieving the image's original dimensionality. This architecture module is called a decoder. The encoder-decoder architectures are intended to encode images in latent space, with low loss of information. For this, the architecture parameters are adjusted in such a way as to minimize the reconstruction error defined from the difference between the original image and the reconstructed image in L_2 norm.

The Ce-Net architecture extends the U-Net architecture by incorporating two processing modules. The Dense Atrous Convolution (DAC) and the Residual Multi-kernel Pooling (RMP) module. Both modules were designed to capture high-level characteristics and also preserve more spatial information throughout the encoder-decoder architecture. We use the encoding of the image generated by the RMP block to build its representation. It is the highest-level encoding generated by the network before entering the decoder. The Ce-Net can be trained for medical image segmentation tasks by showing original-segmented image pairs at the network's input and output. This requires having a set of medical images, together with their segmentation masks generated by specialists.

A second building block of our search system is the Xception architecture [5]. The Xception is based on the Inception architecture used in image classification [10]. The Inception architecture uses modules based on convolutional operators, which manage to capture short-range dependencies in the input image. These characteristics allow learning a new representation of the input image, identifying patterns between the original image's that are useful for a better representation. The Xception architecture extends the Inception architecture, incorporating convolutional layers that allow capturing long-range dependencies.

We combine both architectures trained in different tasks to address the medical image search problem, as we show in Fig. 1. We use the Ce-Net architecture to segment the repository images. The latent representations of the Ce-Net are used as pre-trained vectors to adjust the Xception according to diagnosis. This proposal's rationale is that by segmenting the images and working with their latent representations, we reduce these images' variability by placing them in a common space. This common representation space, the segmenter's latent space, should provide better generalization abilities to the Xception. Instead of working with the original images, it would work with the pre-training carried out in segmentation. The Xception network could work with fewer parameters when solving the diagnostic classification task by reducing the images' dimensionality. This would avoid the risk of overfitting. As we show in Fig. 1,

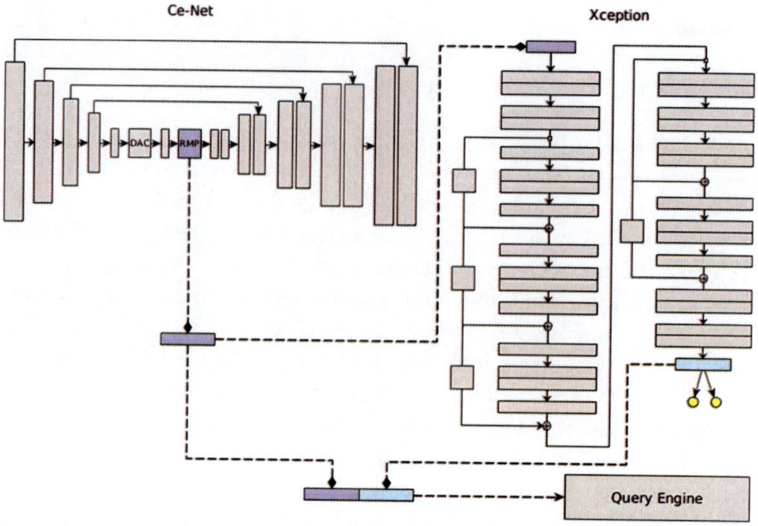

Fig. 1. The Ce-Net is trained to solve a segmentation task. The RMP block is used to get a first image embedding (in purple). This representation is fed in the Xception to solve a SARS-CoV-2 classification diagnosis task. The weights of the last layer are used to get a second image embedding (in green). Finally, both representations are concatenated to feed the query engine.

we use the weights of the last layer of the Xception the generate an image representation. This layer encodes the information required to classify the image according to the diagnostic. Finally, both encodings are concatenated and sent to the query engine.

3.2 System Architecture

We train the Ce-Net segmentation network using CT slices of SARS-CoV-2 patients. Then, the Xception network fits the problem classes using a labeled image dataset. For this purpose, we work with CT datasets with labels available in SARS-CoV-2. Once the Xception network is validated, we retrieve its latent vectors from the last layer of the model. These vectors are concatenated with the RMP Ce-Net embeddings, which are ingested in the query engine.

Once the Ce-Net and Xception models are obtained, and the query engine indexes the repository images' embeddings, a new image can be used to query the system, as shown in Fig. 2. The query engine is implemented using Multiple Random Projection Trees (MRPT) [9], which is considered the state-of-the-art data structure in approximate search for nearest neighbors. MRPT allows building indexes in L2 standard search space. Once the index has been built, the nearest neighbor queries can be run. The queries specify the number of neighbors searched for and return the identifiers of the corresponding images. To specify a query, a new image goes through both models, which provide their embeddings and project the image to the same space in which the images are. The query image is used to retrieve its k-nearest neighbors using the Euclidean distance. The system's final phase allows ordering these results according to proximity.

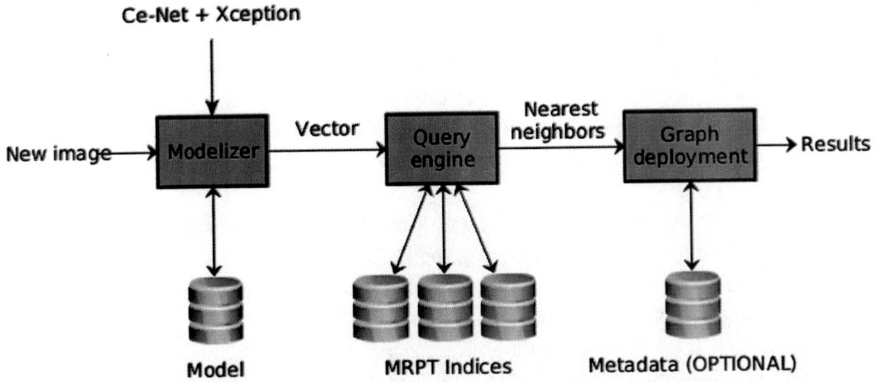

Fig. 2. A new image is processed using the Ce-Net and Xception architectures to obtain its vectorized representation. The query engine accesses the repository indexes, retrieving the nearest neighbors of the image.

The latent representations constructed using the Ce-Net + Xception networks allow obtaining continuous and dense vectors of the same dimensionality for all the repository images. We can also observe that when using the representation obtained by the Xception, the images are expected to be separated by types of images (we owe this to the Ce-Net segmenter) and by diagnosis (we owe this to the Xception). According to image type and diagnosis, the clustering hypothesis is supported by the combination of both architectures in tandem.

4 Experiments

4.1 Datasets

We used the Covid-19 CT segmentation dataset to train the Ce-Net network. The dataset contains 100 axial CTs of more than 40 patients with Covid-19. The images were segmented by a radiologist using 3 labels: ground-glass, consolidation, and pleural effusion. We used 100 CT slices along with their masks for Ce-Net training.

We used the SARS-CoV-2 CT-scan dataset to train the Xception network. The dataset contains 1252 CT slices that are positive for SARS-CoV-2 infection (COVID-19) and 1230 CT slices for patients non-infected by SARS-CoV-2.

We used the Covid-CT dataset as a testing set. The dataset contains 349 CT slices from 216 Covid-19 patients and 463 non-Covid CT slices. The dataset contains images acquired with different media, for example, CT slices post-processed by cell phone cameras and some images with very low resolution. For these reasons, the dataset represents the real conditions of image acquisition for a system of this kind.

To generate a balanced set of queries, the Clinical Hospital of the University of Chile supported us with eight CT scans where half of them suffered from Covid-19. From these CTs, 25 slices with Covid-19 and 25 slices without Covid-19 were extracted. Each of these queries was used to query our system.

4.2 Experimental Design

We evaluate the performance of our search system using precision and recall measures. To compute these metrics, we consider the CT slices' ground labels according to SARS-CoV-2 diagnosis, counting matches between image examples labels and their list results. We validate our proposal considering four alternative methods:

- Ce-Net [6]: It corresponds to a search system based on the encoding of the testing images obtained from the Ce-Net using the RMP block.
- Xception [5]: It corresponds to a search system based on the encoding of the testing images obtained from the Xception using its last layer.
- U-Net-ML [3]: It corresponds to a search system based on the encoding of
- the testing images obtained from the modified architecture of Baur *et al.*, trained for 5 epochs for segmentation, then 5 more epochs for classification. We did tests with several layers of the encoding but the ones that obtained the best results were the embeddings obtained using the last layer of the architecture.
- U-Net-ME [3]: It corresponds to a search system based on the encoding of the testing images obtained from the modified architecture of Baur *et al.*, trained for 5 epochs for segmentation and then 5 epochs with the manifold embedding loss. The embeddings were obtained using the last layer of the architecture.

4.3 Results

We show the results of the experiments in Fig. 3. The performance plots on the whole set of testing queries (at the top of Fig. 3) show that our proposal outperforms the other methods in precision. As we might expect, the precision drops slightly as the list of results grows. The variance around the mean precision also decreases gradually. The recall of all the methods is quite similar, reaching around 20% in lists of length 50.

By separating the testing set between Covid-19 and Non-Covid-19 queries, the results in Fig. 3 show that our method obtains advantages over the rest when using queries of patients with Covid-19, surpassing by a significant margin its most direct competitor, the Xception network. The other methods have lower performances. UNet-ME performs well in the healthy patient class. However, this model exhibits overfitting to this class as its performance in the Covid-19 class is very low. Our proposal surpasses the rest of the methods in Covid-19 images regarding recall rates, while UNet-ME generates a better recall in images of healthy patients. The results confirm that our proposal is suitable for searching for images of Covid-19 patients, surpassing all its competitors in precision and without generating overfitting to any of the classes.

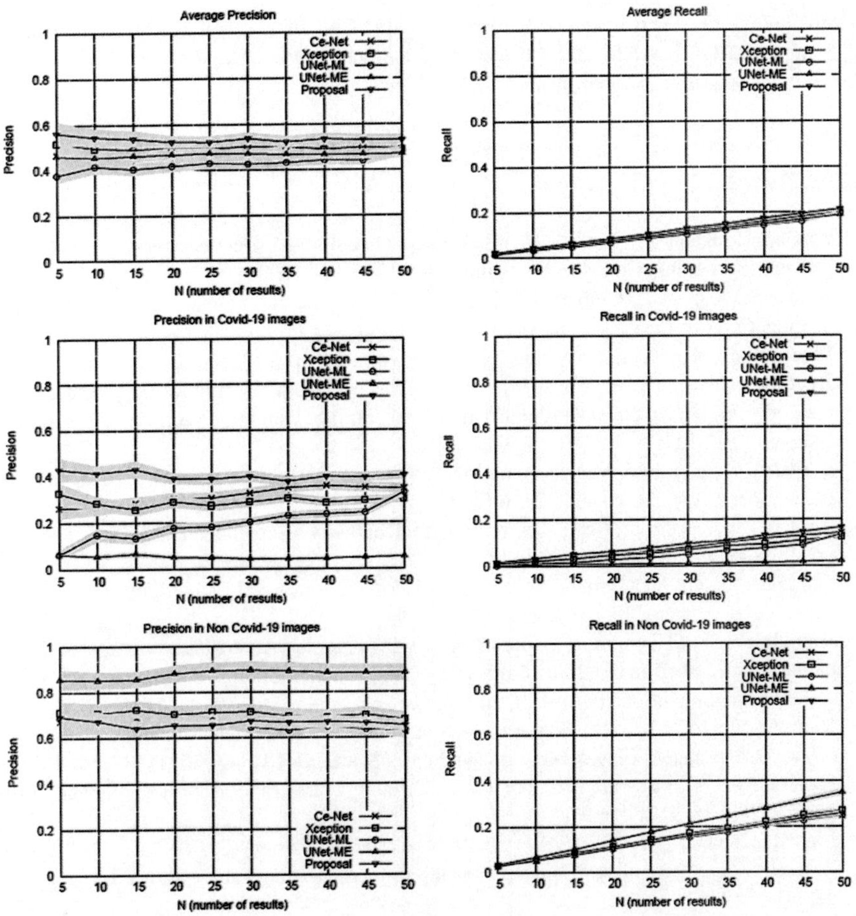

Fig. 3. Precision and recall scores of the methods evaluated in this paper. The plots at the top show the whole set of test images' performance, while the plots at the bottom show the results disaggregated by class.

5 Conclusion

This paper has shown that combining the Ce-Net and Xception architectures, used for segmentation and classification tasks, respectively, is useful in image search. Our experiments conducted on images of patients with Covid-19 show that our method outperforms its most direct competitors in terms of precision, without overfitting to either class of interest.

We are currently expanding our proposal to be able to work with images of different types. This paper has shown results based on CT, but it is interesting to incorporate X-ray images into our search system. We believe that the enabling of precise multi-modal search systems will push the development of these methods in the coming years.

Acknowledgments. This work was funded by ANID FONDEF grant 19I10023, ANID FONDECYT grant 11170475, ANID Basal Project FB0008, and ANID PIA/APOYO AFB180002. Dr. Mendoza acknowledges support from ANID Fondecyt grant 1200211.

References

1. Ahmad, H., Khan, M., Yousaf, A., Ghuffar, S., Khurshid, K.: Deep learning: a breakthrough in medical imaging. Curr. Med. Imaging **16**(8), 946–956 (2020)
2. Anavi, Y., Kogan, I., Gelbart, E., Geva, O., Greenspan, H.: Visualizing and enhancing a deep learning framework using patients age and gender for chest X-ray image retrieval. In: Proceedings of the SPIE on Medical Imaging, vol. 9785, p. 978510 (2016)
3. Baur, C., Albarqouni, A., Navab, N.: Semi-supervised deep learning for fully convolutional networks. In: International Conference on Medical Image Computing and Computer Assisted Intervention, MICCAI, pp. 311–319 (2017)
4. Camalan, S., et al.: OtoMatch: content-based eardrum image retrieval using deep learning. PLoS ONE **15**(5), art. no. e0232776 (2020)
5. Chollet, F.: Xception: Deep Learning with Depthwise Separable Convolutions. CVPR, pp. 1800–1807 (2017)
6. Gu, Z., et al.: Ce-Net: context encoder network for 2D medical image segmentation. IEEE Trans. Med. Imaging **38**(10), 2281–2292 (2019)
7. Hamidinekoo, A., Denton, E., Honnor, K., Zwiggelaar, R.: An AI-based method to retrieve hematoxylin and eosin breast histology images using mammograms. In: Proceedings of SPIE - The International Society for Optical Engineering, vol. 11513, art. no. 1151319 (2020)
8. Haq, N., Moradi, M., Wang, Z.: A deep community based approach for large scale content based X-ray image retrieval. Med. Image Anal. **68**, art. no. 101847 (2021)
9. Hyvonen, V.: Fast nearest neighbor search through sparse random projections and voting. BigData, pp. 881–888 (2016)
10. Lin, M., Chen, Q., Yan, S.: Network in Network. ICLR (Poster) (2014)
11. Litjens, G., et al.: A survey on deep learning in medical image analysis. Med. Image Anal. **42**, 60–88 (2017)
12. Liu, X., Tizhoosh, H., Kofman, J.: Generating binary tags for fast medical image retrieval based on convolutional nets and Radon transform. In: Proceedings of the International Joint Conference on Neural Networks (2016)
13. Muller, H., Unay, D.: Retrieval from and understanding of large-scale multi-modal medical datasets: a review. IEEE Trans. Multimedia **19**(9), art. no. 7984864, 2093–2104 (2017)
14. Ronneberger, O., Fischer, P., Brox, T.: U-net: convolutional networks for biomedical image segmentation. In: Navab, N., Hornegger, J., Wells, W.M., Frangi, A.F. (eds.) MICCAI 2015. LNCS, vol. 9351, pp. 234–241. Springer, Cham (2015). https://doi.org/10.1007/978-3-319-24574-4_28
15. Shah, A., Conjeti, S., Navab, N., Katouzian, A.: Deeply learnt hashing forests for content based image retrieval in prostate MR images. In: Proceedings of the SPIE on Medical Imaging, vol. 9784, p. 978414 (2016)
16. Swati, Z., et al.: Content-based brain tumor retrieval for MR images using transfer learning. IEEE Access **7**, art. no. 8611216, 17809–17822 (2019)
17. Tong, N., Gou, S., Yang, S., Ruan, D., Sheng, K.: Fully automatic multi-organ segmentation for head and neck cancer radiotherapy using shape representation model constrained fully convolutional neural networks. Med. Phys. **45**(10), 4558–4567 (2018)
18. Yu, Y., Li, M., Liu, L., Li, Y., Wang, J.: Clinical big data and deep learning: applications, challenges, and future outlooks. Big Data Mining Anal. **2**(4), art. no. 8787233 288–305 (2019)

Dysplasia Grading of Colorectal Polyps Through Convolutional Neural Network Analysis of Whole Slide Images

Daniele Perlo[1(✉)], Enzo Tartaglione[1], Luca Bertero[2], Paola Cassoni[2], and Marco Grangetto[1]

[1] Department of Computer Science, University of Torino, Torino, Italy
daniele.perlo@unito.it

[2] Pathology Unit, Department of Medical Sciences, University of Torino, Torino, Italy
luca.bertero@unito.it

Abstract. Colorectal cancer is a leading cause of cancer death for both men and women. For this reason, histo-pathological characterization of colorectal polyps is the major instrument for the pathologist in order to infer the actual risk for cancer and to guide further follow-up. Colorectal polyps diagnosis includes the evaluation of the polyp type, and more importantly, the grade of dysplasia. This latter evaluation represents a critical step for the clinical follow-up. The proposed deep learning-based classification pipeline is based on state-of-the-art convolutional neural network, trained using proper countermeasures to tackle WSI high resolution and very imbalanced dataset. The experimental results show that one can successfully classify adenomas dysplasia grade with 70% accuracy, which is in line with the pathologists' concordance.

Keywords: Deep learning · Multi resolution · Colorectal polyps · Colorectal adenomas · Digital pathology

1 Introduction

The cornerstone of conventional histo-pathological examination is the evaluation of hematoxylin & eosin slides by trained pathologists to detect and/or quantify specific features or patterns and provide a diagnostic evaluation. Based on this premise, whole slide image (WSI) analysis approaches based on Deep Learning (DL) are well suited to address the tasks posed by the histo-pathological evaluation [14]. During the last few years, many specific challenges have been tackled: from lymph node metastasis detection [2] to mitotic count [1]. The main aims of these approaches are multiple: i) improve pathologists' accuracy and thus diagnostic sensitivity; ii) speed-up the diagnostic workflow by addressing more

This work has received funding from the European Union's Horizon 2020 research and innovation programme under grant agreement No 825111, DeepHealth Project.

R. Su et al. (Eds.): MICAD 2021, LNEE 784, pp. 325–334, 2022.
https://doi.org/10.1007/978-981-16-3880-0_34

menial, but time-consuming tasks; iii) improve diagnostic agreement by adopting standardized criteria.

Among the multiple fields of surgical pathology, gastrointestinal pathology is one of the most represented [10], thus addressing this specific topic has the potential of significantly affecting the overall workflow of a pathology service. Colorectal polyps, pre-malignant lesions arising from the intestinal epithelium, are one of the most common gastrointestinal specimens submitted to histological examination. These lesions are usually collected during a colonoscopy, which represents the mainstay of colorectal cancer screening programs in many countries [4]. The development of these programs leads to a significant increase in this specific caseload of surgical pathology laboratories: the correct diagnostic assessment has far-reached consequences both for the patient and the public health systems. Indeed, a correct diagnosis is obviously important for the management of the patient, but it is now well acknowledged that different types of polyps are associated with different risks of developing metachronous invasive carcinomas during the following years [13]. For this reason, specific algorithms have been established for tailoring patients' follow-up. Despite such clinical relevance, the concordance rates even among expert pathologists, in the diagnostic assessment of colorectal polyps, is far from optimal [8,9,19,23]. Although the distinction between non-adenomatous and adenomatous tissue is usually reliable, the interobserver agreement between different histological types and dysplasia grades are sub-optimal. For instance, the concordance in assessing a tubulo-villous polyp or low grade dysplasia ranged around 70%.

In this work the main contributions are: i) the design of a deep learning pipeline to tackle the high dimensionality of WSI, working at single patches level; ii) the study on the physical resolutions suitable to deal automatically with the problem of classification of different colorectal polyps; iii) the study of different patch pre-processing approaches, where we find that, for the considered problem, the intensity of the dye present in the scans is the most informative feature of the tissue images.

2 Related Work

Only a limited number of works explored histo-pathological examination through deep learning-based analysis of digital whole slide images [15,22,24]. Among these works, Korbar et al. [12] present a crop-based framework, developed using a ResNet architecture to classify different types of colorectal polyps from whole-slide images. This work provides empirical suggestions the residual network architecture achieves better performance than other models. Following their previous work, Korbar et al. introduce a revised version of Grad-CAM (gradient driven class activation mapping) [21] to visualize the attention map of the network for the annotated whole-slide [15]. Bychkov et al. [5] apply different architectures (convolutional and recurrent neural networks) in order to predict five-years disease survival probabilities for colorectal cancer and estimate the individual risk. This work explores the idea of using spatial information by feeding an LSTM network with the features extracted from image crops by a CNN.

Table 1. Dataset composition.

	HP	NORM	TA.HG	TA.LG	TVA.HG	TVA.LG	Total
Slides	62	30	34	232	44	55	**457**
R_t	158	112	145	777	264	245	**1701**
A_t [cm^2]	9.91	18.38	7.94	71.74	60.45	41.86	**210.29**

Recently, Wei et al. [24] propose an analysis model for annotated tissue and perform a study on the generalization of neural models with external medical institutions. In such work, a hierarchical evaluation mechanism is proposed to extend the classification of tissue fragments to the entire slide.

These efforts show promising results, but the testing data size is small and, most importantly, they do not provide diagnosis based on both histological type and dysplasia grade. Our aim is thus to evaluate the efficacy of a deep neural network for the automatic histo-pathological classification of colorectal polyps employing a large training cohort and assessing both polyp histological type and dysplasia grade.

3 Dataset

In this work we use a collection of 457 WSI biopsies collected within the EU project *DeepHealth* [7], from patients undergoing colorectal cancer screening. Slide scanning is obtained through a Hamamatsu Nanozoomer S210 scanner configured at ×20 magnification (0.4415 µm/px) and stored as `.ndpi` file. Each WSI has been annotated by expert pathologists according to six classes chosen for our study: hyperplastic polyp (HP); normal tissue (NORM); tubular adenoma, high-grade dysplasia (TA.HG); tubular adenoma, low-grade dysplasia (TA.LG); tubulo-villous adenoma, high-grade dysplasia (TVA.HG) and tubulo-villous adenoma, low-grade dysplasia (TVA.LG).

Each slide is associated with some metadata (stored in NanoZoomer Digital Pathology Annotations `.ndpa` file format), including a collection of Region of Interests (RoIs) associated with the corresponding class. Each RoI is determined by the pathologist and is defined by a free-hand contour, identifying the tissue area exhibiting histological findings. The number and the size of RoIs is highly variable and depends on both the tissue availability and the histological analysis. Such heterogeneity unfortunately, leads to dataset unbalancing: the distribution of the data from T tissue classes in our dataset is shown in Table 1. In the table we read the number of WSIs, the number of ROIs R_t and total tissue area A_t for each class t. A subset of the dataset is publicly available [3].

4 Method

In this section we are going to describe and motivate the proposed method. In particular, the use of deep learning for classification already proved, in similar

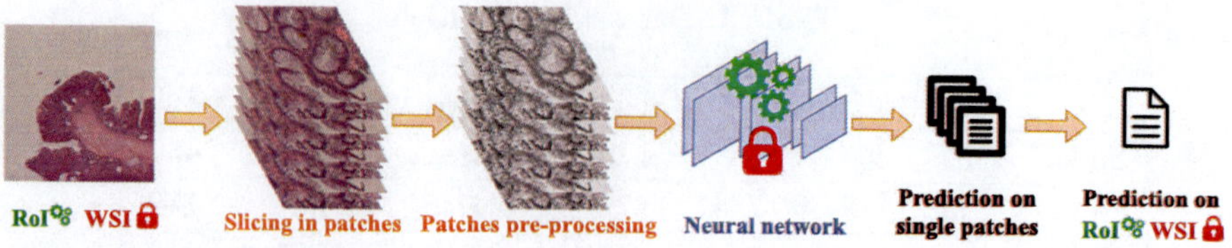

Fig. 1. The neural network is trained on RoI images (gears symbol) and tested on WSI (lock symbol).

Table 2. Dataset composition. Test RoIs are taken from a disjoint set of slides.

	HP	NORM	TA.HG	TA.LG	TVA.HG	TVA.LG	Total
Train slides	50	25	26	203	36	45	**385**
Test slides	12	5	8	29	8	10	**72**
Train RoIs	133	98	113	695	240	208	**1487**
Validation RoIs	5	5	5	5	5	5	**30**
Test RoIs	20	9	27	77	19	32	**184**

learning tasks, to be extremely effective and robust [15,24]. Direct classification on the (high resolution) whole slide, in our context, is unfeasible: the relevant features are local and can be detected at very low image scale. For this reason, the deep learning model is not trained on the full slides, but on some crops we refer to as *patches*. An high-level representation of our approach is depicted in Fig. 1. Once the model is trained on patches' classification, in order to get the whole slide classification (at validation/test time), all the scores from the single patches are averaged on the whole slide. WSIs have large resolution and need to be cropped into patches. The first operation we perform on RoIs (even before slicing them into patches) is re-scaling them to some target resolution φ. using the Lancos-3 filter. Then, we slice the RoIs/WSIs into patches (224×224 pixels large) using sliding windows. These patches can be immediately normalized, using approaches like [17], or simply converting in gray-scale to reduce the expected color shift caused by hematoxylin and eosin.

During training we augment data: we include vertical/horizontal flips and a random operation chosen between rotation, equalization, solarization, inversion and contrast enhancing, as proposed in [6].

In order to perform classification on the patches, we have used ResNet-18: it represents a good trade-off between complexity and performance and is one of the broadly-used to solve similar tasks [15,24]. Pre-trained deep neural networks (on the ImageNet classification task) can be effectively used as initialization for medical classification tasks, showing good performance [15].[1]

[1] The pre-trained model used in all the experiments is available at https://pytorch.org/docs/stable/torchvision/models.html.

5 Results

In this section we show and discuss the classification results obtained on the WSI biopsies dataset described in Sect. 3 with the method proposed in Sect. 4. We can easily expect high error rates, considering that the information about the adenoma type is a visually global information and requires features extracted at different scale than those for the dysplasia grade, which is a more local information. Here we are not interested in distinguishing different adenoma types, but their dysplasia grade. Towards this end, we will follow a hierarchical-like classification approach [25, 26], grouping the adenoma classes into high grade (HG) and low grade (LG) dysplasia.

For all the experiments, we split the data at the whole slide level, in order to maintain the separation of tissues from different patients. For each class, 10% of total patients are considered as test set. We summarise the data split in Table 2. The validation set size is fixed to 5 RoIs for each class from the training set (likewise [24]). We train our model for 250 training epochs, and we choose the best one in terms of balanced accuracy (computed on the validation set). Adam has been used as optimizer, and all the hyper-parameters are tuned via grid-search: weight decay is set to 10^{-4}, learning rate $\eta = 10^{-4}$, exponential learning rate decay 0.99 per epoch, and minibatch size 16. Our algorithms are implemented in Python, using PyTorch 1.5, and training/inference runs over an NVIDIA GeForce GTX 1080 GPU.

5.1 Patches Normalization

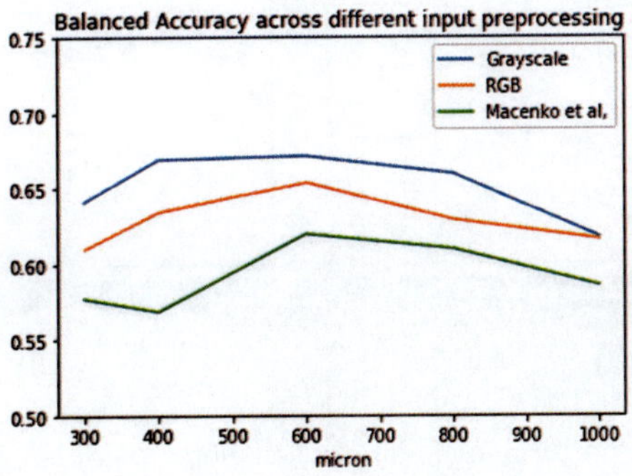

Fig. 2. Patches classification performance.

As a first step, we perform a study at different RoI resolutions: the goal here is to identify the best scale the deep model is able to extract the features. Towards this end, we consider 8 possible patches resolutions $\varphi \in [300; 1000]$ µm, and 3 possible input preprocessing strategies: use of the original patches (RGB), conversion to gray-scale (gray) and the use of a standard slide normalization strategy (Macenko et al. [17]), resulting in 24 training possibilities, which are reported in Fig. 2. For our classification task, the use of gray-scale images does not remove useful information (which might be embedded in the color) and, on the contrary, helps in removing the expected color bias [18,20]. From our results we learn that, for the particular classification task we aim at solving, the relevant features are embed in the image texture and the signal strength, while the direct use of the RGB image does not compensate the color bias, or even standard slide normalization strategies like [17] destroy some useful information which is not embed in the color feature. For these reasons, we will focus our analysis using gray-scale patch images as input for our model.

5.2 Study on Patches Resolution for WSI Classification

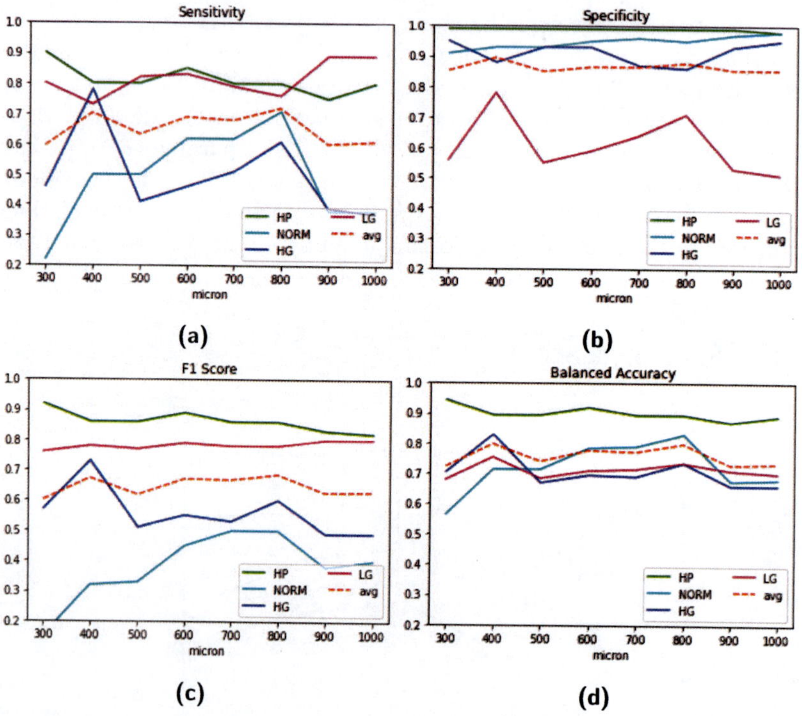

Fig. 3. WSI inference performance comparison between different tissue categories at different patches resolutions: sensitivity (a), specificity (b), F1-score (c) and balanced accuracy (d). Red dashed line is the average performance (avg).

Here we will inspect more in depth the study on WSI classification performance using gray-scaled input. Figure 3 provides a general overview of some metrics evaluated. There is not a clear choice regarding the optimal scale features have to be extracted. If our goal is to maximize the sensitivity for the HG class, we should choose 400 µm: inspecting the HP's specificity for the same scale, we observe a drop which, however, is overall tolerable. F1-score gives us a more

Table 3. Human dysplasia diagnostic performance comparison

		Accuracy	Sensitivity	Specificity
Hyperplastic	Our (400 μm)	0.90	0.80	**0.99**
	Our (600 μm)	**0.92**	**0.85**	**0.99**
	Pathologist [8]	0.79	0.30	0.97
Low grade	Our (400 μm)	**0.76**	0.73	**0.78**
	Our (600 μm)	0.71	**0.83**	0.59
	Pathologist [8]	0.66	0.57	0.69
High grade	Our (400 μm)	**0.83**	0.78	0.88
	Our (600 μm)	0.70	0.46	**0.93**
	Pathologist [8]	**0.83**	**0.81**	0.84

global information: indeed, for the HG class, 400 μm is the best one. However, if we look at average performance on all classes (avg), focusing on F1-score and balanced accuracy, we can observe similar performance for 400 μm and 600–800 μm.

It is important to compare the model performance with the results obtained by human pathologists. Table 3 reports performance comparison for HP, LG and HG in terms of balanced accuracy, sensitivity and specificity. Here, human pathologist's average performance is taken from Denis et al.'s work [8], evaluated on qualitatively similar data. As we observe, our performance is very close to the pathologists'. In particular, HP classification increases of more than 10% in accuracy, showing a quite significant improvement in terms of sensitivity. LG classification improves as well up to 10% in balanced accuracy, yielding a significant improvement both in terms of sensitivity and specificity. HG classification score is in the same order than human pathologists (this finding is likely to be due to HG features that are known to be visually easier to detect).

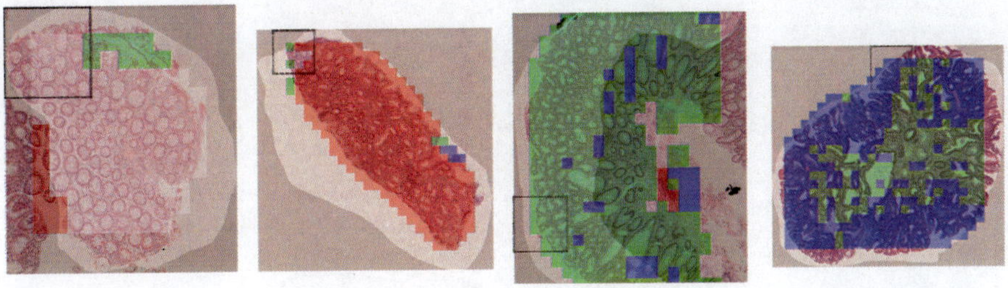

(a) NORM (b) HP (c) LG (d) HG

Fig. 4. Patch classification: each box is located at the center of the corresponding patch with a color representing the predicted class: HP (red), NORM (white), LG (green), HG (blue). The black dashed square visually represents the patch scale ($\varphi = 600\,\mu m$).

Table 4. WSI inferences: confusion matrices.

(a) φ =600 µm, gray-scale

Gr. truth \ Predicted	HP	NORM	HG	LG
HP	**0.85**	0	0.05	0.1
NORM	0.12	**0.75**	0	0.12
HG	0.02	0	**0.63**	0.35
LG	0.03	0.09	0.18	**0.7**

(b) φ =600 µm, RGB

Gr. truth \ Predicted	HP	NORM	HG	LG
HP	**0.75**	0.05	0	0.2
NORM	0	**0.62**	0	0.38
HG	0	0.02	**0.61**	0.37
LG	0.03	0.06	0.15	**0.76**

5.3 WSI Classification with 600 µm Patches

Considering that the overall performance shown by 400, 600, 700 and 800 µm is similar, we decided here on to focus on $\varphi = 600$ µm. Such a scale is a fair compromise, considering that other works in the literature focus on similar scales [15,24]. Figure 4 reports a patch-level classification result for the four possible WSI classes. In particular, we observe that the model finds some HG patches within the LG WSI (Fig. 4c), and viceversa (Fig. 4d). This is an expected behavior, given that the dysplasia grade is provided by the pathologists according to the quantity of tissue (in our case, the number of patches) with high-grade dysplasia. At $\varphi = 600$ µm, the classification between TA and TVA classes in general is poor: this is due to the larger scale required to extract proper features for adenoma classification. This, however, is not our goal, since we are here interested in classifying the dysplasia grade. Hence, we group HG and LG and we obtain the confusion matrix shown in Table 4 on WSI: the score is competitive to the human classification, as described in Sect. 5.2. We also report the confusion matrix for the equivalent model, using RGB images: as also observed in

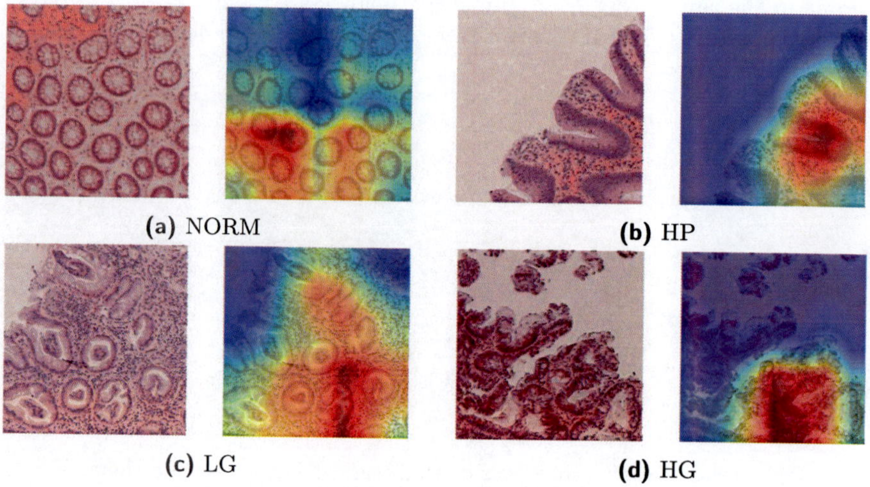

(a) NORM (b) HP (c) LG (d) HG

Fig. 5. Regions where the trained neural network model focuses on 600 µm patches.

Sect. 5.1, the use of gray-scale images positively impacts on the WSI inference task. Additionally, we inspect the areas our deep model focuses in order to perform classification by using Grad-CAM. Figure 5 shows that areas of focus are consistent with the most relevant features of each histo-pathological category. For example, the hot spot of the HP sample is on a serrated gland which is a characteristic finding of this entity.

6 Conclusion

In this work we have designed a neural network-based pipeline for the classification of colorectal polyps in histopathological slides. We found performance benefits by applying grayscale Luma transformation [16] to input tissue patches. We focused on four tissue classes: normal, hyperplastic, high-dysplasia and low-dysplasia adenoma. The dysplasia degree of adenomas is a very important evaluation element for the histopathologist because it leads to different post-polypectomy surveillance protocols [11]. The collected data enable a classification on the dysplasia degree in adenomas. The classification is performed by ResNet-18, inspecting WSI in single patches, and then classified averaging scores on all the patches. Our experiments show a performance which is very close to human pathologists [8]. Future work includes the design of a neural network model able to learn to extract relevant tissue RoIs from the whole slide, evaluated by pathologists' agreement, and the deployment of a multi-scale deep learning pipeline.

References

1. Balkenhol, M.C., et al.: Deep learning assisted mitotic counting for breast cancer. Lab. Invest. **99**(11), 1596–1606 (2019)
2. Bejnordi, B.E., et al.: Diagnostic assessment of deep learning algorithms for detection of lymph node metastases in women with breast cancer. JAMA **318**(22), 2199–2210 (2017)
3. Bertero, L., et al.: Unitopatho (2021). https://doi.org/10.21227/9fsv-tm25
4. Bevan, R., Rutter, M.D.: Colorectal cancer screening-who, how, and when? Clin. Endosc. **51**(1), 37 (2018)
5. Bychkov, D., et al.: Deep learning based tissue analysis predicts outcome in colorectal cancer. Sci. Rep. Nat. **8** (2018)
6. Cubuk, E.D., Zoph, B., Mané, D., Vasudevan, V., Le, Q.V.: Autoaugment: learning augmentation strategies from data. In: 2019 IEEE/CVF Conference on Computer Vision and Pattern Recognition (CVPR), pp. 113–123 (2019)
7. DeepHealth: Deep-learning and HPC to boost biomedical applications for health (2019). https://deephealth-project.eu/
8. Denis, B., et al.: Diagnostic accuracy of community pathologists in the interpretation of colorectal polyps. Eur. J. Gastroenterol. Hepatol. **21**(10), 1153–1160 (2009)
9. Foss, F.A., Milkins, S., McGregor, A.H.: Inter-observer variability in the histological assessment of colorectal polyps detected through the NHS bowel cancer screening programme. Histopathology **61**(1), 47–52 (2012)

10. Gonzalez, R.S.: Updates and challenges in gastrointestinal pathology. Surg. Pathol. Clin. **13**(3), ix (2020)
11. Hassan, C., et al.: Post-polypectomy colonoscopy surveillance: European society of gastrointestinal endoscopy (ESGE) guideline-update 2020. Endoscopy **52**(08), 687–700 (2020)
12. He, K., Zhang, X., Ren, S., Sun, J.: Deep residual learning for image recognition. In: CVPR, pp. 770–778. IEEE Computer Society (2016)
13. He, X., et al.: Long-term risk of colorectal cancer after removal of conventional adenomas and serrated polyps. Gastroenterology **158**(4), 852–861 (2020)
14. Janowczyk, A., Madabhushi, A.: Deep learning for digital pathology image analysis: a comprehensive tutorial with selected use cases. J. Pathol. Informa. 7–29 (2016)
15. Korbar, B., et al.: Deep learning for classification of colorectal polyps on whole-slide images. J. Pathol. Inform. **8** (2017)
16. Luma. https://en.wikipedia.org/wiki/Luma_(video)
17. Macenko, M., et al.: A method for normalizing histology slides for quantitative analysis. In: 2009 IEEE International Symposium on Biomedical Imaging: From Nano to Macro, pp. 1107–1110. IEEE (2009)
18. Mahapatra, D., Bozorgtabar, B., Thiran, J.P., Shao, L.: Structure preserving stain normalization of histopathology images using self supervised semantic guidance. In: Medical Image Computing and Computer Assisted Intervention - MICCAI 2020, pp. 309–319. Springer, Cham (2020)
19. Mollasharifi, T., et al.: Interobserver agreement in assessing dysplasia in colorectal adenomatous polyps: a multicentric Iranian study. Iran. J. Pathol. 167–174 (2020)
20. Roy, S., Kumar Jain, A., Lal, S., Kini, J.: A study about color normalization methods for histopathology images. Micron **114**, 42–61 (2018)
21. Selvaraju, R.R., Cogswell, M., Das, A., Vedantam, R., Parikh, D., Batra, D.: Grad-cam: visual explanations from deep networks via gradient-based localization. In: ICCV, pp. 618–626. IEEE Computer Society (2017)
22. Song, Z., et al.: Automatic deep learning-based colorectal adenoma detection system and its similarities with pathologists. BMJ Open **10**(9), e036423 (2020)
23. Van Putten, P.G., et al.: Inter-observer variation in the histological diagnosis of polyps in colorectal cancer screening. Histopathology (2011)
24. Wei, J.W., et al.: Evaluation of a deep neural network for automated classification of colorectal polyps on histopathologic slides. JAMA Netw. Open **3**(4), e203398–e203398 (2020)
25. Yan, Z., et al.: HD-CNN: hierarchical deep convolutional neural networks for large scale visual recognition. In: Proceedings of the IEEE International Conference on Computer Vision, pp. 2740–2748 (2015)
26. Zhu, X., Bain, M.: B-CNN: branch convolutional neural network for hierarchical classification. arXiv preprint arXiv:1709.09890 (2017)

Deep YOLO-Based Detection of Breast Cancer Mitotic-Cells in Histopathological Images

Maisun Mohamed Al Zorgani(✉), Irfan Mehmood, and Hassan Ugail

Faculty of Engineering and Informatics, School of Media, Design and Technology, University of Bradford, Bradford, UK
M.M.S.AlZoragani@bradford.ac.uk

Abstract. Coinciding with advances in whole-slide imaging scanners, it is become essential to automate the conventional image-processing techniques to assist pathologists with some tasks such as mitotic-cells detection. In histopathological images analysing, the mitotic-cells counting is a significant biomarker in the prognosis of the breast cancer grade and its aggressiveness. However, counting task of mitotic-cells is tiresome, tedious and time-consuming due to difficulty distinguishing between mitotic cells and normal cells. To tackle this challenge, several deep learning-based approaches of Computer-Aided Diagnosis (CAD) have been lately advanced to perform counting task of mitotic-cells in the histopathological images. Such CAD systems achieve outstanding performance, hence histopathologists can utilise them as a second-opinion system. However, improvement of CAD systems is an important with the progress of deep learning networks architectures. In this work, we investigate deep YOLO (You Only Look Once) v2 network for mitotic-cells detection on ICPR (International Conference on Pattern Recognition) 2012 dataset of breast cancer histopathology. The obtained results showed that proposed architecture achieves good result of 0.839 F1-measure.

Keywords: Breast cancer histopathological images · Mitotic cell counting · Deep learning techniques · YOLO-v2 network

1 Introduction

In the World Health Organization, Nottingham Grading System is recommended to use for tumour grading [1]. This system has been widely used to estimate the breast cancer grades based on three morphological features in histopathological images. One of them refers to the deformation occurring in the cell nucleus and it is known as nuclear atypia. The second refers to the cancer cells rate in regular tubule formation and it is known as tubule formation. The third is known as mitotic-cells count and it is used to estimate of mitosis cells from the

R. Su et al. (Eds.): MICAD 2021, LNEE 784, pp. 335–342, 2022.
https://doi.org/10.1007/978-981-16-3880-0_35

division process. Therefore it is the most significant biomarkers among the three morphological features [2].

Recently, Deep learning techniques have proven their ability to achieve a great success in histopathological image analysis tasks. Therefore substituting the visual inspection detection by automated deep learning-based detection for breast cancer prognosis is becoming important. Whereas automated detection techniques could help the pathologists in some tiresome, tedious and time consuming tasks. Moreover, avoiding pathologist inaccurate prognosis, which could have serious consequences. Additionally it can be used in breast cancer prognosis as a second-opinion system. Which in turn improve diagnosis accuracy and treatment plan. Despite this, there are several challenges in automating mitotic-cells detection methods; as in the histopathological images with the high appearance variance, it is rough distinguishing the mitotic cells from normal cells. Therefore the environment of data-preparation must be standard to avoid the issues in slides preparation and their scanning [3].

The traditional methods of mitotic-cells detection depended on the extracted hand-crafted features from the region proposals. These methods require a trained pathologist to identify the features that characterise various cancer severity levels. Whereas deep learning methods can extract the hierarchical features from image without the need of trained pathologist, which avoid us the challenges of manual feature extraction from the images. In analysis of the breast cancer histopathological images for ICPR2012 dataset, the mitotic-cells detection techniques are categorised according into the extracted features from Regions Of Interest (ROIs). In one of the approaches, conventional image-processing techniques [4–7] are utilised to extract the handcrafted features, which after that are employed to train the machine-learning classifiers. In the other approach, convolutional neural networks (CNNs) [8–11] are utilised to extract the deep features from ROIs. These features are capable of self-learning for the different image features.

In the mitotic-cells detection task, some researchers deal with it as a classification task [12,13], while others deal with it as a semantic segmentation [2,14] or object-detection task according to the problem formulation. In classification task, the cells are identified as mitosis or normal cells. In semantic segmentation, the mitotic cells are segmented according in the pixels-based annotations. Whereas in object-detection, the cells are detected and counted. In this work, we deal with the detection of mitotic-cells as an object-detection task.

Up to now, several CNNs [2,15–17] have emerged and proven their ability for mitotic-cells detection in ICPR 2012 dataset. These CNNs composed two stages and depend on generating region proposals, such as Faster Region-based CNN (Faster R-CNN) [18]. In addition to that, there is another methodology composed one stage and based on the regression methods. It integrates components of object classification and object detection together in the same deep learning architecture, such as the YOLO [19] and YOLOv2 [20] models. Such models are characterised by speed and accuracy. In this paper, we leverage the speed and precision of YOLO architecture and propose mitotic-cells detection architecture based on the modified YOLO v2 model. The backbone of proposed architecture is ResNet50 model [21] as feature extractor, then follows by YOLO detector to predict the mitotic-cells of breast cancer in ICPR2012 dataset.

This paper is organized as follows. In Sect. 2, the proposed methodology in this work is briefly described. In Sect. 3, the experiment and its results are presented in detail. Section 4 provides a brief summary of the paper.

2 Methodology for the Proposed Work

In this section, we present a brief explanation of target dataset, data preprocessing, data preparation, anchor boxes choice, detection accuracy metric and finally the proposed architecture that are used in this work.

2.1 Target DataSet

The Hematoxylin and Eosin (H&E) stained images of ICPR 2012 dataset contest [22,23] were acquired by both Aperio XT scanner and Hamamatsu NanoZoomer Scanner. In this paper, we work on the Aperio XT scanner images, which composed 35 training images and 15 testing images. These images were possessed from 10 high-energy fields (HPFs) for five breast cancer biopsies. The HPFs have size of $512 \times 512\,\mu m^2$/pixel at $40\times$ magnification and the dataset images have size of 2084×2084 pixels. The training set images hold 226 mitotic-cells while the testing set images hold 101 mitotic-cells. The annotations were performed by histopathologists in mutual consent.

2.2 Data Pre-processing

In this section, we pre-process dataset images into two steps as follows:

- In the first step, we stain normalise histopathological images of ICPR 2018 dataset as described in [24] to reduce the color variation and standardise the H&E stained images. The stain normalisation toolbox [25] for several techniques of histological images are found the Warwick University website.
- In the second step, we augment training data to enlarge ICPR 2012 MITOSIS dataset. In this paper, we have rotated the training images with angles of 180 degrees, and then flipped them in horizontal and vertical direction to generate an extra augmented image without affecting on the input images quality [8,26] as well as to avoid over-fitting problems [27] and features poorly generation.

2.3 Data Preparation

Data preparation is essential step in our proposed architecture. In this step, we create two tables, one for storing training data information and the other for storing test data information. Each table composed from two columns, where the first column holds the image file storage paths and the other holds dimensions of the mitosis bounding boxes. After that, we store the tables as MATLAB files. Whereas, we prepared the bounding boxes for mitotic-cells manually according to the ground-truth label of images in ICPR2012 dataset. Each bounding box is a vector with four elements in the formula [x y width height]. Whereas, the coordinate (x, y) represents the upper left corner value for bounding box. The other variables represent height of bounding box and its width (pixels).

2.4 Anchor Boxes Choice

Anchor box is essential parameter that has an impact on the deep detectors performance. In this paper, we use Intersection-Over-Union (IoU) distance metric to estimate anchor boxes from training data. IoU distance metric has the ability to clustering similar boxes together, which results in anchor box estimates that fit the data. The ICPR 2012 dataset is annotated by the pixel-level ground truth type which provides us with enough information to estimate bounding boxes for mitotic-cells. From empirical analysis, we determine thirty two anchor boxes with 64 and 128 scale to satisfy YOLO v2 performance requirements.

2.5 Accuracy Metric of Detector

One of the common metrics for evaluating a trained detector on testing images is F1-Score, and it is defined by:

$$F_1Score = \frac{2 \times Precision \times Recall}{Precision + Recall} \quad (1)$$

From the above equation, precision refers to detector's ability to make correct detections, while recall refers to detector's ability to detect relevant objects.

$$Precision = \frac{tp}{tp + fp} \quad (2)$$

$$Recall = \frac{tp}{tp + fn} \quad (3)$$

The above two equations use the following metrics; tp (true positive) is number of the predicted mitotic-cells that intersect with their corresponding mitotic-cells in ground truth, while fn (false negative) is number of the mitotic-cells in ground truth that have not been predicted. Otherwise is fp (false positive) which represents number of the predicted mitotic-cells that wrongly predicted as mitotic-cells.

2.6 Proposed Architecture

The proposed architecture is inspired by YOLO v2 architecture. It is composed from ResNet-50 feature extractor followed by YOLO v2 detector layers as illustrated in the Fig. 1.

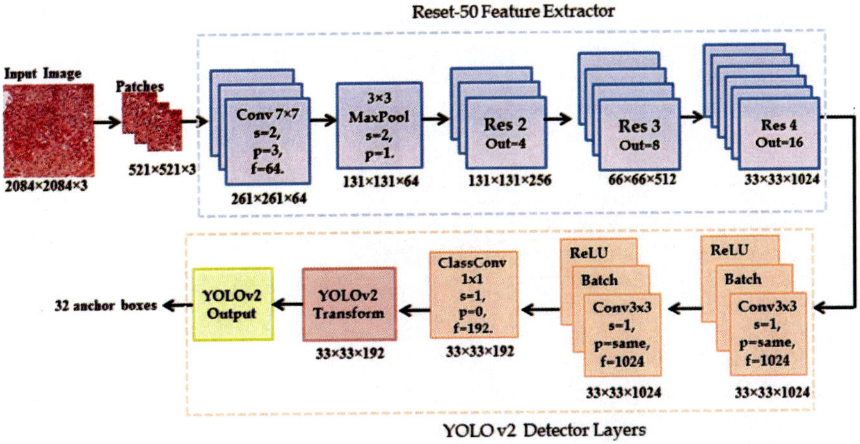

Fig. 1. The proposed detector architecture, where "Conv" represents the convolution block which followed by two layers; Rectified Linear Unit (ReLU) and Batch layers; "f" represents the output number of filters; "s" represents the stride of all convolutions; p is padding.

3 The Experiment and Its Results

The experiment was carried out by using ICPR 2012 dataset. It was implemented in MATLAB R2020a on a desktop computer has a CPU with a 3.60-GHz Intel®Core-i7-7700, GPU wirh NVIDIA GeForce GTX 1070 and RAM with 32 GB.

- **For pre-processing steps**, we stained normalise dataset images, and then divided them into sixteen non-overlapping patches, each patch has a size of 521×521 pixels to cover the whole image. Next, we augmented the patches of training set. After that, we drew out the bounding boxes for mitotic-cells manually according to their ground-truth label to fill in MATLAB tables by dimensions of bounding boxes. Now the data is ready to train our proposed method.
- **For feature extractor model**, the feature extractor was fed by the augmented training patches. So, we change input layer size of ResNet-50 model to $(521 \times 521 \times 3)$. After that, the images were divided into training 80%, and validation 20%.
- **For training deep YOLO detector**, we set Stochastic Gradient Descent with Momentum (SGDM) to 0.90 with mini-batch size of 128, weight learn rate to 20, bias learn rate to 20, and initial learning rate to 0.0001. We validated our model every three iterations, and selected 120 iterations as the maximum number.

The performance results of the modified YOLO v2 decoder were reported in the Table 1. We utilised the standard metrics; precision, recall and F1-score to evaluate the efficiency of our deep decoder for mitotic-cells prediction on the ICPR 2012 dataset. These results have obtained from the three Eqs. 1, 2, 3.

Table 1. The standard evaluation metrics of our model

Metrics	Our detector
Recall	0.7765
Precision	0.8049
F_1 **Score**	0.7903

Table 2 illustrate the comparative analysis of our detector results with some of the works results, which were previously published on the same ICPR 2012 dataset. It can be observed from Table 2 that obtained result of F1-score is 0.7903%. This result confirms that our proposed detector in terms of detection accuracy outweighs the other methods that used the same image dataset.

Table 2. Comparison of the performance of modified YOLO v2 detector with other methods

Methods	F1-Score
[11] Albarqouni and others	0.4330
[9] Wang and others	0.7350
[8] Cireşan and others	0.7820
[17] Li and others	0.7840
[10] Chen and others	0.7880
Our Detector	**0.7903**

In time analysis, the detector velocity to quantify mitotic-cells is an important factor in clinical applications. Our method takes 6 s per image, whereas the proposed methods by Cireşan et al. [8] and Li et al. [2] take 31 and 7 sec/HPF, respectively. So, our detector outperforms some other methods in term of speed.

4 Conclusions

In this study, we have investigated the YOLO architecture to tackle the detection problem of mitotic-cells in breast cancer histopathological images. Therefore we presented a simple detector based on YOLO architecture to leverage of its speed. The proposed detector is the modified YOLO v2 with ResNet-50 backbone network as feature extractor. The results evaluated on ICPR 2012 dataset demonstrated that our detector is robust. It is fast and thus reduces the time that pathologists take for mitotic-cells detection. In future, we will plan to improve the proposed detector to include ICPR 2014 dataset.

References

1. Elston, C.W., Ellis, I.O.: Pathological prognostic factors in breast cancer. I. The value of histological grade in breast cancer: experience from a large study with long-term follow-up. Histopathology **19**(5), 403–410 (1991)
2. Li, C., Wang, X., Liu, W., Latecki, L.J.: DeepMitosis: mitosis detection via deep detection, verification and segmentation networks. Med. Image Anal. **45**, 121–133 (2018)
3. Veta, M., et al.: Assessment of algorithms for mitosis detection in breast cancer histopathology images. Med. Image Anal. **20**, 237–248 (2015)
4. Irshad, H.: Automated mitosis detection in histopathology using morphological and multi-channel statistics features. J. Pathol. Inform. **4**, 1–6 (2013)
5. Tashk, A., Helfroush, M.S., Danyali, H., Akbarzadeh, M.: An automatic mitosis detection method for breast cancer histopathology slide images based on objective and pixel-wise textural features classification. In: KIT 2013, pp. 406–410 (2013)
6. Sommer, C., Fiaschi, L., Hamprecht, F.A., Gerlich, D.W.: Learning-based mitotic cell detection in histopathological images. In: ICPR 2012, pp. 2306–2309 (2012)
7. Paul, A., Dey, A., Mukherjee, D.P., Sivaswamy, J., Tourani, V.: Regenerative random forest with automatic feature selection to detect mitosis in histopathological breast cancer images. In: MICCAI, pp. 94–102. Springer (2015)
8. Cireşan, D., Giusti, A., Gambardella, L., Schmidhuber, J.: Mitosis detection in breast cancer histology images with deep neural networks. In: MICCAI-2013, pp. 411–418. Springer (2013)
9. Wang, H., et al.: Cascaded ensemble of convolutional neural networks and handcrafted features for mitosis detection. In: SPIE Medical Imaging, pp. 1–10
10. Chen, H., Dou, Q., Wang, X., Qin, J., Heng, P.: Mitosis detection in breast cancer histology images via deep cascaded networks. In: 13th AAAI Conference on Artificial Intelligence, pp. 1160–1166 (2016)
11. Albarqouni, S., Baur, C., Achilles, F., Belagiannis, V., Demirci, S., Navab, N.: AggNet: deep learning from crowds for mitosis detection in breast cancer histology images. IEEE Trans. Med. imaging **35**(5), 1313–1321 (2016)
12. Malon, C., Cosatto, E.: Classification of mitotic figures with convolutional neural networks and seeded blob features. J. Pathol. Inform. **4**, 1–5 (2013)
13. Malon, C., Brachtel, E., Cosatto, E., Graf, H.P., Kurata, A., et al.: Mitotic figure recognition: agreement among pathologists and computerized detector. Anal. Cell. Pathol. **35**, 97–100 (2012)
14. Veta, M., Pluim, J.P.W., Diest, V., Paul, J., Viergever, M.A.: Breast cancer histopathology image analysis: a review. IEEE Trans. Biomed. Eng. **61**, 1400–1411 (2014)
15. Cai, D., Sun, X., Zhou, N., Han, X., Yao, J.: Efficient mitosis detection in breast cancer histology images by RCNN. In: IEEE 16th International Symposium on Biomedical Imaging, pp. 919–922 (2019)
16. Dodballapur, V., Song, Y., Huang, H., Chen, M., Chrzanowski, W., Cai, W.: Mask-driven mitosis detection in histopathology images. In: IEEE 16th International Symposium on Biomedical Imaging, pp. 1855–1859 (2019)
17. Li, Y., Mercan, E., Knezevitch, S., Elmore, J.G., Shapiro, L.G.: Efficient and accurate mitosis detection—a lightweight RCNN approach. In: 7th International Conference on Pattern Recognition Applications and Methods, pp. 69–77 (2018)
18. Ren, S., He, K., Girshick, R., Sun, J.: Faster R-CNN: towards real-time object detection with region proposal networks. IEEE Trans. Pattern Anal. Mach. Intell. **39**, 1137–1149 (2016)

19. Redmon, J., Divvala, S., Girshick, R., Farhadi, A.: You only look once: unified, real-time object detection. In: IEEE Conference on Computer Vision and Pattern Recognition, pp. 779–788 (2016)
20. Redmon, J., Farhadi, A.: YOLO9000: better, faster, stronger. In: IEEE Conference on Computer Vision and Pattern Recognition, pp. 7263–7271 (2017)
21. He, K., Zhang, X., Ren, S., Sun, J.: Deep residual learning for image recognition. In: IEEE Conference on Computer Vision and Pattern Recognition, pp. 770–778 (2016)
22. Mitosis Detection in Breast Cancer Histological Images. http://ludo17.free.fr/mitos_2012/download.html. Accessed 23 Nov 2020
23. Roux, L., Racoceanu, D., Loménie, N., Kulikova, M., Irshad, H., Klossa, J., et al.: Mitosis detection in breast cancer histological images an ICPR 2012 contest. J. Pathol. Inf. **4**, 1–7 (2013)
24. Khan, A.M., Rajpoot, N., Treanor, D., Magee, D.A.: Nonlinear mapping approach to stain normalization in digital histopathology images using image-specific color deconvolution. IEEE Trans. Bio. Eng. **61**, 1729–1738 (2014)
25. Stain Normalisation Toolbox. https://warwick.ac.uk/fac/sci/dcs/research/tia/software/sntoolbox/. Accessed 12 Dec 2020
26. Mikołajczyk, A., Grochowski, M.: Data augmentation for improving deep learning in image classification problem. In: 2018 International Interdisciplinary Ph.D. Workshop (IIPhDW), pp. 117–122 (2018)
27. Shorten, C., Khoshgoftaar, T.M.: A survey on image data augmentation for deep learning. J. Big Data **6**, 60 (2019)

Others

Promoting Cardiovascular Health Using a Recommendation System

Ana Duarte and Orlando Belo(✉)

Algoritmi R&D Centre, University of Minho, Campus of Gualtar, 4710-057 Braga, Portugal
pg36084@alunos.uminho.pt, obelo@di.uminho.pt

Abstract. Lifestyle habits have a direct influence on people's health. Regular physical activity, combined with good nutrition, helps to prevent the early onset of diseases such as cardiovascular disease. In fact, a significant number of patients diagnosed with cardiovascular disease is associated with a poor diet and a sedentary routine. However, in today's busy life, it is not always easy to find the motivation for adopting healthy lifestyle habits. Therefore, the existence of a system for recommending healthy meals and workouts can provide the necessary incentive for a healthier life. In this paper, we describe the implementation of a recommendation system following a case-based reasoning approach supported by specific relational databases and ontologies in the field of nutrition and physical activity. The system creates a plan for daily recommendations adapted to the preferences and restrictions of its users, and evaluates the outcome of the recommendations using indexes that quantify cardiovascular health. The success of the recommendations thus depends on a positive evolution of the index after the end of the proposed plan. This system thus presents a new perspective using case-based reasoning and ontologies to propose a diet and exercise plan, evaluating the success of the recommendations objectively through cardiac indexes.

Keywords: Case-based reasoning · Cardiovascular diseases · Ontologies · Recommender systems · Well-being indexes

1 Introduction

Lifestyle habits and daily routine tasks have a direct impact on well-being and Cardiovascular Health. Due to lack of time and motivation, many of the actions people take in their daily lives, especially those related to diet and exercise, are not the result of thoughtful actions and do not reflect healthy choices. At this level, the existence of a recommendation system for diet and physical activity can guide its users towards healthier lifestyle habits. However, conceiving recommendation systems for these areas presents several difficulties due to the complexity of the problems, resulting from the preferences and restrictions of each individual, as well as the high uncertainty associated with the success of the recommendations.

In this domain, the Case-Based Reasoning (CBR) approach, which consists in proposing similar solutions to the previous successful cases, presents itself as a technique

R. Su et al. (Eds.): MICAD 2021, LNEE 784, pp. 345–353, 2022.
https://doi.org/10.1007/978-981-16-3880-0_36

with identical characteristics to the human reasoning. The study of cognitive science has demonstrated that humans do not only learn concepts and tasks, but they also learn to generalize and easily adapt to novel situations. Based on their past experiences, even with few examples, they have the ability to infer new knowledge and new ways of solving problems. The human capacity for generalizing is supported, therefore, in the knowledge of similar cases that have occurred in the past. Human reasoning uses memory and by analogy or association with previous similar successful solutions, it is able to propose solutions to new problems [1]. Due to its ability to propose solutions in areas where the knowledge domain is limited and uncertain, to solve complex problems and to improve the performance of the system with experience, CBR becomes an oriented approach to artificial intelligent systems in the real world [2, 3].

The aim of the present work is to implement a recommendation system based on a CBR approach that helps its users to adopt a healthier lifestyle. The system proposes a 30-day diet and exercise recommendation plan. The paper is divided into five main sections. This first part briefly introduces the case under study and the next chapter gives an overview about different applications of CBR. In its turn, Sect. 3 describes the considered methodology for the implementation of the proposed system, whereas Sect. 4 demonstrates some functionalities of the developed system. Finally, the last section presents the main conclusions and some possible future work.

2 The Evolution of Case-Based Reasoning

The first CBR system mentioned in the literature is the program Cyrus, developed by Janet Kolodner, in 1983 [4]. Cyrus is a software that enables to retrieve events related to the former Secretary of the USA, Cyrus Vance. It acts as a program to answer questions about this political dignitary [5]. In the late 1980s, the first CBR systems for the medical field appeared, such as CASEY, which was introduced by Phyllis Koton in 1988. Casey is a CBR software that uses the United States Heart Failure Program as a model to diagnose heart problems and, as a result, to propose appropriate treatments [6]. In the field of food recommendation systems, [7] proposes Chef, a recipe recommendation system for Szechwan cuisine, based on users requests. In 2003, [8] created Mikas, a menu recommendation system, based on CBR, that takes into account the needs and preferences of the users.

An important evolution in the food recommendation systems occurred with the integration of ontologies. One of the examples of this inclusion was proposed by [9], in 2008, as part of the first Computer Cooking Contest. The authors presented ColibriCook, a CBR system that uses an ontology to adapt culinary recipes according to the requests of the users. In general, the vast amount of the developed CBR systems do not analyse the evaluation of the success of the recommendations based on quantifiable metrics. Instead, these systems typically use the feedback given by the users or experts to classify the results. In addition, there are few examples in previous research integrating ontologies with CBR presenting a comprehensive view of health and well-being, such as proposing joint recommendations of nutrition and physical exercise.

3 Methodology

3.1 The Proposed System

The developed system consists in a CBR approach that is supported by cardiovascular well-being indexes. These indexes are calculated based on a set of personal and clinical data, using an adapted methodology from QRisk2 [10], and support the evaluation of the success of the recommendations. For the implementation of the system, each case is represented by a description, containing a set of relevant attributes, a justification, a solution and a result, as listed in Table 1.

Table 1. Case representation structure.

	Id	Age	Gender	Ethnicity	Family history	Systolic blood pressure	Total cholesterol	HDL cholesterol	Diabetes	Abdominal circumference	BMI	Eating habits	Smoking habits	Physical exercise	Stress	Index	Justification	Solution	Result
Description	x	x	x	x	x	x	x	x	x	x	x	x	x	x	x	x			
Justification																	x		
Solution																		x	
Result																			x

Regarding the data, we considered a mixed persistence with two MySQL databases [11], to store and retrieve the data (a case base and a general archive), an ontology created with Protégé 5.5 [12], for adapting the solutions of the cases, and a set of Semantic Web Rule Language (SWRL) rules, for inferring knowledge based on the individual restrictions of each user. The ontology represents the available knowledge about nutrition, physical exercises, and restrictions. Since it stores the most important properties and values in these domains, the ontology serves as a basis for recommending the best options regarding diet and exercise. Considering the specificities of each user, it enables to calculate the similarity between menus and between exercises and to recommend the most similar ones. The option for a single ontology encompassing these knowledge domains allows to separate the different concepts, on the one hand, and to integrate all the knowledge required for the implementation of the system in the same structure, on the other hand.

In the food domain, the ontology is organised according to the classes Dish, Type of Dish, Type of Meal, Season, Ingredients and Nutrients. On the other hand, in the field of physical exercise, the ontology is divided considering the main types of exercises: Flexibility, Resistance, Strength and Balance [13]. Moreover, the ontology also contains the "UserRestriction" class, which is divided into two subclasses related to the dietary and physical restrictions of the users. In addition to these aspects, the ontology has a set of object and data properties that, together with SWRL rules, allow inferring knowledge. For example, in the case of a user who is lactose intolerant, it is necessary to ensure that none of the proposed menus contains any type of dairy ingredients. To address this limitation, the following rule was defined:

```
hasIngredient(?m,?d)^Dairy(?d)->cannotEat(intolerantLactose,?m)
```

To infer knowledge from the ontology, axioms and rules, Pellet was the chosen reasoner.

3.2 Case-Based Reasoning Steps

Retrieve. The process of retrieving the most similar cases starts by applying the k-Nearest Neighbors (k-NN) algorithm and selecting the *k* cases from the case base that are most similar to the query (new case). For this purpose, the local similarities between the attributes of the query and the attributes of the cases from the case base are calculated and the global similarity for each case with respect to the query is returned. With the goal of eliminating cases that have a low global similarity with the query, we de-fined a minimum threshold and only considered the cases with a similarity above this value. Consequently, there may be Cold Start (CS) situations, in which no case is re-turned. In these cases, it is necessary to consider fixed rules to do the recommendations. Therefore, depending on whether any cases are returned, there are two different methods to consider in the process: the CS problem and the determination of the most similar case. Figure 1 schematically illustrates the main steps to retrieve the cases.

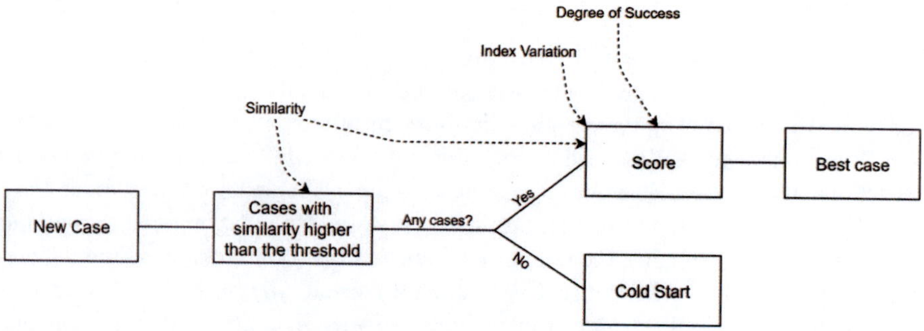

Fig. 1. Considered methodology for case retrieval.

The rules to be applied in CS situations have been defined based on the recommended dietary intakes indicated in [14], and vary according to the characteristics of the users.

Regarding the determination of the best case, we established Eq. 1, considering that the index variation corresponds to the average variation of the cardiovascular well-being index, and that the degree of success reflects the confidence in a successful result. Using this equation these values can be converted into a score and the best case corresponds to the returned case with the highest value.

$$Score = Similarity \times Index\,Variation \times Degree\ of\ Success \tag{1}$$

Reuse. The solution obtained in the previous step must be adapted to the new case, considering the restrictions, preferences and specificities of the new user. More concretely, to adapt the diet plan, the dietary restrictions, food preferences and recommended caloric intake of the new user must be taken into account. In this case, the methodology for adapting the solution begins with the execution of the following steps:

1. Retrieving the available menus: all the menus that satisfy the recommended calories intake for that user, according to the type of meal (breakfast, lunch, snack and dinner).
2. Retrieving the restricted menus: i.e. menus that contain at least one ingredient to which the user has an intolerance or is allergic.
3. Identifying the possible menus: i.e. menus that the user can eat (menus retrieved in step 1. but not indicated in step 2.).

After these steps, the methodology varies depending on the type of retrieval. Thus, towards a CS situation, the methodology is completed by the following procedures:

4. a) Retrieving the menus that comply with the CS rules: i.e. menus that respect the CS applicable rules.
5. a) Proposing menus: first, the similarity between the menus from 4.a. and the preferences of the user is calculated. Then, the results are sorted in descending order according to the similarity values obtained. Finally, the three most similar menus are selected and proposed.
6. a) Selecting the recommended menu: the recommended menu corresponds to the menu selected by the user among the three suggestions and becomes part of the meal plan.

Conversely, when a similar case (best case) is retrieved, the first three steps are followed by:

4. b) Retrieving the equivalent menus: the nutrients of each possible menu from 3. are compared to the nutrients of the reference menu (best case) using similarity measures. Only the menus with a similarity higher than a predefined threshold are returned.
5. b) Proposing menus: first, the similarity between the menus from 4.b. and the preferences of the user is calculated. Then, the values of similarity in terms of nutritional values and similarity in terms of preferences are weighted and the results are ranked in descending order. Finally, the top three menus are selected and presented to the user.

6. Selecting the recommended menu: the user selects a menu from the available options and that menu is included in the meal plan.

For the execution of these steps, we developed code in Java and constructed SPARQL statements in order to execute the connection to the ontology and to return the menus to recommend.

The adaptation process of physical activities involves a similar methodology. The first step consists in retrieving the available exercises for the user, considering his/her restrictions. These restrictions are related to injuries or physical limitations in specific parts of the body, equipment availability, and the time and intensity that the user is willing to dedicate to the exercise.

In a next step, to define the methodology for the CS problems, we followed the recommendations of [15, 16] and converted them into rules. Thus, we created SPARQL statements in order to filter only the exercises that comply with the CS rules. After, for each returned exercise, the similarity with the user's preferences is calculated, and the exercises with the higher values are proposed for selection. On the contrary, when the best case is returned, the similarity is determined considering the proximity between the types of exercises and the user's preferences. Again, the exercises with the highest similarities are proposed for selection.

Revise. Since in CBR approaches the correspondences between cases are not completely equal, and there is no guarantee that all cases behave the same towards the same solutions, the system requires a later validation of the proposed solutions. First, the result of the case must be classified as a success or a failure, depending on the variation of the index calculated by Eq. 2, where Vfinal is the value of the index after the end of the plan and Vinitial is the value at the beginning of the plan.

$$Index\,variation = \frac{V_{final} - V_{initial}}{100} \tag{2}$$

As there is no linear correspondence between a solution and the result of each user, it is possible that successful and unsuccessful results regarding the same case exist simultaneously in the case base. Therefore, an important metric to take into account is the degree of success of the cases in the case base. This metric reflects the probability of the solution to produce a successful result, considering the ratio between the number of successes and the total number of cases, as given in Eq. 3.

If the result is successful, 1 unit is added to the number of successful cases and the degree of success is updated according to the equation. On the other hand, if the outcome is not successful, 1 unit is added to the number of unsuccessful cases. In this case, if the degree of success is high, the next step is performed and, if it is low, the case is removed from the case base. This occurs because the case already contains a significant number of unsuccessful cases and, for this reason, it must not support the recommendation system.

$$DS = \frac{numSuccess}{numSuccess + numUnsuccess} \tag{3}$$

Retain. At the end of the review phase, the new successful cases are stored in the case base and/or in the archive, as summarized in Fig. 2. In these situations, it is necessary to verify whether the 30-day plan is similar or significantly different from the plan of the best-case solution. If it is similar, the attributes of the new case are added to the best-case attributes. If not, the case is only inserted into the archive and when that case represents a considerable number of records it is inserted into the case base as a new case. The same methodology is followed when the retrieval is done using CS rules.

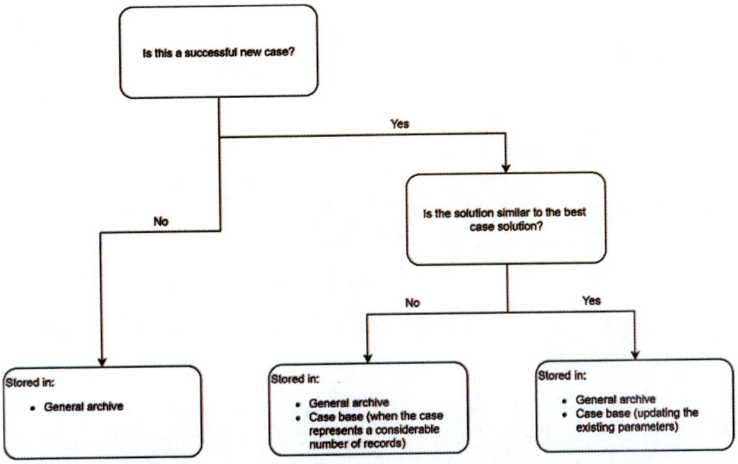

Fig. 2. Considered methodology for retaining cases.

The inclusion of a new record into one of the existing cases in the case base is done in a weighted way, taking into account the number of cases that are represented by the existing record in the case base. Considering that the case record represents *n* cases, then, each of its parameters will assume new values, according to the Eq. 4, where NV_i represents the new value of parameter i, NC_i is the value of parameter i of the new record, and IV_i is the initial value of parameter i in the case base.

$$NV_i = \frac{NC_i + n \times IV_i}{n + 1} \tag{4}$$

4 The Developed System

To implement the proposed system, we developed an application using Java and JavaFX in order to enable the interaction with the users. For evaluating the created program, we performed some tests inserting new queries. Each time a new case is introduced, the program asks for some personal and clinical attributes of the user, which are required for the CBR steps. In the next phase, the application performs the retrieval and the reuse stages. At the end of this step, the window depicted in Fig. 3 appears to the user indicating three alternative dishes for each meal. At this point, the user must specify his/her preferences by selecting a single option for each meal.

After choosing the preferred menus, three types of exercises are presented. Similarly, the user should select one of the available options. Once confirmed this second choice,

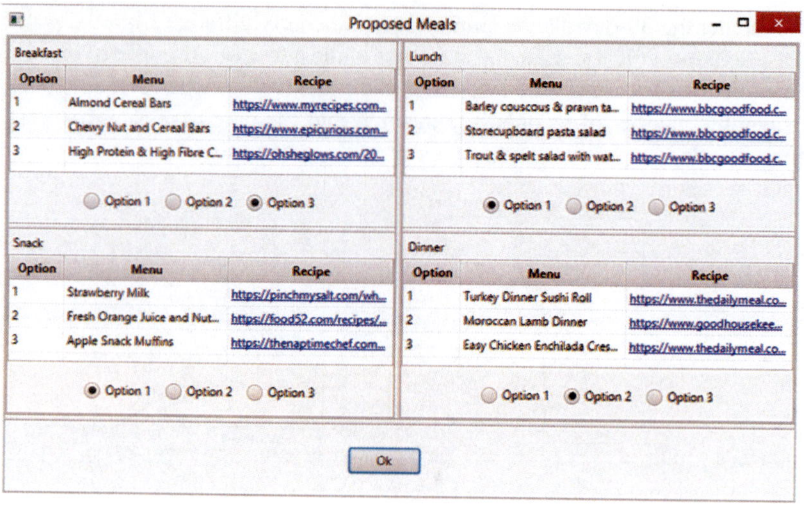

Fig. 3. Graphical interface displayed after inserting the values of the query.

the system stores these data in the archive. This recommendation procedure is repeated daily until the plan is completed. At the end of the 30-day plan, the user is asked to update his/her clinical values in order to determine the success/failure of the proposed solution.

5 Conclusions and Future Work

This paper describes the development of a recommendation system in the field of nutrition and physical activity, following a CBR approach supported by databases and an ontology to adapt the cases. This work leads to the conclusion that it is possible to implement a recommendation system in the domain of Health, without requiring human intervention to verify the success/failure of the recommendation. Furthermore, the present work has highlighted that the knowledge integrated in an ontology permit an efficient adaptation of cases.

In summary, since it is not always possible to dedicate much attention to our daily choices, the proposed system can promote the adoption of healthier lifestyle habits, by proposing personalized recommendations for food and exercise. However, there are some important issues that need to be examined in future research. The most obvious is data limitation. Since no real data were used, the effectiveness of the system in promoting cardiovascular health could not be tested. Moreover, further studies in this area should consider additional aspects that were not contemplated in the present work, such as remote communication and security issues. Another opportunity for improvement in future work would be to consider the quantities of the ingredients and propose different portions of each menu according to the nutritional needs of the users. It would also be interesting to explore the combination of different workouts in the same exercise recommendation.

Acknowledgements. This work has been supported by FCT – Fundação para a Ciência e Tecnologia within the R&D Units Project Scope: UIDB/00319/2020.

References

1. Thrun, S., Pratt, L. (eds.): Learning to Learn. Springer US, Boston, MA (1998). https://doi.org/10.1007/978-1-4615-5529-2
2. Pal, S.K., Shiu, S.C.K.: Foundations of Soft Case-Based Reasoning. John Wiley & Sons, Inc., Hoboken (2004)
3. Clifton, J.R., Frohnsdorff, G.: Applications of computers and information technology. In: Handbook of Analytical Techniques in Concrete Science and Technology, pp. 765–799. Elsevier (2001). https://doi.org/10.1016/B978-081551437-4.50021-7
4. Aamodt, A., Plaza, E.: Case-based reasoning: foundational issues, methodological variations, and system approaches. Artif. Intell. Commun. **7**, 39–59 (1994). https://doi.org/10.3390/s120811154
5. Kolodner, J.: What Is Case-Based Reasoning? In: Case-Based Reasoning, pp. 3–31. Elsevier (1993). https://doi.org/10.1016/B978-1-55860-237-3.50005-4
6. Koton, P.: Reasoning about evidence in causal explanations. In: AAAI'88: Proceedings of the Seventh National Conference on Artificial Intelligence, pp. 256–261 (1988)
7. Hammond, K.: CHEF: a model of case-based planning. In: AAAI'86: Proceedings of the Fifth National Conference on Artificial Intelligence, pp. 267–271 (1986)
8. Khan, A.S., Hoffmann, A.: Building a case-based diet recommendation system without a knowledge engineer. Artif. Intell. Med. **27**, 155–179 (2003). https://doi.org/10.1016/S0933-3657(02)00113-6
9. DeMiguel, J., Plaza, L., Díaz-Agudo, B.: ColibriCook: a CBR system for ontology-based recipe retrieval and adaptation. In: ECCBR - 9th European Conference on Case-Based Reasoning, pp. 199–208. Trier, Germany (2008)
10. QRISK2. https://qrisk.org/2017/. Accessed on 18 Dec 2020
11. MySQL. https://www.mysql.com/. Accessed on 18 Dec 2020
12. Protégé. https://protege.stanford.edu/. Accessed on 18 Dec 2020
13. Corbin, C.B.: Concepts in Physical Education, with Laboratories and Experiments. W.C. Brown Co, Dubuque, Iowa (1983)
14. Stallings, V.A., Harrison, M., Oria, M. (eds.): Dietary Reference Intakes for Sodium and Potassium. National Academies Press, Washington, D.C. (2019). https://doi.org/10.17226/25353
15. WHO Guidelines on physical activity and sedentary behaviour. World Health Organization, Geneva (2020)
16. Physical Activity Guidelines for Americans. U.S. Department of Health and Human Services (2018)

Unsharp Masking with Local Adaptive Contrast Enhancement of Medical Images

Ivo Draganov(✉) and Veska Gancheva

Technical University of Sofia, 8 Kliment Ohridski Blvd, 1756 Sofia, Bulgaria
{idraganov,vgan}@tu-sofia.bg

Abstract. In this paper we present a generalized algorithm for unsharp masking of medical images which takes as one of its inputs a high contrast image underwent local adaptive contrast enhancement. Selection of optimal values of the number of histogram bins, processing window size and intensity lower and upper limits in iterative manner is part of applying Contrast Limited Adaptive Histogram Equalization (CLAHE). Experimental results reveal higher quality of the output images both in terms of root mean square contrast and sharpness. Achieved quality, both visually and quantitatively, is compared to that from the Adaptive Histogram Equalization (AHE) algorithm, limited histogram stretching and ordinary histogram equalization which proves its applicability. The algorithm is considered appropriate for processing a number of types of images, such as CT, X-ray, etc.

Keywords: Unsharp masking · Contrast enhancement · CLAHE · CT · X-ray

1 Introduction

Medical images contrast plays extremely important role during visual inspection of the internal structure of the human body for issuing correct diagnosis and further treatment of patients. Over the years there are many proposed techniques for contrast enhancement [1–3].

One of the more recent studies related to the CT image analysis, using deep learning, also include an aspect of predicting the contrast enhancement [4]. A number of maps, such as class activation, its gradient-weighted variant, saliency and backpropagation modifications are combined in a new type of a map which further eases the prediction process. As a result voxel visualization is reported to be more clear and allows for more precise feature selection to improve overall accuracy. Prediction probability for some of the modifications tried goes over 90% with registering higher specificity for the saliency map in particular.

Kallel and Hamida [5] rely on more direct approach, that is the discrete wavelet transform with singular value decomposition in order to implement adaptive gamma correction. Singular values are found from the low-low frequency sub-band and then modified by a factor, followed by classification of the whole sub-band into low and average contrast types. Adaptive gamma correction is applied over the low contrast

R. Su et al. (Eds.): MICAD 2021, LNEE 784, pp. 354–363, 2022.
https://doi.org/10.1007/978-981-16-3880-0_37

areas. All these steps take place in wavelet domain prior restoring the final enhanced image. Increased efficiency is reported over other well-known methods.

Another recent approach for CT contrast enhancement [6] employs clustering-based algorithm where the input image is at first converted through one-dimensional separation on a column basis. Then, data sorting of the elements follows prior the clustering of subsequent elements, ending with a labeling in order to get the output image. As main benefit of the approach, it is pointed out its lower processing time with regards to 5 other algorithms.

Enhancement of X-ray images also has its own development in the recent years. Irrera et al. [7] apply multiscale contrast enhancement after patch-based filtering of X-ray images. Noise presence is estimated in a parametric fashion in order to optimize the level of contrast increase without corrupting intolerably the quality of output images. Visual evaluation, as well as the signal and contrast to noise ratios, prove the proposed approach applicable. Kushol et al. [8] achieve contrast enhancement of X-ray images by morphological operators. They apply the top-hat and bottom-hat operations and the parameters of the structuring element are autonomously estimated from the intensity gradient over processed area. Visual comparison of resulting images with the contrast-limited adaptive histogram equalization (CLAHE) proves the applicability of this technique. Another autonomous algorithm [9] making use of CLAHE at the addition of noise and high-pass filters aims to adapt its performance based on few tunable parameters to the modality being registered. Around 48% of the test database involved in the study got highest evaluation score of 5 as a subjective measure, given by medical personnel and other experts.

The aim of the study presented in this paper is to evaluate the performance of the three of the most popular image contrast enhancement algorithms – histogram equalization, image adjustment and CLAHE when applied on CT and X-ray images for unsharp masking. Based on experimental results, simple general purpose algorithms for selecting the optimal parameters of all input arguments for these algorithms are proposed in Sect. 2. Their efficiency is presented in Sect. 3 where the experimental results are reported. In Sect. 4 a conclusion is made.

2 Algorithms Description

The well-known unsharp masking algorithm for general purpose images [3], especially in photography, is given in Fig. 1. In its form here, it takes a grayscale input image *I(i,j)*, where *i* and *j* are the spatial coordinates of the pixels. In order to get a better contrast and details, a Gaussian kernel [10] blurs it to *G(i,j)* and by subtracting with the original a contour mask *C(i,j)* is found. After applying any contrast enhancement algorithm the resulting image *E(i,j)* is combined with *I(i,j)* and *C(i,j)* to get the final result *O(i,j)*.

According to the purpose of the current study, three of the most popular contrast enhancement algorithms are tried within the unsharp masking scheme – the histogram equalization (histeq) [1], image intensity adjustment (imadjust) [2] and the contrast-limited adaptive histogram equalization (CLAHE, adapthisteq) [11].

Since histeq has the number of histogram bins ($2^n, n = 1, 2, 3, \ldots$) as input argument, the imadjust – the clipping limit *cl* of the intensity level in the range of low intensities

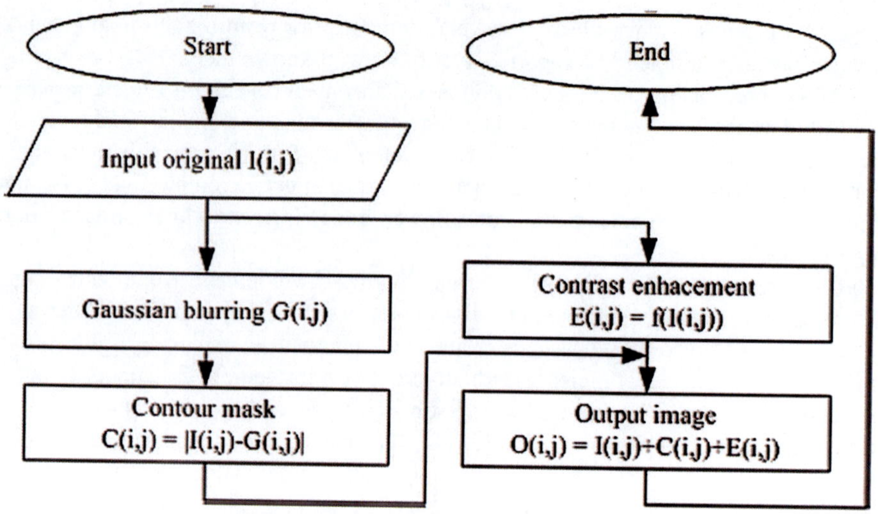

Fig. 1. General unsharp masking scheme

and $(1 - cl)$ – in the high, and the CLAHE – the tile size over one dimension m, again the clipping limit cl, and the number of histogram bins 2^n, there is a need to select those based on certain criteria. A simple way of doing so, is to seek for the highest possible root mean square contrast $RMSC$ [12]:

$$RMSC = \sqrt{\frac{1}{MN}\sum_{i=0}^{M-1}\sum_{j=0}^{N-1}\left(O(i,j) - \overline{O}\right)^2}, \tag{1}$$

where M and N are the number of rows and columns of the resulting image O with its mean intensity $\overline{O}$. In addition to that one would expect also as high as possible sharpness ($Shrp$) [13] of the image which could be found over particular direction (d), according to:

$$Shrp_d = \frac{1}{P}(T_1 - T_2)\sum_{p=1}^{P} S_p^2, \tag{2}$$

where T_1 and T_2 are the maximum and minimum densities of an area of the image over which the $Shrp_d$ is sought; P – the number of points through which the change of the intensity profile S_p (slope) is traced. More generally, the sharpness as a vector filed could be found from the gradient of the intensity in all image points. The norm of that vector is what is used as a scalar in this study.

It may turn out that both the RMSC and Shrp could rise or fall monotonically without any expressed maximum and in the same time the quality of the processed image decrease significantly, rendering it unusable. In order to avoid that, the peak signal-to-noise ratio (PSNR) [3] and the structural similarity index (SSIM) [3] are used as limiting factors into the selection of appropriate input arguments for the contrast enhancement algorithms. Optimal selection for histeq and imadjust is given in Fig. 2.

The three input arguments for the CLAHE algorithm could be found, following the iterative approach, presented in Fig. 3.

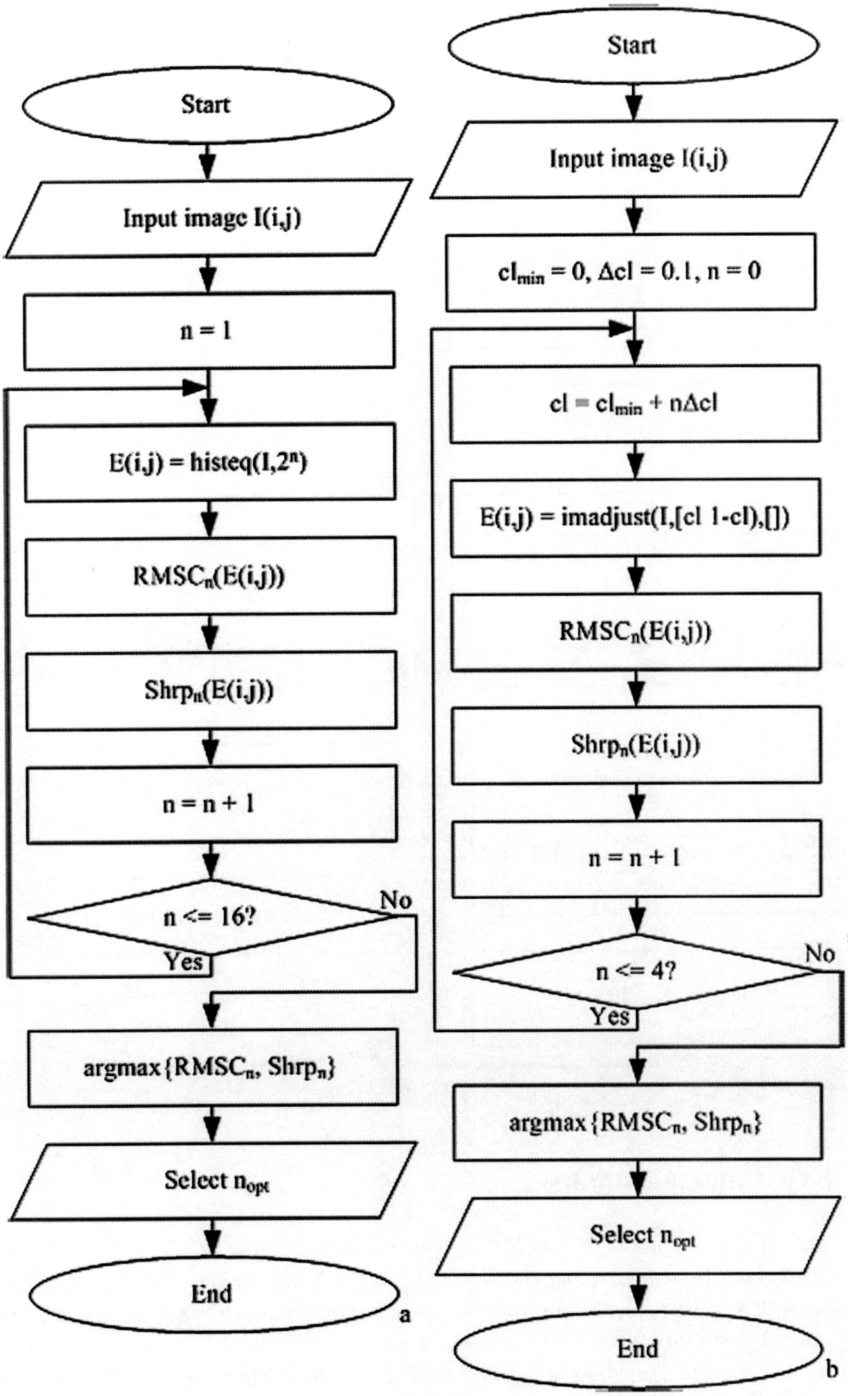

Fig. 2. Finding optimal parameters for histogram equalization (a) and image adjusting (b)

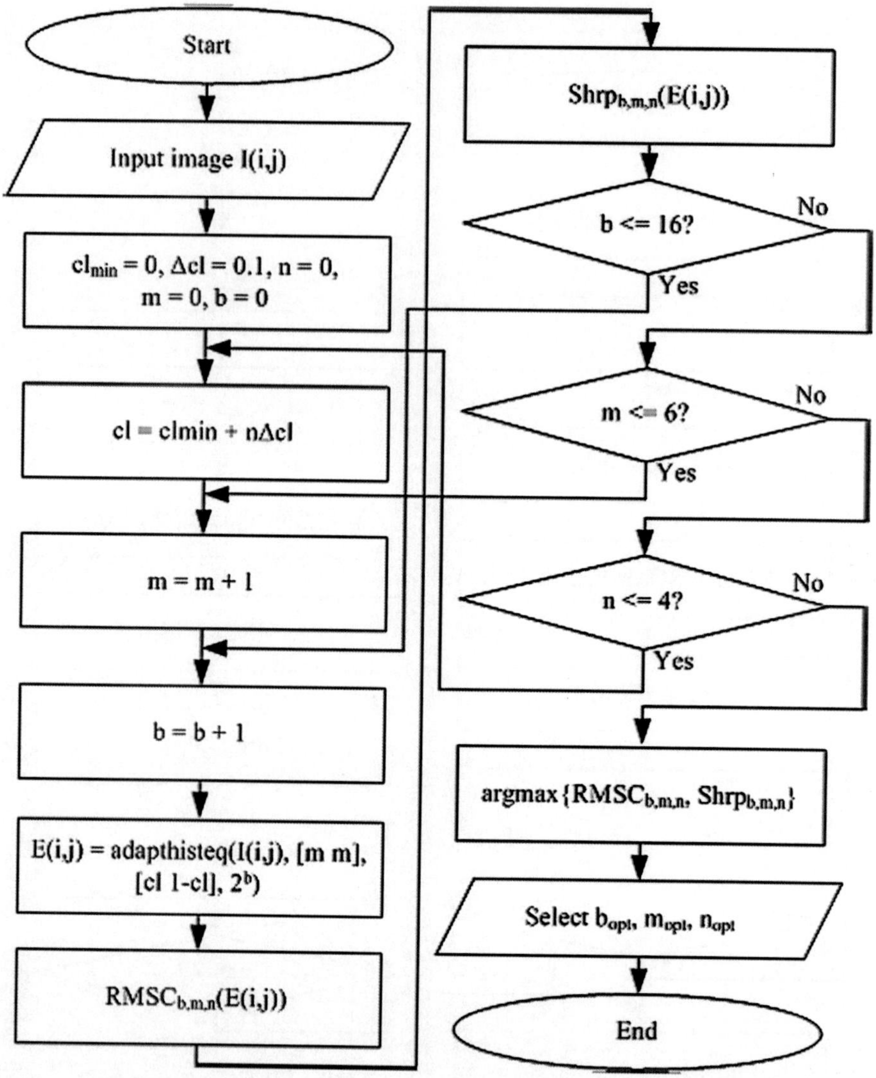

Fig. 3. Finding optimal parameters for contrast-limited adaptive histogram equalization

3 Experimental Results

The test database consists of 103 CT images with dimensions 512 × 512 pixels each, 16 bpp, part of the DeepLesion gathering [14] and 105 X-ray images, 1024 × 1024 pixels in size, with 8 bpp representation, which come from the ChestX-ray8 [15] collection. All experiments are implemented on a desktop computer with Intel Core i5 x64 processor, having 4 cores and operating at 3.1 GHz, 12 GB of RAM under the control of Linux Ubuntu LTS 14.04. The simulation environment is Matlab R2016a.

The only adjustable parameter for the histeq algorithm, being the number of bins to process from the histogram of the input image 2^n, is found to be 64, that is $n = 6$. While the average RMSC and Shrp from all CT images are high for $n = 1$, around 0.5 and 0.028, respectively (Fig. 4), the PSNR and SSIM for the processed images are too low, below 10 dB and 0.3 in the same time. A saturation for the similarity from above between the original image and enhanced one is observed for $n = 6$ and higher, where SSIM reaches around 0.6. That bound is thought to define the optimal n. Similar results are obtained for the X-ray images.

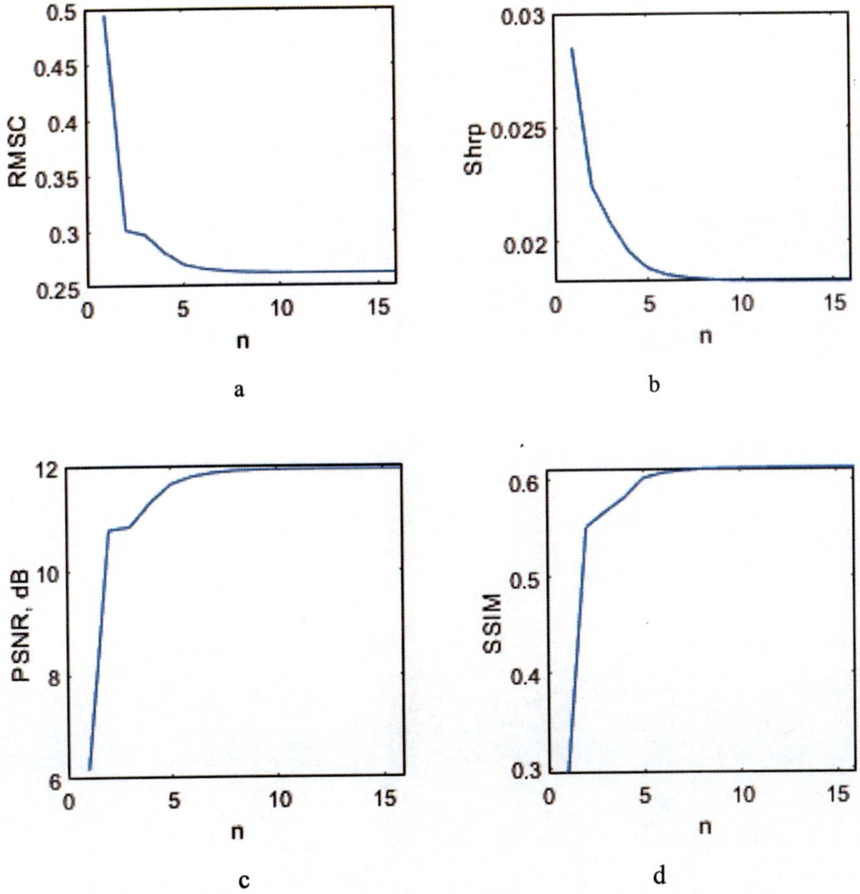

Fig. 4. Finding the optimal number of bins for the histogram processed by histeq

Analogous approach is undertaken when estimating the optimal clip limit for the imadjust algorithm. Both the RMSC and Shrp parameters rise monotonically but SSIM starts to fall from almost 1 after $cl = 0.01$ and PSNR drops significantly below 50 dB after that value which means significant deterioration of the image structure. Hence, cl_{opt} is selected to be 0.01. This result is true for both CT and X-ray images.

CLAHE supports high RMSC and Shrp for 2 histogram bins ($n = 1$) – around 0.18 and 0.016, respectively, which decrease gradually to 0.02 and 0.002 for $n = 8$ in the case of CT enhancement. PSNR and SSIM however constantly rise close to 35 dB and 0.99, respectively. The observed change of RMSC for X-ray images is from around 0.195 up to 0.245, and Shrp changes from 0.01 up to 0.022 in the interval [1, 8] for n. SSIM is above 0.8 when $n\ n = 8$. That's why all subsequent experiments use $n\ n = 8$. In Fig. 5 the mutual influence of the clip limit (cl – from 0 to 0.3) and tile size (m – from 2×2 to 64×64 pixels) reveals significant change in RMSC and Shrp of enhanced CT images.

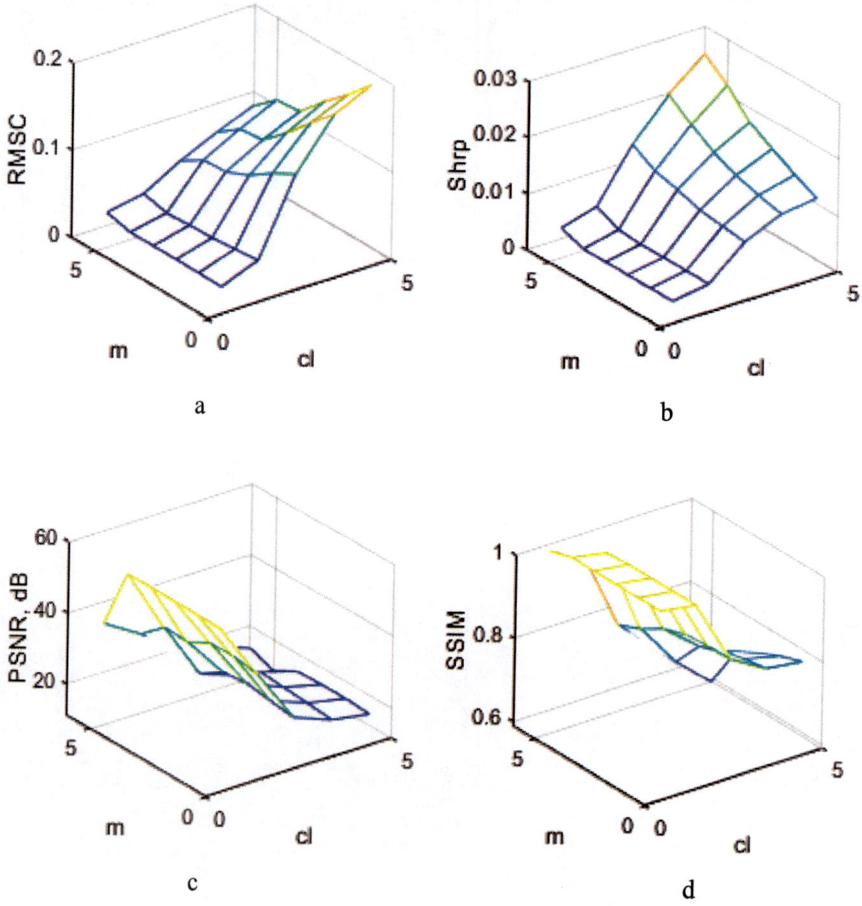

Fig. 5. Finding the optimal clip limit and tile size for the adapthisteq

The highest RMSC is obtained for $cl = 0.3$ (Fig. 5a) but PSNR drops below 20 dB (Fig. 5c) and SSIM is around 0.7 (Fig. 5d). There is almost none dependency on the tile size for all four parameters at fixed cl. In order to get most of the details in the image preserved the following selection is made – $cl_{opt} = 0.01$ and $m = 1$ (2×2 tile).

The average RMSC, Shrp and processing time for each of the tested contrast enhancement algorithms, when applied separately outside the complete unsharp masking procedure, are presented in Table 1. It seems that histeq and adapthisteq are close one to each other and better than imadjust with regards to all 3 registered parameters. The adapthisteq leads to higher sharpness in X-ray images but is slower than histeq for both types of images. The fastest algorithm is imadjust.

Table 1. Average performance for histeq, imadjust and adapthisteq alone.

Algorithm	CT images			X-ray images		
	RMSC	Shrp	Time, s	RMSC	Shrp	Time, s
Input images	0.0084	0.0005	N/A	0.2320	0.0099	N/A
histeq	0.2656	0.0185	0.0026	0.2926	0.0142	0.0071
imadjust	0.0210	0.0012	0.0012	0.2363	0.0101	0.0029
adapthisteq	0.1850	0.0108	0.0159	0.2832	0.0156	0.0183

Table 2 contains the final average RMSC, Shrp and processing time, which represents the period needed for the Gaussian blurring, finding the contour mask and the fusion of it with the original and the contrast enhanced image (Fig. 1). The optimal parameters of the Gaussian kernel, found empirically based on highest RMSC and Shrp in a separate experiment carrying out test unsharp masking, are $\sigma = 10$ for the CT and $\sigma = 0.8$ for the X-ray images. Naturally, the Time is higher for the X-ray images due to their higher resolution. The histeq algorithm has the peak values of RMSC but comparable to those for adapthiseq and for the X-ray photos Shrp is higher for the adapthisteq. Both parameters are considerably lower for the imadjust algorithm.

Table 2. Unsharp masking average evaluating parameters.

Algorithm	CT images			X-ray images		
	RMSC	Shrp	Time, s	RMSC	Shrp	Time, s
Input images	0.0084	0.0005	N/A	0.2320	0.0099	N/A
histeq	0.1220	0.0086	0.0087	0.2232	0.0118	0.0207
imadjust	0.0155	0.0011	0.0076	0.1992	0.0102	0.0196
adapthisteq	0.0851	0.0051	0.0076	0.2162	0.0125	0.0191

The visual comparison between input and processed images (Fig. 6) show more details in the range of the low and high intensities from the human body when employing adapthisteq algorithm in the unsharp masking. Slightly lower contrast and some more difficult to distinguish areas appear in images, obtained with the histeq algorithm. The overall contrast and some of the details' visibility are lower for the imadjust with comparison to the other two algorithms.

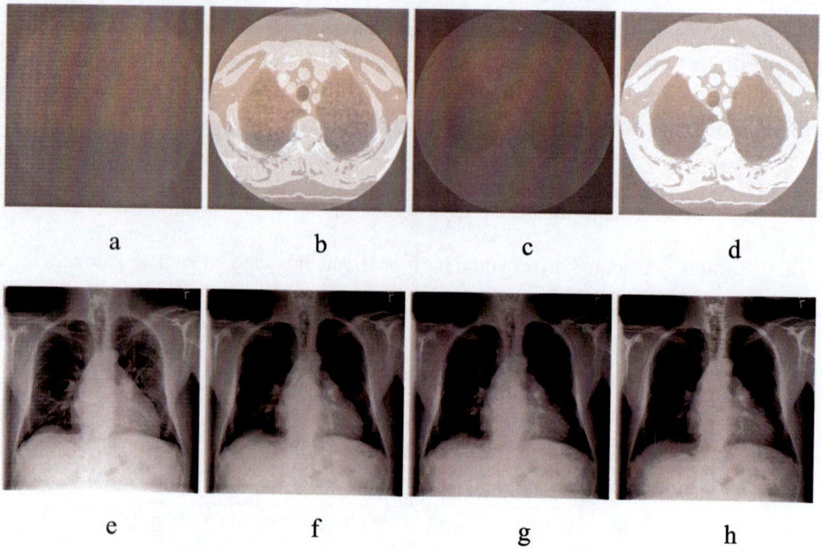

Fig. 6. Original – a (CT), e (X-ray), and processed by histeq – b, f, imadjust – c, g, and adapthisteq – d, h images

4 Conclusion

In this paper simple optimization procedures are presented for the histogram equalization, intensity adjusting and the contrast-limited adaptive histogram equalization algorithms in order to find optimal parameters for them. The root mean square contrast, the sharpness and structural similarity between the contrast enhanced and original image play the role of target parameters. Tests with CT and X-ray images confirm the plausibility of the undertaken approach and the applicability of resulting images for the unsharp masking algorithm to use them as input. The contrast-limited adaptive histogram equalization yields more detailed and contrast enhanced final images, followed by the histogram equalization and the image adjusting algorithms at the price of more computational time. The unsharp masking in this general and easy to implement form is thought to be an useful tool for medical imaging purposes.

Acknowledgement. This work was supported by the National Science Fund at the Ministry of Education and Science, Republic of Bulgaria, within the project KP-06-PN-37/55 "Innovative integrated platform for smart management and big data flow analysis for biomedical research".

References

1. Gonzalez, R., Woods, R.: Digital Image Processing, 4th edn. Pearson, New York (2018)
2. Burger, W., Burge, M.J.: Principles of Digital Image Processing: Core Algorithms. Springer Science & Business Media, London (2010)
3. Beutel, J., Kundel, H.L., Van Metter, R.L.: Handbook of medical imaging, vol. 1. Spie Press, Washington (2000)

4. Philbrick, K.A., et al.: What does deep learning see? Insights from a classifier trained to predict contrast enhancement phase from CT images. Am. J. Roentgenol. **211**(6), 1184–1193 (2018)
5. Kallel, F., Hamida, A.B.: A new adaptive gamma correction based algorithm using DWT-SVD for non-contrast CT image enhancement. IEEE Trans. Nanobiosci. **16**(8), 666–675 (2017)
6. Mehmood, A., Khan, I.R., Dawood, H., Dawood, H.: Enhancement of CT images for visualization. In: ACM SIGGRAPH 2019 Posters, pp. 1–2 (2019)
7. Irrera, P., Bloch, I., Delplanque, M.: A flexible patch based approach for combined denoising and contrast enhancement of digital X-ray images. Med. Image Anal. **28**, 33–45 (2016)
8. Kushol, R., Raihan, M., Salekin, M.S., Rahman, A.B.M.: Contrast enhancement of medical x-ray image using morphological operators with optimal structuring element. arXiv preprint arXiv:1905.08545 (2019)
9. Qui, J., Li, H.H., Zhang, T., Ma, F., Yang, D.: Automatic x-ray image contrast enhancement based on parameter auto-optimization. J. Appl. Clin. Med. Phys. **18**(6), 218–223 (2017)
10. Blinchikoff, H.J., Zverev, A.I.: Filtering in the Time and Frequency Domains. Wiley, New York (1976)
11. Pizer, S.M., et al.: Adaptive histogram equalization and its variations. Comput. Vis. Graph. Image Process. **39**(3), 355–368 (1987)
12. Peli, E.: Contrast in complex images. J. Opt. Soc. Am. A **7**(10), 2032–2040 (1990)
13. Präkel, D.: The Visual Dictionary of Photography. AVA Publishing, Lausanne (2010)
14. Yan, K., Wang, X., Lu, L., Summers, R.M.: DeepLesion: automated mining of large-scale lesion annotations and universal lesion detection with deep learning. J. Med. Imaging **5**(3), 036501 (2018)
15. Wang, X., Peng, Y., Lu, L., Lu, Z., Bagheri, M., Summers, R.M.: ChestX-ray8: Hospital-scale chest X-ray database and benchmarks on weakly-supervised classification and localization of common thorax diseases. In: 2017 IEEE Conference on Computer Vision and Pattern Recognition (CVPR), pp. 2097–2106. IEEE, Honolulu, HI, USA, 21–26 July 2017

Check for updates

Building a COVID-19 Literature Knowledge Graph Based on PubMed

Hualing Liu(✉), Yi Sun, and Shijie Cao

Shanghai University of International Business and Economics, Shanghai, China
liuhl@suibe.edu.cn

Abstract. COVID-19, the most destructive global event in 2020, poses gigantic challenges to global medical systems. Meanwhile, the useful concepts and newly-emerging technical terms in medical field generate ambiguity and bring difficulties in extraction, which would set immense obstacles to anti-epidemic actions. To solve this problem, we built a knowledge graph by extracting six kinds of medical entities from titles and abstracts related to COVID-19 in PubMed. Then, we eliminated author name ambiguity and integrated articles' publication information as well as authors' affiliation information into the graph. By this way, connections are established between authors, articles, entities and affiliations. Our model which aims at named entity recognition achieved an F1 score of 92.57% on average. This graph not only allows us to seek out hotspots, utilize specific knowledge and transfer research results quickly, but also helps us understand the research development process. It can also aid scholars to focus on specific authors and entities. This method of a knowledge graph is extensible and transplantable, which means it will not be limited to COVID-19 research in the future.

Keywords: COVID-19 · Knowledge graph · PubMed

1 Introduction

At the beginning of 2020, COVID-19 has swept the world as a sudden epidemic, disrupting the peace of every family in every country in the world. The spread of COVID-19 is so fast and infectious that it is beyond everyone's imagination. As a result, it has had a catastrophic impact on the world's population, economy, environment, and education. The severity of the epidemic problem quickly drew a response from scientific researchers in most countries, and academic research on vaccine development, drug research, and disease transmission trend prediction on COVID-19 was quickly launched. Papers from various fields and angles have been included on PubMed.

PubMed is an abstract database developed by the National Center for Biotechnology Information (NCBI) under the National Library of Medicine (NLM). As one of the most influential databases in the biomedical field, PubMed has the advantages of timely update, free access, and high coverage rate. Therefore, we choose PubMed and LitCovid (dataset in PubMed [1, 2]) as our data source.

R. Su et al. (Eds.): MICAD 2021, LNEE 784, pp. 364–373, 2022.
https://doi.org/10.1007/978-981-16-3880-0_38

In this context, a complete and efficient retrieval approach is particularly important. It must meet two requirements: on the one hand, it can enable researchers to quickly obtain research progress in a specific research field, and on the other hand, it also needs to provide a way for researchers to find research partners in the same direction. The powerful information extraction capabilities and intuitive visualization functions of the knowledge graph perfectly meet our needs, so we chose to construct the COVID-19 literature knowledge graph to summarize existing research.

In the research field of bio-entity recognition and knowledge graph, lots of scholars has been fruitful. Song HJ used Word2Vec to complete Bio-NER, and got F1 score of 72.82% [3]. Ling, Luo added attention mechanism on BiLSTM-CRF model to enforce tagging consistency and recognize CHEMDNER corpus and CDR task corpus [4]. Roderic mapped local identifiers to shared global identifiers. He constructed a knowledge graph based on this [5]. Xu trained Bio-BERT model to build a PubMed knowledge graph, and achieved an F1 score of 86.04% [6]. The goal of our study is building a knowledge graph about COVID-19 by extracting valuable information from literatures and integrating multi-source data.

2 Building Methods

2.1 Named Entity Recognition

NER is an important issue in natural language processing and it also plays an important basic role in building a knowledge graph. It can be said that if the problem of NER cannot be resolved reasonably, our follow-up works won't be possible. Our article uses the BERT-BiLSTM-CRF model to complete the extraction of biological entities in COVID-19 related literature, our process of the model can be shown as Fig. 1.

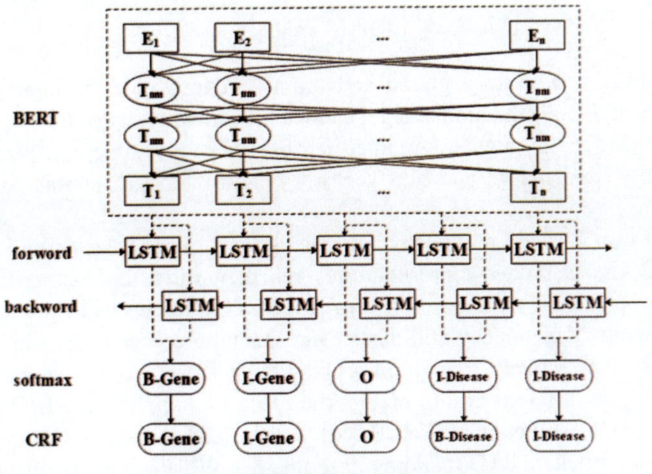

Fig. 1. BERT-BiLSTM-CRF model

Bidirectional Encoder Representation from Transformers (BERT) is an Encoder which is based on Bidirectional-Transformer. The Transformer model can be seen as a text sequence architecture depended on the self-attention mechanism. With this transformer, not only could we consider the contextual relationship more clearly and make parallel calculations, but also allow the prediction sequence with no length limit which means we can better capture the semantic features of the context. So, the multi-layer Bidirectional-Transformer in BERT makes the sequence be constrained by the left and right context at the same time. Compared with the ELMo model which was proposed by Matthew E. Peters and others in 2018 [7], Bert can obtain contextual semantic information better.

So, our first step is using the BERT pre-training language model to get the semantic representation of each token. However, the basic BERT is based on common corpus training and cannot be directly applied to our target medical field. It is necessary to fine-tune the existing parameters of the model. We use WordPiece embedding to supplement the missing words, which is an algorithm that decomposes a word into several different units and expresses each unit. The results prove that this method can improve the effect of extracting semantic features of uncommon words.

After getting the vector representation of each token, we input the vector into the BiLSTM model. The structure of basic LSTM can be formalized as follows:

$$i_t = \sigma\left(x_t W_x^i + h_{t-1} W_h^i + b_i\right) \tag{1}$$

$$f_t = \sigma\left(x_t W_x^f + h_{t-1} W_h^f + b_f\right) \tag{2}$$

$$o_t = \sigma\left(x_t W_x^o + h_{t-1} W_h^o + b_o\right) \tag{3}$$

$$\widetilde{c_t} = tanh\left(x_t W_x^c + h_{t-1} W_h^c + b_c\right) \tag{4}$$

$$h_t = o_t * \tanh(f_t * c_{t-1} + i_t * \widetilde{c_t}) \tag{5}$$

In the formula, σ is the sigmoid activation function, x_t is the input word at the current moment, h_{t-1} is the hidden layer state at the previous moment,i_t, f_t, o_t represent the values of the input gate, forget gate, and output gate at time t respectively. W, b represent the weight matrix and bias vector, $\widetilde{c_t}$ is an intermediate state, and h_t is the output at time t.

BiLSTM uses forward and backward calculations on the basis of LSTM to obtain two different sets of hidden representations and then stitch the vectors to obtain the final hidden representation. The improvement of LSTM allows us to better capture the two-way semantic dependency and master the semantic co-occurrence information of the context more effectively, thereby improving the performance of named entities.

We also set up different tags to predict the type of token, they are BIO (Beginning, inside, out-side), X (subtoken of WordPiece), [CLS] (leading token of sequence), [SEP] (delimiter of a sentence), PAD (padding in sequence). What's more, the BIO annotation is subdivided into six categories: Gene, Disease, Chemical, Mutation, Species, CellLine. Input the word vector obtained by BERT into BiLSTM and pass through the softmax classification, we can get the probability distribution of each token belonging to different labels.

In order to solve the problem that BiLSTM does not consider the relationship between labeled entity sequences, we introduce Conditional Random Field (CRF) to obtain the globally optimal labeled sequence.

We define matrix P as the output of the BiLSTM layer, and the size of P is $n \times m$, n is the number of words, m is the label category. $P_{i,j}$ represents the probability of the word i in the sentence belonging to the label j. The probability of the entire prediction sequence $y = \{y_1, y_2, \cdots, y_n\}$ can be expressed as follows:

$$K(X, y) = \sum\nolimits_{i=0}^{n} A_{y_i, y_{i+1}} + \sum\nolimits_{i=1}^{n} P_{i, y_i} \tag{6}$$

Matrix A is the transition matrix, A_{ij} represents the probability of transferring from tag i to tag j.

$$y^* = \underset{\tilde{y} \in Y_X}{\operatorname{argmax}} K(X, \tilde{y}) \tag{7}$$

$\tilde{y}$ represents the true value of tag, and Y_X represents all possible tag sets. The sequence y^* with the largest overall probability which is output by formula (7), is also the best labeling result obtained after our model training.

2.2 Validation of BERT-BiLSTM-CRF

For the NER model, we need to perform a validity test. All of our data in this article come from PubMed, a website which contains almost all papers in the medical field. The data published on this website has been physically labeled, but the latest published and included articles have not yet labeled information. Therefore, we set 70% of the labeled articles in PubMed as the training data set, 20% as the test set, and 10% as the verification set. The quality of our model is evaluated by the indicators of recall, accuracy and F1 score. In order to verify the effect of the model, we used the unfine-tuned Bert model, Word2Vec, and Att-BiLSTM-CRF to compare and verify the data set. The results are shown in Table 1.

Table 1. Performance of different models

Model name	Precision%	Recall%	F1%
BERT	82.61	84.00	83.25
Word2Vec			72.82
Att-BiLSTM-CRF	91.65	90.04	90.84
BERT- BiLSTM-CRF	91.78	93.35	92.57

2.3 Author Name Disambiguation

It is common for researchers having the same name or surname, while the names and affiliations of an individual changes over time. Therefore, when constructing a knowledge graph, it is important to disambiguate different authors. So far, the commonly used methods are mainly divided into three categories. The first one is manual disambiguation, searching for the author's information and comparing the author's message to make judgments. The advantage of this method is its high accuracy, but it is time-consuming and labor-intensive, which makes it impossible to be applied in huge data sets. The second method is accessing public scholar registration platforms such as ORCID, Google Scholar, and Semantic Scholar to get author's information. This method can quickly and easily obtain high-precision author identity information, but sometimes the coverage of the research field is limited. The third method is to evaluate the similarity of two same-name authors through algorithms to determine whether they belong to the same author. The acquisition of author's feature usually depends on the authors' affiliation information, titles and keywords of the published article, the information of the collaborators, the type of journal, etc. In recent years, with the rapid development of machine learning, the accuracy of such methods has reached a high level.

In our research, we integrate the data and information in Semantic Scholar and Google Scholar to complete the disambiguation and mark the authors. First, we use a two-classifier trained by the Semantic Scholar database to disambiguate each group of authors with the same name, and add the processed authors as increments to the created author dataset. Then use the corresponding author's information obtained in Google Scholar as a supplementary information source. Finally, we correct false disambiguation results manually, while supply the affiliation information of authors not covered.

3 CLKG Construction Process

CLKG is built based on python3.7 and networkx. The output is stored as gpickle. Anyone can get CLKG in https://github.com/spicycock/CLKG. The construction process of CLKG is shown as Fig. 2. Up to the date of writing, we obtained 82365 articles related to COVID-19 on PubMed. First, we use BERT-BiLSTM-CRF model to solve the NER problem and get the entity and its corresponding type from the abstract of each article. In this step, we extract 26,458 entities in total (including 15,437 Disease tags, 3783 Gene tags, 4832 Chemical tags, 316 Mutation tags, 1975 Species tags, and 115 CellLine tags). Then use the method mentioned in 2.3 to extract and disambiguate scholar names, and finally obtain 294655 disambiguated author names. In the third step, construct a knowledge graph based on three types of relationships: entity-entity, author-author, and entity-author. Make a further explanation, we use entity or author as a node. If there is an association between the two nodes, add an undirected edge to connect. In this way, the basic architecture of CLKG can be constructed.

After establishing the basic graph, we integrate the author's affiliation information from Google Scholar into the node information of the graph. At the same time, for each entity-author connection, we added the publication information of the related articles obtained from PubMed, Including journal name, issue time and issue number. By this way, we can expand the information of the knowledge graph to construct CLKG completely.

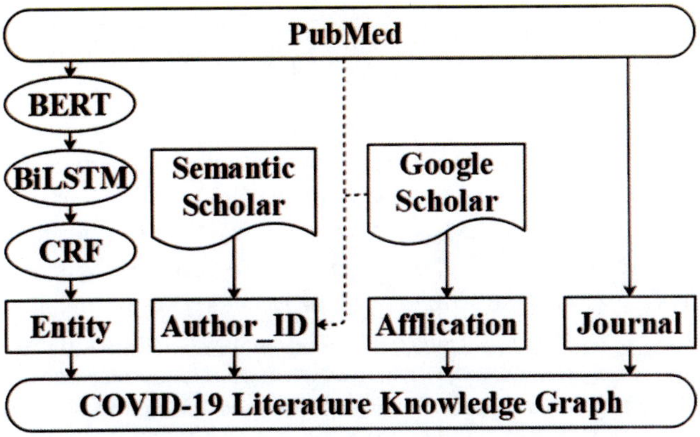

Fig. 2. Construction process of CLKG

4 CLKG Visualization

Since CLKG is constructed based on all 82365 documents related to COVID-19, it contains a huge amount of information and the relationship between nodes is also complicated, which means it is difficult to visualize it with general methods. CLKG provides a convenient search interface, allowing us to extract only the relevant fields of interest

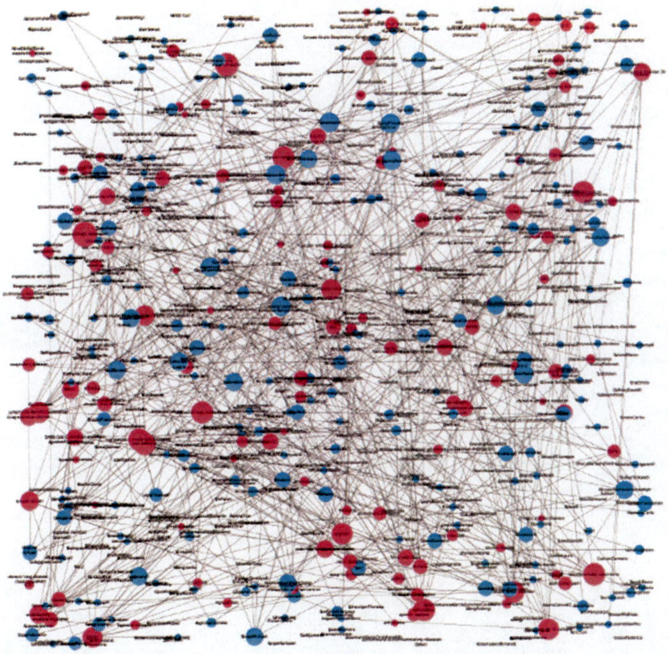

Fig. 3. Select some nodes in the overall graph for visual expression, the pink node is entity, and the blue node represents author.

and reduce the amount of information to the extent that the two-dimensional image can carry. An example of the visualization result is shown in Fig. 3, where the size of the author node is determined by the number of articles published by the author, and the size of the entity node is determined by the number of times mentioned.

Not only could we focus on the overall research status in a certain academical area, but also can conduct more refined searches. On one hand, we can locate a specific well-known scholar to find out what he has said about COVID-19. On the other hand, we can also focus on a specific research entity, listen to other people's opinions on this issue or look for the future potential partners. We have made two examples to show how it works, Anthony S. Fauci is a well-known infectious disease expert in the United States, who has made great contributions to the control, treatment, and research of the epidemic. We can quickly extract the relevant research content, co-collaborators and other related information from CLKG, and the sub-graph constructed is shown in Fig. 4.

Sinefungin is a medicinal ingredient that is often mentioned in the research on the treatment of COVID-19. As a professional scholar in the medical field, you may be concerned about whether it is proven to be effective. Figure 5 takes sinefungin as an example, and extracts relevant information from CLKG. With Fig. 5, we can clearly see the current status of published research and the clustering relationship among various nodes.

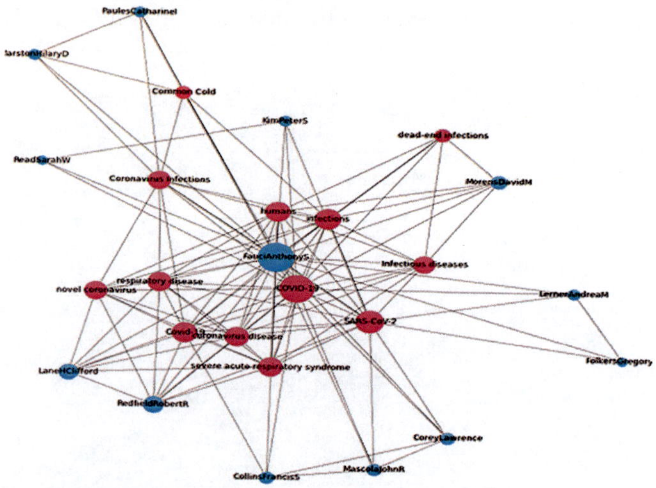

Fig. 4. The subgraph extracted with Dr. Fauci as the center, the pink nodes are related entities, and the blue nodes are the collaborators of Dr. Fauci

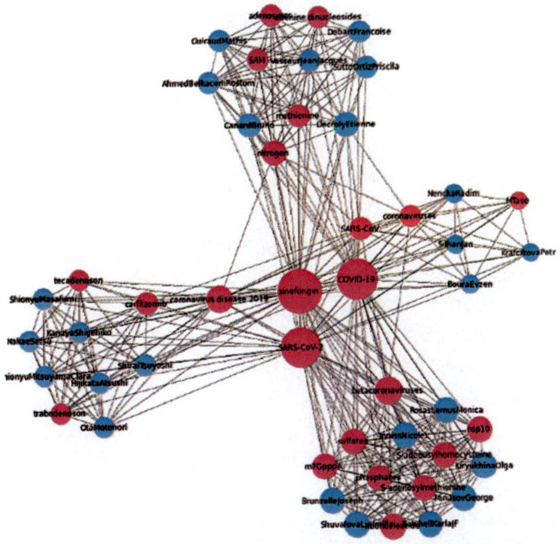

Fig. 5. The subgraph extracted with sinefungin as the center, the pink nodes are the entities related to it, and the blue nodes are the authors who studied sinefungin in the paper

5 Conclusion

As stated at the beginning of this article, COVID-19 is a severe test for each family in every country in the world. We should be one mind to overcome this disaster together. Our article uses all COVID-19 related papers in PubMed as the basis, applies the BERT-BiLSTM-CRF model to solve the key NER problem, disambiguates the researcher with the same name, and finally establishes a comprehensive and complete CLKG based on the relationship across authors and entities. As a knowledge map, CLKG collects and summarizes the research results of the world's top scientists, pharmacists and other experts on COVID-19 from all over the world and then visualizes the output. Through CLKG, we can not only quickly query the research status, frontier hotspots and research process of COVID-19, but also allows researchers find their academical partners in specific subject areas more quickly and efficiently. This timely and accurate information sharing and sincere cooperation among top scholars will undoubtedly play a key role in overcoming the epidemic, reducing unemployment, restarting the economy and restoring education.

At the same time, CLKG has excellent scalability in both vertical and horizontal directions. Vertically, CLKG can quickly extract the biological entities and add new information to the knowledge map when new literature appears, without complex and time-consuming reconstruction. Horizontally, the CLKG construction method in this article can be easily applied to any field of the same type (such as cancer, heart disease, etc.). Even not only limited to the medical field, global issues such as global warming and environmental pollution can also be extended well.

References

1. Chen, Q., Allot, A., Lu, Z.: Keep up with the latest coronavirus research. Nature **579**(7798), 193 (2020)
2. Chen, Q., Allot, A., Lu, Z.: LitCovid: an open database of COVID-19 literature. Nucleic Acids Res. **49**(D1), D1534–D1540 (2020)
3. Song, H.-J., Jo, B.-C., Park, C.-Y., Kim, J.-D., Kim, Y.-S.: Comparison of named entity recognition methodologies in biomedical documents. BioMed. Eng. OnLine **17**, 158 (2018). https://doi.org/10.1186/s12938-018-0573-6
4. Luo, L., et al.: An attention-based BiLSTM-CRF approach to document-level chemical named entity recognition. Bioinformatics **34**(8), 1381–1388 (2018)
5. Page, R.D.M.: Ozymandias: a biodiversity knowledge graph. PeerJ **7**, e6739 (2019). https://doi.org/10.7717/peerj.6739
6. Xu, J., et al.: Building a PubMed knowledge graph. Sci. Data **7**, 205 (2020)
7. Devlin, et al.: BERT: Pre-training of deep bidirectional transformers for language understanding (2018).
8. Yoon, W., et al.: Collaboration of deep neural networks for biomedical named entity recognition. BMC Bioinform. **20**(249), 55–65 (2019)
9. Peters, M.E., Neumann, M., Iyyer, M., et al.: Deep contextualized word representations. In: Proceedings of the Conference of the North American Chapter of the Assocition for Computational Linguistics, pp. 2227–2237 (2018)
10. Wang, Y., et al.: Named entity recognition in Chinese medical literature using pretraining models. Sci. Program. **2020**, 1–9 (2020)
11. Lee, J., et al.: BioBERT: a pre-trained biomedical language representation model for biomedical text mining. Bioinformatics **36**, 1234–1240 (2019)
12. Habibi, M., et al.: Deep learning with word embeddings improves biomedical named entity recognition. Bioinformatics **33**, 37–48 (2017)
13. Liao, F., Ma, L., Yang, D.: Research on construction method of knowledge graph of US military equipment based on BiLSTM model. In: 2019 International Conference on High Performance Big Data and Intelligent Systems, pp. 146–150. Shenzhen, China (2019)
14. Hakala, K., Kaewphan, S., Salakoski, T., Ginter, F.: Syntactic analyses and named entity recognition for PubMed and PubMed Central—up-to-the-minute. In: Proceedings of the 15th Workshop on Biomedical Natural Language Processing, pp. 102–107 (2016)
15. Rossanez, A., dos Reis, J.C., Torres, R.d.S., et al.: KGen: a knowledge graph generator from biomedical scientific literature. BMC Med. Inform. Decis. Mak., 20(Suppl. 4) (2020)
16. Tosi, M.D.L., dos Reis, J.C.: SciKGraph: a knowledge graph approach to structure a scientific field. J. Inform. **15**(1), 101109 (2021)
17. Berven, A., Christensen, O.A., Moldeklev, S., et al.: A knowledge-graph platform for newsrooms. Comput. Ind. **123**, 103321 (2020)
18. Cho, M., Ha, J., Park, C., et al.: Combinatorial feature embedding based on CNN and LSTM for biomedical named entity recognition. J. Biomed. Inform. **103**, 103381 (2020)
19. Luo, L., Yang, Z., Cao, M., et al.: A neural network-based joint learning approach for biomedical entity and relation extraction from biomedical literature. J. Biomed. Inform. **103**, 103384 (2020)
20. Song, Y., Tian, S., Yu, L.: A method for identifying local drug names in Xinjiang based on BERT-BiLSTM-CRF. Autom. Control. Comput. Sci. **54**(3), 179–190 (2020)
21. Song, M., Kim, E.H.-J., Kim, H.J.: Exploring author name disambiguation on PubMed-scale. J. Informet. **9**(4), 924–941 (2015)
22. Milojević, S.: Accuracy of simple, initials-based methods for author name disambiguation. J. Informet. **7**(4), 767–773 (2013)

23. Veloso, A., Ferreira, A.A., Gonçalves, M.A., et al.: Cost-effective on-demand associative author name disambiguation. Inf. Process. Manage. **48**(4), 680–697 (2012)
24. Ferreira, A.A., Gonçalves, M.A., Almeida, J.M., et al.: A tool for generating synthetic authorship records for evaluating author name disambiguation methods. Inf. Sci. **206**, 42–62 (2012)
25. Schulz, C., Mazloumian, A., Petersen, A.M., Penner, O., Helbing, D.: Exploiting citation networks for large-scale author name disambiguation. EPJ Data Sci. **3**(1), 1–14 (2014)
26. D'Angelo, C.A., van Eck, N.J.: Collecting large-scale publication data at the level of individual researchers: a practical proposal for author name disambiguation. Scientometrics **123**(2), 883–907 (2020)
27. Mu, X., Wang, W., Xu, A.: Incorporating token-level dictionary feature into neural model for named entity recognition. Neurocomputing **375**, 43–50 (2020)
28. Gligic, L., Kormilitzin, A., Goldberg, P., et al.: Named entity recognition in electronic health records using transfer learning bootstrapped Neural Networks. Neural Netw. **121**, 132–139 (2020)

Moving Target Tracking Algorithm Based on Color Space Distribution Information

Na Wang(✉)

LiaoNing Construction Vocational College, LiaoYang 111000, China

Abstract. A new method for target tracking in video images is proposed. The method firstly detects and extracts the target to be tracked based on the motion information, and then obtains the color area object characteristics according to the color space distribution information of the target to be tracked. Then the current frame image and background are detected by difference to extract the candidate target. Finally, the candidate target is matched with the target to be tracked to get the correct target. Experimental results show that the algorithm can track the target effectively and accurately in multi-object scene.

Keywords: Target tracking · Color space distribution model · Color area object

The performance of extracting moving objects from video sequences is a basic and important problem in many computer vision systems. These visual systems include video surveillance, traffic monitoring, teleconferencing or moving target tracking, face recognition, iris recognition, and so on [1]. The main task of moving target detection is to detect moving target from video image. After detecting the target, it is often necessary to trace one or more targets of interest. This is especially important in video surveillance system and military target tracking system [2].

This paper mainly discusses an algorithm for detecting and tracking moving objects in the surveillance video shot by a static camera. The algorithm is to exercise more color and their combination structure for the description of the main features of the search target, to color quantitative statistical analysis technology and high-speed image processing algorithm for the implementation of technology, which can realize real-time monitoring of suspected targets in video streams of search, greatly improve the search efficiency, bring new applications for traditional video monitoring system.

1 Moving Target Extraction

In video sequences, motion makes the target different from the background, and motion information becomes an important basis to extract the target from the background. Common moving object detection algorithms mainly include the algorithm based on the difference between adjacent frames and the algorithm based on the difference between the background image and the current frame [3, 4]. In this paper, the background image and the current frame difference algorithm are used to detect and extract the moving target when the camera is still.

R. Su et al. (Eds.): MICAD 2021, LNEE 784, pp. 374–379, 2022.
https://doi.org/10.1007/978-981-16-3880-0_39

(1) Construct the background frame. This paper adopts the threshold segmentation method based on image chromaticity deviation under THE *RGB* color model to process the three CHANNELS of *RGB* respectively. For A pixel point in the video stream, the pixel value (R, G, B) of the point will change greatly only when the foreground moving target passes through the point. Use $Pixel(x, y, c, n)$ to represent a pixel. Where, (x, y) represents the position of pixels in the image, c represents the three channels $(c = 1, 2, 3)$ of *RGB* in the color image, and n represents the frame number of the image. For each pixel point, the *Pixel* pixel value of the continuous k frame image is sorted. The middle value is taken as the background pixel value, and the size of the k value is determined by factors such as the passing speed of the moving target and the sampling rate when the camera is shooting. Use the middle value instead of the average value as the background value, because the value of a pixel may change greatly when the foreground operational target passes through it. If the average value is used as the background value, the value of the pixels through which the foreground target passes will be distorted.

Let $\lambda(x)$ and $\sigma(x)$ be the median value and mean square deviation of pixels in a continuous N frame image. The background is constructed by taking $\lambda(x)$ as the pixel value of the background image, that is, in the initialization background, the initial background pixel point $B(x) = \lambda(x)$.

However, due to the influence of unmeasurable factors such as illumination change and camera shake, the background will change and error will occur in the detection of operational targets. Therefore, the background model must be updated to make it robust and adaptive.

The first-order Kalman filtering model is used to update the background, as shown below:

$$\begin{aligned} B_{t+1}(x) &= (1-\alpha)B_t(x) + \alpha F_t(x) \\ \sigma_{t+1}^2(x) &= (1-\alpha)\sigma_t^2(x) + \alpha(F_t(x) - B_t(x))^2 \end{aligned} \tag{1}$$

Where, $\mathrm{B}_t(x)$ is the background pixel value at point x at time t, $F_t(x)$ is the current pixel value at point x at time t, $\sigma_t(x)$ is the mean square error value at point x on the background image at time t, and α is the update factor.

(2) After obtaining the background image of the video image sequence and knowing the pixel value of a point on the current frame image, the differential image value can be calculated. The binary mask of the difference image is determined by the following formula:

$$\mathrm{M(x)} = \begin{cases} 1 \ abs(F_t(x) - B_t(x)) > Th \\ 0 \ \text{other} \end{cases} \tag{2}$$

Where, $\mathrm{T}h = 2.5\sigma_t(x)$.

However, as pixels with similar colors may exist between the target and the background area, the extracted foreground area may be cracked or empty, and isolated noise will also occur in the background area. To filter the obtained binomial mask image, morphological operator is applied to treat the fracture or cavity. Meanwhile, morphological filtering can also make the boundary of the moving target area more smooth. In addition, the pixels that make up the independent moving parts are interconnected, while the independent pixels are isolated strings. Based on this feature, the area threshold method based on the foreground region is adopted to remove the noise, that is, if the total number of pixels of the interconnected parts exceeds the set threshold, the part is an independent moving part, and the rest is random noise.

(3) After obtaining the accurate object binary template, according to the object template, the segmentation result of moving object can be obtained by clearing the pixel points that are not in the template in the current frame. For a multi-target scene, multiple targets can be divided into a single moving target area and the targets can be extracted.

2 Target Tracking

2.1 Establishment of Target Color Space Distribution Model

The objects (people, vehicles, etc.) contained in the image sequence obtained by the video surveillance system often have a certain obvious color distribution [5, 6]. It is easy for the human eye to give one or several main tones of the moving object and distinguish the position of the object of interest. In fact, the target color can be represented by a limited number of primary colors. The target is usually composed of these main color regions, which constitute a fixed distribution relationship at the same time. For example, taking a person in a video image as a moving target, the main color can be distinguished as black hair, yellow coat on the upper body and black trousers on the lower body. Therefore, the target can be represented by one or more color region objects *RO*, and the regions can be numbered in relative position. *RO* includes the representative color of the region, the ratio of the region area (the ratio of the number of pixels in the region to the total pixels of the target) and the numbering of the region, that is, $RO = (color, ratio, number)$.

In this experiment, a single target is tracked. Before tracking, the initial target is obtained by difference between the initial frame and the background, and the target of interest, that is, the target to be tracked, is selected by human-computer interaction. At this point, the color distribution model of the target to be tracked can be obtained by the region growth method. In the case of multi-target tracking, the color space distribution model can be established for each target in the initial state.

This paper defines the distance threshold between colors as T1. If the color distance of two pixels adjacent to each other in space (using eight-connected mode) is lower than the threshold T1, then these two pixels can be combined into a region, which grows until no adjacent pixels can be combined. In order to avoid pixels with too big color difference in the same area, another threshold T2 is set. In the process of region growth, if the distance between the color of a pixel and all the pixels in the region is greater than the threshold T2, the pixel is not merged. If the target still has unmerged pixels, the new region continues to grow until all pixels belong to a region for comparison and are grouped into the region with the smallest color distance. Calculate the average color of each area and the ratio of the number of pixels contained in the area to the total number of target pixels, so as to obtain the final several color area object RO. According to the experimental requirements, we extracted two color area objects and numbered them according to the relative positions of the areas, $RO_1 = (avc_1, r_1, 1)$ and $RO_2 = (avc_2, r_2, 2)$. The color region feature vector *VOP* of theof the $S_{vop} = (RO_1, RO_2)$ target of interest is established. Calculate the central coordinate $(\overline{x}, \overline{y})$ of the target. Where A_{vop} is the number of pixels contained in the target $r_1 = n_i/A_{vop}, i = 1, 2$.

$$\overline{x} = \frac{1}{A_{vop}} \sum_{x \in vop} x, \overline{y} = \frac{1}{A_{vop}} \sum_{y \in vop} y \tag{3}$$

3 Target Tracking

In this experiment, people in the video scene were tracked. Before tracking, the target interested in the first few frames of the video was extracted, and the color space distribution model of the target was established by using the regional growth method. Starting from the initial pixel point of the target, all pixels are merged into two large areas to obtain two color area object RO, and the color area feature vector is established to enter the tracking state. It is assumed that the target tracked in frame $i - 1$ is represented as vop^G_{i-1}, and the feature vector $S_{vop_{i-1}} = (RO^G_1, RO^G_2)$ in the color area and the center coordinate $(\overline{x}^G, \overline{y}^G)$ of the target are obtained. The image of the current frame *i* is differenced from the background, *n* candidate targets are extracted and the central coordinate $(\overline{x}_i^k, \overline{y}_i^k)$ of each candidate target k is calculated. Calculate the central coordinate distance $d = \sqrt{(\overline{x}_i^k - \overline{x}^G)^2 + (\overline{y}_i^k - \overline{y}^G)^2}, k = 1, \ldots, n$ between the target to be tracked and all the candidate targets, and select the candidate target vop^D_i with the minimum distance.

According to the average color (avc^G_1, avc^G_2) of object (RO^G_{i-1}, RO^G_{i-1}) in the color area of target vop^G_{i-1} tracked by frame $i - 1$, all pixels of target vop^D_i with the minimum distance between the current frame and target vop^G_{i-1} are traversed. Combine all points similar to color avc^G_1 and adjacent points in space into a large area, record the number of pixels n_1 in the area, calculate the average color value avc^D_1 of the area, and number it as 1. Combine all points similar to color avc^G_2 and adjacent in space into a large area, record the number of pixels n_2 in the area, calculate the average color value avc^D_2 of the area, and number it as 2. In this way, the two color area objects $RO^D_1 = (avc^D_1, r_1, 1)$ and $RO^D_2 = (avc^D_2, r_2, 2)$ of candidate target vop^D_i are obtained, and the eigenvector $S^D_{vop} = (RO^D_1, RO^D_2)$ is obtained.

For two targets *i* and *j*, define the color area object distance between them as

$$d_m(i,j) = \begin{cases} (r_m(i) - r_m(j))^2 & s(avc_m(i), avc_m(j)) > Th \\ +\infty & other \end{cases} \tag{4}$$

Where, *m* is the region number, $s(avc_m(i), avc(j))$ is the similarity measure of color $avc_m(i)$ and color $avc_m(j)$, and *Th* is the threshold of color similarity. For a target with two color region objects, define the union distance as $d_{joint}(i,j) = d_1(i,j) \times d_2(i,j)$.

In the current frame i, if $d_{joint}(vop_{i-1}^{G}, vop_{i}^{D})$ is less than the corresponding distance threshold η_d, the two are considered to match, and this candidate target is the target tracked. Otherwise, it is considered mismatched, and the next candidate target with a smaller distance from target vop_{i-1}^{G} is selected to make the same match. This continues until the target is matched or the trace fails.

vop tracking of two adjacent frames has the following three results:

(1) For the *vop* obtained from the previous frame tracking, if there is only one *vop* in the current frame *vop* candidate set, it is directly matched; if successful, it is the target tracked.
(2) For the *vop* obtained from the previous frame tracking, the most matching *vop* is found in the current frame *vop* candidate set, and the tracking is successful.
(3) If the current frame *vop* candidate set does not match the appropriate target, it may be because the target has disappeared. Continue to process the next few frames; if the successive frames (usually five) do not match the appropriate target, the target is considered to have disappeared. If the target can be found, the normal target tracking stage will be re-entered.

3.1 Update of Color Area Objects

Once the tracked target is found in the current frame, the target color space distribution model is updated. As time goes by, the tracked target color model may change due to the influence of external factors. If the target color model is not updated, the target may be lost soon. For the principal color component *color* of the color region object $RO = (color, ratio, number)$, this paper uses an adaptive color update model: $c_i = (1-\alpha)\overline{c} + \alpha c_{i-1}$. Where, c_i is the area color value of the i frame, c_{i-1} is the area color value of the $i-1$ frame, and $\overline{c}$ is the area color mean value of the previous i frame. This adaptive region represents the color update model formula. By adjusting the ratio of the previous Frame $i-1$ to the color, the representative color of the target of frame i is updated, where α is the weight factor. For the *ratio* component, the corresponding *ratio* component of the target color area object correctly tracked by the current frame is used as the new value. And the corresponding number *number* stays the same. The color area object is updated with each new frame.

4 Conclusion

In this paper, a moving target detection and tracking scheme based on motion and color information with fixed background in surveillance video scenes is proposed, and experiments are carried out in a large number of video sequences shot indoors and outdoors respectively. The experimental results are satisfactory. From the experimental results, it can be seen that the proposed scheme can effectively detect and track moving targets in video scenes when moving targets have significant color characteristics.

References

1. Fan, M., Fan, Y., Ren, F.: Moving target tracking algorithm based on improved TLD. Adv. Laser Optoelectr. **57**(12), 121021-1–121021-6 (2020)
2. Wang, J.Y., et al.: Fast TLD visual tracking algorithm with kernel correlation filter. J. Image Graph. **23**(11), 1686–1696 (2018)
3. Jian-peng, L., Zhen-hong, S., Hui, L.: Visual object tracking algorithm based on correlation filters with hierarchical convolutional features. Comp. Sci. **46**(7), 252–257 (2019)
4. Danelljan, M., et al.: Discriminative scale space tracking. IEEE Trans. Pattern Anal. Mach. Intell. **39**(8), 1561–1575 (2017)
5. Chen, L.: Research on tracking algorithm of fast human motion target in video image. Modern Electr. Tech. **42**(3), 49–51 (2019)
6. Zhang, S., et al.: Exploring human vision driven features for pedestrian detection. IEEE Trans. Circ. Syst. Video Technol. **25**(10), 1709–1720 (2015)

Predicting Neurostimulation Responsiveness with Dynamic Brain Network Measures

Jin-Wei Lang[1,2], Wen-Juan Wang[2], Yan-Fei Zhou[3], Zong-Tao Hu[3], Xiao Fu[3], Chen Gan[3], Hong-Zhi Wang[1,3], Li-Zhuang Yang[1,3](✉), and Hai Li[1,3](✉)

[1] Anhui Province Key Laboratory of Medical Physics and Technology, Institute of Health and Medical Technology, Hefei Institutes of Physical Science, Chinese Academy of Sciences, Hefei 230031, China
lzyang@ustc.edu.cn, hli@cmpt.ac.cn

[2] University of Science and Technology of China, Hefei 230026, China

[3] Hefei Cancer Hospital, Chinese Academy of Sciences, Hefei 230031, China

Abstract. Transcranial direct current stimulation (tDCS) shows great promise in enhancing neurocognitive abilities. However, the neurostimulation responsiveness varied hugely. Our previous work demonstrates that people receiving tDCS stimulation over Temporoparietal Junction (TPJ) fall into two heterogeneous groups: the positive responders who benefit and the negative responders who hurt from tDCS. The present study investigated whether dynamic brain network properties of resting-state fMRI could predict the pattern. We calculated each subsystem of the default mode network's dynamic attributes using the multilayer community detection algorithm. Results indicated that the recruitment indexes were significantly different in bilateral aMPFC, PCC, Rsp, and PHC regions between positive responders and negative responders. Our results also confirm the advantages of the dynamic network measures over the static network measures. The study provides a feasible protocol in establishing the pre-stimulation screening procedure using resting-state fMRI.

Keywords: tDCS · Temporoparietal junction · Neurostimulation responsiveness · Dynamic functional connectivity · Default mode network · Community detection

1 Introduction

Transcranial direct current stimulation (tDCS) is a non-invasive brain stimulation technique in which a specific low-intensity current is applied to a specific brain region to modulate neural activity. Recent years have witnessed growing research evidences on the promises of tDCS in enhancing neurocognitive abilities in healthy, neurological, and psychiatric populations [1, 2]. However, it is also notorious that the neurostimulation responsiveness from tDCS varied enormously among participants. Our previous work demonstrates the necessity of pre-stimulation screening by showing that people receiving stimulation could be classified into two heterogeneous groups: the positive responders

R. Su et al. (Eds.): MICAD 2021, LNEE 784, pp. 380–389, 2022.
https://doi.org/10.1007/978-981-16-3880-0_40

whose performance was improved by tDCS, and the negative responders whose performance was impaired by tDCS [3]. Besides, our study also demonstrates the feasibility of pre-stimulation screening based on simple and interpretable brain measures, such as functional lateralization index [3]. However, the functional lateralization index was calculated with task-based fMRI, which might not be suitable for patient populations.

Resting-state fMRI (RS-fMRI) is a quick and convenient neuroimaging protocol that records brain activations for several minutes during which participants 'do nothing' in the scanner. It has been shown that RS-fMRI contains rich patterns of brain activity, which can be quantified with graph theory and network science, such as static and dynamic functional network measures. Compared with static measures, Dynamic Functional Connectivity (DFC) can indicate the flexible reorganization of brain networks, which might be useful measures to predict brain plasticity. Recent studies supported DFC measures as powerful neuroimaging markers of neurological and psychiatric disorders [4–9].

Using structural imaging scans and a non-linear brain dynamic model, one recent study verified the relationship between regional controllability and the stimulation effect [10]. However, whether DFC calculated from RS-fMRI could predict neurostimulation responsiveness from tDCS is not directly tested yet. Moreover, static functional network measures have been used successfully in predicting the non-invasive brain stimulation effect [11]. It is still ambiguous whether DFC has some advantages over static functional connectivity measures.

The present study investigated whether DFC measures calculated from RS-fMRI were effective predictors of neurostimulation responsiveness and directly compared the usefulness of DFC and traditional static network measures. Specifically, we tested whether DFC could successfully classified positive responders versus negative responders using our neurostimulation responsiveness dataset [4]. The default mode network because it was selected is theoretically related to the TPJ stimulation effect [12,13]. We adopted a dynamic community algorithm to quantify the flexible reorganization within the DMN (see Fig. 1 for an illustration). The recruitment, integration, flexibility, and promiscuity indexes were calculated for each node of DMN. The results show that DFC measures could successfully predict neurostimulation responsiveness and indicate DFC's unique value over static brain network measures.

2 Methodology

2.1 DataSet

The dataset included 45 young adults [24 females, mean age (SD) = 22.44 (2.24)], who were recruited from the USTC campus by advertisement. All participants attended one MRI scan session and three tDCS sessions [3]. The MRI session included functional images of the false-belief task, resting state, and anatomical T1 images. In this study, only RS-fMRI images were used to construct dynamic functional networks to predict the effectiveness of tDCS. The preprocessing of RS-fMRI data was same as our previous study [3].

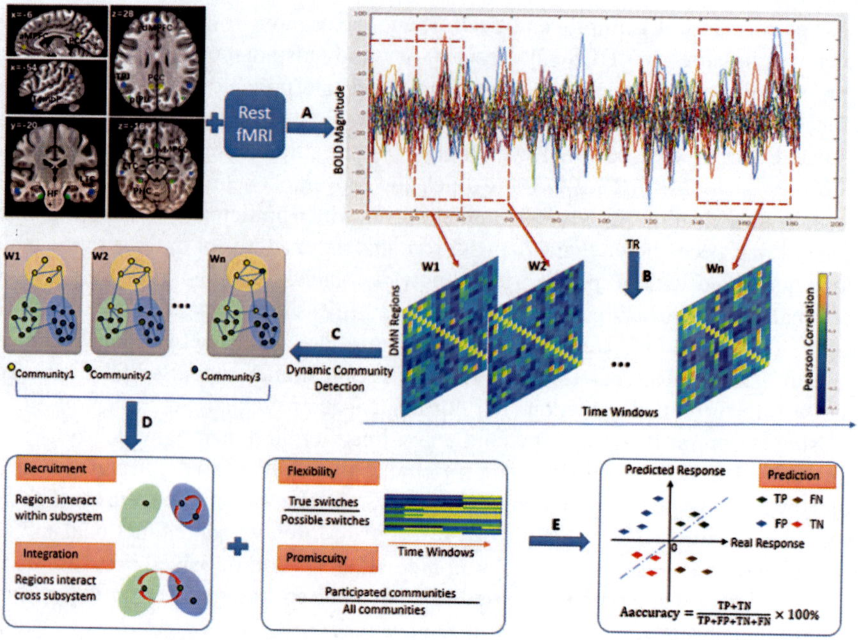

Fig. 1. Schematic overview of the analysis.

2.2 Region of Interest

The region of interest (ROI) was constructed using Andrews-Hanna's DMN template [13, 14]. The DMN was fractionated into three networks: (i) The core hubs (include the bilateral aMPFC and PCC), which are closely related to the processing of self-referential information; (ii) The dMPFC subsystem (include the midline dMPFC and bilateral TPJ, LTC, and TempP), which contribute to memory-based scene construction; (iii) The MTL subsystem (include the midline vMPFC and bilateral pIPL, Rsp, PHC, and HF +), which supports social cognition. We created sphere ROIs (diameter = 10 mm) using the Montreal Neurological Institute coordinates listed in Table 1. Then the time series of ROI was extracted using AFNI's 3dNetCorr command (see Fig. 1(A)).

2.3 Multilayer Community Detection

First, an overlapping sliding window strategy was used to construct the DFC matrix for each participant based on the fMRI time series (see Fig. 1(B)). Here we used the time window length of 40, 50, and 60 TRs, respectively, and the sliding step length was set as half of the time window length (namely 20, 25, and 30 TRs). Then, the Pearson's correlation between regions was calculated, and the Fisher's z-transform was performed to obtain the static functional connection strength of each window. Finally, for the functional connectivity matrix of all time windows for each subject, the generalized Louvain

Table 1. Coordinates of DMN ROIs used in this study.

Region	Abbreviation	x	y	z
dMPFC subsystem				
Dorsal medial prefrontal cortex	dMPFC	0	52	26
Temporal parietal junction	TPJ	−/+54	−54	28
Lateral temporal cortex	LTC	−/+60	−24	−18
Temporal pole	TempP	−/+50	14	−40
MTL subsystem				
Ventral medial prefrontal cortex	vMPFC	0	26	−18
Posterior inferior parietal lobule	pIPL	−/+44	−74	32
Retrosplenial cortex	Rsp	−/+14	−52	8
Parahippocampal cortex	PHC	−/+28	−40	−12
Hippocampal formation	HF+	−/+22	−20	−26
Core hubs				
Anterior medial prefrontal cortex	aMPFC	−/+6	52	−2
Posterior cingulate cortex	PCC	−/+8	−56	26

algorithm is used to obtain the maximum modular multilayer community network (see Fig. 1(C)). The algorithm is defined as follows[15]:

$$Q = \frac{1}{2\mu}\sum_{ijlr}\left\{\left(A_{ijl} - \gamma_l N_{ijl}\right)\delta_{lr} + \delta_{ij}\omega_{jlr}\right\}\delta\left(G_{il}, G_{jr}\right) \tag{1}$$

Where Q is the multilayer modularity index; A_{ijl} is the edge weight between region i and j in layer l; N_{ijl} is the corresponding edge weight in a null model matrix; G_{il} is the community assignment of region i in layer l; G_{jr} is the community assignment of region j in layer r; $\delta\left(G_{il}, G_{jr}\right) = 1$ if $G_{il} = G_{jr}$; otherwise, it equals 0. γ_l is the structural resolution parameter of layer l, which determines the number of modules within a given layer; ω_{jlr} is the temporal resolution parameter between region j in layer l and region j in layer r, which controls the consistency of modules detected across layers. Respectively, these two constant parameters ω and γ control the size of communities with a given layer and the number of communities detected across layers. We tested a serial of combinations of ω and γ. Finally, we chose $\gamma = 1$ and $\omega = 0.4$ for balance between community number and nodal flexibility [16].

2.4 Dynamic Network Statistics

The following four dynamic network statistics of each ROI was calculated: (i) recruitment, which provides the probability of ROIs assigned to the same community with its peers [17], (ii) integration, which provides the probability of ROIs assigned to the same community with regions other than its peers [17], (iii) flexibility, which provides the frequency of an ROI change its assigned community [18], (iv) promiscuity, which provides the frequency of one ROI participates in different communities [19]. See more information about the mathematical details below:

Recruitment and Integration. To quantify the dynamic role of regions in each subsystem, we calculate two coefficients: recruitment and integration. For system S, the recruitment coefficient of region i is defined as:

$$R_i^s = \frac{1}{n_s} \sum_{j \in S} P_{ij} \tag{2}$$

Where n_s is the size of system S, calculated as the number of regions is S. P_{ij} represents the probability that region i and j were assigned to the same functional community. R_i^s corresponds to the average probability that the i_{th} brain region is located in the same community as the rest of the system. The high areas of system S are typically the regions found in S across many time windows. The integration coefficient of region i is defined as:

$$I_i^S = \frac{1}{N - n_s} \sum_{j \notin S} P_{ij} \tag{3}$$

Where N is the total number of brain regions. Accordingly, I_i^S corresponds to the average probability that the i_{th} brain region is the same community as any other region in the system except S. Regions with high integration in system S tend to interact with regions in another system rather than its own.

Flexibility and Promiscuity. A node's flexibility f_i is defined as the probability that changes its community allocation within the continuous-time window. Flexibility is the number of times each node changes module loyalty divided by the total number (i.e., one less than the number of time windows) of possible changes. Then, the flexibility F of the entire network is defined as the average of all nodes:

$$F = \frac{1}{N} \sum_{i=1}^{N} f_i \tag{4}$$

Promiscuity ψ_i is defined as the probability that a node i traverses all communities in the network layer at least once. The promiscuity clarifies whether a particle is simply switching between a few communities (high f but low ψ) or truly participating in many different communities (both high ξ and high ψ) throughout compression. As with the flexibility, we define the network promiscuity ψ to be the average overall particles.

$$\psi = \frac{1}{N}\sum_i \psi_i \tag{5}$$

2.5 Dynamic and Static Predictive Parameters

To construct the prediction model of neurostimulation responsiveness, the dynamic network parameters adopted include four dynamic statistical parameters for every subsystem of the DMN, a total of 12 dynamic network statistics (see Fig. 1(D)). For comparison, the introduced static network parameters include graph theory and static functional connectivity characteristics of the DMN subsystem. FC within the entire DMN and the subsystem is obtained by directly calculating the Pearson correlation, such as the strength of FC between the subsystem. The network's graph theory parameters include the global network metrics and the nodal or modular network metrics. For the global metrics, we calculated the small-word property and global efficiency. We calculated the clustering coefficient, shortest path length, nodal efficiency, nodal degree centrality, and betweenness centrality for the modular network metrics. Above all, we have 37 parameters to construct the predictor, 12 for dynamic and 25 for static. We selected five machine learning models (random forest, decision tree, KNN, neural network, SVM) to predict the neurostimulation responsiveness. And experiments were carried out in static, dynamic, and combined, respectively (see Fig. 1(E)). Three-time window schemes, 40, 50, and 60, were tested for each group of experiments, and the top five prediction factors were selected in these models.

3 Results

3.1 Statistical Differences of DFC Characteristics

The participants in our study can be classified into positive responders (n = 17) and negative responders (n = 28) according to their neurostimulation responsiveness profile [3]. The group difference on the DFC measures was tested using two-sample t-test for each network node. The multiple comparisons were performed using the False Discovery Rate (FDR) method. See Table 2 for a summary of significant results.

3.2 Prediction of Neurostimulation Responsiveness

We compared the effectiveness of DFC and static network measures in identifying positive responders from negative responders. Five different machine learning algorithm was selected, as shown in Table 3. For each algorithm, we compared the prediction accuracy for the model using static measures alone, using DFC alone, and using a combination of static and dynamic measures. The leave-one-out cross-validation method was used

Table 2. Significant differences in brain regions between positive and negative responders

Window/step length (TRs)	Dynamic features			
	Integration	Recruitment	Flexibility	Promiscuity
40/20	–	aMPFC,PCC,Rsp,PHC	–	–
50/25	–	aMPFC,PCC,Rsp,PHC	–	–
60/30	–	aMPFC,PCC,Rsp,PHC	–	–

to balance the robustness of the prediction and the small sample size. The analysis was performed using the Caret package in the R environment [20].

The results were shown in Table 3. The effectiveness of static measures was not related to window length selection but only varies under different machine learning models. The advantage of DFC over static network measures was manifested by all five modeling approaches.

Table 3. Prediction accuracy of neurostimulation responsiveness

Method	Window/Step	Static	Dynamic	Static & dynamic
Random forest	40/20	64.44%	68.89%	62.22%
	50/25		68.89%	62.22%
	60/30		73.33%	60.00%
Decision tree	40/20	71.11%	77.78%	88.89%
	50/25		71.11%	73.33%
	60/30		77.78%	80.00%
KNN	40/20	62.22%	77.78%	64.44%
	50/25		66.67%	62.22%
	60/30		66.67%	62.22%
Neural network	40/20	62.22%	75.56%	68.89%
	50/25		77.78%	73.33%
	60/30		77.78%	64.44%
SVM	40/20	62.22%	80.00%	62.22%
	50/25		68.89%	62.22%
	60/30		71.11%	62.22%

The artificial neural network, random forest, and support vector machine models showed a good performance among five machine learning models. The best choice of window width step size was the 40/20 group. Moreover, we calculated the ranking of feature importance in all mixed features and found that dynamic features accounted for

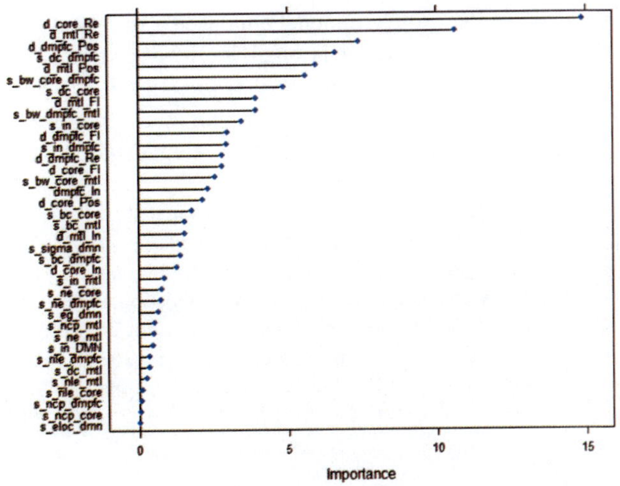

Fig. 2. Rank the importance of static and dynamic features

four among the top five features when applied neural network model (see Fig. 2). Other machine learning models have produced similar results.

4 Discussion and Conclusions

The brain plasticity originates from flexible and dynamic network reorganization. The present study investigated whether dynamic functional connectivity measures could predict neurostimulation responsiveness. To characterize dynamic reorganization within DMN, four DFC measures, including recruitment, integration, flexibility, and promiscuity of each node, were used. Our results suggested that positive responders differed from negative responders in the core subsystems (bilateral aMPFC, PCC) and MTL subsystems (bilateral Rsp and PHC) on the dimension of recruitment. Moreover, the DFC alone shows advantage over static network measures in identifying positive responders from negative responders, which was verified by a cross-validation model comparison approach using several state-of-art statistical learning algorithms. A combination of static and dynamic measures did not outperform the models with DFC alone, except for the decision tree model.

The dynamic community detection algorithm, a methodology borrowed from social network analysis, is more suitable for brain network analysis than traditional static functional brain connectivity analysis. The static brain network measures neglect that the brain was not organized as stationary network components. In fact, the network nodes in the brain reallocate themselves regarding the task demand. The dynamic community analysis can comprehensively consider the rapid interactions among nodes and subsystems, which might help explain the advantage of DFC measures over static measures in predicting the neurostimulation responsiveness in the present study.

Although models with DFC measures alone outperform models combining static and dynamic measures in general, the model based on the decision tree algorithm yielded inconsistent findings. The decision tree model only used a small number of trees in the classification task. When the sample size is small, it might be vulnerable to over-fitting.

In general, our study supports the feasibility of pre-stimulation screening program using DFC measures from RS-fMRI. Future studies may optimize the community detection algorithm to best characterize the network reorganization during RS-fMRI.

Acknowledgments. This work was supported by the National Key R&D Program of China (2017YFB1300204), the Key R&D Program of Anhui Province (201904a07020104), the Natural Science Fund of Anhui Province (2008085MC69), Hefei Foreign Cooperation Project (ZR201801020002), Hefei Municipal Natural Science Foundation (2021033), Health Commission of Anhui province (AHWJ2021b150), Collaborative Innovation Program of Hefei Science Center, CAS (2020HSC-CIP001). Anhui Province Key Laboratory of Medical Physics and Technology (LMPT201904), Director's Fund of Hefei Cancer Hospital of CAS (YZJJ2019C14, YZJJ2019A04).

References

1. Das, N., et al.: Cognitive training and transcranial direct current stimulation in mild cognitive impairment: a randomized pilot trial. Front. Neurosci. **13** (2019)
2. Srivastav, A.K., et al.: tDCS combined with cognitive training in a patient with chronic traumatic head injury. Neurophysiol. Clin. **50**(2), 133–134 (2020)
3. Yang, L.-Z., et al.: Neural and psychological predictors of cognitive enhancement and impairment from neurostimulation. Adv. Sci. **7**(4) (2020)
4. Du, Y., et al.: Dynamic functional connectivity impairments in early schizophrenia and clinical high-risk for psychosis. Neuroimage **180**(Pt B), 632–645 (2018)
5. Fiorenzato, E., et al.: Dynamic functional connectivity changes associated with dementia in Parkinson's disease. Brain **142**(9), 2860–2872 (2019)
6. Faghiri, A., et al.: Changing brain connectivity dynamics: from early childhood to adulthood. Hum Brain Mapp. **39**(3), 1108–1117 (2018)
7. Sendi, M.S.E., et al.: Multiple overlapping dynamic patterns of the visual sensory network in schizophrenia. Schizophr Res. **228**, 103–111 (2021)
8. Braun, U., et al.: Dynamic reconfiguration of frontal brain networks during executive cognition in humans. Proc Natl Acad Sci U S A. **112**(37), 11678–83 (2015)
9. He, C., et al.: Dynamic functional connectivity analysis reveals decreased variability of the default-mode network in developing autistic brain. Autism Res. **11**(11), 1479–1493 (2018)
10. Muldoon, S.F., et al.: Stimulation-based control of dynamic brain networks. PLoS Comput Biol. **12**(9), e1005076 (2016)
11. Hartwright, C.E., et al.: Resting state morphology predicts the effect of theta burst stimulation in false belief reasoning. Hum Brain Mapp. **37**(10), 3502–14 (2016)
12. Anticevic, A., et al.: When less is more: TPJ and default network deactivation during encoding predicts working memory performance. Neuroimage **49**(3), 2638–2648 (2010)
13. Wen, T., et al.: The functional convergence and heterogeneity of social, episodic, and self-referential thought in the default mode network. Cereb Cortex. **30**(11), 5915–5929 (2020)
14. Andrews-Hanna, J.R., et al.: Functional-anatomic fractionation of the brain's default network. Neuron **65**(4), 550–562 (2010)
15. Mucha, P.J., et al.: Community structure in time-dependent, multiscale, and multiplex networks. Science **328**(5980), 876–878 (2010)

16. He, X., et al.: Disrupted dynamic network reconfiguration of the language system in temporal lobe epilepsy. (2018)
17. Mattar, M.G., et al.: A functional cartography of cognitive systems. PLoS Comput. Biol. **11**(12), e1004533–e1004533 (2015)
18. Bassett, D.S., et al.: Dynamic reconfiguration of human brain networks during learning. Proc. Natl. Acad. Sci. U. S. A. **108**(18), 7641–7646 (2011)
19. Papadopoulos, L., et al.: Evolution of network architecture in a granular material under compression. Phys. Rev. E **94**(3–1), 032908 (2016)
20. Kuhn, M.: Building predictive models in r using the caret package. J. Stat. Softw. Articles. **28**(5), 1–26 (2008)

Visualization of Continuous and Pulsed Ultrasonic Propagation in Water

Lishan Zhi, Heng Zhang, Weiping Liu, Bin Ni, Fan Yu, Bin Xu(✉), Jichuan Xiong(✉), and Xuefeng Liu(✉)

School of Electronic and Optical Engineering, Nanjing University of Science and Technology, Nanjing 210094, China
jichuan.xiong@njust.edu.cn

Abstract. Imaging the distribution and propagation of sound fields in water is important for applications of ultrasound in water. In this paper, a stroboscopic polarization parameter imaging method was implemented to visualize and quantify ultrasonic wave propagation in water. A k-space numerical method was used to simulate the propagation of the ultrasonic wave and verify the relationship between the pressure distributions of ultrasonic wave and the optical parametric images. Ultrasonic wavefield generated by continuous sinusoidal and pulsed signals were visualized experimentally. The results demonstrated high sensitivity and spatial resolution for visualization of the ultrasound field distribution in water.

Keywords: Ultrasonic · Visualization · Polarization imaging · Liquid

1 Introduction

An ultrasonic wave is a kind of sound wave with a frequency higher than 20000 Hz. It has the advantages of good directivity, strong permeability and easy to obtain concentrated sound energy. Therefore, it was widely used in applications for solid medium, such as metal cutting and welding in the industry [1], non-destructive testing (NDT) [2], etc. In medium like water or biomedical tissues, the utilization of ultrasonic waves is also well developed, such as medical diagnosis and treatment [3], photoacoustic imaging (PAI) [4], ultrasonic cleaning [5], etc. Among these applications in liquid, ultrasonic cavitation [6] is an important group.

Ultrasonic cavitation is that the propagation of the ultrasonic wave in the liquid will cause the local increase or decrease of the internal pressure of the liquid, small bubbles begin to form and grow in the low-pressure region, and break in the high-pressure region, accompanied by high temperature and high pressure to form a strong impact force. It is usually used as the driving force in the liquid related ultrasonic processing technology, such as preparation of metal oxide nanoparticles by ultrasonic-assisted plasma discharge [7], ultrasonic-assisted electrocoagulation to remove organic matter in water [8], ultrasonic-assisted water confinement laser micromachining [9], etc.

L. Zhi and H. Zhang contributed equally to the manuscript.

R. Su et al. (Eds.): MICAD 2021, LNEE 784, pp. 390–401, 2022.
https://doi.org/10.1007/978-981-16-3880-0_41

In the ultrasonic cavitation process, not all the cavities in liquid can go through the whole process of rapid growth, enlargement and collapse. The frequency, intensity and field distribution of ultrasonic waves play an important role in the cavitation effect of ultrasonic waves [10], which will affect the efficiency of ultrasonic applications in water. The frequency and intensity of the ultrasonic wave can be controlled accurately by the generation source, typically an ultrasonic transducer, while the distribution and propagation of the ultrasonic wave are influenced by many other parameters. A better understanding of the ultrasonic wave generation and propagation in liquids is fundamental for many applications of ultrasound in water, including the ultrasonic cavitation-based techniques. Visualizing the distribution and propagation of sound fields in water is a necessary for this purpose. To address this issue, imaging methods based on diffraction and interferometry polarimetry have been developed to visualize the propagation of acoustic waves [11–21].

In previous work of the group, a parametric indirect microscopic imaging method (PIMI) was developed, with the capability of measuring the phase retardation and polarization orientation angle induced by stress in medium [22, 23]. Later, we adapted it to a stroboscopic polarization imaging method to visualize the ultrasonic wave and has detected the ultrasonic wave in quartz glass, with high spatial and temporal resolution [24]. In this paper, we mainly utilize this stroboscopic polarization imaging technology to image ultrasound distribution and propagation in water. The distribution and propagation properties of continuous and pulsed ultrasonic wave in water were investigated both numerically and experimentally.

2 System and Theory

The sound field visualization system consists of two parts: the polarization imaging optical path and the stroboscopic controlling system, as shown in Fig. 1.

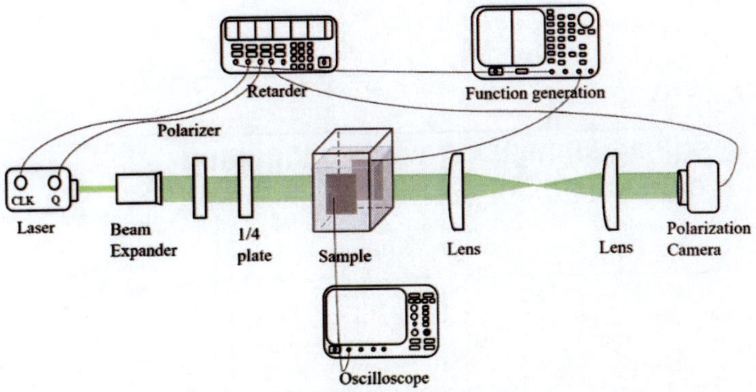

Fig. 1. The visualization system of ultrasonic propagation in water.

2.1 Polarization Imaging Optical Path

The polarization imaging optical path is very sensitive to small changes caused by ultrasound, and can visualize the ultrasound with optical polarization parameters. The propagation of ultrasonic wave will affect the polarization state and phase of the detection light, through the stress-induced refractivity change of the medium. The resulting changes in optical parameters can be converted into changes in light intensity by polarization detection and recorded by a charge-coupled device (CCD).

The polarization imaging optical path includes a pulsed laser, a beam expander, a polarizer, a quarter-wave plate, a plano-convex lens and a polarization camera (PCCD), as shown in Fig. 1. The wavelength of the pulsed laser is 532 nm, with a pulse duration of 10 ns, and triggered by an external signal from the delay generator. Through the beam expander, the polarizer and quarter-wave plate form an angle of 45 degrees to form a circularly polarized light incident on the sample. The sample is a quartz glass tank filled with water. Two faces of the quartz glass tank are pasted with piezoelectric ceramics, one of the piezoelectric ceramics is used as the ultrasonic excitation source, and the other piezoelectric ceramics is used to detect the ultrasonic signal after propagating in water. The 4F system consists of two planoconvex lenses with a focal length of 75 mm. A 1:1 image of a plane located in the water tank was projected on a PCCD by the 4F system. PCCD is a polarized charge-coupled element device, which can take images at four different polarization angles (0°, 45°, 90° and 135°) in one snapshot.

2.2 Stroboscopic System

The propagation speed of the ultrasonic wave in the medium is fast compare to the exposure time of an ordinary camera, which makes it difficult to image the propagation of ultrasonic wave instantaneously. The purpose of the stroboscopic imaging system is to make the time of the image taken by the camera is at the nanosecond level, to ensure that the ultrasonic wave propagation in the medium can be captured.

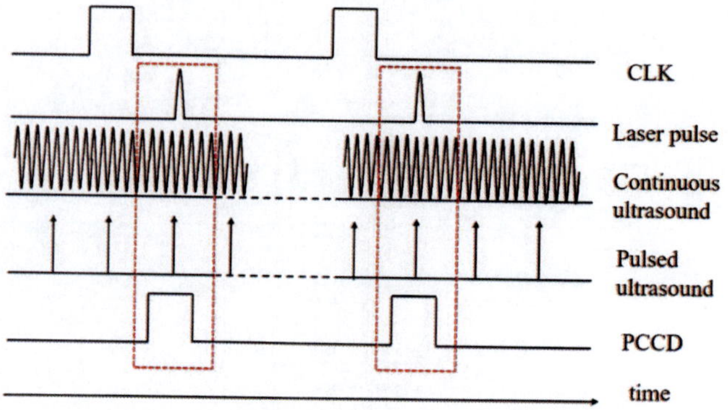

Fig. 2. The timing diagram of the stroboscopic system.

The stroboscopic system consists of a pulsed laser, a function generator, signal delay generator and a PCCD. The pulse width of the pulsed laser is 10 ns, and the exposure time of the PCCD is 30 μs. The purpose of the stroboscopic system is to control the relative delay time of the pulsed laser and the exposure of PCCD so that each laser pulse emission is included in the camera exposure time. The timing diagram of the stroboscopic system is shown in Fig. 2.

The CLK signal in Fig. 2 is the trigger signal of the xenon pumping lamp in the laser, with a repetition frequency of 10 Hz. The laser pulses were generated when the Q-switch in the cavity was triggered, with a delay of 220 μs relative to the CLK signal. The triggering frequency of the PCCD is the same as that of the CLK signal, and the delay is 200 μs relative to the CLK signal so that the emission time of each laser pulse is included in the exposure time of the camera. Two kinds of ultrasonic waves were generated, i.e. continuous sinusoidal and pulsed waves. The continuous sinusoidal ultrasonic waves are generated continuously at the pizeo transducer attached to the face of water tank and can always be captured in the medium during the exposure time of the camera. The pulsed signal, with a period of 200 μs, emits an ultrasonic excitation wave repetitively. By controlling the function generator and the delay generator, the ultrasonic excitation signal can be synchronized with the laser pulse, and the relative delay time can be controlled to allow the camera to take pictures of ultrasonic at different positions in the medium.

2.3 Theory of Sound Field Visualization

Under the effect of pressure or tension, the dielectric constant or refractive index of the transparent isotropic medium will change due to the photoelastic effect, thus affecting the propagation characteristics of light in the medium. Using the polarization imaging system, the stress distribution can be analyzed.

When circularly polarized light passes through an isotropic transparent material with stress and strain, the stress-induced birefringence leads to different phase retardation of the two orthogonal polarization components decompose along with the two principal stress directions. When the light propagates through the sample, the polarization state of the output light can be expressed as:

$$\frac{E_x^2}{E_{ox}^2} + \frac{E_y^2}{E_{oy}^2} - \frac{2E_xE_y}{E_{ox}E_{oy}} cos\delta = sin^2\delta \tag{1}$$

Among them, E_x and E_y are electric vectors in two orthogonal directions, and E_{ox} and E_{oy} are the amplitudes of the electric vectors, and δ is the phase delay.

According to the above polarization imaging system, the formula for determining Stokes parameters is as follows:

$$\begin{cases} S_0 = E_{ox}^2 + E_{oy}^2 = I_0 + I_{90} \\ S_1 = E_{ox}^2 - E_{oy}^2 = I_0 - I_{90} \\ S_2 = 2E_{ox}E_{oy}cos\delta = I_{45} - I_{135} \\ S_3 = 2E_{ox}E_{oy}sin\delta = I_{RCP} - I_{LCP} \end{cases} \tag{2}$$

The phase delay is equal to the sum of the initial phase of the incident polarized light and the phase difference caused by the change of the acoustic-induced refractive index. The Stokes parameter and the polarized light intensity of the output beam can be expressed as follows:

$$\delta = arccos\left(\frac{S_2}{(2I_0I_{90})^{\frac{1}{2}}}\right) \tag{3}$$

According to Eq. (1) and Eq. (2), the azimuth of polarized light can be expressed as follows:

$$\varphi = \frac{1}{2}tan^{-1}\left(\frac{2E_{ox}E_{oy}}{E_{ox}^2 - E_{oy}^2}cos\delta\right) = \frac{1}{2}tan^{-1}\left(\frac{S_2}{S_1}\right) \tag{4}$$

Assuming the ultrasonic wavefield propagating in the sample (transmission imaging mode) is $u(x, y, z, t)$ expressed with displacement, the strain tensor is:

$$\varepsilon_{ij} = \frac{1}{2}\left(\frac{\partial u_i}{\partial x_j} + \frac{\partial u_j}{\partial x_i}\right) \quad i, j = x, y, z \tag{5}$$

The anisotropic photoelastic relationship between the strain and the refractive index of the detection light is [25]:

$$\Delta\left(\frac{1}{n^2}\right)_{ij} = \sum_{kl} P_{ijkl}\varepsilon_{kl} \tag{6}$$

Where P_{ijkl} is the photoelastic tensor and $\Delta\left(1/n^2\right)_{ij}$ is the tensor describing the change of refractive index.

In isotropic medium, there are only two independent constants P_{11} and P_{12} in P_{ijkl} tensor. The relationship between the change of refractive index and the change of stress can be simplified as follows:

$$\Delta n_i = \frac{n_0^3}{2}(P_{11} - P_{12})\Delta\varepsilon_i \quad i = x, y, z \tag{7}$$

where n_0 is the initial refractive index.

In this optical path, the beam is propagating in the z-axis. The phase retardation δ can thus be expressed as:

$$\delta = \frac{2\pi}{\lambda}\int_0^d \Delta n dz \tag{8}$$

Where Δn is the change of refractive index; λ is the wavelength of the detection light wave; d is the thickness of the sample. If the refractive index changes uniformly along the Z-axis and Eq. (8) is substituted by Eq. (7), the phase delay can be simplified as:

$$\delta = \frac{\pi d n_0^3}{\lambda}(P_{11} - P_{12})\left(\frac{\partial u}{\partial y} - \frac{\partial u}{\partial x}\right) \tag{9}$$

The above equation gives the relationship between the ultrasonic pressure field and the optical phase delay.

2.4 Simulation of Sound Field Propagation

The k-wave toolbox [26] of MATLAB software is used to simulate the stress distribution of ultrasonic propagation in the medium. The grid points in X, Y and Z directions are 64, 64 and 64 respectively, and the grid interval is 0.1 mm. A 3-D simulation model of 6.4 mm × 6.4 mm × 6.4 mm is established. A square ultrasonic signal source with the size of 0.5 mm × 0.5 mm is set at the Y-Z plane (x = 0.5 mm). A continuous sinusoidal signal with the frequency of 5 MHz is used as the ultrasonic signal, and a group of Cartesian points are set to collect data. The medium parameters of the model mainly include sound velocity and density. The k-space pseudospectral method is used to simulate the time-varying pressure source in three-dimensional homogeneous medium. The pressure distribution of the sound field on the X-Y plane is observed. The relationship between pressure distribution and optical phase delay is discussed, and the propagation of ultrasonic wave in water is simulated.

3 Results and Discussion

3.1 Sound Field Simulation

The relationship between acoustic pressure distribution and optical phase delay is simulated in quartz glass at first. The final pressure distribution of acoustic field is shown in Fig. 3(a). Through Eq. (9), the pressure distribution of the sound field can be converted into an optical phase delay diagram, as shown in Fig. 3(b). As can be seen from the two curves in Fig. 3(c), there is a displacement along the propagation direction between the ultrasonic field pressure distribution diagram and the optical phase delay diagram, but the general trend does not change. Therefore, there is a certain equivalent relationship between the ultrasonic field pressure distribution diagram and the optical phase delay diagram.

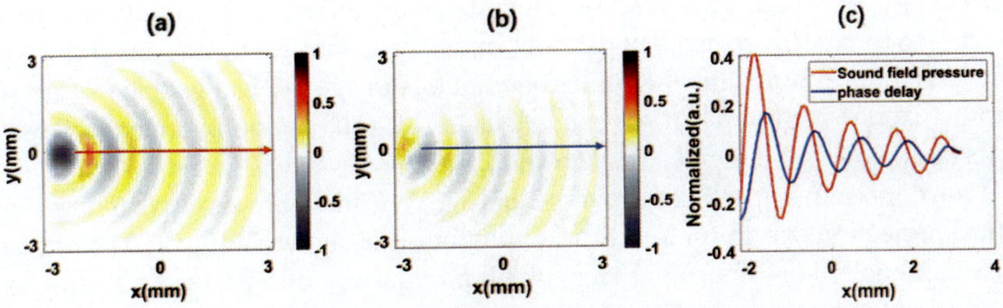

Fig. 3. Relationship between pressure distribution of ultrasonic field and optical phase delay diagram. (a) The figure shows the final pressure distribution of 5 MHz ultrasonic wave in quartz glass, (b) the phase delay figure corresponding to figure (a), (c) the two lines are the intensity distribution curves along the arrow (x = −2.2 mm ~ 3.2 mm, y = 0 mm) in figure (a) and (b).

Then, based on the same three-dimensional model and the same ultrasonic signal, the ultrasonic wave in water is simulated. As shown in Fig. 4, ultrasound energy is mainly concentrated in the main lobe, but there are also side lobes. As shown in Fig. 4(b), the wavelength of sound waves in water is very small, which is 0.3 mm, and the attenuation of the ultrasonic wave in water is also weak. Therefore, in the next experiment, a large enough ultrasonic transducer was set to observe the propagation of the main lobe of ultrasonic waves in water.

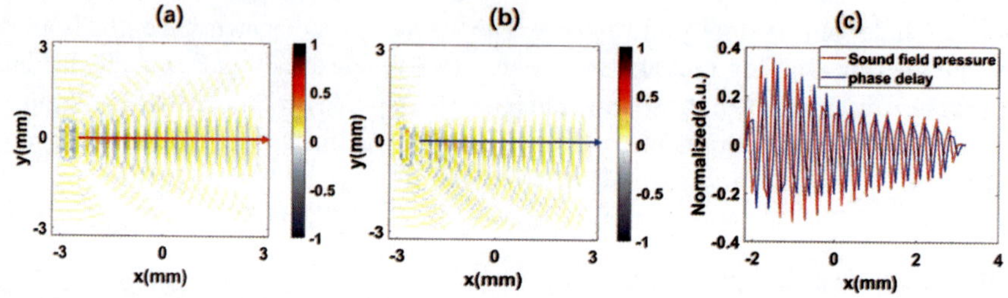

Fig. 4. Pressure distribution of continuous ultrasonic signal with a frequency of 5 MHz in water. (a) Final pressure distribution of continuous ultrasonic wave in water, (b) the phase delay figure corresponding to figure (a), (c) The intensity distribution curves along the arrow (x = −1.2 mm ∼ 3.2 mm, y = 0 mm) in figure (a) and (b).

3.2 Visualization of Continuous Ultrasound

In the experiment, the piezoelectric ceramic excitation signal is a continuous sinusoidal signal with an amplitude of 4 V and frequency of 5 MHz, as shown in Fig. 5(a). The ultrasonic signal received on the other side of the sample is shown in Fig. 5(b). From the above system in Fig. 1, we can get a picture of the sound field in water by PCCD, as shown in Fig. 5(c). In this picture, we can find that the reflection and scattering of some light caused by the tiny suspended particles in the water lead to strong background noise in the image. After removing the background of this image, we can get the pictures with four polarization angles. Then we can calculate the polarization parameters to get the results of S_0, S_1, S_2, S_3, δ and ϕ, as shown in Fig. 6.

It can be seen in Fig. 6 that the parameters S_0, S_3, δ and ϕ are sensitive to ultrasound. Vertical projection curves for S_0, δ and ϕ diagrams are shown in Fig. 7. The ultrasonic source is a continuous sinusoidal signal with a frequency of 5 MHz. According to the sound velocity in water of 1500 m/s, the wavelength should be $s = v / 2f = 0.15$ mm in theory. From the vertical projection curve of S_0, the wavelength is about 0.1508 mm, and the error between the two values is 0.533%. This proved that the imaging result is the propagation of the ultrasonic wave. It can be seen from the vertical projection curve of S_0 that the distribution of the ultrasonic wave can be clearly visualized, while it is influenced by nonuniformity of light distribution. The curves of δ and ϕ are rough, which shows that the noise of δ and ϕ is larger than that of S_0, but the influence of nonuniform light spot on δ and ϕ is smaller.

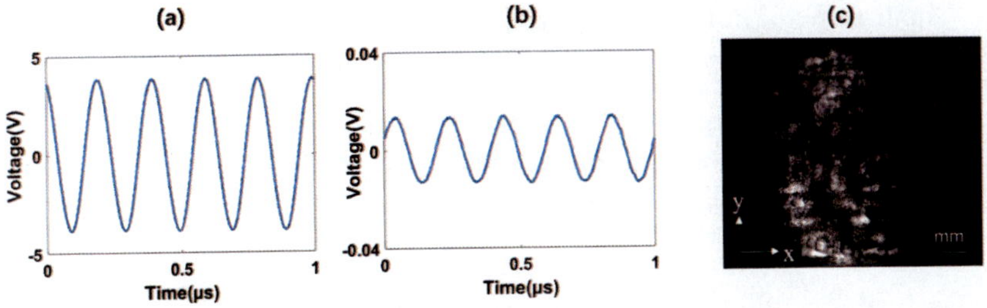

Fig. 5. Ultrasonic signal. (a) Signal of exciting piezoelectric ceramics to produce ultrasonic wave, (b) Ultrasonic signals received by piezoelectric ceramics after propagation in water, (c) Original image.

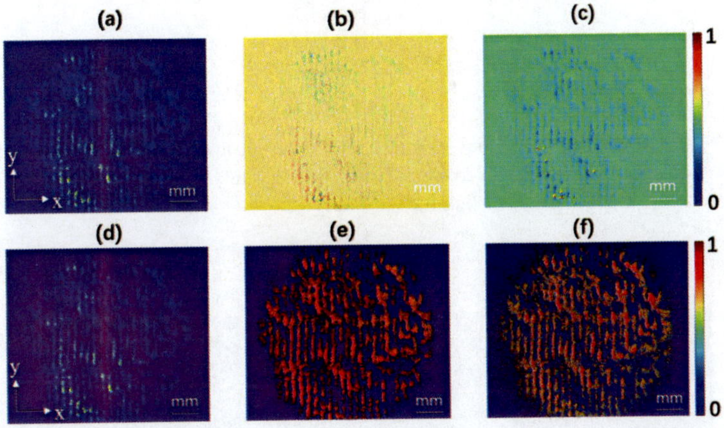

Fig. 6. The results of Stokes parameters image. (a) - (f) Stokes parameters, respectively S_0, S_1, S_2, S_3, δ, ϕ.

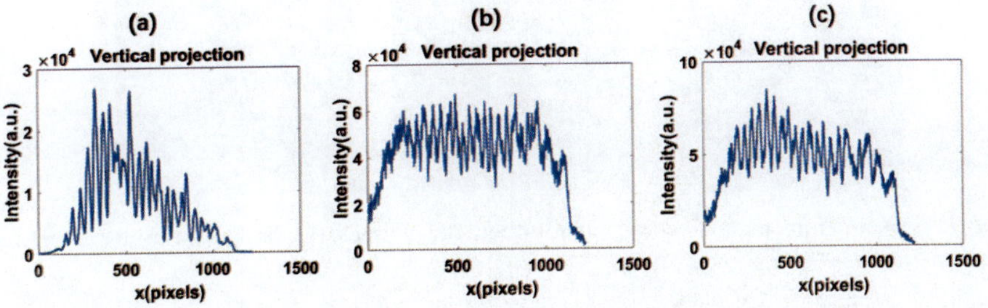

Fig. 7. Vertical projection curves. (a) Vertical projection curves of Stokes parameters S_0, (b) Vertical projection curves of Stokes parameters δ, (c) Vertical projection curves of Stokes parameters ϕ. (Vertical projection curves: The abscissa is the pixel in the X direction, and the ordinate is the sum of all the pixel values in the Y direction).

3.3 Visualization of Pulsed Ultrasound

The pulse signal is a trapezoidal pulse with a duration of 170 ns, as shown in Fig. 8. By changing the relative delay time of ultrasonic wave and laser pulse, the ultrasonic wave propagation diagram in water at different delay time can be visualized. A group of S_0 graphs with a time interval of 0.5 μs are shown in Fig. 9. And vertical projection curves of S_0 were shown in Fig. 10.

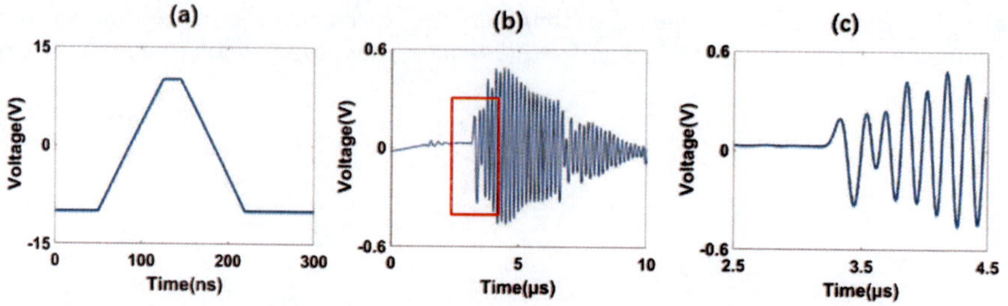

Fig. 8. Ultrasonic signal. (a) Signal of exciting piezoelectric ceramics to produce ultrasonic wave, (b) Ultrasonic signals received by piezoelectric ceramics after propagation in water, (c) The enlarged part in the red box of figure (b).

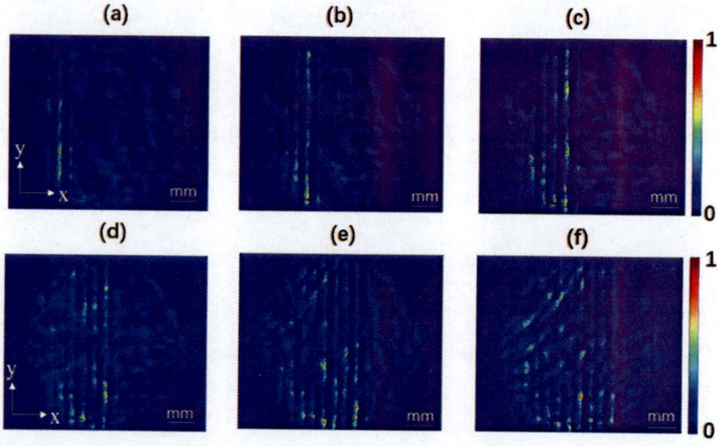

Fig. 9. Stokes parameter S_0 diagram with different delay times. (a)–(f) The time interval between the two graphs is 0.5 μs.

The wavelength of the pulsed ultrasonic wave was found to be 0.3 mm, which is twice that of a 5 MHz continuous ultrasonic wave. In Fig. 9, ultrasonic waves propagate from left to right, and the boundary of ultrasonic wave field is obvious. In Fig. 10(f), there is a fuzzy boundary between peaks in the red frame. This is due to the reflection of ultrasonic wave pulses at the wall of water tank.

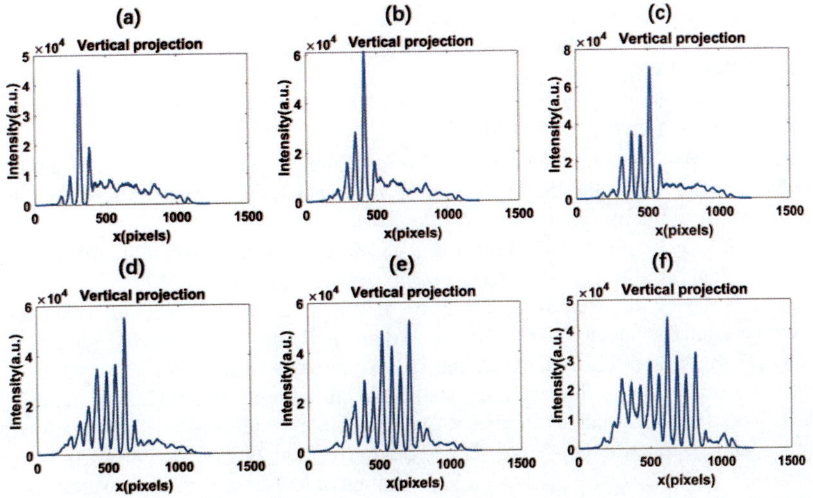

Fig. 10. The vertical projection curve of the S_0 diagram in respective Fig. 9. (a)–(f) The time interval between the two graphs is 0.5 μs.

4 Conclusion

In this paper, a stroboscopic polarization parameter imaging method is used to visualize the propagation of ultrasound in water. Based on the theoretical model, images with different polarization parameters are obtained by image processing. These images prove that polarization parameter images are sensitive to ultrasound and can detect the propagation of ultrasound in the water at a certain depth. Moreover, the propagation of pulsed ultrasound in water is clearer than that of continuous ultrasound, and the propagation distance can be controlled. However, the impurities in the sample will cause the reflection and scattering of ultrasound and light in the transmission process, which will affect the contrast and imaging depth of the visualization results of ultrasonic propagation in water.

Acknowledgement. This work was supported by the National Major Scientific Instruments and Equipment Development Project under Grant No. 61827814, National Key Research and Development Program of China under Grant No. 2017YFF0107100), Beijing Natural Science Foundation under Grant No. Z190018, the Fundamental Research Funds for the Central Universities under Grant No. 30920010011, the Postdoctoral Foundation of Jiangsu Province under Grant No.2020Z331, and the Ministry of Education collaborative project B17023.

References

1. Ni, Z.L., Wang, X.X., Li, S., Ye, F.X.: Mechanical strength enhancement of ultrasonic metal welded Cu/Cu joint by Cu nanoparticles interlayer. J. Manuf. Process. **38**, 88–92 (2019)
2. Chatillon, S., et al.: Ultrasonic non-destructive testing of pieces of complex geometry with a flexible phased array transducer. Ultrasonics **38**(1–8), 131–134 (2000)
3. Sumi, C.: Ultrasonic diagnosis and treatment equipment using lateral modulation. Jpn. J. Med. Ultrason. **35**, S277 (2008)
4. Weber, J., Beard, P.C., Bohndiek, S.E.: Contrast agents for molecular photoacoustic imaging. Nat. Methods **13**(8), 639–650 (2016)
5. Anonymous: Ultrasonic cleaning technology helps SoCalGas achieve greater efficiency. Pipeline Gas J. **242**(12), 73–74 (2015)
6. Lippert, T., Bandelin, J., Schlederer, F., Drewes, Jörg. E., Koch, K.: Impact of ultrasound-induced cavitation on the fluid dynamics of water and sewage sludge in ultrasonic flatbed reactors. Ultrason. Sonochem. **55**, 217–222 (2019)
7. Ivanov, A.V., et al.: Properties of metal oxide nanoparticles prepared by plasma discharge in water with ultrasonic cavitation. Int. J. Nanotechnol. **14**(7/8), 618–626 (2017)
8. Zanki, A.K., et al.: Removal of organic matter from water using ultrasonic-assisted electrocoagulation method. IOP Conf. Ser.: Mater. Sci. Eng. **888**(1), 012033 (2020)
9. Zhou, J., Xu, R., Jiao, H., Bao, J.D., Long, Y.H.: Study on the mechanism of ultrasonic-assisted water confined laser micromachining of silicon. Optics Lasers Eng. **132**, 106118 (2020)
10. Cui, F.L., Ji, W.: Dynamic simulation of ultrasonic cavitation bubble and analysis of its influencing factors. Ed. Off. Trans. Chin. Soc. Agric. Eng. **29**(17), 24–29 (2013)
11. Miao, R., Yang, Z., Zhu, J., Shen, C.: Visualization of low-frequency liquid surface acoustic waves by means of optical diffraction. Appl. Phys. Lett. **80**(17), 3033–3035 (2002)
12. Kakue, T., et al.: High-speed phase imaging by parallel phase-shifting digital holography. Opt. Lett. **36**(21), 4131–4133 (2011)
13. Xiong, J., Xu, X., Glorieux, C., Matsuda, L., Cheng, O.: Imaging of transient surface acoustic waves by full-field photorefractive interferometry. Rev. Sci. Instrum. **86**(5), 053107 (2015)
14. Kimmo, K., Lauri, L., Igor, S., Steffen, N., Matti, K., Hanne, L.: Characterization of surface acoustic waves by stroboscopic white-light interferometry. Opt. Express **23**(8), 9690–9695 (2015)
15. Hargather, M.J., Settles, G.S., Madalis, M.J.: Schlieren imaging of loud sounds and weak shock waves in air near the limit of visibility. Shock Waves **20**(1), 9–17 (2010)
16. Chitanont, N., Yaginuma, K., Yatabe, K., Oikawa, Y.: Visualization of sound field by means of Schlieren method with spatio-temporal filtering. In: Proceedings of IEEE International Conference on Acoustics, Speech and Signal Processing, pp. 509–513 (2015)
17. Glorieux, C., Beers, J.D., Bentefour, E.H., Van, dR.K., Nelson, K.A.: Phase mask-based interferometer: operation principle, performance, and application to thermoelastic phenomena. Rev. Sci. Instrum. **75**(9), 2906–2920 (2004)
18. Washimori, S., Mihara, T., Tashiro, H.: Investigation of the sound field of phased array using the photoelastic visualization technique and the accurate FEM. Mater. Trans. **53**(4), 631–635 (2012)
19. Yamamoto, K., Sakiyama, T., Izumiya, H.: Visualization of acoustic evanescent waves by the stroboscopic photoelastic method. Phys. Procedia **70**, 716–720 (2015)
20. Nam, Y.H., Lee, S.S.: A quantitative evaluation of elastic wave in solid by stroboscopic photoelasticity. J. Sound Vib. **259**(5), 1199–1207 (2003)
21. Date, K., Udagawa, Y.: Visualization of ultrasonic waves in a solid by stroboscopic photoelasticity and image processing techniques. Review of Progress in Quantitative Nondestructive Evaluation. Springer, Boston, MA, pp. 1755–1762 (1989)

22. Liu, X., et al.: Characterization of graphene layers using super resolution polarization parameter indirect microscopic imaging. Optics Express **22**, 020446 (2014)
23. Liu, W., Xiong, J., Zhang, H., Liu, X., Liu, G., Zhao, H.: Characterization of Komagataeibacter xylinus by a polarization modulation imaging method. J. Phys. D: Appl. Phys. **53**, 125403 (2019)
24. Liu, G.S., et al.: Visualization of ultrasonic wave field by stroboscopic polarization selective imaging. Opt. Express **28**, 27096 (2020)
25. Cao, Y., et al.: Sensing of ultrasonic fields based on polarization parametric indirect microscopic imaging. Chin. Opt. Lett. **17**(4), 93–98 (2019)
26. Treeby, B.E., Cox, B.T.: k-wave: MATLAB toolbox for the simulation and reconstruction of photoacoustic wave fields. J. Biomed. Opt. **15**(2), 021314 (2010)

An Infrared Imaging Method that Uses Modulated Polarization Parameters to Improve Image Contrast

Min Sun, Heng Zhang, Weiping Liu, Bin Ni, Fan Yu, Bozhi Liu, Huizheng Tang, Bin Xu(✉), Jichuan Xiong(✉), and Xuefeng Liu(✉)

School of Electronic and Optical Engineering, Nanjing University of Science and Technology, Nanjing 210094, China
jichuan.xiong@njust.edu.cn

Abstract. In infrared imaging techniques, overcoming the interference of complex background reflections is a challenge for obtaining sub-surface information of samples. The polarization indirect parameter imaging (PIMI) method can characterize the polarization property of samples by modulating the polarization states of the illumination light and highlight the anisotropic details of the sample through parametric images. In this paper, a far-infrared PIMI imaging system and the inversion model of the properties of the sample were established. A composite structure plate made of carbon fiber plate and aluminum alloy with internal defects was measured. The experimental results demonstrated that the polarization parameter images can sense the structures of the sample beneath the surface and improve the contrast between the target area and the background area, which implies that the system has the potential for non-destructive evaluation applications.

Keywords: Infrared imaging · PIMI imaging · Polarization parameter images · Image contrast evaluation

1 Introduction

Infrared imaging technology is based on the temperature difference between the target and the background radiation power to achieve the target detection [1]. With its advantages of strong penetration capability, it has been widely used in industrial, military, aviation, remote sensing, medicine [2], etc. In practical applications, due to the background reflections from the sample and random noise introduced in the image processing, the signal-to-noise ratio and contrast of infrared images could be degraded [3]. Thus, suppressing background noise is of great significance for improvement of the infrared imaging techniques. There are generally two ways to improve the quality of infrared imaging. One is to develop high-resolution and high-precision infrared detectors, which is difficult and the cost is high. Another method is to develop advanced image enhancement algorithm.

M. Sun and H. Zhang—Contributed equally to the manuscript.

R. Su et al. (Eds.): MICAD 2021, LNEE 784, pp. 402–410, 2022.
https://doi.org/10.1007/978-981-16-3880-0_42

Jaspreet [4] proposed a non-training contrast enhancement algorithm for infrared image improvement. Cao Mei [5] developed an infrared image enhancement method based on the improved histogram equalization and non-sub sampled contourlet transform (NSCT) to enhance the global contrast. Chen Chaoqi [6] proposed a fusion method of infrared image and visible image based on multi-scale low-rank decomposition and it is proved to be able to improve the resolution of infrared image and enhance the target area. These works can supress the imaging noise and improve the contrast of the infrared images. However, limitations still exist, including the lack of universality of particular algorithms, and the complexity and computation costs.

Therefore, it is of great practical significance to find a method that can suppress background noise, improve global contrast of images and simplify the processing complexity. In this paper, we proposed a parametric imaging method of far-infrared radiation, which can obtain high contrast and resolution images of sub-surface information of the sample with minimum post-processing of images.

The method is based on the utilization of polarization indirect parameter imaging (PIMI) in the far-infrared range. It mainly depends on the inversion of near-field information based on the coupling of electromagnetic waves with the sample and variation of reflection light in the far-field [7, 8]. When interacting with the target, the electromagnetic wave will couple the near-field information into the polarization parameters of the scattered light, including phase retardation, polarization orientation angle, and Stokes parameters. The precisely controlled modulation leads to predictable change of the far-field optical wave parameters, in addition to the variation caused by the sample properties. This far-field variation can be utilized to inversely calculate the optical properties of the sample and high contrast images can be obtained.

Theoretically, objects with a temperature above 0 K will emit infrared radiation and the asymmetry of radiation results in the polarization characteristics of the object's thermal radiation [9, 10]. In this paper, the advantages of this method were fully exploited by employing the far-infrared detection. The sub-surface information can be carried by the far-infrared light to the far-field through the PIMI imaging process. Results shows that this imaging method achieved the enhancement of the contrast between the target and the background, highlight the details of sub-surface structure of the sample.

2 Acquisition of Polarization Parameter Images

2.1 Infrared Polarization Parameter Imaging System

The infrared polarization parameter imaging system for internal defect detection of carbon fiber-aluminum alloy composite plate is shown in Fig. 1. The light source in the system is a continuous laser with a wavelength of 532 nm and the maximum power of 1 W (LWGL532 series), which is used to heat the sample. The laser is collimated and the beam diameter is expanded by a continuous zoom beam expander (GCO-25 series). After the illumination of the 532 nm laser, the sample emits far-infrared radiation and the radiation was collected and passed through a silicon substrate infrared grating polarizer working in the 7–15 micron spectrum range (WP25M-IRC). Then it is received by the infrared camera with a detection range of 8–14 microns (PLUG617R). The resolution of the imaging sensor is 640×512 and the pixel size is 17 microns. In the experiment, a motor is used to rotate the polarizer, and the infrared camera is controlled for synchronous acquisition of images at different rotation angles of the polarizer.

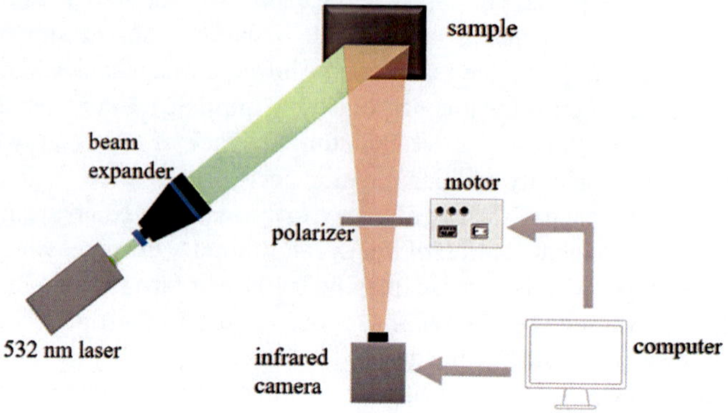

Fig. 1. The schematic of the infrared polarization parameter imaging system.

2.2 Sample Preparation

To simulate the defects beneath the sample surface, a four-layer PTFE film was used to mimic the defects buried between the carbon fiberboard and the aluminum plate. A X-shaped defect was composed of two rectangular thin films with lengths, widths and thickness of 20 mm, 4 mm and 0.18 mm, respectively. The aluminum plate, PTFE film and carbon fiberboard were bonded together with the mixed epoxy resin adhesive. And the samples were pressed uniformly to avoid the generation of bubbles at the bonding place, as shown in Fig. 2.

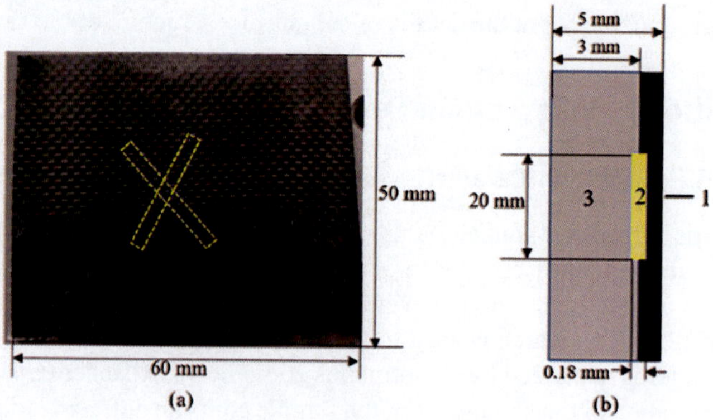

Fig. 2. Sample schematic. (a) Top view of sample, (b) cross-section diagram of the sample (1. Carbon fiberboard, 2. Teflon, 3. Aluminum alloy).

2.3 Measurement Procedure of the Experiment

As shown in Fig. 1, a laser in the visible spectrum (532 nm) was used for thermal excitation of the sample and the far-infrared radiation in the far-field was imaged with an infrared camera. The polarization angle of the polarizer was rotated and the infrared emission from the sample was fitted and filtered to a theoretical model. The polarization direction of the incident laser is ensured to be perpendicular to the fiber axis of carbon fiber to maximize the optical absorption [11]. It has been proved that the infrared radiation of the target has polarization characteristics, and the polarizability is related to the emission angle (the angle between the detector and the normal line of the sample) [12]. The smaller the emission angle is, the lower the polarization degree of the sample is. The laser illumination direction is parallel to the horizontal plane to irradiate the sample surface at a certain angle to improve the polarization characteristics of the sample. The polarizer is rotated from 0° to 360° with a step length of 20° to obtain 19 images of different polarization states.

2.4 Theoretical Model of the Imaging System

The infrared images of multiple polarization angles are collected, fitted and filtered to the theoretical model. Polarization parametric images including the phase retardation between orthogonal components, polarization ellipticity orientation angle and Stokes parameters were calculated with the model.

a) Calculation of theoretical model.

The principle of the whole system is that the incident polarized light acts on the Mueller matrix of the sample and the polarizer, and its output light can be expressed as [13]:

$$S_{out} = M_{pol} M_{sample} S_{in} \tag{1}$$

$$M_{sample} = \begin{pmatrix} 1 & 0 & 0 & 0 \\ 0 & cos2\varphi & sin2\varphi & 0 \\ 0 & 0 & -cos\delta sin2\varphi & -sin\delta cos2\varphi \\ 0 & -sin\delta sin2\varphi & sin\delta cos2\varphi & cos\delta \end{pmatrix} \tag{2}$$

Where M_{pol}, M_{sample}, S_{in} represent the Mueller matrix of the polarizer, the sample and the Stokes vector of the linearly polarized input beam, respectively. In the sample Muller matrix, δ represents the phase difference between two orthogonal polarization components, and φ is the polarization ellipticity orientation angle.

The calculated intensity of each pixel detected on the detector is:

$$I = \frac{1}{4} S_0 [1 + (-cos\delta sin2\varphi sin2\alpha) sin2\theta + cos2(\alpha - \varphi) cos2\theta]$$

Where S_0 is Stokes vector, and α and θ are the polarization angles of the incident light and the polarizer respectively.

a_0, a_1 and a_2 are respectively represented as:

$$a_0 = \frac{1}{4}S_0,\ a_1 = -\frac{1}{4}cos\delta sin2\varphi sin2\alpha S_0,\ a_2 = \frac{1}{4}cos2(\alpha - \varphi)S_0 \tag{4}$$

If the polarizer obtains a picture at each rotation angle, the image intensity collected at the n_{th} time is:

$$I_n = a_0 + a_1 sin2\theta_n + a_2 cos2\theta_n \tag{5}$$

The corresponding parameters can be obtained by Fourier series analysis:

$$a_0 = \frac{1}{N}\sum_{n=1}^{N} I_n,\ a_1 = \frac{2}{N}\sum_{n=1}^{N} I_n sin2\theta_n,\ a_2 = \frac{2}{N}\sum_{n=1}^{N} I_n cos2\theta_n \tag{6}$$

Where N is the total number of rotations, and θ_n represents the angle of rotation. Combining Eq. (4) and Eq. (6), the final equation can be deduced as:

$$\begin{gathered} I_{dp} = a_0,\ \varphi = \alpha - \tfrac{1}{2}arccos\tfrac{a_2}{a_0}, \\ cos\delta = -a_1\left(a_0 sin2\alpha \sin\left(2\alpha - arccos\tfrac{a_2}{a_0}\right)\right)^{-1} \end{gathered} \tag{7}$$

Where I_{dp} is the average light intensity of all polarization intensity images. The Stokes parameters can be denoted by the Muller matrix as:

$$\begin{gathered} S_0 = I_{dp}(1 + sin\delta),\ S_1 = I_{dp}(1 + sin\delta)cos2\varphi, \\ S_2 = \sqrt{2}I_{dp}(1 + sin\delta)\sqrt{sin2\varphi}\,cos\delta,\ S_3 = \sqrt{2}I_{dp}(1 + sin\delta)\sqrt{sin2\varphi}\,sin\delta \end{gathered} \tag{8}$$

b) Modification of theoretical model.

The polarization characteristics of the sample, such as carbon fiber microstructure materials, are ignored in the above calculation, which are anisotropic and have a certain regularity in this experimental arrangement. The strong polarization properties have an impact on absorption of the illumination light and the emission of far-infrared radiation. Therefore, a method of introducing the polarization into the Muller matrix of the sample is proposed, to adapt the above theoretical model and the optimization of the polarization parameter image of the far-infrared radiation.

The modified sample Muller matrix can be described as:

$$M'_{sample} = \begin{pmatrix} 1 & 0 & 0 & 0 \\ 0 & cos2\varphi & sin2\varphi & 0 \\ 0 & 0 & -cos\delta sin2\varphi & -sin\delta cos2\varphi \\ 0 & -sin\delta sin2\varphi & sin\delta cos2\varphi & cos\delta \end{pmatrix} \times M_{pol1} \tag{9}$$

The detected light intensity of each pixel is:

$$I = \frac{S_0}{8}[1 + cos(2\alpha - 2\beta)]$$

$$\times\ [1 + (-cos\delta sin2\varphi sin2\beta)sin2\theta + cos(2\beta - 2\varphi)cos2\theta] \tag{10}$$

Where β represents the polarization angle when the sample is in a certain polarization state and the corresponding expressions for a_0, a_1 and a_2 are:

$$a_0 = \tfrac{S_0}{8}[1 + cos(2\alpha - 2\beta)],\ a_1 = \tfrac{S_0}{8}[1 + cos(2\alpha - 2\beta)](-cos\delta sin2\varphi sin2\beta),\\ a_2 = \tfrac{S_0}{8}[1 + cos(2\alpha - 2\beta)]\,cos(2\beta - 2\varphi) \tag{11}$$

The polarization parameters are obtained:

$$I_{dp} = a_0,\ tan\varphi = \tan\left(\beta - \frac{1}{2}arccos\frac{a_2}{a_0}\right),\\ cos\delta = -a_1\left(a_0 sin2\beta sin\left(2\beta - arccos\frac{a_2}{a_0}\right)\right)^{-1} \tag{12}$$

Then the corresponding Stokes parameters can be calculated according to Eq. (8).

3 Experimental Results and Analysis

3.1 Comparison of the Two Processing Models

A series of polarization parameter images are obtained by theoretical calculation of the raw images with different polarization states. Comparison of the original image I_0, depolarization intensity figure I_{dp}, Stokes parameter S_0, S_1, S_2, S_3, δ before and after modification of the theoretical model are shown in Fig. 3, 4.

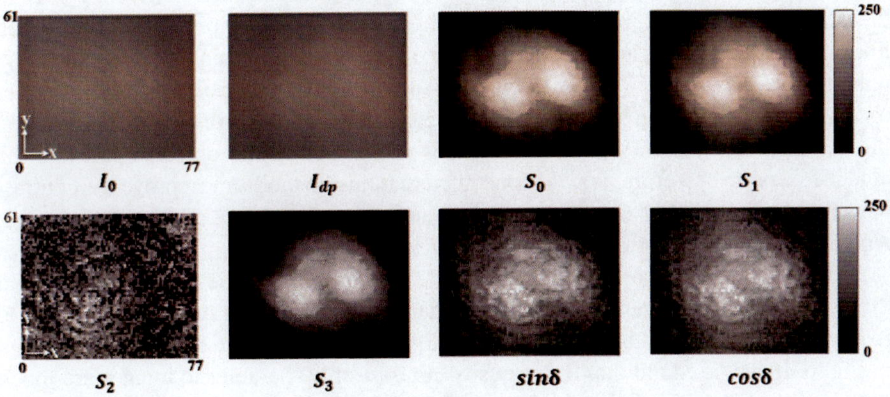

Fig. 3. Polarization parameter image before algorithm correction.

It can be seen intuitively that the image contrast and clarity of the polarization parametric images of the two algorithms are improved compared with the conventional intensity image. And contour of internal defects buried in the sample is also shown clearly, indicating that two algorithms for the system are both feasible. It is also found that

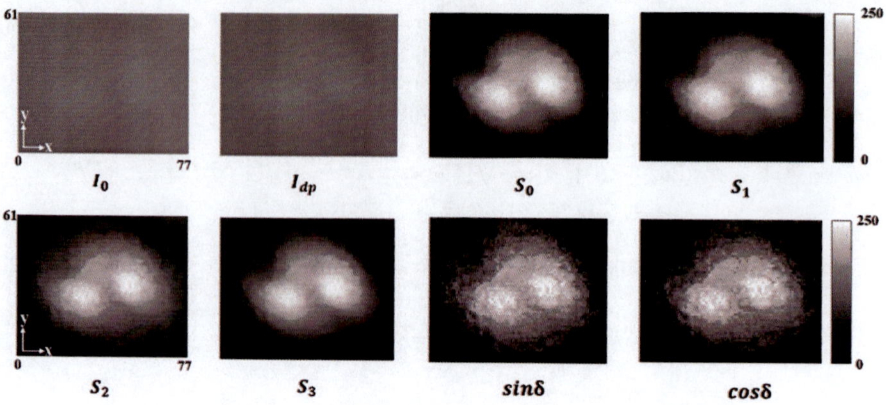

Fig. 4. Polarization parameter image after algorithm modification.

the image results with the modified algorithm is much better than that of the one before the correction. The defects in the δ and S_2 image with the model before modification was almost invisible. Generally, the modified model introducing polarization parameters not only complements the information of Stokes S_2 image but also improves the contrast of other Stokes parameter image and the δ image of the sample.

3.2 Polarization Parametric Imaging of Subsurface Structure

The contours of the "X" defects can be seen in S_0 and S_1 Stokes parameter images, as shown in Fig. 4. A low-temperature region was shown due to fast heat transferring speed in aluminum and large thermal resistance (poor thermal conductivity) of PTFE. In the defect-free part, this indicates that the emissivity of different regions on the carbon fiber surface is different, and the morphology of internal defects can be characterized by polarization parameters. The results suggested that in a certain polarization parameter image, such as S_0, S_1, the polarization parameter can enhance the difference of radiation in each area of the surface, which allows us to distinguish the defected part and the defect-free part. Therefore, it is demonstrated that this method can improve the contrast between the defect area and the non-defect area through the Stokes parameter image. And the internal defect morphology can be visualized.

To make a more accurate comparison, the same area from the direct image I_0 and the S_0 image were selected for analysis, as the marked by the red straight line in Fig. 5. Intensity profiles along the line for I_0, S_0, S_1, S_2, S_3, $\sin\delta$, $\cos\delta$ images are shown in Fig. 6. It can be found that the intensity contrast of all parametric images are much greater than that of the I_0 image. It is evident that polarization parameter images can increase the contrast between the defect and its background.

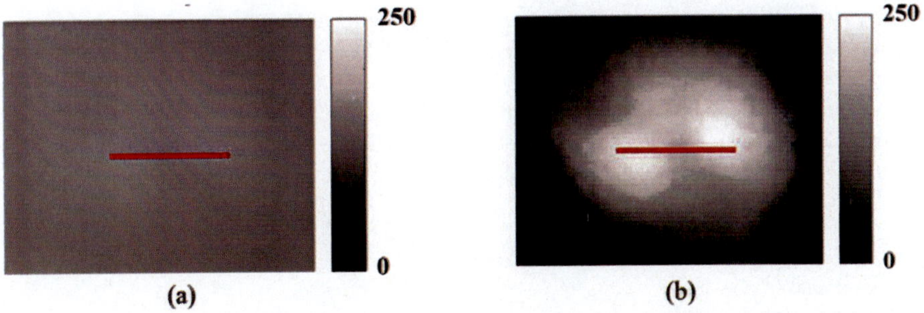

Fig. 5. Comparison of original image and polarization parameter image. (a) Original image I_0, (b) Polarization parameter image S_0.

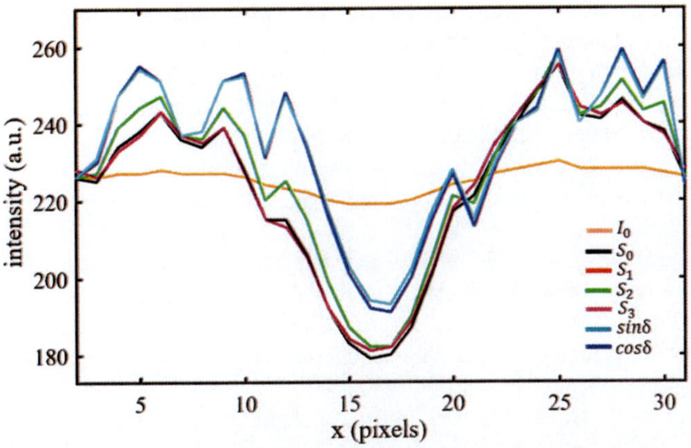

Fig. 6. Comparison of intensity distribution perpendicular to defect in I_0, S_0, S_1, S_2, S_3, $sin\ \delta$, $cos\ \delta$ images

4 Conclusion

In this paper, the infrared polarization indirect parameter imaging method is used to characterize the sub-surface structure of the sample. The carbon fiber-aluminum composite plate with internal defects was thermally excited by a laser in the visible spectrum, and the infrared emission from the sample was recorded when rotating the polarizer in the infrared radiation path. The images were fitted and filtered to the theoretical model to obtain the polarization parameter images. The experimental results manifest that the method can detect structures beneath the sample surface, suggesting capability of the detection of near-surface defects of composite materials. It is further confirmed that the imaging method can suppress background noise and improve the contrast of target area and background area. The far-infrared imaging method based on polarization parameters is not only a supplement to improve the quality of infrared imaging, but also has great potential for non-destructive evaluation of samples.

Acknowledgement. This work was supported by the National Major Scientific Instruments and Equipment Development Project under Grant No. 61827814, National Key Research and Development Program of China under Grant No. 2017YFF0107100), Beijing Natural Science Foundation under Grant No. Z190018, the Fundamental Research Funds for the Central Universities under Grant No. 30920010011, the Postdoctoral Foundation of Jiangsu Province under Grant No. 2020Z331, and the Ministry of Education collaborative project B17023.

References

1. Jedrasiak, P., Shercliff, H.R.: Finite element analysis of heat generation in dissimilar alloy ultrasonic welding. Mater. Des. **158**, 184–197 (2018)
2. Xingyu, C., Hao, L.: Application analysis of infrared thermal imaging technology in intelligent manufacturing field. J. Phys: Conf. Ser. **1693**(1), 12129 (2020)
3. Ashiba, H.I., Mansour, H.M., Ahmed, H.M.: Enhancement of infrared images based on efficient histogram processing. Wirel. Pers. Commun. **2**(6), 619–636 (2018)
4. Wang, F.B., Sun, F., Zhu, D.R., et al.: Metal fatigue damage assessment based on polarized thermography. Acta Optica Sinica **40**(7), 1412002 (2020)
5. Cao, M., Cheng, Y.L., Sheng, H.X., et al.: Application of improved histogram equalization and NSCT transform algorithm in infrared image enhancement. Appl. Sci. Technol. **43**(2), 24–27 (2016)
6. Chen, C.Q., Meng, X.C., et al.: Infrared and visible image fusion method based on multiscale low-rank decomposition. Acta Optica Sinica **40**(11), 72–80 (2020)
7. Liu, X., Qiu, B., Chen, Q., Ni, Z., et al.: Characterization of graphene layers using super resolution polarization parameter indirect microscopic imaging. Opt. Express **22**(17), 20446 (2014)
8. Ullah, K., Liu, X., Habib, M., et al.: Subwavelength far field imaging of nanoparticles with parametric indirect microscopic imaging. ACS Photonics **5**(4), 1388–1397 (2018)
9. Liu, F., Shao, X.P., Gao, Y., et al.: Polarization characteristics of objects in long-wave infrared range. J. Opt. Soc. Am. A: **33**(2), 237 (2016)
10. Li, N., Zhao, Y.Q., Pan, Q., et al.: Removal of reflections in LWIR image with polarization characteristics. Opt. Express **26**(13), 16488 (2018)
11. Freitag, C., Weber, R., Graf, T.: Polarization dependence of laser interaction with carbon fibers and CFRP. Opt. Express **22**(2), 1474 (2014)
12. Niu, J.Y., Li, F.M., Ma, L.X.: The theoretical analysis of thermal infrared emission polarization and experimental verification. Opto-Electron. Engin. **41**(2), 88–93 (2014)
13. Collett, A.E.: Field Guide to Polarization, pp. 115–118 (2015)

The Overview of Medical Image Processing Based on Deep Learning

Qing An[✉], Bo Jiang, and Jupu Yuan

Wuchang University of Technology, No. 16 of Jiang Xia Avenue, Wuhan 430223, Hubei, China

Abstract. With the rapid development of artificial intelligence technology, deep learning is being applied to the field of medical image analysis. This paper summarizes the deep learning models related to medical image analysis, and the application results of these models in medical image classification, detection, segmentation and registration. It specifically involves the image analysis tasks of nerve, retina, lung, digital pathology, breast, musculoskeletal and other aspects. Finally, it summarizes the current research status of deep learning related to medical image analysis, and discusses the challenges and direction of future research.

Keywords: Deep learning · Clinical application · Image detection · Image segmentation · Image registration

1 Introduction

Deep learning is a hot research field and a branch of machine learning. Compared with traditional artificial neural network, the depth and the number of parameters of the model have increased significantly. Convolutional neural network (CNN) and recurrent neural network (RNN) are the two most important models in deep learning. The former is mainly used in image recognition, object detection, speech recognition and other tasks, while the latter is mainly used in sequence data. Convolutional neural network was first proposed to recognize handwritten numbers, and achieved high accuracy. In the 2012, large-scale visual recognition challenge finally won the first place by using GPU acceleration training. A variety of CNN models have been proposed and applied in a variety of tasks, which promote the development of convolutional neural network to a deeper and broader level. Direct connection is added between layers to simulate identity mapping. The application of deep learning to medical field is a hot topic recently, especially in the recognition of some medical detection images. For example, in the machine learning competition platform, the application of deep learning in medical image recognition has a wide range of application prospects. The theme of this year's annual competition is to detect lung cancer based on the chest CT scan data of patients diagnosed with cancer within one year. Because some patients diagnosed with lung cancer may not be ill in fact, and the size of nodules is different on the CT images of patients' lungs. The larger the nodules, the higher the probability of lung cancer. Therefore, the use of deep learning to assist doctors in noninvasive detection can avoid many unnecessary surgical detection.

R. Su et al. (Eds.): MICAD 2021, LNEE 784, pp. 411–417, 2022.
https://doi.org/10.1007/978-981-16-3880-0_43

At present, artificial intelligence technology based on machine learning algorithms such as deep learning has been deeply integrated into all aspects of the medical field. From the development of new drugs to auxiliary clinical diagnosis and treatment, medical big data analysis is gradually becoming an important factor affecting the development of the medical industry. The market scale of artificial intelligence in medical industry in China was 13.65 billion yuan in 2017 and 21 billion yuan in 2018, with a year-on-year growth of 54%. It is estimated that the contribution rate of artificial intelligence application to the annual compound growth rate of the medical industry will reach 40% from 2017 to 2024. By the end of 2019, the annual compound growth rate of the medical industry will reach 40%. There are more than 80 AI medical enterprises in China. AI analysis of medical images is a research hotspot of digital medical industry, involving more than 40 enterprises, including Alibaba, Tencent, Baidu, iFLYTEK and other famous companies. AI technology has gradually become an important factor affecting the development of medical industry, especially in the field of medical image analysis.

2 Analysis of Medical Image Research

Artificial analysis of medical images not only takes a long time, but also is limited by the experience of analysts. It takes a lot of time and cost to cultivate a qualified professional of medical image analysis. Therefore, artificial intelligence has entered people's vision. In 1963, American radiologist Lodwick proposed the digitization method of X-ray film. In 1966, the method of X-ray film digitization was put forward. American scholar Ledley formally put forward the concept of "computer-aided diagnosis", hoping to reduce the workload of doctors through computer. In 1972, CT was applied in clinical practice, creating a precedent of digital medical imaging. In 1982, the American College of Radiology decided to jointly establish a committee called ACR-NEMA, which is dedicated to developing communication specifications between medical imaging devices. In 1985 and 1988, ACR-NEMA issued a set of specifications (ACR-NEMA 1.0 and ACR-NEMA 2.0). In 1993, ACR-NEMA issued a new set of specifications named DICOM 3.0, which specifies the transmission standard of medical images and related information.

Although medical image storage and transmission standards have developed, it is still difficult for artificial intelligence to be used in medical image analysis. The main reasons include blurred image of visual system, complexity of human tissue, structure, function, and limitations of traditional machine learning algorithm. In 2006, depth algorithm appeared, which made a breakthrough in image recognition research. Some researchers use the structure of multi-layer convolutional neural networks (CNN) to reduce the error rate of image recognition from 26.2% to 3%, and the deep machine learning algorithm has entered the application stage in medical industry.

Supervised deep learning models commonly used in medical image analysis include CNN, CNN based transfer learning and recurrent neural networks (RNN), while unsupervised deep learning models include automatic encoder, restricted Boltzmann machines (RBM) and general adaptive networks (GaN) [1]. CNN is the most commonly used machine learning algorithm in medical image analysis at present. Its advantage is that it can save the spatial relationship features of the image, and this feature is very important for medical image analysis. For example, in histological examination, the proportion of DNA and cytoplasm of cancer cells on the slide is higher than that of normal cells. Therefore, if strong DNA features are detected in the first few layers of CNN, CNN can predict the existence of cancer cells. Through medical image analysis, transfer learning is often used to transfer the weights learned by CNN during the training of one dataset to another CNN, and then use these weights to receive the training of the marked medical dataset. RNN is often used to analyze sequence data, and image segmentation in medical image analysis. The main difference between RNN and CNN is that the output of one layer of RNN will not only become the input of the next layer, but also feedback to this layer. That is to say, RNN can learn to use the past information. Automatic encoder is mainly used for data dimension reduction or feature extraction, which does not need labeled data sets. In deep learning, the automatic encoder can transform the input data into another form, and then carry out a series of learning on this basis. The generative model continuously learns the real probability distribution in the training set, and converts the input random noise into the true image. In addition to the models introduced above, there are many variant models based on these models.

3 Application of Deep Learning in Medical Image Analysis

There are four main application ways of deep learning in medical image analysis, which are image classification, detection, segmentation and registration. Among them, classification is to distinguish different types of objects according to the different features reflected in the image information; detection is to determine the boundary box around each object, and these objects may come from different classifications; Segmentation is to determine the contour of the object at the edge and mark it semantically; Matching criterion is to fit one image to another one.

In fact, in clinical practice, it is not very necessary to distinguish these tasks accurately. In fact, in some of the studies described below, these tasks are more or less confused or mixed. The most ideal machine learning system is to unify these tasks, such as detecting lung tumor from CT image, and then to locate and segment it. From the perspective of big data, training a robust deep learning model needs to use a lot of high-quality medical data.

3.1 Medical Image Classification

From 2015 to 2017, a total of 47 papers on medical image analysis based on multi classification tasks were published, including 36 papers using CNN model, 6 papers using RBM model, and 5 papers using automatic encoder model. In general, CNN is still the standard model for multi classification tasks.

As early as 1995, Lo et al. [2] tried to use CNN model to detect pulmonary nodules on chest X-ray images. They used 55 chest X-ray images and established a CNN with two hidden layers to detect the presence of pulmonary nodules in the image area. Rajkomar [3] enhanced the data set with 1850 chest X-ray images. The image is divided into front image and side image by using a pre-trained CNN googlenet. The results show that the classification accuracy is nearly 100%. Rajpurkar [4] used an improved densenet to classify 14 diseases (including pneumonia) of 112000 chest X-ray images from chest x-ray dataset. The improved densenet has 121 convolution layers. The area under curve of receiver operating characteristics (AUC) is 0.763. The researchers also use the test set to compare the receiver operating characteristics of the diagnosis results. Radiologist Shen used CNN combined with support vector machine and random forest to classify 1010 labeled lung CT images from data set for benign and malignant pulmonary nodules. They used three parallel running CNN, and each CNN was used for classification. CNN has two layers of convolution layer. Different CNN uses different scale image blocks to extract features, and then combines the learned features to construct a feature vector. Finally, support vector machine or random forest with radial basis function as kernel function is used as classifier for classification. The classification accuracy of their model reaches 86%, and the model shows strong robustness. Kallenberg [5] combined the unsupervised convolution layer as the training of automatic encoder with the supervised layer to classify mammogram images according to different textures and densities. It was found that the AUC of the convolution stack self encoder model was 0.57. Van Tulder used convolution RBM to classify lung tissue according to normal, emphysema, fibrosis, micronodule and ground glass tissue. The data set is composed of 128 CT images of patients with interstitial lung disease in ILD database. Convolution RBM generates filters through pure discrimination, pure generation, mixed discrimination and target generation. Then these filters are used to extract features. Finally, random forest is used for classification. The classification accuracy of their model is 41%–68%. In addition, Khatami used depth belief network to classify X-ray images into five categories according to anatomical region and direction.

Li [6] proposed a three-dimensional CNN model to complete multimodal data. Hosseini used deep 3D CNN to learn and capture the common features of Alzheimer's disease and adapt to different data set domains. 3D CNN is based on 3D convolution automatic encoder, which can capture the anatomical shape changes in structural brain MRI after pre training. Then for each task specific classification of Alzheimer's disease, fine tune the fully connected upper layer of 3D CNN. Korolev proposed a residual neural network architecture based on vggnet. This architecture can make the neural network model with 100–1000 layers and also get good training. They use the data from ADNI database, and use voxnet and RESNET to classify the brain MRI images of healthy people and patients with Alzheimer's disease. The results show that the classification accuracy of the model is 79% and 80% respectively. But their modeling process is simpler.

Pratt trained a CNN with 10 convolution layers and three full connectivity layers to process 90000 fundus images. They divided diabetic retinopathy into five categories according to the severity, and the classification accuracy of the model was 75%. Deep belief network is used to extract features from fMRI images.

3.2 Medical Image Detection

It is an important step in medical image analysis to detect and locate the lesion site of anatomical objects. The task of 2017 kaggle "data science bowl" competition includes the detection of cancerous pulmonary nodules in lung CT images, and the data set used 2000 CT images. The 3D CNN model used by the winner of the competition is inspired by the u-net architecture. First, the sub image block of the image is used to detect the pulmonary nodules, and then the output is used as the input of the second stage. The second stage is composed of two fully connected layers, which are used to output the probability of cancer. Shin et al. used five famous CNN models to detect the thoracic and abdominal lymph nodes and pulmonary interstitial lesions on CT images. They used googlenet to detect mediastinal lymph nodes, and the AUC of the model was as high as 0.95, which was a very good result. In addition, they also summarized the benefits of transfer learning, Ciompi combined simple support vector machine with random forest classifier, and used two-dimensional slices of coronal plane, axial plane and sagittal plane of lung CT image for training to detect whether there were pulmonary nodules in and around the lung space. In addition to lung disease detection, it is also used for other disease detection, such as malignant skin cell detection.

At present, the images of histopathological examination are more and more digital, and there are more and more related researches. A piece of histopathological section may contain hundreds or even thousands of cells. Ciresan used CNN with 11–13 convolution layers to identify mitotic images in 50 breast tissue images from the MITOS data set. Yang [7] used CNN with 5–7 layers of convolution layer to classify the pathological examination images of renal cell carcinoma into tumor and non tumor. The accuracy rate was 97%. Sirinukunwattana [8] used CNN to detect the nuclei of colon adenocarcinoma in 100 staining histopathological images of colon adenocarcinoma. Xu [9] used stacked sparse self encoder to detect breast cancer cell nucleus in breast cancer tissue section image, and the results showed that the accuracy of the model was 89%, which also proved that unsupervised learning can be used in this aspect of detection.

3.3 Medical Image Segmentation

CT and MRI image segmentation research covers liver, prostate, knee joint cartilage and other organs and tissues, but a large number of studies focus on brain, including brain tumor image segmentation. Therefore, it is very important to determine the exact boundary of brain tumor for guiding the implementation of resection surgery. In the traditional treatment process, this boundary is drawn layer by layer by brain surgeons through CT or MRI images. Akkus summarized various CNN architectures and their performance used in brain MRI image segmentation.

Moeskops used three parallel running CNN to classify brain MRI images of 22 children and 35 adults according to different tissues, such as white matter, gray matter and cerebrospinal fluid. The smallest sub image block focuses on the local texture features of the captured image, while the larger sub image block focuses on the spatial features of the captured image. The results show that the Dice coefficient of the model is between 0.82 and 0.87. Tajbakhsh analyzed four different types of medical images using transfer learning. It includes polyp detection on colonoscopy images, frame classification of colonoscopy images, pulmonary embolism detection on pulmonary angiography CT images and intima-media interface segmentation of ultrasound scanning carotid artery wall images. Their research also found that compared with CNN trained from scratch, transfer learning can better improve the performance of CNN. Chen et al. combined CNN with RNN, and the structure of neuron and fungus was segmented from the microscope image.

Most of the research on medical image segmentation is carried out on two-dimensional images, but milletari used three-dimensional CNN to segment prostate MRI images from promise 2012 dataset. Their v-net has u-net architecture, and the Dice coefficient of the model is 0.869. Pereira [10] used a 3 × 3 matrix filter, and a CNN model with 11 convolution layers was designed and trained with 274 brain MRI images with glioma. He won the first prize in the "multimodal brain tumor segmentation" challenge held by the International Association for medical image computing and computer aided intervention in 2013. Havaei also studied the image segmentation of glioma. Their CNN model uses a cascade architecture, that is, the output of the first CNN is used as the input of the second CNN. The running time of the algorithm is reduced from 100 min to 3 min. Chen [11] proposed a deep lab architecture, which performs well in Pascal voc-2012 image segmentation. Casamitjana compared the performance of various 3D CNN architectures in image segmentation tasks. It is found that the model modified by deepmediccnn [12] performs best in image segmentation of brats 2015 brain tumor dataset. They advocate using smaller receptive field and multi-scale architecture. Stollenga uses long-term and short-term memory network to segment three-dimensional electron microscope images. There are various methods for medical image segmentation. For the purpose of subdivision, RNN is also commonly used. Xie [13] used clockwork RNN model to segment the sarcolemma in the histopathological examination image stained by hematoxylin eosin.

3.4 Medical Image Registration

Medical image registration is a common image analysis task, which is usually carried out in a specific (non) parameter conversion type of iterative framework. At present, there are two main strategies for image registration: the first is to use deep learning network to estimate the similarity of two images, and then drive the iterative optimization strategy; the second is to use deep learning network to calculate the similarity of two images; Neurosurgeons or spinal surgeons use image registration to locate tumor or spinal bone "landmarks" for surgical resection of tumor or implantation of spinal screw. Image registration involves two images, namely reference image and perceptual image, in which the reference image is preoperative brain magnetic resonance imaging image. The perceptual image can be the brain MRI image after the first tumor resection. The perceptual image is used to determine whether there is residual tumor and whether secondary resection is needed. Yang used the brain MRI image in oasis data set to stack convolution layers in the way of encoding and decoding. They used LDDMM registration model, which greatly reduced the calculation time. Miao used CNN model with five layers of convolution layer to register the three-dimensional models of knee joint implant, hand implant and esophageal probe on the two-dimensional X-ray images, so as to evaluate their posture. Compared with the traditional registration method, it has significant progress.

4 Conclusion

Deep learning is one of the hotspots in the field of artificial intelligence. In machine learning, a key problem is the data problem. High quality data can effectively improve the performance of the algorithm. But in fact, especially in medical images, there is a serious lack of high-quality labeled data. Therefore, researchers hope to avoid the limitation of limited data through better model architecture. Some generating models in deep learning, such as Gan and variational self encoder, can also avoid the problem of data shortage by synthesizing medical data. This paper introduces some traditional applications of deep learning in medical image analysis. But now deep learning also has many new applications, such as using Gan to generate CT images with higher resolution from the original image. This method can also be used to generate high-quality MRI images to reduce medical costs.

Machine learning is developing rapidly in medical image analysis. In general, although there are some important problems to be solved in the application of artificial intelligence in medical image analysis, such as interpretability, robustness and so on. The existing artificial intelligence has surpassed human beings. I believe that in the future, artificial intelligence system will be able to assist or even replace doctors in film reading and diagnosis to a great extent, and intelligent medical image analysis products will be used widely in clinical practice.

References

1. Lecun, Y., Bottou, L., Bengio, Y., et al.: Gradient - based learning applied to document recognition. Proc. IEEE **86**(11), 2278–2324 (1998)
2. Krizhevsky, A., Sutskever, I., Hinton, G.E.: Imagenet classification with deep convolutional neural networks. Adv. Neural Inf. Process. Syst., **25**, 1097–1105 (2012)
3. Li, R., Zhang, W., Suk, H.I., et al.: Deep learning based imaging data completion for improved brain disease diagnosis. Med. Image Comput. Assist. **17**(3), 305–312 (2014)
4. Khatami, A., Khosravi, A., Nguyen, T., et al.: Medical image analysis using wavelet transform and deep belief networks. Expert Syst. Appl. **86**, 190–198 (2017)
5. Van Tulder, G., de Bruijne, M.: Combining generative and discriminative representation learning for lung CT analysis with convolutional restricted Boltzmann machines. IEEE Trans. Med. Imaging **35**(5), 1262–1272 (2016)
6. Hinton, G.E., Srivastava, N., Krizhevsky, A., et al.: Improving neural networks by preventing co - adaptation of feature detectors. Comput. Sci. **3**(4), 212–223 (2012)
7. Han, H., Xie, L., Ding, F., et al.: Hierarchical least - squares based iterative identification for multivariable systems with moving average noises. Math. Comput. Model. Inter. J. **51**(9–10), 1213–1220 (2010)
8. Girshick, R., Donahue, J., Darrell, T., et al.: Rich feature hierarchies for accurate object detection and semantic segmentation. In: Proceedings of the IEEE Conference on Computer Vision and Pattern Recognition, pp. 580–587 (2014)
9. Erhan, D., Bengio, Y., Courville, A., et al.: Why does unsupervised pre – training help deep learning. J. Mach. Learn. Res. **11**(3), 625–660 (2010)
10. Wan, L., Zeiler, M., Zhang, S., et al.: Regularization of neural networks using drop connect. In: International Conference on Machine Learning, pp. 1058–1066 (2013)
11. Futoma, J., Morris, J., Lucas, J.: A comparison of models for predicting early hospital readmissions. J. Biomed. Inform. **56**, 229–238 (2015)
12. Han, H., Xie, L., Ding, F., et al.: Hierarchical least - squares based iterative identification for multivariable systems with moving average noises. Math. Comput. Model. Int. J. **51**(9–10), 1213–1220 (2010)
13. Ross, G.J., Adams, N.M., Tasoulis, D.K., et al.: Exponentially weighted moving average charts for detecting concept drift. Pattern Recognit. Lett. **33**(2), 191–198 (2012)

Typical Fault Classification and Recognition of Photovoltaic Modules Based on Deep Learning and Thermal Imaging Picture Processing

Shijie Xu(✉)

Harbin, China

Abstract. In order to solve the problems of high cost and low efficiency of manual fault detection of photovoltaic modules in real life, a typical fault classification and recognition system for photovoltaic modules based on thermal imaging photography and machine processing was proposed. Feature extraction network is used to extract features from thermal imaging images. Classify different types of faults and make training sets; The YOLOV5 target detection algorithm was used to train the model through subset pre-training, weight allocation, multi-group multi-number training and other methods, and the test set was used for multiple tests. The test results show that the system has a strong ability to identify faults, and the average accuracy of network detection in the task of fault classification reaches 84.2%. In the complex area images including the target photovoltaic modules, the accuracy of the result reached 79.1% after the test set tested the training model. It is judged that the system can replace manual work to complete the typical fault classification and identification of photovoltaic modules.

Keywords: Deep learning · Image processing · PV module failure · YOLOv5 · Target classification

1 Introduction

Today, with the development of scientific and technological civilization, the global energy crisis has become increasingly serious, and environmental pollution has become one of the fundamental problems threatening the survival and development of human society. Correspondingly, countries around the world are paying more and more attention to the problem of energy crisis, and more and more material resources and manpower have been invested in the research and development of new energy. In this regard, many countries in the world have introduced many corresponding policies and issued many official documents. Such problems have attracted people's attention to environmental pollution and energy crisis, and the search for new energy with sustainable development and strong alternative has become an important research topic in the scientific community.

R. Su et al. (Eds.): MICAD 2021, LNEE 784, pp. 418–425, 2022.
https://doi.org/10.1007/978-981-16-3880-0_44

At the end of the 20th century, with the idea of taking the sun as the core of energy in the world's strong support and positive development, many new energy technologies were developed, such as solar thermal energy, wind energy, water conservancy, geothermal energy and so on. It is worth mentioning that the photovoltaic power generation technology has been widely used in the world because of its wide illumination area and low energy consumption and high efficiency. Many world-class large-scale solar power stations have been set up. However, due to time, environment, force and other factors, many faults will occur in the use of this technology, including strip battery faults, hot spots, junction box damage, whole component faults, etc., which will reduce power generation efficiency, affect capacity, and cause great losses to economic benefits. How to quickly and accurately identify these faults has become the key to efficiently and rapidly repair the photovoltaic power generation system to ensure its normal power generation. This key point has also constantly attracted the attention of scholars at home and abroad.

Thermal imaging is a non-contact infrared energy detection to display thermal images and temperature values. Under normal circumstances, different faults show different abnormal conditions in the thermal imaging images, so the type of faults can be inferred backwards. This detection method is easy to use and avoids the risk of disassembly inspection. Therefore, the working mode of carrying the camera system by UAV and checking it manually has been used in many places now. However, compared with the convenience and quickness of photovoltaic fault shooting by thermal imaging, the method to complete the identification of photovoltaic system fault by manpower shows the problem of huge cost and low efficiency. Compared with the ability of a large number of mechanical calculations, the artificial backward method will obviously be eliminated by the rapid development of society. Therefore, a set of machine can replace the human and practical system has a very important significance.

Based on the above situation, this paper proposes a typical fault classification and recognition algorithm of photovoltaic modules based on YOLO neural network. The algorithm classifies different fault types by labeling the images in the training set, and gives four values of each image, which are X_center/image_width, Y_center/image_height, width/image_width, and height/image_height, and integrates them into a data set. The model is obtained by training the data set through YOLOV5 neural network. This method has the advantages of high precision, low error detection rate and strong anti-interference, and can complete the task of fault classification and recognition well.

2 Typical Fault Classification and Analysis of Photovoltaic Modules

2.1 Heat Spot

Cause of failure: battery damage in the module, or dirt and dust accumulated on the surface of the photovoltaic module causing a shadow, resulting in heat spots.

Judgment method: If a single or multiple heating battery pieces present patchy and scattered distribution, they are judged as hot spots.

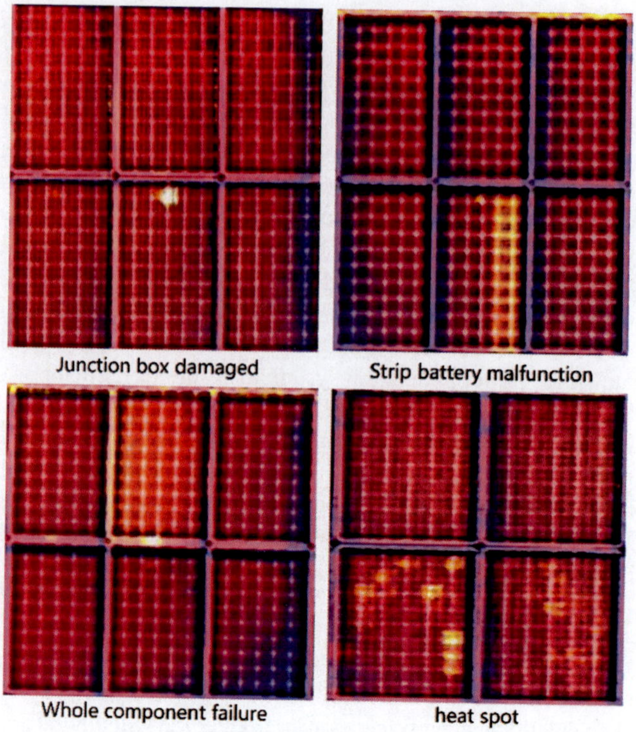

Fig. 1. Thermal imaging display diagram of PV module faults

2.2 Whole Component Failure

Cause of fault: all the diodes are on, the component process is not up to standard or the bus bar is falsified, resulting in heating of the whole component.

Determination method: If all the batteries of a component are abnormally hot and the temperature is obviously higher than that of other components in the same group, the whole component is judged to be faulty.

2.3 Strip Battery Malfunction

Fault cause: junction box exists welding phenomenon or diode fault causes strip distributed heating phenomenon.

Judgment method: If the two ends of the abnormal components are distributed in strip shape and several batteries are heated at the same time, it is judged as strip battery fault.

2.4 Junction Box Damaged

Cause of the fault: the installation of the junction box is not up to standard or the internal contact of the junction box is not good.

Judgment method: If the two ends of the abnormal components are distributed in strip shape and several batteries are heated at the same time, it is judged as strip battery fault. If the temperature at the junction box of the component is significantly higher than that of other components in the same group, the junction box is judged to be damaged.

3 Inspection System Framework

3.1 The Structures

The typical fault classification and recognition algorithm framework of photovoltaic modules designed in this paper consist of two parts. The first part is image feature extraction based on OpenCV, which is used to label the RGB original image selected by the box and give coordinate data, to generate an appropriate training set and use it in the subsequent YOLOV5 network training model. The second part is the operation processing based on the YOLOV5 Network structure (as shown in Fig. 1). The Focus structure and CSP structure of the Network ensure a large number of convolutional kernel operations and reduce the operation cost. When sampling, FPN (Feature Pyramid Network) and PAN (Pyramid Attention Network) are adopted, and YOLOV5 uses the CSP2 structure designed by CSPnet (Cross Stage Partical Network) for example. Enhance the ability of network feature fusion. Therefore, this system adopts this network structure, whose function is to consider the different fault characteristics of different types of photovoltaic modules for regression classification, and at the same time to improve the computing capacity of the system.

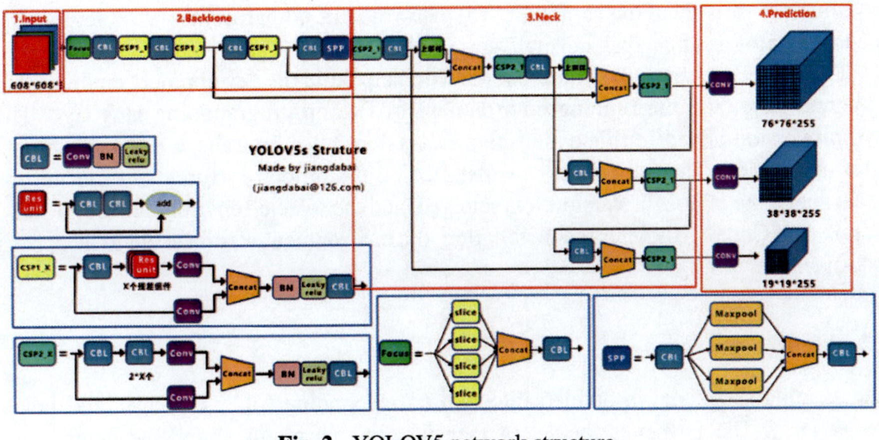

Fig. 2. YOLOV5 network structure

Figure 2 describes the network structure of YOLOv5. The recognition model of the system uses this structure to train the model. For different models of YOLOv5, the system uses YOLOv5X model to replace YOLOv5S model to build.

3.2 YOLOv5 Principle

YOLOv5 YOLOv3 Darkent based network migrated to Pytorch development environment, the framework of the overall network structure is still the old version of the one - stage structure, compared with YOLOv4 of promotion in the COCO dataset, YOLOv5 compared to ascend is not big, but the accuracy is higher, and the reasoning speed has reached 140 FPS, its weight (weight) file size, however, is only 1/9 of the four generations. The same with Yolov4, the network structure of Yolov5 still uses four parts: Input, Backbone, Neck and Prediction. The difference between Yolov5 and Yolov4, however, is the addition of adaptive anchor box and adaptive image scaling code at the input end. Meanwhile, Focus structure and CSP structure are adopted in the Backbone, and the SSP of YOLOV4 is moved to the Backbone. Compared with the CIOU_LOSS and DIOU_NMS operations of YOLOV4 at the output end, the GIOU_LOSS algorithm is added.

4 Environment and Models

4.1 Environment Setting

For the convenience of development, the system is built on Linux computer system. After installing the Ubuntu system (version 18.04 is installed in this experiment), download and install the RUN file from the official website of NVIDIA. The system selects the latest version RUN file, and the resolution of the monitor is normal after installing the RUN file. Then install CUDA to the environment, this system uses CUDA version 11.0, after the installation of ' ~ /.bashrc' command, through this command can set the environment variable of the computer; Then download Cudnn from the website; Finally, the test environment can run normally.

Then you can use the software tool Anaconda to build the development environment PyTorch. First, add the running environment of Python programming language. The Python version added in this experiment is version 3.9.1, and check the environment after installation. Then, PyTorch was installed on the official PyTorch website. In this experiment, the 1.71 GPU version was selected, and the selected environment was Linux, Conda, and Cuda 11.0. After the installation, the environment was detected to be correct by Anaconda.

4.2 Model Training

The training set model is divided into two corresponding folders, images and labels respectively. The former is the set of thermal imaging pictures, and the latter is the label file corresponding to each image. Since the algorithm of YOLO series supports the label of Text file TXT (Text), the labels and the corresponding four information of images, x_center/image_width, y_center/image_height, width/image_width, and height/image_height, are stored in Text files, and images and labels are stored in trains folder, which is called training set. After the installation of YOLOV5 program, trains of the training set will be stored in the statistics folder of YOLOV5 project. Modify the data.yaml file under trains file to "nc:2", and then modify the nc value of yolov5x.yaml file under “yolov5/models/” to “nc = 2”. Since there are four training algorithms with different specifications and different performances given by the authorities, the X algorithm with the highest performance is selected for this system. The PT file generated after training is the typical fault classification and identification model of photovoltaic modules to be detected.

5 Experimental Analysis

5.1 Experimental Data

Figure 3 describes the effect display of classification and labeling of different thermal imaging problems, including thermal imaging extraction of four kinds of problems including Heat spot, Whole component failure, Strip battery malfunction and Junction box damaged. After extracting the coordinates of the corresponding features, as shown in Fig. 4, the similarity percentages of each feature are marked, and the photovoltaic module faults corresponding to these features are classified. Based on the above process, the detection results of single thermal imaging can be obtained finally.

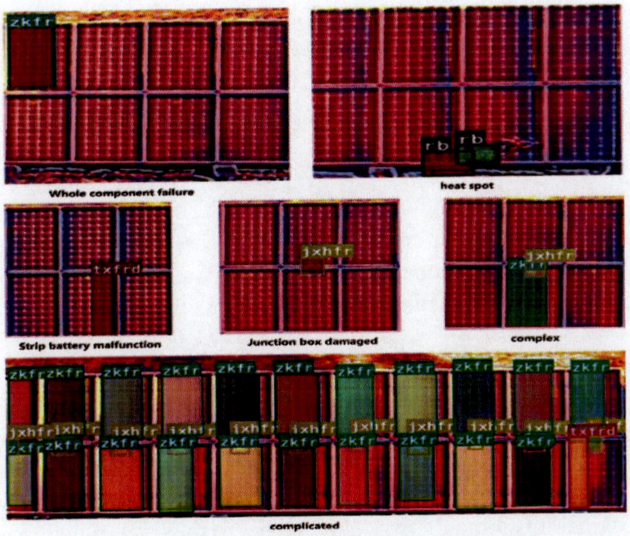

Fig. 3. Visual effect display of training results

Through the study, it is found that the training times of an image set as 300, the step size of training as 1, and the effect of training with the same training set for 3 times is better than that of other training models, and the curve of its fitting parameters is also more regular. Finally, the detection result of simple image test set is 84.2%, while the detection result of complex image test set is 79.1%. (to one decimal point).

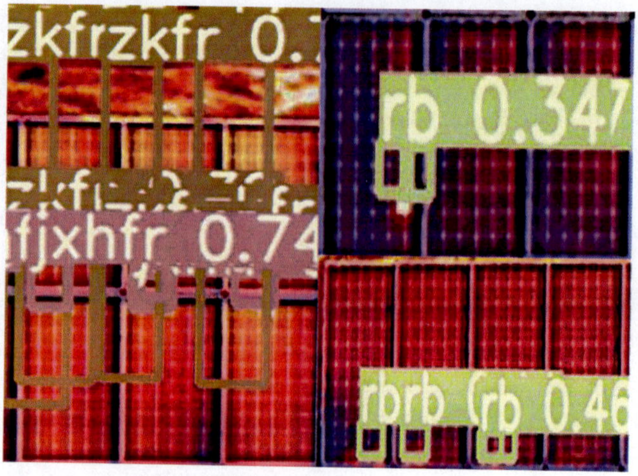

Fig. 4. Testing effect diagram of test set

5.2 Experimental Environment

The hardware environment built in this experiment is as follows: CPU model of Intelcore i7-9700K, the memory capacity of 8GX2, GPU model of NVIDIA GeForce RTX-2080TI 11G video memory. The algorithm program of the experimental system is trained based on the PyTorch framework YOLOV5 training model.

5.3 Evaluation Criterion

In this paper, T (true) is set for correctly classified cases, F (false) is set for wrongly classified cases, and PR (precision rate) is set for classification accuracy. The value of PR is taken as the standard for evaluating the model. The calculation formula of classification accuracy PR is as follows:

$$PR = \frac{\mathrm{T}}{\mathrm{T} + \mathrm{F}} \tag{1}$$

The accuracy rate reflects the quality of the correct classification of the model, that is, the higher the accuracy, the more powerful the performance of the model can be proved. Generally speaking, it is difficult to train the model to the level of high accuracy, which requires a lot of practice. Different training times, training amount, and training set will affect the direction of the final effect. If only certain samples are trained, the actual performance of the model will fluctuate. At the same time, there may be a variety of faults on a photovoltaic panel. Whether the model can be fully judged also needs repeated debugging. As mentioned earlier, a good model should have the following characteristics: the PR value should be as high as possible while ensuring the identification of multiple faults in complex scenarios. MAP (Mean Average Precision) used in the target detection experiment has the same meaning as PR in this paper and is a conventional index. It is the average value of various categories. There are multiple detection targets in this paper, so PR can be used to replace the MAP index.

6 Conclusion

This paper proposes a typical fault classification and recognition system for photovoltaic modules based on deep learning and thermal imaging image processing. The whole system is built based on YOLOV5 algorithm for model training. By using different quality training sets, the fault categories of different photovoltaic modules can be identified effectively and accurately. The experimental results show that the system proposed in this paper can accurately classify and identify different faults of photovoltaic modules based on YOLOV5 algorithm, and has achieved excellent detection results.

References

1. Lecun, Y., Bengio, Y., Hinton, G.: Deep learning. Nature **521**(7553), 436 (2015)
2. Ren, S., He, K., Girshick, R., et al.: Faster R-CNN: towards real-time object detection with region proposal networks. IEEE Trans. Pattern Anal. Mach. Intell. **39**(6), 1137–1149 (2017)
3. Wang, W., Wu, B., Yang, S., et al.: Road Damage Detection and Classification with Faster R-CNN. In: 2018 IEEE International Conference on Big Data (Big Data). IEEE (2018)
4. Ren, S., He, K., Girshick, R., et al.: Faster R-CNN: towards real-time object detection with region proposal networks. IEEE Trans. Pattern Anal. Mach. Intell. **39**(6) (2015)
5. Chen, Z., Wang, H., Zhang, L., et al.: Visual saliency detection based on homology similarity and an experimental evaluation. J. Vis. Commun. Image Repres. **40**(pt.A), 251–264 (2016)
6. Li, X., Zhao, L., Wei, L., et al.: DeepSaliency: multi-task deep neural network model for salient object detection. IEEE Trans. Image Process. Publ. IEEE Signal Process. Soc. **25**(8), 3919 (2016)
7. Nian, B., Fu, Z., Wang, L., et al.: Automatic detection of defects in solar modules: image processing in detecting. In: International Conference on Wireless Communications Networking & Mobile Computing. IEEE (2010)
8. Laganiere, R.: OpenCV 2 computer vision application programming cookbook : over 50 recipes to master this library of programming functions for real-time computer vision (2011)

An Obstacle Avoidance Method for Agricultural Plant Protection UAV Based on the Fusion of Ultrasonic and Monocular Vision

Kunlin Yu(✉)

Department of Aeronautical Mechanical and Electrical Equipment Maintenance, Changsha Aeronautical Vocational and Technical College, Changsha 410124, China

Abstract. Monocular vision obstacle avoidance technology has some defects, such as low accuracy of obstacle detection, difficult to directly detect the distance and position information of obstacles, In this paper, an obstacle detection method of agricultural plant protection UAV Based on ultrasonic and monocular vision is proposed. Firstly, the obstacles in the flight direction of UAV are detected quickly by ultrasonic sensor, When the dangerous distance between the obstacle and UAV is detected, The monocular vision sensor is triggered to collect the obstacle image, and the collected obstacle image is transmitted to the image processing module for image processing. Through the simulation experiment and effect comparison of six automatic threshold edge detection algorithms, a better algorithm is found to detect the edge of the image. The contour information of the image is detected, and the flight path of the UAV is planned according to the obstacle avoidance strategy and algorithm, so as to realize the autonomous obstacle avoidance of the agricultural plant protection UAV.

Keywords: Fusion of ultrasound and monocular vision · Agricultural plant protection UAV · Obstacle avoidance methods

1 Introduction

At present, The plant protection UAV has the advantages of uniform application, high efficiency and low cost. However, in China's farmland, there are many complex obstacles, such as houses, power poles, trees and so on, which seriously threaten the flight safety of UAV. Therefore, it is necessary to realize the autonomous control of plant protection UAV Obstacle avoidance can significantly improve the safety of operation. Automatic obstacle avoidance technology is of great significance to ensure the flight safety and automatic flight of plant protection UAV, and obstacle detection is one of the key problems in the use of plant protection UAV.

2 Common UAV Obstacle Avoidance Methods

2.1 Ultrasonic Obstacle Avoidance Method

Ultrasonic obstacle avoidance is to measure the distance of the surrounding obstacles with the help of ultrasonic sensors. Ultrasonic sensor can measure the distance of the

R. Su et al. (Eds.): MICAD 2021, LNEE 784, pp. 426–435, 2022.
https://doi.org/10.1007/978-981-16-3880-0_45

surrounding obstacles, but it can not measure the azimuth angle of the surrounding obstacles.

2.2 Obstacle Avoidance Method of Lidar

The principle of laser radar obstacle avoidance is that the transmitter and the receiver transmit and receive specific light pulses respectively, and use the ranging method to calculate the distance information. Lidar has the advantages of long measurement range, high precision, light weight and small volume, but it is expensive and vulnerable to strong light interference.

2.3 Millimeter Wave Radar Obstacle Avoidance Method

There is a time delay between the radar echo signal and the transmitted signal. The beat signal is obtained by mixing the echo signal with the mixer local oscillator signal. The frequency of the beat signal is proportional to the distance between the obstacle and the radar. The distance between the obstacle and the radar can be calculated from the frequency of the beat signal. Millimeter wave radar has high ranging accuracy, but it can't get the angle information of obstacles in space.

2.4 Obstacle Avoidance Method of Machine Vision

Machine vision obstacle avoidance method uses camera to capture the image of obstacles, and gets the position and contour information of the surrounding obstacles through image processing [1]. Vision sensor passively receives the information of light source, which is rich in information. However, machine vision obstacle avoidance requires camera calibration, image processing, geometric operation and other operations, which requires a large amount of calculation and high performance of hardware processing.

3 UAV Obstacle Avoidance Algorithm Flow Based on the Fusion of Ultrasonic and Monocular Vision

The ultrasonic sensor can measure the distance of the surrounding obstacles, and has the advantages of high precision, small volume, simple method, cheap price, not easily affected by light wave, but it can not measure the azimuth of the surrounding obstacles. Although the monocular vision sensor has low accuracy in measuring the distance of obstacles, it can measure the orientation and position of the surrounding obstacles, At the same time, compared with the multi vision sensor, it has the advantages of small amount of calculation and low requirement of hardware processing capacity. Therefore, the combination of ultrasonic sensor and monocular vision sensor installed on the plant protection UAV can not only obtain high-precision distance information of obstacles, but also obtain the orientation and position information of obstacles, The advantages of the two sensors complement each other, and the scheme involves less computation, requires less processing power of embedded microprocessor, and can realize the automatic obstacle avoidance function of UAV with lower cost and computational cost, which is suitable for installation and use on plant protection UAV.

At present, there are mainly two types of vision image sensors in the market: CCD and CMOS. Considering that the imaging quality of CCD is better than that of CMOS, and the anti noise ability of CCD is better than that of CMOS, the monocular vision sensor here is CCD image sensor.

The obstacle detection method of agricultural plant protection UAV Based on ultrasonic and monocular vision firstly uses ultrasonic sensor module to measure the distance of obstacles around the flying UAV, When the distance between the UAV and the surrounding obstacles is 5 m, the visual sensor is activated to collect the image of the obstacles, and then the distorted image is preprocessed by correction, histogram equalization, image filtering, and then the edge of the preprocessed image is detected. Finally, the orientation of the obstacles is recognized according to the edge information and recognition algorithm of the obstacles, The whole obstacle detection flow is shown in Fig. 1.

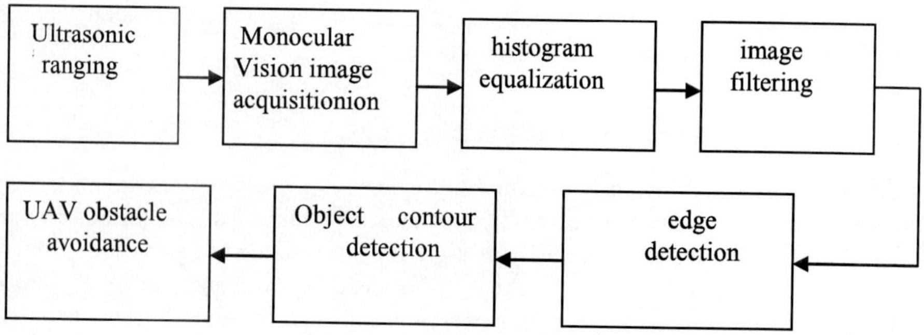

Fig. 1. Obstacle detection flow

4 UAV Obstacle Avoidance Algorithm Based on Ultrasonic and Monocular Vision Fusion

4.1 Ultrasonic Ranging

The principle of ultrasonic distance measurement is to send ultrasonic wave to a certain range of measuring beam angle through ultrasonic transmitter, and calculate the distance according to the time difference of ultrasonic round trip [2]. In general, the ranging formula is adopted when the application requirements are not high.

$$s = \frac{c \times t}{2}$$

Where, “c”is the propagation velocity of sound wave in the air, generally 340 m/s, and “t” is the propagation time.

4.2 Histogram Equalization

Because the gray distribution of the original image is concentrated in a narrow range, the contrast is very small when calculating the contrast, which leads to the details of the image is not clear enough. In order to make the details of the image more clear, it is necessary to make the gray distribution of the image wider and the gray value distribution more uniform. Histogram equalization is to stretch the image to be processed nonlinearly, so that the histogram distribution of the transformed image is uniform [3]. Because there are many obstacles in our country's farmland, such as houses, poles, trees and so on, so we select houses as obstacles for image processing. The image histogram equalization experiment is shown in Fig. 2.

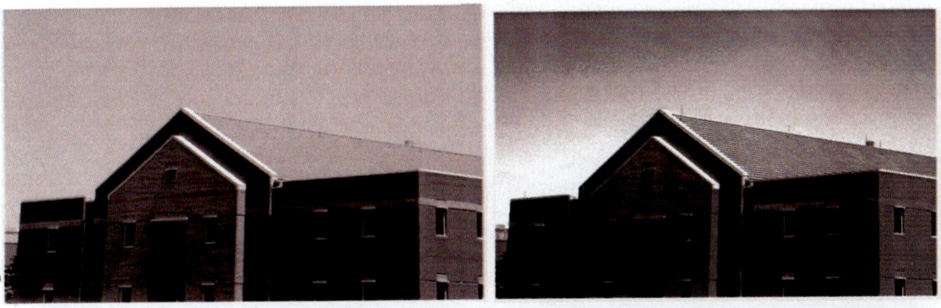

(a) original image (b) Histogram equalization image

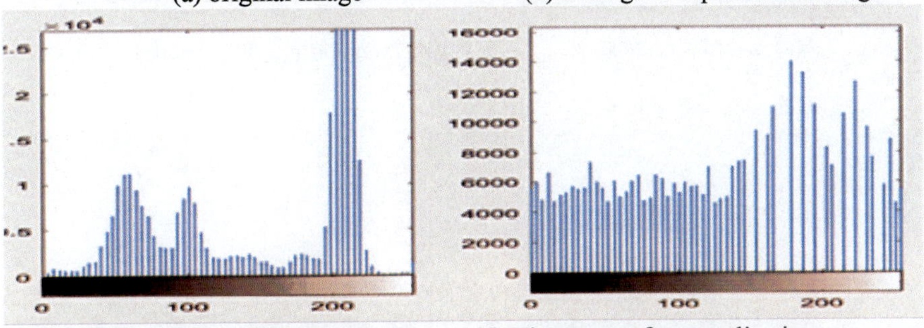

(c) original image histogram (d) Histogram after equalization

Fig. 2. Histogram equalization experiment

It can be seen from the experiment that the gray range occupied by the original image histogram is relatively narrow. After histogram equalization of the original image, the histogram occupies the allowable gray range of the whole image. Histogram equalization increases the dynamic gray range and the contrast of the image, so many details of the image are clearer.

4.3 Image Filtering

Because the obstacle image contains a lot of noise, if the noise in the image is not removed, it is easy to misjudge the noise points with large gray value of the image as false edges, resulting in inaccurate edge detection, so the noise must be eliminated before edge detection. Image filtering is to eliminate the noise in the original image. There are many methods of image smoothing filtering, among which the commonly used methods are mean filtering and median filtering. Mean filtering is a typical linear filtering algorithm. It refers to giving a template to the target pixel on the image, which includes the adjacent pixels around it, and then replacing it with the average value of all the pixels in the template Replace the original pixel value. Mean filtering is also called linear filtering, and its main method is domain averaging. Median filtering is a non-linear smoothing technique, which sets the gray value of each pixel to the median value of all pixels in a neighborhood window [4].

The experiment of using mean filter and median filter to filter the obstacle image of plant protection UAV in flight is shown in Fig. 3.

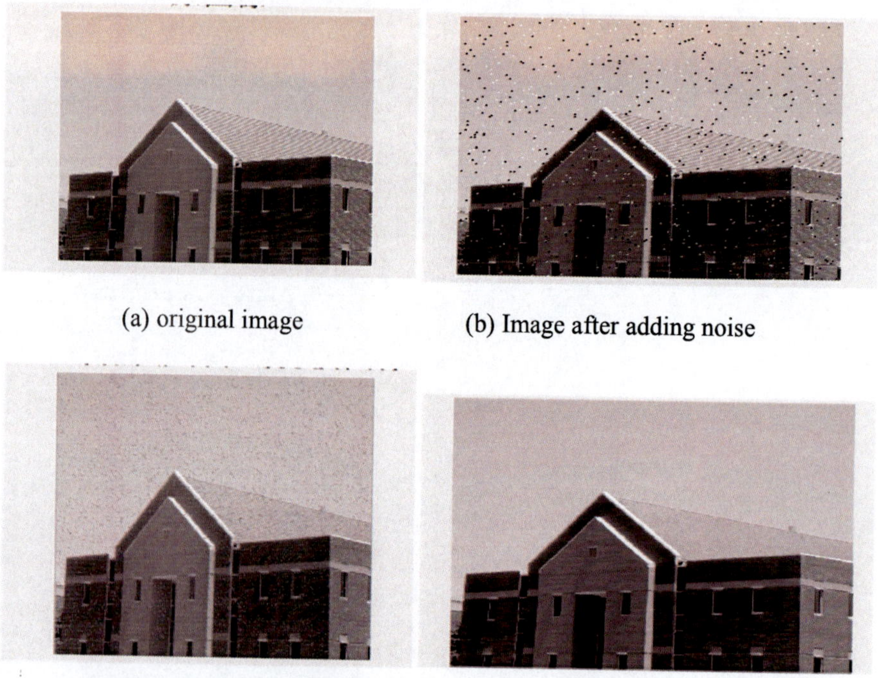

(a) original image (b) Image after adding noise

(c)3X3 Window mean filtering (d) 3X3 Window median filter

Fig. 3. Obstacle image filtering experiment

From the experiment, it can be seen that the mean filtering method can effectively suppress the noise of the image, but the edge of the filtered image becomes more fuzzy, while the median filtering method is obviously less fuzzy, which is very effective in dealing with salt and pepper noise, and the filtering effect is better.

4.4 Edge Detection

4.4.1 Common Edge Detection Methods

Image edge is often caused by the change of the physical characteristics of the scene in the image. There is a direct relationship between the image edge and the physical characteristics of the image content. The image edge contains most of the information of the image. Traditional image edge detection methods mostly extract edge information from high-frequency components of the image, and differential operation is the main means of edge detection and extraction.

Edge detection methods usually use edge detection operators to detect. The commonly used first-order differential edge detection operators include Roberts operator, Sobel operator, Prewitt operator, Canny operator and so on [5]. The commonly used second-order differential edge detection operators include Laplacian operator, LOG operator and so on.

4.4.2 Canny Operator Edge Detection Algorithm

Canny operator uses templates in different directions to convolute the given image and obtain the optimal edge. Canny operator has the advantages of high detection accuracy, high signal-to-noise ratio and poor real-time performance.

The steps of Canny operator edge detection are as follows:

(1) Gaussian filtering
Gaussian function is used to denoise the source image which needs edge detection, The Gauss function is

$$G(x, y) = \frac{1}{2\pi\delta^2}\exp\left[-\frac{x^2 + y^2}{2\delta^2}\right] \tag{1}$$

(2) The gradient amplitude and direction of the filtered image are calculated

$$M(x, y) = \sqrt{G_x(x, y)^2 + G_y(x, y)^2} \tag{2}$$

$$\theta(x, y) = \arctan\frac{G_y(x, y)}{G_x(x, y)} \tag{3}$$

$$G_X(x, y) = G(x, y + 1) - G(x, y - 1) \tag{4}$$

$$G_Y(x, y) = G(x + 1, y) - G(x - 1, y) \tag{5}$$

The gradient and direction of the image are obtained by using the first-order partial derivative in the neighborhood of 2×2.

(3) The gradient amplitude is not maximally suppressed, The non maximum points in the gradient are set to zero to get the thinning edge.
(4) Edge detection and connection with double threshold method.

High and low thresholds are used to detect the results after non maximum suppression, and two threshold edge images, T h and T l, are obtained. The points whose gradient amplitude is greater than T h are regarded as edge points, and the points whose gradient amplitude is less than T l are regarded as non edge points, and T l is used to connect the edges [6].

4.4.3 Edge Detection Simulation Experiment

In order to improve the accuracy of obstacle edge detection, adaptive threshold is set for six kinds of edge detection operators, and the edge detection operator with adaptive threshold is used for image edge detection. The contrast experiment is shown in Fig. 4.

In the above experiments, six kinds of automatic threshold edge detection operators are used to detect the edge of the obstacle image. Through the experimental comparison, it can be seen that the obstacle edge detection accuracy in figure (f) is the highest, and the edge detection effect is the best. In figure (f), canny operator with automatic threshold is used for edge detection. Canny edge detection operator is an optimal edge detection operator, and its edge detection effect is the best Edge detection image contains rich image edge details. Canny edge detection operator in order to avoid the detection of false edges, it uses the non maximum suppression method. In order to avoid false edge points in the detection process, and also in order to avoid missing edge detection, Canny edge detection algorithm uses the double threshold technology. The key of using Canny operator to detect image edge is to select the appropriate threshold, so it is used here Canny operator of automatic threshold is used for edge detection. The double thresholds of Canny operator edge detection calculated by the program are 0.0188 and 0.0469 respectively.

4.5 Obstacle Contour Detection

After completing the edge detection of the obstacles in the monocular camera image, the edge information of the obstacles has been obtained. After the implementation of the edge detection step, the edge detection results are searched by the contour matching algorithm, and the position coordinates of the obstacle target contour and the number of extracted contours are searched in the binary image.

5 Obstacle Avoidance Strategy

In this paper, the plant protection UAV adopts two kinds of obstacle avoidance strategies: vertical obstacle avoidance and left and right obstacle avoidance. When the plant protection UAV detects obstacles in the front during flight operation, it is necessary to calculate the height of the obstacles in front, and then judge whether the maximum flight height of the plant protection UAV is greater than the height of the obstacles. If the maximum flight height of the plant protection UAV is greater than the height of the obstacle, the vertical obstacle avoidance mode of the UAV will be started to avoid the obstacle. If the maximum flight height of the plant protection UAV is less than the height of the obstacle, the left and right obstacle avoidance mode will be started. This is the first

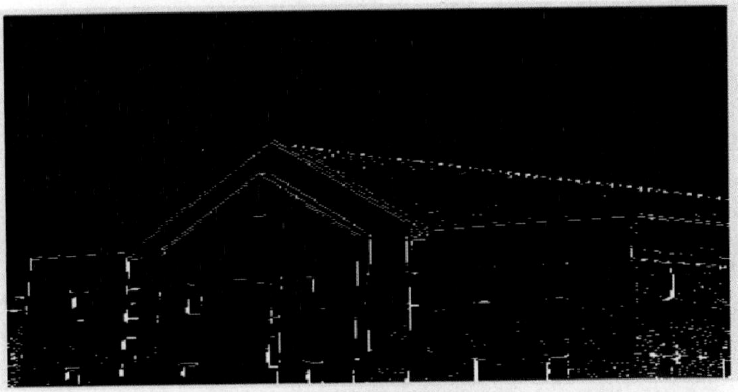

(a) original image

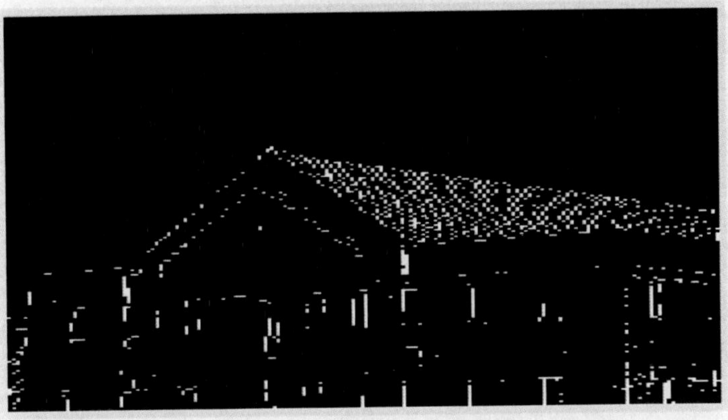

(b)Sobel edge detection with threshold of 0.0738

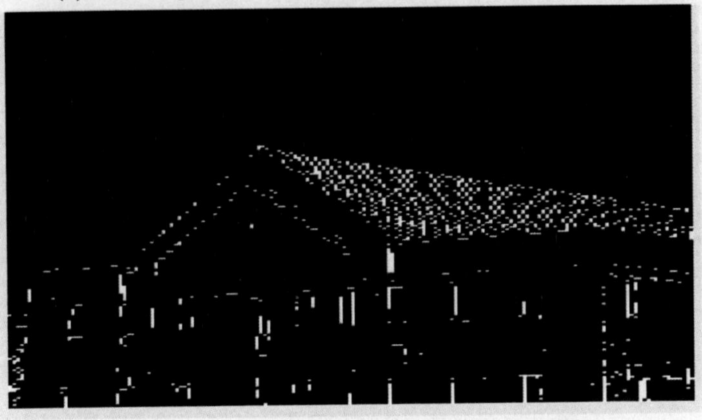

(c) Prewitt edge detection with threshold of 0.0722

Fig. 4. Edge detection experiment of obstacle image

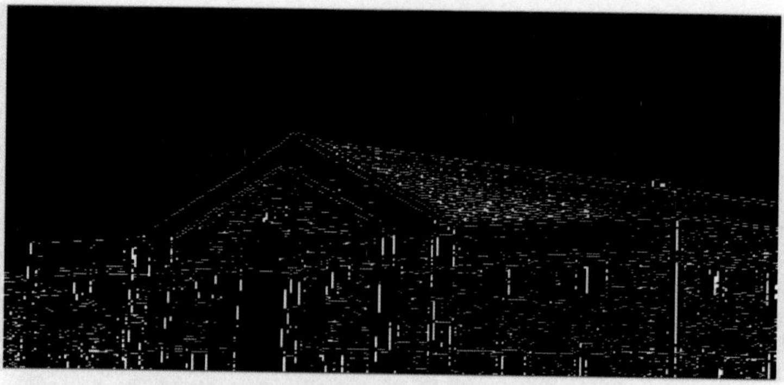

(d) LOG edge detection with threshold of 0.002

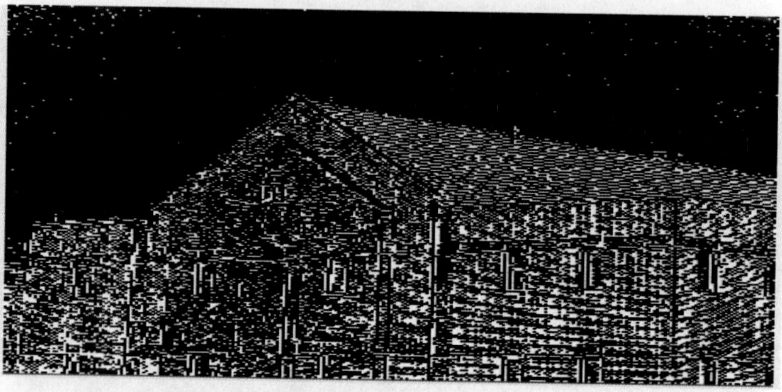

(e)Zero cross detection with threshold of 0.0109

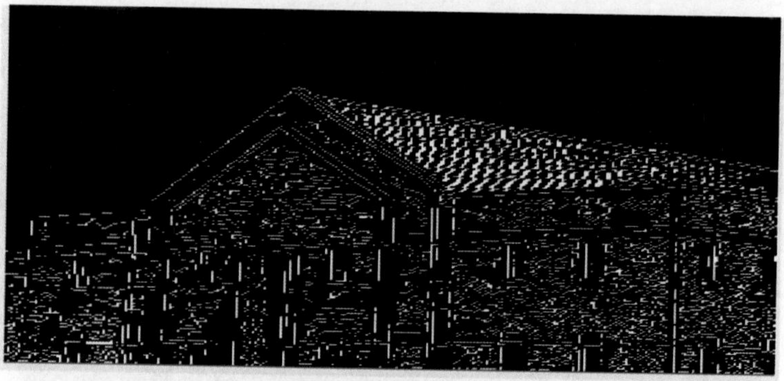

(f) Canny edge detection with threshold [0.01880.0469]

Fig. 4. (*continued*)

step to calculate the distance between the plant protection UAV and the left and right boundary of the obstacle. When the plant protection UAV is close to the left boundary of the obstacle, it will fly around the obstacle from the left side of the obstacle. When the UAV is close to the right boundary of the obstacle, it will fly around the obstacle from the right side of the obstacle [7].

6 Conclusion

In this paper, the obstacle detection algorithm based on ultrasonic and monocular vision is analyzed in detail and simulated. The experimental results show that the method greatly improves the detection accuracy of obstacle image edge. The algorithm provides a new method for obstacle detection of agricultural plant protection UAV, and provides a technical basis for UAV automatic obstacle avoidance technology, which has very high application value.

Acknowledgement. This work was supported by the joint project of science and education of Hunan Provincial Natural Science Foundation of China "Research on the technology of agricultural plant protection UAV simulating autonomous flight based on machine vision" (Project No. 2018JJ5061). This paper is the phased research achievement of this subject.

Fund Project:. This paper comes from the joint project of science and education of Hunan Natural Science Foundation "Research on the technology of agricultural plant protection UAV simulating autonomous flight based on machine vision" (Project No. 2018JJ5061). This paper is the phased research achievement of this subject.

References

1. Inoue, K., Kaizu, Y., Igarashi, S., et al.: The development of autonomous navigation and obstacle avoidance for a robotic mower using machine vision technique. IFAC-PapersOnLine **52**(30), 173–177 (2019). https://doi.org/10.1016/j.ifacol.2019.12.517
2. Kim, H.-W., Joo, Y.-S., Park, S.-J., et al.: Ultrasonic ranging technique for obstacle monitoring above reactor core in prototype generation IV sodium-cooled fast reactor. Nucl. Eng. Technol. **52**(4), 776–783 (2020)
3. Magudeeswaran, V., Fenshia Singh, J.: Contrast limited fuzzy adaptive histogram equalization for enhancement of brain images. Int. J. Imag. Syst. Technol. **27**(1), 98–103 (2017). https://doi.org/10.1002/ima.22214
4. Lakshmi, A., Arivoli, T., Rajasekaran, M.P.: A novel M-ACA-based tumor segmentation and DAPP feature extraction with PPCSO-PKC-based MRI classification. Arab. J. Sci. Eng. **43**(12), 7095–7111 (2018). https://doi.org/10.1007/s13369-017-2966-4
5. Punarselvam, E., Suresh, P.: Investigation on human lumbar spine MRI image using finite element method and soft computing techniques. Cluster Comput. **22**(S6), 13591–13607 (2019). https://doi.org/10.1007/s10586-018-2019-0
6. Song, R., Zhang, Z., Liu, H.: Edge connection based Canny edge detection algorithm. Pattern Recognit. Image Anal. **27**(4), 740–747 (2017)
7. Ming, Y.: A vision based obstacle avoidance method for plant protection UAV. Electron. World **22**, 141–142 (2018)

Author Index

R. Su et al. (Eds.): MICAD 2021, LNEE 784, pp. 437–439, 2022.
https://doi.org/10.1007/978-981-16-3880-0